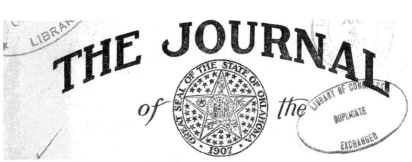

THE JOURNAL

of the

Oklahoma State Medical Association.

VOL. 2, NO. 1   JUNE, 1909.   Annual Subscription $1.00

PUBLISHED MONTHLY AT MUSKOGEE, OKLAHOMA, UNDED DIRCTION OF THE COUNCIL.

CONTENTS.

Chairman's Address on the Section of State Medicine, J. M. McComas, M. D., Elk City, Oklahoma.................... 1

Cancer of the Breast, Some General Considerations, Dr. Jabez N. Jackson, Kansas City, Mo. 5

Ilio-Colitis, Diagnosis and Treatment of, in Rural Practice, Dr. H. M. Williams, Wellston 12

Editorial 17

County Societies 21

Exchanges 25

Miscellaneous 24

A PRIVATE SANITARIUM

FOR the treatment of Nervous and Mental Diseases, Drug and Alcohol Addictions. Conducted by Drs. Duke & Rucks. Special attention given Baths, Dietetics, Massage and Rest Cure. A Strictly Ethical Institution. We invite the investigation of every reputable physician.

For Rates and further particulars, address

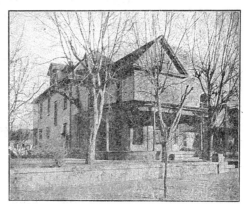

DRS. DUKE & RUCKS   310 N. Broad Street, GUTHRIE, OKLA.

Arlington Heights Sanitarium

(Incorporated under the Laws of Texas)

For Nervous Diseases, Selected Cases of Mental Diseases, Drug and Alcohol Addictions.

Postoffice Box 978   FORT WORTH, TEXAS

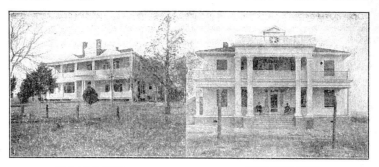

OLD BUILDING   NEW BUILDING

A New and Modern Institution Built Especially for the Homelike Care and Scientific Treatment of Its Patients

Separate buildings for Male and Female, comprising 40 rooms, heated by steam, lighted by electricity and furnished with artesian water—hot and cold. All rooms are outside rooms.

Patients Under Care of Specially Trained Nurses Day and Night

The Sanitarium is located in beautiful Arlington Heights, 150 feet above and five miles from the city of Fort Worth, and within three blocks of Lake Como—the most popular pleasure resort in the vicinity—to which convalescent patients have access. Pure, fresh, invigorating air, sunshine and shade in abundance; pleasure walks and drives. A quiet retreat, yet convenient to car line and city. Institution strictly ethical.

WILMER L. ALLISON, M. D.,
Supt. & Resident Physician,
For several years first
Asst. Supt. of Insane
Asylum at San Antonio.

BRUCE ALLISON, M. D.,
Resident Physician,
Formerly Assistant Phy-
sician of San Antonio
Asylum.

JNO. S. TURNER, M. D.,
Consulting Physician,
Late Superintendent of Terrell
Asylum.

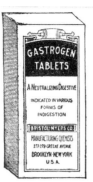

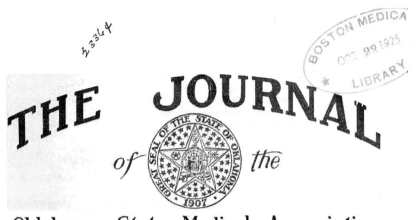

Oklahoma State Medical Association.

VOL. 2.   MUSKOGEE, OKLAHOMA, JUNE, 1909.   No. 1.

CLAUDE A. THOMPSON, Editor-in-Chief.

ASSOCIATE EDITORS AND COUNCILLORS.

DR. J. A. WALKER, Shawnee.
DR. CHARLES R. HUME, Anadarko.
DR. F. R. SUTTON, Bartlesville.
DR. G. W. ROBERTSON, Dustin.

DR. JOHN W. DUKE, Guthrie.
DR. A. B. FAIR, Frederick.
DR. W. G. BLAKE, Tahlequah.
DR. H. P. WILSON, Wynnewood.

DR. J. S. FULTON, Atoka.

Entered at the Postoffice at Muskogee, Oklahoma, as second class mail matter, June, 1909.

This is the Official Journal of the Oklahoma State Medical Association and every member of that organization is entitled to a copy and if, through accident or oversight, you fail to receive a copy notification of that fact to this office will receive prompt attention. All communicaions should be addressed to the Journal of the Oklahoma State Medical Association, English Block, Muskogee, Oklahoma.

CHAIRMAN'S ADDRESS.

SECTION ON STATE MEDICINE
Dr. J. M. McComas Elk City, Oklahoma

When one examines closely into the history of state medicine and sanitary science he is very soon impressed with the fact that progress seems to be constantly evident. Authorities tell us that in the sixteenth century the average life covered a period of eighteen or twenty years. In the eighteenth century it had been lengthened to approximately thirty years and today the span of human life is about forty years. Since the year 1880 man's average life has been extended by nearly six years. For such splendid humanitarian and economic benefits progress in state medicine and sanitary science is beyond doubt, directly responsible.

The year that has elapsed since last we met has, I think, been marked by unusual interest throughout our country in the problems of public health. This interest has been manifested by legislators, by medical men and best of all by the people at large. The great majority of medical men have in the past quarter century been unremitting in their ardent zeal for better measures concerning public hygiene and sanitation. Legislators have shown but intermittent interest in such questions and the people up to seven years ago were scarcely more than lukewarm in matters pertaining to their health as communities in need of sanitary regulations.

And while still today there is much to be desired, very much in the matter of public interest in health regulation and state medicine, nevertheless, the signs of the times are hopeful. There seems to be a general and increasing appreciation of the fact among all classes of society that on state medicine depends the happiness of our people and our national success. Not the hordes of barbarians but the degeneracy of her citizens caused the fall of Rome.

There are several facts pointing to better things and still greater progress in public health measures. Notice first, the wide prevalence of the agitation for a national department of Public Health with a medical man at its head who should have a seat in the President's cabinet. With greater or less completeness all political parties of any claim to national importance incorporated into their platforms last summer a plank favoring such a step. Surely, the pressure of public opinion is strong when political parties are practically uniform in proclaiming the need for a reform not usually carried into the political arena.

President Taft has recently declared himself emphatically in favor of a National Board of Health though he has not committed himself as to what he believes should be its composition and its status. Medical societies and medical journals have recently waxed eloquent and forceful in their arguments in behalf of a National Board with extensive powers. Incidentally I may say that those same journals have at the same time brought out clearly the highly commendable work done by the present federal organization known as the Public Health and Marine Hospital Service. See, for instance the New York Medical Journal, volume 88 (1908) page 1,024, where is an excellent article by Dr. C. E. Wood.

Public hygiene has become a kind of social quest. An excellent campaign of education stressing the importance of official sanitary work is being carried on by such societies as the Public Health Defense League, the American Public Health Association and the American Association for the Advancement of Science which through its committee of One Hundred is doing and has been doing for three years noble service in a strenuous warfare against tuberculosis. Professor Irving Fisher of Yale University, at the head of this committee, has made his voice heard far and wide in the plea for proper treatment of consumptives.

One reason for the recent awakening of the people to the great merits of state medicine and sanitary science has been the growing realization of the economic value to the country of a general raising of the average health. Professor Fisher and others have calculated in dollars and cents what preventable illness means to the country. Newholme has estimated the economic burden of sickness in startling concreteness. He postulates nine days of average illness per year. At this rate two million years of life are lost each twelfth month. Estimating wages at one dollar per day and all other expenses at one dollar a day, a loss of $1,144,000,000 a year is registered by illness. Could days of illness be cut down one-third, nearly five hundred million dollars would be saved. Higgins has estimated that six hundred million dollars are now spent on criminality in the United States. If the criminality is largely the product of social environment, such as overcrowding, alcoholism, etc., measures which would decrease this only fractionally are worthy of consideration.

At the last conference of the governors at the White House, Dr. George M. Kober in a speech on "Conservation of Life and Health by Improved Water Supply," showed that the decrease in the "vital assets" of of the country through typhoid fever in one year is more than $350,000,000. The death rate from typhoid being frequently directly traceable to polluted water, the purification of the city water of Albany by means of filtration plants was accomplished and this reduced the death rate from one hundred to twenty-six in one hundred thousand inhabitants. This Dr. Kober calculated was equivalent to a real increase of $350,-000 per year in the "vital assets" of the city.

In view of the wide heralding of such facts by organized societies and by medical and lay journals, we cannot wonder greatly at the increasing popular interest in the needs of public health regulation. Rather do we note such an awakening with approval and much satisfaction.

Besides noting progress in our observation of state medical and sanitary science, one is impressed with the growing need of specialists in this branch of medical work. The three medical specialties of the future, due to the new importance of state control of health, probably will be curative medicine, supervision of personal hygiene and the direction of public hygiene. The problems of sanitation, it has been said, are essentially as attractive as those of curative medicine and effective public recognition seems the one thing at present withheld. But it seems to me that the time will surely come when physicians will, by special courses of study in medical colleges, qualify as experts in public sanitation and public hygiene. Preventative medicine is assuredly of as much value as remedial medicine. After all there can be no absolute distinction between personal and public hygiene. A physician's services are surely as valuable to a man in showing him how to maintain good health and prevent disease as in making him whole when disease fastens itself upon him. Popular opinion might not support this statement, but men of medical training doubtless uniformly believe it. The knowledge of matters of health among the masses should be of far

greater extent than the early smattering of health laws obtained in school days. The trained physician is needed always to advise and instruct.

Another phase of the question of public health is suggested in the truth that all general advancement in this direction is conditioned absolutely upon law, upon sanitary legislation. And laws that are passed should first of all be wise, and secondly should be, not persuasive, but compulsory. Wise laws! How we long for them in every line of activity! The usual complaint from which we suffer in this respect is not entirely the indifference of legislators to matters of state medicine and public health, but more frequently it is hasty and ill-advised medical legislation of which we physicians must complain. In many states sanitary measures are passed by state law makers without previously consulting, either at all or sufficiently, competent medical advisers. Legal men are good advisers in many or most matters of proposed legislation but they cannot possibly render the service that physicians and scientific men can in regard to legislation affecting state medicine. Nor can legislators afford to listen to quacks and visionaries when the health of the people is in question Two much crude, half digested and even nefarious legislation attributable to one cause or another, has been passed in nearly every state legislature.

As to th eneed of sanitary legislation being made compulsory, evidence is overwhelmingly in support of such a contention. Written law, with stringent penalties attached, is necessary if state medicine is to be practical. As Dr. Samuel G. Dixon said before the American Medical Association, "The great majority of men are not wise enough to submit themselves to requirements of sanitary laws or righteous enough to be willing to exercise self-denial and repress cravings of avarice to save others from sickness and contagion." We have compulsory education laws in many states that are quite rigid. Certainly more rigid should be the laws that regulate the control of the health of the commonwealth.

As citizens of a young state whose career has but begun doubtless we have much to learn of the older states in matters of state medicine. It is true, however, that in most respects we have laws that pretty adequately fit our own particular needs At the same time it is of profit to us to examine briefly what some of the other members of the Union accomplished the past year in legis-sanitation.

The excellent system of state control set up by Pennsylvania in 1905-06 is in smooth, successful operation. The plan of making the state Health Commissioner a state officer with a seat in the governor's cabinet and with absolute power of initiative has been more than justified. Oklahoma's State Commissioner of Health exercises a similar prerogative.

Rhode Island has continued her remarkable activity in public sanitation begun in 1905.

South Carolina in the past year provided for the first time in history for a state Health Officer although it had previously had a state Board of Health. It also enabled cities of more than twenty thousand population to establish and maintain public baths. It also authorized its Board of Medical Examiners to revoke the license of any physician guilty of a felony or gross immorality or so addicted to the liquor or drug habit as to be unfit to practice medicine, or in case he has been convicted of illegal practices.

Louisiana created a Board of Osteopathy and provided regulations for the practice of osteopathy.

Kentucky passed a pure food law and an act to encourage the establishment of a Tuberculosis Sanitarium.

Ohio was very active in sanitary legisla-tion. Among other measures it provided for cumpulsory fire drills in every public and private school having an average daily attendance of fifty or more pupils; the establishment of county hospitals for the care and treatment of inmates of county infirmaries and other residents suffering from tuberculosis; the organization of a State Dental Board, with regulations as to the licensing of practitioners of dentistry; severe statutes affecting production of and traffic in milk; the regulation of the manufacture and sale of "renovated" and "process" butter and requirements for the branding of drugs and foods.

Virginia was a close second to Ohio in the quantity of medical legislation passed. This state effected extensive tuberculosis measures; a provision for a Dairy and Food Commissioner having extended powers and supported by laws with hard penalties attached; a statute prohibiting all dispensing or traffic in cocaine, alpha or beta eucaine except on a physician's order; the regulation of the practice of pharmacy and the composition, branding and sale of drugs.

Alabama provided for the establishment of an Epileptic Colony "to secure the humane, curative, scientific and economical care of epileptics. exclusive of violently insane persons who may require treatment at an insane hospital."

Kansas passed laws prohibiting the use of sulphites and any preparation containing sulphar dioxide in the manufacture of meat products. This legislation is expected to insure purity in the packing house products of Kansas City.

Louisiana passed an act regulating the swinging of scaffolding in cities of thirty thousand or over and also made obligatory the equipping of the doors of all public buildings and factories with outward swinging doors. Rhode Island passed a similar law.

Massachusetts authorized towns to appropriate money for public gymnasium and swimming baths and required that every town or city of ten thousand or over shall provide a public play ground for minors and one additional for every additional twenty thousand of population provided such towns or cities shall accept the provisions of the act by a vote. This state also provided for instruction in public schools as to tuberculosis and its prevention.

Maryland brought professional Christian Science within the legal provisions affecting medical practitioners.

New York provided for reports from physicians of persons known by them to have tuberculosis. Any person afflicted with this disease not exercising proper care may be declared guilty of a misdemeanor.

This is the major portion of the health legislation passed by the various states during 1908. Oklahoma, with the exception of a new pure food and drug law, is conspicuous by its absence from the list and it cannot be because of the entire sufficiency of present statutory provisions in such matters. Federal law is necessary in many instances, whereas state law and municipal regulation are needed in others. Our state could be benefited, I believe, by certain health regulations that I might suggest had I time.

But Oklahoma is alive to all questions of public interest and I am confident that at more pressing need and when our wants shall in the course of time become more clearly known, the people, the medical profession and the legislators of the state will rise to the occasion.

Meanwhile let us in season and out of season cherish and further the cause of state medicine and sanitary science.

CANCER OF THE FEMALE BREAST.

By Jabez N. Jackson, M. D., Kansas City, Missouri.

Statistics seem to indicate that the prevalence of cancer is continually on the increase. It is stated that the annual death rate from cancer in England is today, four times as great as it was fifty years ago. And this despite the fact that millions of dollars have been expended on laboratories for cancer research and the entire lives of many of the ablest and most scientific investigators in our profession have been devoted exclusively to this problem. Some day perhaps in the golden future the secret will be solved and this scourge will yield as others have and are to the banishing dictates of preventive medicine. As yet today, however, we must contend with its increasing prevalence and bend our efforts as practicing physicians and surgeons to secure a cure of that which we are as yet powerless to prevent. Even here alas, our efforts are too often of little avail, though year by year with increasing thoroughness of work and earlier recognition of the disease our results are showing greater encouragement.

Next to the uterus the mammary gland is of all organs of the woman most prone to malignant disease. And here likewise should be the most favorable field for early recognition of the disease and accordingly earlier institution of radical therapeutic measures. The mammary gland being the most superficial of all epithelial glandular organs and subject ever to much attention and observation affords great opportunity for the earliest possible recognition of the beginning of any diseased process, and a correct diagnosis of its pathological character.

At the very outset it is of utmost importance to remember that from eighty to ninety per cent of all tumors of the breast are malignant. According to B. Hillroths Statistics embracing 440 cases, eighty-two per cent of all tumors of the breast are cancers. Scmidt (Heidelberg) found 82.66 per cent malignant; Bryant 83.16; Cross 82.47. The author of the Chapter on Breast Tumors in Von Bergman's Surgery states that in his clinic of 359 tumors of the breast, 306 were carcinoma or 80.9 per cent; 34 were sarcoma, 9.1 per cent, making the net percentage of malignancy 90 per cent; while but 19 of the series were benign growths. Jonas, of Omaha, in a recent report embracing 260 cases from his experience found 218 cases or 87 per cent malignant and 42 or 13 per cent benign.

When it is further remembered that many cases apparently benign at the outset finally undergo or manifest malignant development the figures become most impressive. C. H. Mayo in his clinic, tersely remarks "that 80 per cent of all breast tumors are primarily malignant; that of the remaining 20 per cent of primarily benign growths, one-half ultimately become malignant, raising the final percentage of malignancy to 90 per cent, and that the remaining 10 per cent must be viewed with great suspicion."

Diagnosis.—The correct diagnosis of breast cancer is therefore of vast importance, and to the first attending physician one of gravest responsibility. For as William Francis Campbell of Brooklyn has so forcibly said, "Given a patient with cancer of the breast in the first stage, consulting a physician on its first detection, the fate ot that woman is in the hands of the doctor whom she first consults, provided she follows his counsel."

Of most suggestiveness at the outset are certain general etiologic facts pertaining to cancer of the breast, (1) *Age* cancer of the breast is, generally speaking, a disease of middle life, the average age according to Crile being 49. The complete statistics of the Massachusetts General Hospital show of a total of 309 cases, five occuring between the age of 20 and 30, fifty-six be-

tween 30 and 40 years, 120 between 40 and 50 years; 107 between 50 and 60 years, and twenty-one between 70 and 80. It is also noteworthy here that while cancer of the breast is quite rare under 30 yet it does occur. On the other hand it is quite probable that most benign tumors show themselves at an early age in the woman's life. Indeed I feel that we may generally assume that a tumor in the breast of a woman under 30 years of age except with pathognomonic evidence of malignancy, is probably benign, while after we pass this age the probability of cancer becomes so much greater that we will be much safer in assuming malignancy as a fact. (2) *Heredity*, on which in the past much stress has been laid is of little importance and in only about one-third of our cases can a hereditory history of cancer be found. (3) *Lactation* factors likewise are of little significance since according to Crile, 59 per cent of his cases had not borne children and in but 11 per cent was there distinct a history of lactation complications. It is quite probable, however, that chronic mastitis has something to do in producing a favorable nidus for carceer as is true in chronic inflammations elsewhere. (4) *Injury* likewise has some influence but is of too little importance to be significant. In fact it is too easy to find a history of injury antecedent to any condition to which the human flesh is heir, if we but ask for it

Physical Evidences. — Giving whatever weight we wish however to etiologic factors, we are finally forced back to physical finding for correct diagnosis in a given case. (1) *Tumor.* It is undoubtedly a fact that almost without exception the finding of a tumor in the breast is the first sign that calls the patient's attention to the existence of disease. This was true in 94 per cent of Crile's cases, while subjective symptoms such as pains, tensions, stinging, etc., preceded in but 6 per cent. It is furthermore worthy of note that in but one-third of these cases was pain a symptom at all while two-thirds of them were free from pain. This should warn us forcibly against the folly of waiting for pain as an evidence of cancer. It is generally a quite late symptom, one only manifest often when the disease has so far advanced, "that a wayfaring man though a fool, could not err" in diagnosis.

2. *Palpation,* therefore becomes probably our most accurate resource in diagnosis. The intelligent manipulation of a hand trained in the sense of touch becomes therefore of paramount importance For the exercise of this faculty it is essential that the flat of the fingers and palm of the palpating hand should be pressed gently down upon the breast and the tumor thus defined between the hand and the unyielding chest wall behind. inching up the breast between the fingers has doubtless led to many fallacies, oftimes I am sure leading to the removal of mammary glands in which there was actually no disease present whatsoever. When we remember that the breast is a lobular organ, it follows that in pinching up as breast, as I have seen many done we can find an apparent tumor, certainly a mass in all. With the hand or finger flatly applied to the chest however and gently compressing the breast between it and the bony wall, then moving the breast beneath horizontally over the underlying ribs with the skin fixed by contact with the hand, any existing tumor even though small can be detected with surprising ease and accuracy. The nodule may be exceedingly small, yet the stony hardness of a cancer growth will be striking and characteristic. Careful comparison in all manipulations should be made with the healthy breast, though here it should be remembered that bilateral disease while infrequent and therefore improbable is not impossible. A Carcinomatous tumor is generally single and multiple tumors speak against malignancy. The can-

cerous growth likewise infiltrates the normal breast tissue and thus not being circumscribed, it moves with the breast in which it is definitely fixed. It is also quite apt to become early fixed either to the skin overlying in superficial growths, or to the pectoral fascia beneath in deep seated growths. The skin attachment is easily recognized. The fascial attachment may only become evident when the arm is carried upward and outward rendering the pectoral muscles tense. Then oftimes the tumor and with it the breast becomes absolutely immovable on the chest wall. "Dividing the breast into a central or areolar portion and four quadrants, we find the frequency of location in the following sequence: upper outer, central, upper inner, lower outer, lower inner." It is also important to observe the relative amount of normal gland remaining outside the area of the tumor. Inasmuch as the cancer grows at the expense of the breast, and fibrous tissue contraction accompanies the process, there is oftimes but little normal gland tissue left. The extent of this ratio is oftimes also an evidence of the rate of growth which may be of service in prognosis as well as in diagnosis. In simple tumors on the other hand the normal breast tissue is pushed aside but not consumed.

(3) *Trabecular Shortening.*—The tendency of the fibrous tissue trabeculae to shorten and thus to fix the breast, may also give visual evidence even at a very early stage of the disease, in the slight dimpling of the overlying skin evidenced by moving the breast over the chest wall, producing also a sensation of tugging to the examining hand. Halstead especially lays great stress on this sign, even going so far as to say that "the faintest conceivable trace of a difference on the two sides in a minor pectoral crease, for example, may suffice for the diagnosis. Frequently there is no sign but this almost imperceptible sugges-

tion of pull, which when the faintest possible is, of course, elicited by dislocation in one direction only. This sign, however slight, is all that is needed for the diagnosis." Surely, however, we must remark, extreme care must be taken in this test and only an experienced examiner of breast tumors could follow the refinement of Halstead's test in its entirety. When well developed however it is surely trustworthy. Minute compression of both breasts is of course essential.

(4) *Retraction of Nipple.*—The sign of retraction of the nipple on which so much reliance was formerly put, is not now given quite so much prominence. In some subjects it will be found that this characteristic is normally found and is then present in both nipples. When present in one nipple alone it is still a highly significant sign. Its absence, however, is of little value in negating a diagnosis. In fact Crile found it present in only 33 per cent of his cases. It must be remembered that this sign is likewise dependent upon shortening of the troabeculae, and unless the growth is in the central area or quite near the nipple no retraction will occur except in a large or well advanced cancer.

(5) *Absorption of Overlying Fat.*— The fat overlying a cancerous nodule, if it be superficial, is oftimes absorbed also lessening the freedom with which the skin moves over the tumor and oftimes making the tumor stand out so prominently as to be at once apparent to the inspecting eye. In early diagnosis, particularly in that of deeply seated nodes, it is valueless.

(6) *Glandular Enlargement.*—The involvement of the axilliary glands and their enlargement comes sooner or later, alas often too soon. It is to be remembered that acute inflammations, tuberculosis, etc., can likewise produce enlargement of the axilliary glands. The local evidences of infection and inflammation however are usually so easily recognized in these diseases as to lead to no confusion in their differential diagnosis. When these inflammatory causes can be set aside the evidence of enlarged axilliary glands is quite conclusive of cancerous disease. In fact the diagnosis should be made before this symptom is evident.

As to the evidences of (7) Ulceration, (8) Emaciation, (9) Cachexia, we will only say that they are such late evidences as to be of no service to a clinician. By the time these symptoms are manifest a housemaid could make a diagnosis.

Finally as to diagnosis I would say with Crile, "An undurated invading, solid somewhat irregular mass when gently pressed against the chest, with or without retraction of the nipple, with or without discharge from the nipple, with or without absorption of fat over the tumor, with or without dimpling, with or without pain, with or without hereditory history, with or without cachexia, ulceration or metastasis should be surgically treated, either explored or execised."

Operative Diagnosis.—After, however, all is said as to physical diagnosis, and all the various diagnostic signs have been fully exhausted we must yet admit the fact that in many cases preoperative absolute diagnosis is impossible. This is particularly true in the earliest stages of the disease. And here is to be found therefore the somewhat plausible excuse for a course of hesitation, palliation and delay so fatal in the end to the fate of the unfortunate woman. When however, we reflect that even a benign tumor never disappears except by removal; when we remember that from the aspect of general probabilities alone the chances are nine out of ten in favor of malignancy; when we realize that a simple incision will make a diagnosis absolutely clear; is there then left any possible excuse for the responsible physician to counsel a course of procrastination which as we shall later see probably robs the sufferer of one-half her chances of life. Certainly not. Exploratory diagnosis must therefore in doubtful cases be insisted upon. If the tumor prove benign, without harm or risk to the patient in the least, local excision alone has at least removed a course of menace which should be removed anyway. On the other hand should the evidence of malignancy be found, the operator should be prepared to at once push his operation to immediate complete amputation. With Bloodgood we believe that the experienced surgeon should have relatively no difficulty or doubt in the diagnosis, and secondary operation once in mere gross appearance of the tumor tissue. If in doubt, however, a competent pathologist must be at hand for immediate microscopic diagnosis from the frozen section, a proceeding which adds exactness with a delay of less than ten minutes at the farthest. We cannot too strongly condemn the policy of excision, delay for fixed specimen diagnosis, and secondary operation once in vogue, since Halstead has shown that in cases of cancer of the breast where this course has been pursued not one single case has ever been finally cured. Fortunately immediate diagnosis is now the practice of all operating surgeons, and such fatal mistakes will not occur.

Treatment.—Once an absolute diagnosis is made or even a probable diagnosis, the treatment becomes the responsible question between patient and physician. Is it too much to say today that radical surgical treatment is absolutely the only treatment?

Certainly no physician today would for a moment consider salves, caustics or local applications of like nature, methods now happily employed only by absolute ignorance or quackery.

Thus far, moreover, the writer has never known nor heard of nor read in scientific literature of a single case of breast cancer

cured by the X-Ray. Injection of trypsin or allied preparations have not a single record of cure to their credit. It is of course easy to find reports of cases when from such various methods temporary shrinkage or apparent disappearance of the growth has occured. But does this prove a cure? Volkman many years ago established the dictum, since universally recognized in surgery, that to class a case of cancer cured at least three years must elapse with absolutely no evidence of recurrence either local or remote. Even this limit is ofttimes transgressed in apparent safety with yet later recurrence until today we are rather inclined to push our limit of time standard forward to five years. If this be the criterion by which the cure of cancer is to be measured, how ridiculous the often bombastic claims of methods based on apparent results of but a few months test at best. Undoubtedly all honest surgeons look forward with earnest hope to some time when we can cure cancer of the breast without the horrors of the knife. Likewise undoubtedly most all honest physicians admit that up to the present hour there is nothing but surgery which offers the faintest hope of success.

At this point possibly the patient or her sceptical attendant will ask: "and what can surgery offer?" I must confess that during many years of our earlier work, before accumulative evidence was at hand, our answer would needs have been, faith. But time and evidence have converted faith into very encouraging facts, some of which I beg now to record.

End Results.

Halstead reporting the final results in 210 fully traced cases from the records of John Hopkins Hospital, all passed the three year period of time since the operation, shows eighty-nine permanent cures, a percentage of 42.4, in detail as follows:

PATHOLOGICAL VARIETY	NO. CASES	NO. CURED 3 YEARS)	PER CENT
Cancer cysts	6	2(19)	33 3
Adeno carcinoma	52	24	75
Medullary	25	12	4 3
Circumscribed scirrhus	28	13	46 4
Small infiltration scirrhus	80	30	35 5
Large infiltration scirrhus	39	8	20 5
Total	210	89	42 4

It is furthermore worthy of note that from this gross number there were sixty cases operated upon in which there was no glandular metastasis and of this number forty-five, (75 per cent) were permanent cures and fifty-one or 85 per cent were free from recurrence on the three-year limit. This clearly demonstrates the absolute importance of early diagnosis and early operation whereby the chance of cure is absolutely twice as good.

GLANDULAR INVOLVEMET	NO. CASES	PERMT CURE	PER CENT	3 YRS CURE	PER CENT
Axilla and neck negative	60	45	75	51	85
Axilla positive, neck negative	111	27	24 8	34	31
Axilla and neck positive	40	3	7 5	4	10

Massachusetts General Hospital, Boston.

Between the years 1894 and 1898 inclusive (first five years), there were 160 cases operated, of which twenty-six were cured, or 16.2 per cent. In the years 1899 to 1903 (second five years) of 157 cases forty-one were cured, or 26 per cent, almost double the percentage of the first five years, surely a convincing evidence of improving results. Here also we find that whereas the percentage of cures where the axillary glands were enlarged was but 12 per cent when the axilla was negative the percentage was 29

PATHOLOGICAL VARIETY	CASES	SURVIVING OPERAT'N	CURES	PER CENT
Medullary	136	104	19	18 2
Scirrhus	46	45	10	25
Adeno carcinoma	24	21	10	47 6
Colloid	4	3	2	666
Cancer	127	107	18	16 8
No. Path. report	39	31	8	25 8

Crile, of Cleveland, in a traced record of ninety-one cases, found that in cases with

grandular involvement his percentage of cures was 14 per cent while in cases where no glands could be found prior to operation his percentage of cures was raised to 80 per cent.

Cabot, of Boston, in an experience of forty-two cases has had nine or 21 per cent of cures.

Dennis, of New York, in a series of 116 cases reported before the American Surgical Society in 1891 showed 45 per cent of three-year cures. In 1895 in the report of a smaller series the same society, he recorded 77 per cent cures.

Willy Myer, of New York, in a series of eighty cases reported twenty-eight or 35 per cent cures. Of these there were sixteen cases operated on 10-12 1-2 years, or which three (18.75 per cent) alive today; twenty-seven cases operated on 5-10 years, of which six (22.2 per cent) alive today; twenty cases operated on 3-5 years, of which 10 (50 per cent) alive today; seventeen cases operated on last three years, of which nine (50 per cent) alive today.

Vander Veer, of Albany, N. Y., in a series of 103 cases, reports seventy cured, or 68 per cent.

Ochsner, of Chicago, in ninety-eight fully traced cases. reported fifty-four or 43 per cent cured.

Oliver, of Cincinnati, of thirty-five cases reports twelve cured from three to ten and one-half years or 34 per cent cures. Here also we learn that in cases where the tumor has been known to exist for one year or more, the per cent of cures was 28.5, whereas in cases where tumor had existed over from six months to one year the percentage was 50.

Jonas, of Omaha, in 177 traced cases found 105 cured three years or over or 56 per cent.

Rodman, Philadelphia, reports that in cases from his private practice 70 per cent were cured.

Cheyne, of England, in thirty-tour private cases, had seventeen or 50 per cent of cures alive after six to sixteen years.

Childe, in forty-six cases, had seventeen, or 36.9 per cent well after from five to twenty years.

Dowd's analysis of 199 cases from the clinics of Bull, Rotter, Helfreich, Cheyne, Dennis, and may shows 39.6 per cent cured.

A summary of this rather extended evidence shows a percentage of cures ranging from 25 per cent at the lowest to 75 per cent at the best. This in a disease otherwise absolutely fatal is certainly most encouraging and has furnished a magnificent proof for the faith of surgery. Two other facts likewise stand out prominently. First, that in cases of early diagnosis and early operation the percentage of cures is practically doubled. Surely the responsibility resting on the first attendant is enormous. Second, the results in private cases are vastly better than in those selected from crowded tenements of pauper population. Have we not therefore particular ground for encouragement with a class of patients to whom fresh air. glorious sunshine, and good food is not a luxury but an every day possession.

But perhaps again some doubting Thomas or some timid subject may inquire, is there not great risk to life in a formidable surgical procedure which furbishes such results. To this, we reply, Halstead had but four deaths in 232, 1.7 per cent mortality. Crile in ninety-one cases had no deaths. At the Massachusetts General Hospital in 416 cases operated on by over twenty various surgeons there was but 3.6 per cent mortality and in the later years (1899-1903) but 2 per cent. Cabot in his forty-two cases had no deaths. Ochsner had five deaths in 164 cases. Jonas had six deaths in 255 cases. According to Haggard on the analysis of 600 operations in the hands of twenty-one different surgeons

the mortality was but 9 per cent. The writer in his personal experience has had no deaths from operation nor has he known of one in the service of colleagues.

In conclusion permit me to epitomize the following conclusions:

First. At least 90 to 95 per cent of all tumors of the breast are malignant and no possible intelligence can proclaim which of the remaining 10 per cent will remain benign.

Second. There is no known cure for any tumor of the breast, benign or malignant, except through surgical removal.

Third. From 25 to 50 per cent of cases of breast cancer are permanently cured by radical surgical removal. With early diagnosis this per centage could be raised to 80 per cent.

Fourth. Every tumor of the breast, therefore, should be considered malignant and treated as such at the very first moment of its detection, unless incision has proven it benign, in which instance, local excision should at least be insisted upon.

To trifle with tumors of the breast is therefore, practically nothing short of criminal.

Read before the 1909 meeting of the Oklahoma State Medical Association, of Oklahoma City, Oklahoma.

DISCUSSION.

Dr. Blesh was called upon to open the discussion.

Dr. A. L. Blesh:

I was very very much pleased to hear the paper. We owe a good deal to Dr. Jackson on this breast operation. He has made a valuable invention in the way of an instrument for this operation. He has an indisputable array of facts showing that surgery offers the only means of dealing with the disease and is to the patient the only remedy. It seems criminal to wait for

—diagnosis in many cases. By resorting to the laboratory findings we can tell in ten minutes the exact nature of the case. We can do a simple enucleation if the tumor is benign and in case of a malignant one a more thorough enucleation.

———

Dr. U. L. Russell, Oklahoma City:

Dr. Russell urged the education of the public by the profession as to the character of this trouble and its more evident manifestations, to the end that operation might be resorted to while there was still chance of cure.

———

Dr. George A. Boyle, Enid, Okla.:

Dr. Boyle spoke of the late statistics in these cancer cases, and of the matter of reaching the people to inform them of the necessity of early action.

ILEO-COLITIS OR DYSENTERY.

By Dr. H. M. Williams, Wellston, Okla.

The subject of this paper is one of unusual importance to the rural practitioner, as well as one that is looked upon by the laity with less seriousness by far than should be. A disease that so oft times proves fatal, and which requires as careful attention from the onset as ileo-colitis.

The purpose of this discussion shall be to deal with the causes, diagnosis and treatment as confined to the rural practitioner. Giving prominence or special consideration to the latter. When taken into consideration the many disturbances to which the gastro-intestinal tract is subject during the first few years of the average child's life, the number of attacks and the almost miraculous recoveries that are made, with but little attention ,there may be some allowance for the progress which this disease has made when first met with by the physician. There is a prevailing, erroneous, opinion that gastro-intestinal disturbances are essential to normal dentition. People who live in the country and especially those who live at a distance, do not as a rule, summon a physician as quickly as those who live in towns or cities or convenient to medical aid. The physician is called after the "Granny" doctor of the neighborhood, as each and every neighborhood has from one to a dozen, has tried all her "sure remedies" without their usual success, and she reluctantly yields to the calling of a physician, after expounding the virtues of her various teas, that never had failed before. The unfortunate child whom this class of would-be doctors seek as their victims is now placed in the hands of a physician, either to cure or sign a death certificate, of which the latter is often the case.

The history of these cases as a rule, are very similar and that received from the mother or those in charge is usually the following: Having previously taken improper food which is followed by vomiting, sudden rise in temperature, bowels acting freely, with watery stools, which may be yellowish, brown or green or mixed with blood of mucous and acting from six to a dozen times in twenty-four hours. If containing blood the physician is summoned early, as the laity consider these cases more serious. When sleeping the child's eyes are only partly closed and may lay as in a stupor. If this condition has continued for a few days, will show evidence of loss of flesh, a flabby condition of the muscles and weak pulse.

Causes: The predisposing causes of ileo-colitis are many. Those most common are due to improper food. Either the child or the mother, if a nursing child, eating unmatured vegetables, unripe fruits, or an excess amount of sweets or over-loading the stomach with undigestible foods. Milk may be the cause when cows are allowed to feed upon improper food, such as corn or hay that is spoiled or pastures that are filled with poisonous weeds, the juices of which find their way into the milk. While dysentery may occur at any season of the year, for the past nine years we have found more cases occuring during the latter part of May, all of June and continuing throughout the month of July, at the beginning of the vegetable and fruit seasons. During this season we also find the greatest number of gastro-intestinal disturbances, and fermental diarrhoes, which in many cases are predisposing causes of ileo-colitis. It is also said to follow diphtheria, measels and bronchopneumonia. I have no knowledge of ever having a case following the latter named diseases. Poorly nourished or bottle fed children are the most frequent subjects.

The generally accepted opinion is that the direct cause of ileo-colitis is due to the Bacillus Shiga which lives and grows in all seasons of the year and in all climates that is inhabited by man, but found most frequently in the tropics and sub-tropical climates during the summer months.

There are three varieties met with which are determined by the extension of the lesion.

First: The simple catarrhal form which involves the lymph nodules of the mucosa.

Second: The Follicular or ulcerative type which does not only involve the lymph nodules of the mucosa but destroys them as well.

The third of membranous type involves both the mucosa and the sub-mucosa and is the most severe form met with.

These lesions are usually found in the colon and the ileum but the latter type has been known to extend through the entire intestinal tract and even involving the stomach. These different varieties can best be described by a case of each that has come under my own observation.

Case: Child; male, age three, taken suddenly sick after overloading the stomach, high temperature from the onset, rapid pulse, frequent stools mixed with blood and mucous, suppresed urine, general depressed condition. After the first twenty-four hours temperature declined, at the end of seventy-two hours both temperature and pulse normal. Stools less frequent, with little or no blood, gradual return to appetite which was previously lost. At the end of one week's time stools had assumed a normal condition. Child apparently well with the exception of an indication of loss of flesh, weak and pallid countenance. At the end of the second week there was no evidence of sickness, apparently recovered. Indications pointed that the lesion involved only part of the colon and was that of the catarrhal variety.

Case 2: Child, female, eighteen months old, having cut both eye and stomach teeth. Previous to attack had been taken from the breast. Taken to sudden vomiting about 1 o'clock in the night, which consisted of particles of undigested food with a sour odor. Being deprived of its nurse, caused an increased appetite for food, it had been allowed on the day previous to attack, to eat chowchow, nuts, and a small quantity of ice cream. When on the following morning the bowels were flushed, the rectum was filled with hard normal faeces; after this there was passed a large quantity of undigested foods, which had been eaten during the previous day. Following this irrigation the bowels acted seven to eight times before they checked which was the case throughout the entire sickness. The character of the stools were yellowish brown in color which became green after remaining on the napkin for a short time. This condition continued for four days. During this time, patient took very little nourishment. There was a loss of flesh with a temperature ranging from normal to 101 with very little sleep at any time.

On the fourth day there was a sudden rise of temperature with an increased pulse, a refusal to take any nourishment at all, stools assumed a green color, mixed with a considerable mucous, and acted more frequently. There was a considerable bloating, and tenderness throughout the region of the colon. Urine scant. This condition continued with a gradual decrease in temperature until the end of the twelfth day when the stools assumed a more yellowish color. The mucous less, bloating and tenderness disappeared from the colon, temperature became normal, patient less peevish, and continued to slowly improve upon a restricted diet. 'At the end of four weeks stools had become practically normal. Appetite having returned at the end of the second week made the task very difficult to keep the patient on a restricted diet. At the end of the fourth week there was a considerable weakness and evidence of great loss of flesh. This case was diagnosed as follicular type.

Case 3: Child a female, age two years. During the month of July, taken suddenly sick, with high fever, frequent and bloody stools moving every one-half to one nour with a history of having overloaded the stomach with green peaches. The discharges contained both blood and mucous from the beginning, with a considerable pain and tenesmus. After the fourth or fifth day the blood disappeared from the stools, only excepting at short intervals, the stools were mixed with threads of mucous, which increased and decreased from time to time throughout the entire sickness, which lasted for a period of fourteen weeks. During the time there would pass particles of membrane especially in the latter part of sickness. Through the entire sickness there was a considerable bloating, in the in-

testinal tract and even at times involving the stomach, this condition we were unable to wholly relieve. At times there was a prolapsus of the rectum. At the end of 104 days the child died greatly emaciated with a general dropsical condition which was due to acute nephritis. This case represented the membranous type.

Diagnosis.

The diagnosis of a case of ileo-colitis when accompanied by bloody mucous stools is not difficult, but the absence of this condition, which is sometimes the case requires a more careful study. Mucous and bloody stools eliminates acute milk infection. Some of our text books point out the fact that Gastro-Enter-colitis and Entero-colitis have a greenish spinach like or brown muddy stool with very foetid odor, while in dysentery the stools are smaller in quantity." Dr. Holt says that typhoid fever or intussusception might be taken for dysentery, but when we remember the slow gradual rise of temperature of the former, and the entire absence of temperature of the latter the task of discriminating should not be so difficult. The diagnosis by the rural practitioner is made wholly from clinical symptoms, not having access to a patholigical laboratory, and those of us who have access to microscopes are not accustomed to using them as often as we should and especially in this class of cases, because of the pronounced clinical symptoms and the immediate demand for action. While a student in college a quotation of Dr. Osler made a very vivid impression on my mind when he said that, "No case of dysentery should be lightly considered as he considered it one of the four epidemic diseases of the world." In my opinion when a case is met with that has the cardinal symptoms of ilio-colitis it should be considered and treated as such, and if we err at all we should err upon the side of safety. As to the diagnosis of the different varieties of lesions it is almost impossible and not altogether essential from the onset, but is very important to know that the case is ileocolitis. The variety can be determined by the extent of the involvment. A few points may be mentioned which is characteristic of the different types. The catarrhal variety, the symptoms are more marked from the onset with high temperature, rapid pulse and frequent stools. While in the follicular type the progress is more gradual and frequently follows gastro-enteric intoxication or any derangement of the gastro-intestinal tract, which was the case in the one above described. While in the membranous form the symptoms are not so pronounced at the beginning and might be diagnosed as some other disease.

Treatment.

The treatment of ileo-colitis is one of unusual importance and from the rural practitioner's standpoint can best be considered in the following manner:

First: Sanitary or general surroundings.

Second: Medicinal.

Third: Dietetic.

Each point is of importance in itself and closely related to each other. In many homes a physician meets with very unsanitary conditions. Houses poorly ventilated. Rooms damp and dark and filled with foul air. Especially is this the condition in the log cabin and undeveloped communities where these cases are frequently met. Bed clothing and gowns are unclean, many parents little realizing the importance of cleanliness in these cases. It is necessary if this condition does exist that it be corrected at once. Those in charge are to be given to understand, if results are expected in the case that everything must be kept clean and also that it must be explained this is an infectious disease. And instructed that the diapers and sheets must be boiled when changed. The floors must be scrubbed with carbolic acid or bichloride solu-

tion. All linens must be kept absolutely clean. For nursing we have to depend on the anxious mother or the mercy of the neighbors who will lend assistance at short intervals, as home duties prevent them from coming to stay for a few hours only. Between the physician's visit the little patient has passed into three or four different hands and as many different remedies may be given which you have not prescribed, and will never learn of in case the child should die. If recovery should be the outcome this remedy is given the credit of cure. A trained nurse, especially in this class of patients, is looked upon as an unnecessary luxury. Unfortunately the majority of cases met with are in families who have not the means to secure the services of an experienced nurse, and this makes the physician's duty of double importance.

The drug remedies in these cases are many. Each physician after having tried the regular routine, selects those on which he can best rely.

The profession is about a unit, however, that both castor oil and calomel are essential, early in these cases. For cleansing a way as far as possible the pathogenic organism. A child two years old should be given one to two drams of castor oil together with three to five calolactose tablets on first seeing the case. In the event that the stomach will not tolerate oil, calomel should be given at once in broken doses, until the stomach is settled, which is usually the case after thoroughly flushing the bowels by passing a rectal tube as high as is safe in doing. For this use a normal saline solution to which may be added two drams of borate of soda to the quart, allowing the flow of water as soon as the tube passes the sphincter so as to cleanse the lower bowel. This should be repeated in six or eight hours for the first day or two. I make it a practice to give this first en'ema myself in the presence of some one who is instructed as to sterilizing, lubricating, position and passing of tube. For sterilizing hot water is used; for lubricating either castor oil and carbolated vaseline. Position, the child is placed on left side with hips elevated. The flushing aids in relieving gases and pain and will in most cases cause vomiting to cease and reduce temperature if high. If the bowels are acting frequently with blood and mucous, which is often the case, this may be controlled by giving bismuth and cerium oxlate in large doses, one to two drams of the former and one-half dram of the latter in twenty-four hours. As an intestinal antiseptic sulpho-carbolate of zinc or salol may be given. As for me I use the former in one-half grain doses every three or four hours. For pain give the tincture of camphorated opium in ten to fifteen miniums or one-half teaspoonful of papine every two or three hours. As a corrective give one-half teaspoonful of neutralizing cordial every three or four hours. As a stimulatnt brandy may be given in one to two teaspoonfuls every three or four hours unless pronounced weakness of the pulse is manifested then the strychnine should be given instead. As a tonic the pepto manganate of iron should be added a teaspoonful three or four times daily. This is well borne by the stomach. Malaria is associated with a majority of these cases in malarial districts. For this condition quinine should be administered by inunction or applied in a dilute solution of alcohol. Hemorrhage may be controlled by irrigating the rectum and colon three or four times daily with one to one thousand solution of nitrate of silver. Tenesmus of the rectum may be relieved by irrigating the rectum with a starch solution to which one-half dram of laudanum has been added or painting the rectum with 2 per cent solution of cocaine. If prolapsus of the rectum is present may be controlled by mechanical means.

The diet in these cases is of all importance and should receive most careful attention when taking in consideration the nature and extent of the lesion. In many cases the colon alone is affected but the lesions frequently extend in the first two or three feet of the ileum. In severe types may extend through the entire intestinal tract. The question of nourishment becomes one of importance. The diet that would be of most service to the patient, is that class which is acted upon most quickly by the secretions of the stomach and intestines. In my judgment milk is one of the most valuable diets in the majority of these cases and should be taken from the upper half of the vessel after having stood for a few hours. Animal broths are valuable, rice, oat meal and barley water are usually well tolerated. The liquid of beef peptonoids has proved of service to me in these cases. As to the different varities of proprietary foods I have had but little experience. Horlick's Malted Milk I have uesd during convalescence to some advantage. Eggs properly prepared, fresh sweet buttermilk can also be used to some advantage. The milk must be from a cow that has been placed upon proper food or pasture.

Anti-dysentery serum has been recomemnded as of service in the treatment but has not yet been sufficiently developed to know of its real merit. But it is to be hoped that it will prove a success when fully developed.

Case 1 was placed on the following: Oil two drams and calomel in one-half grain doses until six doses were given, lower bowel irrigated three times during the first twenty-four hours with normal saline and borate of soda solution. On the following day oil and calomel was repeated with one-half of the amount for the next two or three days which was then discontinued. Bismuth and cerium oxlate and sulpho carbolate of zinc, together with neutrolizing cordial was given from the onset. After the third day pepto manganate of iron was added. Patient was placed upon a milk and animal broth diet with the results as above stated.

Case 2 was treated largely as one, less bismuth was given owing to the inactivity of the bowels, calomen and oil were given daily for the first ten days. In addition to high rectal irrigations turpentine stupes were used over the region of the colon for relieving gases. The diet consists of milk to which was added oat meal water and liquid beef peptonoids, and chicken broths. During convalescence was given dry toasts, fresh butter, poached eggs and malted milk.

Case 3 was treated in like manner as one and two with addition heart stimulants strychnae, diuretics, and opium. Hemmorrhage was controlled by nitrate of silver solution tenesmus with a cocaine solution with results as above stated.

In conclusion would add that the family physician should carefully investigate all cases of gastro-intestinal derangements that comes to his attention. Do not agree with the misguided mother that the disturbance is due to teething only, but thoroughly impress upon her mind that the child may be seriously sick though the patient does not manifest grave symptoms. From general appearances we are unable to tell the extent of these lesions which may have already advanced beyond our control.

Read before the 1909 meeting of the Oklahoma State Medical Association, of Oklahoma City, Oklahoma.

EDITORIAL

TO MEMBERS OF THE OKLAHOMA STATE MEDICAL ASSOCIATION.

On assuming the management of the Secretary's office and the Journal of the Association the undersigned wishes to thank his friends for the honor conferred in his election and to outline the policy he proposes to follow during the year.

I shall at all times endeavor to continue the interest in the association's affairs that I have evinced in the past. Having been a rather constant attendant on meetings of the old Indian Territory Association and afterwards a worker in the organization of the Western Ditsrict Society—being its first Secretary and later its President—this attendance dating from before my graduation in medicine, I naturally have some ideas of organization I hope to carry out for our benefit. This matter of organization is one of co-operation and enthusiasm on the part of all our membership. I want to try to persuade each member to help in increasing our growth; in each community you know some one who should affiliate with his county society and it is to the mutual interest of all that he be induced to join. Try to get him in.

I want each reader to understand that I am working in the interest of no particular or individual interest of the Association, but for the entire organization and with this in view I want the suggestions of every one in making the year a successful one. With a united and critical membership there is no reason why we should not have the best Association in the Mississippi valley and our Journal should be in keeping with it. I will therefore appreciate your suggestions as to management and receive them in the spirit they are given.

It is not amiss here to make public acknowledgment of the kindness and efficient help given me by the retiring Secretary, Dr. E. O. Barker. He gave me many helpful suggestions and every assistance possible in the removal and installation of the office and its complexities and I take this means to thank him for his kindness.

Reiterating my interest in the Association and also in the personal welfare of all the members, I am,

Very truly,

CLAUDE A. THOMPSON,

Secretary.

One of the most important matters taken up by the State Association at Oklahoma City and one which, if carried out, will have a far reaching influence eventually, was the adoption of the following resolution read and introduced by Dr. H. M. Williams, of Wellston:

Whereas, According to statistical reports, tuberculosis, which is known to be an infectious disease, is causing thousands of deaths annually, and its unfortunate victims are permitted daily to come in contact with the public in general, thereby spreading the dread disease,

Therefore, Be It Resolved, That a committee of three be named by the chair whose duty it shall be to study plans and methods as to the best policy for both physician and state to pursue relative to tubercular patients, and that this committee report at our next annual meeting.

Resolved, Further, That we favor the taking of a census of the tubercular patients of this state by the State Board of Health.

The President appointed the following committee to take the matter in hand:

Dr. H. M. Williams, chairman, Wellston; Dr. R. H. Harper, Afton; Dr. J. M. Postelle, Oklahoma City.

Dry words cannot express the importance to the state and the people of this matter, which so far as Oklahoma is concerned, has heretofore been only considered in an abstract way and looked upon in an apathetic manner.

While Oklahoma is spending many millions for the construction and maintenance of schools and for the building of cities and modern improvements of various kinds, and all of which are needed and proper in their place, our greatest infectious troubles are, comparatively speaking, not receiving the attention they deserve.

Of course it is difficult for a layman to appreciate the importance of such conditions and the only hope that they will ever be brought to consider them and act for their prevention along sane and intelligent lines is through the forcible and strong co-operative aid of the medical profession of the state.

It is to be sincerely hoped that this move will be productive of great good and that the medical men of the State will give it careful consideration.

DID YOU MISS YOUUR JOURNAL?

Subscribers who come up short the Journal of the Oklahoma State Medical Association this month are requested to drop a card to the editor and the deficiency will be supplied at once.

During the rush of transferring the records and papers of the Secretary's office many names may be omitted through oversight and we will be glad to remedy the mistakes thus made.

On the advice of the retiring Secretary, which we consider good and business-like, many names who were in arrears for dues and who have previously received the Journal, were omitted from the mailing list.

This was a necessary move for several reasons; printing and other bills in connection with the Journal must be promptly met and we see no reason for carrying a name on the subscription list at the expense of a fellow member.

OUR ANNUAL NATIONAL HOLO- CAUST.

Physicians of Oklahoma may well take a lesson from the pages of the past on the frivolities of the 4th of July now nearly upon us and try to do something along the line of preventive medicine or rather "preventive foolishness."

Each year adds to the list of victims of this day, until instead of being our national celebration it is fast becoming our national holocaust.

Many of the larger cities have hospitals and dispensaries where these cases receive immediate and proper treatment without cost to the injured person, the system is good as can be under the circumstances, but it irritates one to know that the initial trouble could be prevented by enactment and enforcement of proper laws.

Oklahoma has received so much criticism on account of its newly made laws that another departure from the usual might well be made in this case and laws passed prohibiting the use of unnecessary fireworks, or at least limiting their use to certain places and times. While in certain quarters this law would probably be received as was our nine-foot sheet regulation, with derision, that would not prevent it from being timely legislation, in keeping with the trend of modern advancement and not a stinging reflection on our civilization as it is today.

A movement by our various city and county medical organizations should be inaugurated in order to secure the legislation necessary to remedy this evil.

THE SANITARY SITUATION.

As we have been in office a month we must be pardoned for wanting to reform everything about us. Perhaps we cannot do much toward the regulation of the festive fire cracker and the toy pistol, but we feel that there is not a physician in the state who cannot do more or less toward the prevention of our greatest plagues— malarial infection, typhoid and dysentery. The first mentioned is of far greater importance from an economic standpoint, they are all bad enough and are all preventable. The loss to the state annually due to these preventable diseases cannot be computed, any attempt to arrive at it leads one to a staggering summary. From the banker's desk to the man in the field pitching hay malaria yearly collects its toll.

The writer has observed that as his home town becomes more civilized in respect to drainage of ponds and oiling those that cannot be drained the malarial indicator falls lower. Every physician in the state has observed the same conditions and many have taken advantage of their knowledge of the sources of infection to insist publicly and privately that the proper remedy be applied.

A written communication to your city council backed up by a strong personal appearance of the virile men of the profession of your locality before the authorities, showing them by argument and illustration the good to be accomplished in a general cleaning up and how it may be done goes far toward the solution of the problem.

Personally each physician should find it within his province to show the family who know him as attendant how to do their share. The intelligent already know, the thoughtless have not thought and the ignorant do not know how to think about it. They will appreciate your intervention in their sanitary affairs; those who do not need not be worried much with your consideration.

"For ways that are dark and tricks that are vain"

Some insurance companies are peculiar.

An agent of the Metropolitan Life Insurance Company approached the editor not long since with a proposition that in politeness should be termed unique, however we must call it by some other name if the vocabulary contains it. He wanted an examiner, his blank was right up to date calling for more than the usual number and kinds of endorsements and information. For his high class examinations they would pay three dollars and then he pulled out what he called an "Inspector's Report," this report was to be filled out at the residence of the applicant. if necessary, and contained questions as to age, occupation. appearance, when ill and what with during the past five years or so and besides other requirements it was necessary to make an examination of the heart and lungs in the event his history indicated it. For this mere effort on our part we were to receive the princely sum of twenty-five cents per capita.

The gentleman assured us that he could and did get good men to undertake the work everywhere else, going so far as to name men in other states, whom he considered representative men in the profession, who would do this work under the terms and at that time were doing it.

We declined the honor about to be conferred and say nothing more about it on account of a peculiarity in the postal law referring to profanity being circulated in the mails.

Muskogee is just now experiencing its annual visitation of smallpox and this year the malady seems more widely distributed than in many years past.

The situation is in the efficient hands of Dr. Sessler Hoss, the newly appointed City Physician

---

In the case of Pennington vs. Goeske, tried before Justice M. G. Bailey of Muskogee county some time since the decision of Justice Bailey fixes the status of the CHIROPRACTOR, at least for the time being, so far as he is concerned.

Pennington, who advertises to the public that he is a Chiropractic Physician and Surgeon, sued Goeske for a balance of ninety odd dollars for professional services and on trial the verdict was given the defendant, Goeske, on the grounds that the plaintiff was not a legally registered physician within the meaning of the laws of Oklahoma and therefore could not recover.

An appeal was taken by Pennington's attorney and the final outcome will be observed with great interest by the profession generally throughout the state.

A remarkable fact concerning this cult, which may have escaped some of the regular profession, is this: Osteopathy, which at the most and under the most liberal interpretation, can only be beneficial to a certain class of ailments and in many of these is liable to cause damage in view of their meagre diagnostic attainments is one of the most strenuous objectors to their recognition.

It is certainly a case of being "hoist by one's own petard" the osteopath has long contended that his was the only branch worth considering and now comes the chiropractor with his special claims of manipulating certain obscure and harmless nerves and discarding the gross anatomy of the osteopath, selecting only a small part, of the goodness of their parent body and alledging to the public that here is the solution of all human difficulties.

But for that loyalty which actuates the minds of most medical men one is almost forced to wish the chiropractor good luck on the theory that one fraud will get retributive justice at the hands of the other one.

Our only fault to find with the various schisms and cults aggravating the medical field today is that they are sadly deficient in that most important of all things, that Holy of Holies, without which there can be no success, a proper schooling in DIAG-NOSIS.

The idea that a person can attend an alleged school for six months or so and then be competent to make a diagnosis as between gall stones, appendicitis, volvulus, intusseption or even between smallpox, typhoid and pneumonia is repulsive to say the leats and when he further insults the intelligence of man by proposing to regulate these various evils by pinching a spinal nerve one is inclined to commiserate all concerned. L

TO SECRETARIES OF ALL COUNTY SOCIETIES.

You are requested to· please forward to the editor the names of the officers of your society, and all changes in them as they occur.

This is found necessary on account of changes that are constantly taking place; and will enable the Journal to give information of the various counties as it is requested.

In some instances the blank "Memoranda for Permanent Record" has not reached this· office; you are requested to forward this blank to the Secretary as soon as application has been acted upon, together with all completed blanks now on hand.

In the event this record has not been completed for your members kindly complete it and send it in.

If you are needing blanks, accurately describe them or send one of the old ones in and a new supply will be sent you.

The Journal will appreciate all items of interest occuring in the state affecting the profession generally; scientific papers read before your society will also be given consideration.

DEWEY COUNTY.

Physicians of Dewey county perfected a permanent organization in June.

Dr. D. C. Adams, of Taloga, was electea President.

Dr. Boyce, of Cestos, was elected Vice President.

Dr. J. B. Leake, of Taloga, was elected Secretary and Treasurer.

GREER COUNTY.

Greer County Medical Society met in the court house at Mangum, Okla., June 8th, at 2 o'clock p. m.

A general discussion of the subject, "The Heart," was held and this was followed by a quiz prepared by Dr. DeArman.

President, M. M. DeArman; Secretary, T. J. Dodson.·

M'INTOSH COUNTY.

The McIntosh County Medical Society held its monthly meeting in Eufaula, 2 p. m., June 8th, 1909.

A general discussion on the subject of infantile diarrhoea was held, the discussion being opened by Dr. Geo. W. West, Eufaula.

President, Dr. A. B. Montgomery, Checotah.

Secretary, Dr. W. A. Tolleson, Eufaula.

OKMULGEE COUNTY.

The Okmulgee County Medical Society held its monthly meeting June 7th in Okmulgee in the parlors of the Parkinson hotel.

Program.

Report of Delegate to State Society, Dr. Breese, Henryetta.

Etiology of Pneumonia, Dr. Stephanson.

Treatment of Pneumonia, Dr. Shankle.

Clinic.

Paper, Dr. Cott.

POTTAWATOMIE COUNTY.

On Saturday evening, May 22, the Potawatomie County Medical Society enteretained at an informal banquet in honor of those members of the society who had received recognition at the hands of the State Association meeting at Oklahoma City,; viz.

Doctor W. C. Bradford, President of the State Association.

Doctor J. A. Walker, Councillor for the First District.

Doctor Charles Blickensderfer, Chairman of Section on Surgery.

The Journal is in receipt of the program of the Hughes County Medical Society which outlines the work for the remainder of the year 1909.

The officers of this organization are to be congratulated in this work, on account of its neatness and good arrangement. It is an innovation in society work in this state, which may well be imitated by all other county societies.

The program contains a roster of the members and officers, outlines the work for each meeting and contains pertinent extracts from the Constitution and By-Laws and Code of Ethics of the American Medical Association.

Following is a list of officers: President, Dr. I. W. Robertson; Vive President, Dr. J. D. Scott; Secretary, Dr. A. M. Butts; Board of Censors, Drs. J. W. Lowe, A. J. Williams, H. A. Howell; Committee on Scientific Program, Drs. A. M. Butts, I. W. Robertson, J. D. Scott; Delegates to State Association, Drs. I. W. Robertson, W. D. Adkins; Committee on Public Health and Legislation, Drs. H. A. Howell, F. E. Warterfield, T. J. Cagle.

This county may well be imitated in another respect; it has forty physicians, thirty-nine of whom are members of the county society. This condition is almost the millenium when one reflects on it.

Dr. B. K. Wood, of Anadarko, has retired from the practice of medicine. This was necessitated on account of ill health

LIST OF COUNCILLORS WITH THEIR RESPECTIVE COUNTIES.

1st District, Dr. J. A. Walker, Shawnee. Canadian, Cleveland, Grady, Lincoln, Oklahoma, Pottawatomie and Seminole.

2nd District, Dr. John W. Duke, Guthrie. Grant, Kay, Osage, Noble, Pawnee, Kingfisher, Logan and Payne.

3rd District, Dr. Charles R. Hume, Anadarko. Roger Mills, Custer, Dewey, Blaine, Beckham, Washita and Caddo.

4th District, Dr. A. B. Fair, Frederick. Greer, Kiowa, Jackson, Comanche, Tillman, Stephens and Jefferson.

5th District, ..., ... Cimarron, Texas,. Beaver, Harper, Woodward, Alfalfa, Ellis, Woods, Major and Garfield.

6th District, Dr. F. R. Sutton, Bartlesville. Washington, Nowata, Ottawa, Rogers, Mayes, Delaware, Tulsa and Craig.

7th District, Dr. W. G. Blake, Tahlequah. Muskogee, Creek, Wagoner, Cherokee, Adair, Okmulgee, Okfuskee and McIntosh.

8th District, Dr. G. W. Robertson, Dustin. Sequoyah, LeFlore, Haskell, Hughes, Pittsburg and Latimer.

9th District, Dr. H. P. Wilson, Wynnewood. McClain, Garvin, Carter, Love, Murray, Pontotoc, Johnston and Marshall.

10th District, Dr. J. S. Fulton, Atoka. Coal, Atoka, Bryan Pushmataha, Choctaw and McCurtain.

OFFICERS OF THE OKLAHOMA STATE MEDICAL ASSOCIATION.

President, Dr. Walter C. Bradford, Shawnee.

First Vice President, Dr. C. L. Reeder, Tulsa.

Second Vice-President, Dr. D. A. Myers, Lawton.

Third Vice-President, Dr. J. W. Duke, Guthrie.

Secretary, Dr. Claude Thompson, Muskogee.

DELEGATES TO AMERICAN MEDI-CAL ASSOCIATION.

Dr. L. A. Hahan, Guthrie.

Dr. Chas. L. Reeder, Tulsa.

Place of meeting for year 1910, Tulsa.

TRANSACTIONS OF THE COUNCIL MEETINGS IN OKLAHOMA CITY.

May 11, 1909, 8 p. m.

Dr. A. L. Blesh was elected Chairman and Dr. E. D. Ebright Secretary pro tem. Councillors present: Drs. G. A. Wall, E. S. Lain, A. L. Blesh, E. B. Mitchell, E. B. Ebright, F. R. Sutton, C. A. Thompson, LeRoy Long, and H. P. Wilson. A report and general discussion of the condition of the districts was held. The action of Dr. Sutton in withholding the charter of Delaware county was sustained, with the recommendation that he grant the charter when certain objectionable features were corrected.

Bills of the Councillors were presented and ordered paid, as follows:

Dr. G. A. Wall _____

Dr. E. S. Lain _____$16.50

Dr. E. D. Ebright _____ 7.90

Dr. C. A. Thompson _____

Dr. H. P. Wilson _____ 10.30

Dr. A. L. Blesh _____ 32.51

Dr. E. B. Mitchell _____ 9.20

Dr. F. R. Sutton _____ 10.10

Dr. LeRoy Long _____

Motion prevailed to adjourn until 8 a. m. Tuesday morning.

May 12, 1909, 8:30 a. m.

Chairman, LeRoy Long; Secretary, E. D. Ebright, pro tem. Drs. Sutton and Ebright were appointed an auditing committee to audit books of the Secretary. They report the books are correct.

F. R. SUTTON,

E. D. EBRIGHT.

Motion made and seconded to allow Dr. E. O. Barker $50.00 for stenographer's fees; carried.

Motion to adjourn; carried.

May 13, 1909, 8:30 a. m.

Chairman, Dr. A. L. Blesh. Dr. G. H. Thrailkill, of Chickasha, presented matter of Dr. Peters, of Chickasha, preferring charges against the latter; a motion prevailed that the Secretary of the Council advise the Grady County Medical Society that the Council recommends that it investigate the charges and take proper action.

Council adjourned until called together by the Chairman.

May 13, 1909, 1:30 p. m.

Dr. Charles R. Hume, Chairman; Dr. J. W. Duke, Secretary. Moved by Dr. J. S. Fulton, seconded by Dr. J. H. Walker, that the President appoint a committee on the revision of the Constitution, the committee to consist of three members.

Moved by Dr. A. B. Fair and seconded by Dr. J. S. Fulton that Dr. Claude Thompson assume the publication and editorship of the Journal; carried. Moved by Dr. Thompson and seconded by Dr. Duke that a bill for $18.90 be paid to Dr. B. J. Vance for expenses.

Moved by Dr. Fair that we adjourn subject to call of the President; carried.

The report of the condition made at the first council meeting discloses the following condition with reference to unorganized counties:

1st District—Seminole.

2nd District—Osage.

3rd District—Dewey (since organized).

5th District—Five unorganized counties.

6th District—Three unorganized counties.

8th District—One unorganized.

Dr. I. B. Oldham, of Muskogee, will spend most of the month of July with the Mayo Brothers in Rochester, Minn.

Dr. O. T. Robinson, of Hydro, has located in Oklahoma City.

OBITUARY.

Dr. H. J. Hughes.

Doctor Hugh Jones Hughes was born in Wrexham, Wales, November 5th, 1868. Came to America in May, 1869, with his parents, and settled on a farm in Champaign county, Illinois. There he attended the district school and later attended Chaddock College at Quincy, Illinois. Taught school for two years. Attended Northwestern Un versity at Evanston, Illinois. Graduated from the National Medical College at Chicago in 1894. Served as house physician and surgeon for the following two years in the Cook County Hospital, Chicago. In 1896 he located in Mount Carroll, Illinois, where he practiced medicine and surgery for eight years. Married on December 31st, 1902, to F. Dora Bucher, of Mount Carroll, Illinois. In 1904 he moved to Muskogee, Oklahoma, where he practiced until his death on June 6th, 1909, from peritonitis accompanying appendicitis. Left surviving him his widow and two brothers, Henry W. Hughes and John L. Hughes, both of North Yakima, Wash.

Dr. O. D. Reed, of Frederick, Oklahoma, died on May 3rd, 1909, from an attack of acute endocarditis accompanying rheumatism.

The Secretary must strongly call the attention of the Secretaries of county societies to the great virtue of promptness in answering communications and reporting the state of affairs in their counties.

It is only by strict promptness that we can successfully issue a good Journal, and each Secretary should see to it that his end of the work is finished and all his reports in on time.

It has been necessary already to send telegrams in some cases in order to get information that could have been supplied by one minute's time on a one-cent postal card.

One of the most convenient and economical means for the instantaneous manufacture of oxygen ever devised is being put on the market by the Booth Oxyyen Generator Company, Ashtabula, Ohio. This device is simple and very compact, its principal parts being a small cylinder and cartridge, which contains a compound of fused sodium peroxide, this cartridge is placed in the cylinder and after being punctured and allowed to come in contact with water, resulting in the immediate production of oxygen.

This apparatus should especially appeal to all physicians in the smaller towns as well as the large, as great difficulty is at times experienced in securing oxygen without delay.

Dr. E. D. Ebright announces that he will remove from Carmen, Oklahoma, his present location, some time in the near future. The editor has known Dr. Ebright for several years and we feel sure that his removal will be felt as a distinct loss to the citizens of his community.

The Journal, with his many professional friends, wishes him success in whatever he may undertake.

The Baptist Hospital Association of Muskogee announces that they expect to have their hospital ready for occupancy about July 15th. This institution will contain only one wing, of twenty rooms at present, and later an addition will be made as demands justify it. It will be open to all reputable physicians.

The Muskogee Hospital Association has advertised for bids for the construction of a three story hospital building in Garrett Heights, Muskogee.

EXCHANGES

FOOD INTOXICATION IN INFANCY.

J. Brennemann (Jour. Amer. Med. Ass'n., Feb. 27, 1909,) discusses Fingelstein's theory that disturbances of the alimentary tract, such as indigestion, summer complaint, ileocolitis, cholera infantum, etc., commonly accompanied by more or less profound nervous symptoms that in their totality make up the clinical picture of an intoxication, are not due to the absorption of bacterial toxins, but are the result of a perversion of food metabolism. They are thus rather to be classed with uremia or diabetic coma than with pneumonia or typhoid, for instance. The exact nature of the toxins is not yet known. The condition is probably analogous to an acid intoxication. The idea that the toxic substances are apparently of alimentary, not of bacterial or intestinal origin is supported by the following considerations: 1. In many cases of fatal intoxication coming to autopsy no demonstrable pathologic lesions are found in the alimentary canal, though the evidences are so manifest in the known inflammatory lesions, such as ileocolitis, enteritis, typhoid, etc. In an intoxication the abnormal conditions that may be present are those of the condition on which it may be engrafted. 2. If a symptom-complex, so alike under all circumstances under which it may arise, were due to a microorganism, one would expect that there would be a certain specific organism, or group of organisms, with which it would be associated constantly. There is apparently no such connection. 3. It hardly seems possible that in any bacterial invasion of the intestinal wall, we could remove all symptoms within twenty-four or forty-eight hours by any process, and certainly not by simply withdrawing food. In a known infection starvation will not prevent it from running its course. Furthermore, we would not expect different food elements to have so different an action under such anatomic conditions. It is hard enough to see how food could have any influence much less one so selective. And yet here the course of the disease can be influenced at will, can be made better or worse to any degree, by simply increasing or diminishing or eliminating the fat and the sugar of the food. 4. The fact that these intoxications occur in such widely different infections as pneumonia or sepsis or other nonalimentary affections, yet have in all the same characteristics, are in all influenced in exactly the same way by different food elements, can certainly be accounted for more easily by assuming of food intoxication than by assuming a secondary intestinal infection, of which there is not pathologic evidence. 5. From the known behavior of an intoxication, under the influence of different amounts of certain food elements, it is likewise hard to believe that we have here to deal with the absorption or putrefactive or fermentative or other products that are the result of bacterial activity within the intestine. The appearance and odor of the bowel movements do not suggest such a condition. Furthermore, we ordinarily associate putrefaction and toxic products of bacteria activity with proteids, not with sugar and fat; yet here the proteids are innocuous or unimportant, and the fat and the sugar all-important. The treatment of these intoxications is simply to withhold all food, even human milk, for a sufficient period of time.

THE ANTISEPSIS OF ABORTION.

J. Lucas-Championniere, (Annals of Gynecology and Obstetrics, Feb., 1909,) says that we may consider a normal labor as a fresh wound, a labor of the contact with hands and instruments as a dirty wound which will often become infected. He puts us on our guard against wounding the uterus by curettings which produce a site for the entrance of infection. Intrauterine injections continue these abusive measures. Lastly, the uterus is left distended with tampons of iodoform or sterilized gauze. All this is defective and often causes infection. The author's treatment consists in the injection into the uterus of a few cubic centimeters of strong carbolized solution, in cleansing the vagina thoroughly with the speculum in place, and allowing no injection. Abortion should be treated in the same way. Injections are of value neither before nor after abortion. The author detaches the ovum with his fingers, makes the same small injection of a strong solution, and allows no injection. This procedure is possible only when the case has not been much handled. Infection caused by abortive measures should not be confounded with puerperal fever. When there is infection already present with a retained ovum or only debris, we must first cleanse the uterus through the speculum with a small tampon soaked in carbolic acid solution. Chloroform should be given for this cleansing to allow of thoroughness and that dilation may be placticed. We may use both carbolic and peroxide of hydrogen on small tampons, pushed up to the fundus. Having made your cavity antiseptic, remove all debris with the nail. There is generally no need of curetting. When infection is present curettage sufficient to remove debris, but not to wound the uterus is necessary.

Then cleanse the cavity with carbolic or peroxide on a sound; next push up to the fundus a small tampon soaked in creosote and glycerine, 2 to 5 per cent. This cauterizes but leaves no slough that will putrefy. Use no other tampon or injection, and have nothing in the vagina. Creosote is an admirable, nontoxic antiseptic.

THE NEW YORK POLYCLINIC.

Every progressive physician will be glad to hear that this well known educational institution has had within recent date opened up to it a new era of prosperity. Organized in 1881, and open for students in 1882, it was the pioneer post-graduate medical school in America. It may be safely said that the faculty of the Polyclinic has played an important part in raising the standard of requirements for the practice of medicine and surgery, and in making available for instruction to the busy practitioner the large clinical material and laboratory facilities which the great metropolis offers. After twenty-seven years of experience obtained in the struggle against abstracts which were formidable the Polyclinic has through the generous approbation of the profession and the public received a gift of money which will enable the trustees to erect a large new hospital and school and laboratory building. In addition to the wards for charity patients which will furnish material for demonstration it is announced by Prof. Wyeth that there will be a large number of private rooms which will be placed at the service of the visiting physicians and surgeons who can thus treat their patients in New York. The building is to be of steel and brick with concrete floors of modern construction and absolutely fire-proof. We congratulate the faculty of the Polyclinic and the profession as well upon this happy turn in the affairs of this great and deserving institution.

ACCURACY IN THERAPEUTICS.

The efficiency of a medical agent cannot be determined by mere physical appearance. Two specimens of fluid extract of digitalis, for example, may look precisely alike. One, upon administration, may exhibit a wholly satisfactory therapeutic action; the other, given under precisely the same conditions, may prove to be practically inert. Lack of uniformity in the crude drug, and absence on the other hand of an adequate method of assay, account for the singular discrepancy. And this serves to show the necessity of standardized remedial agents if we would proceed in the treatment of disease with any assurance of success. It emphasizes, too, the futility of trusting to chance that the extract of a crude drug contains what the practitioner supposes it to contain and what it ought to contain.

It is a healthy sign that manufacturers of medicines—some of them at least—are giving serious thought to this matter of standardization. It is cause for gratulation that the largest producers of medical products in the world consider the subject of sufficient importance to make it the basis of an expensive promotion campaign. We have in mind a series of announcements which have been published from time to time in practically the entire medical press of the country, the later appearing under the significant title, "Who is the Keeper of Your Reputation?" In their plea for greater accuracy in therapeutics Messrs. Parke, Davis & Co. are doing vastly more than to exploit the products of their manufacture—they are rendering a lasting service to medicine.

It is to the physician's own interest, and to the interests of his patients, to prescribe self with the most trustworthy agents that standardized preparations; to provide him the market offers. The best is none too good for his purpose.

Announcement is made that the State Board of Examiners of Oklahoma will meet in Guthrie July 15th for the purpose of examining all applicants for license to practice medicine in the state.

The following is copied from the June issue of the California State Journal of Medicine and needs no comment:

TO THE EDITOR.

Dr. Philip Mills Jones,
San Francisco, California.

Dear Doctor:

"In Human Life," a magazine of which I never heard until I received the April copy, there appears a writeup of father, Charlie and I, which is substantially a reproduction of the article published broadcast about two years ago, and about which we wrote a letter to the medical journals at that time. This particular issue is written so fulsomely as to hold us up to derision and has been sent as a marked copy to a large proportion of the regular medical profession in Wisconsin, Minnesota and Iowa. Not only has this marked copy been sent, but a few days after a follow-up letter came, again calling particular attention to this article under the guise of asking for subscriptions.

So far as we can learn it has been sent only to physicians, and evidently maliciously, with a view of injuring our standing with the medical profession, as every practitioner receiving such a copy would take it as a personal insult. Many physicians with whom we are not acquainted might believe that we knew of it or could have prevented it.

The animus lying behind this attack is evidently the same as is trying to secure a change in the management of the Journal and the Association; evidently the idea is to discredit the Association through attacks upon those who have been influential in its management. I was president of the American Medical Association when some of these reform movements were initiated.

Can you tell me whether there has been the same distribution of the "Human Life" magazine in your state? If you can learn anything which will be useful to us in protecting ourselves please let us know.

Yours very truly,
W. J. MAYO.

Dr. J. C. Mahr, State Superintendent of Public Health, attended the meeting of the National Public Health Association which met in Washington.

THE PHTHISICAL CHEST.

W. L. Niles, New York (Journal A. M. A., June 12), notices the old teaching that the consumptive chest is flat and says that it remained for Woods Hutchinson to show that, instead of being flat it is abnormally round. Since his first publication on the subject others have confirmed, to a more or less degree, his findings. Niles takes up the subject of the cause of this peculiarity, and shows how an examination of the human chest from fetal to adult life gives us, in the earlier stages of development, a chest considerably deeper than it is broad, i. e., a tendency to the type of the quadrupedal animal. With only two exceptions (whales and bats) all animals below the anthropomorpha have chests that are deeper than they are broad. At birth the chest is practically round in man, after birth it gradually flattens out until the normal index of seventy is reached at about the eighteenth year. It seems a fair conclusion that the typical tuberculous chest is one that has been arrested in its development at puberty, and Hutchinson seems to think that this has some influence on the prognosis of pulmonary tuberculosis. Niles states his conclusions as follows: "1. The typical tuberculous chest is more nearly round than the normal chest. 2. The increased index precedes development of tubercle infection in the lungs. It is due to an arrest of development at or about puberty and predisposes to pulmonary tuberculosis. 3. Abnormally high-indexed chests in children should be corrected by proper exercises."

In the eye the chief causes of headaches are congenital in origin, yet the patient may not suffer from this reflex until maturity is reached, or even until later in life, perhaps after an attack of general illness. Anything which lessens vitality is likely to betray the existence of previously hidden faults in these organs.—*Graef.*

Dr. John A. Wyeth, President of the New York Polyclinic, one of the best known surgeons of the United States and a writer of note on the history of the Confederate States and its leaders, spent a week visiting in Oklahoma in June.

Dr. Wyeth visited in Nowata, Tulsa, Muskogee and Ardmore.

Dr. E. O. Baker attended the meeting of the American Medical Association at Atlantic City, visiting New York and Boston while in the East.

Epistaxis.—Before resorting to a plugging of the nares to check nosebleed it is best to apply a small ball of cotton saturated with peroxide of hydrogen, or with a 10 per cent solution of antipyrin. If at hand, a solution of adrenaline chloride may be likewise tried, generally with success.—*Lanphear.*

Dr. Paul Sanger, of Dutton, has returned from Chicago where he has been taking an extended post-graduate course in surgery.

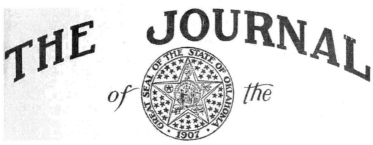

THE JOURNAL of the

Oklahoma State Medical Association.

VOL. 2.	MUSKOGEE, OKLAHOMA, JULY, 1909.	No. 2.

CLAUDE A. THOMPSON, Editor-In-Chief.

ASSOCIATE EDITORS AND COUNCILLORS.

DR. J. A. WALKER, Shawnee.

DR. CHARLES R. HUME, Anadarko.

DR. F. R. SUTTON, Bartlesville.

DR. G. W. ROBERTSON, Dustin.

DR. JOHN W. DUKE, Guthrie.

DR. A. B. FAIR, Frederick.

DR. W. G. BLAKE, Tahlequah.

DR. H. P. WILSON, Wynnewood.

DR. J. S. FULTON, Atoka.

Entered at the Postoffice at Muskogee, Oklahoma, as second class mail matter,.June, 1909.

This is the Official Journal of the Oklahoma State Medical Association and every member of that organization is entitled to a copy and if, through accident or oversight, you fail to receive a copy notification of that fact to this office will receive prompt attention. All communications should be addressed to the Journal of the Oklahoma State Medical Association, English Block, Muskogee, Oklahoma.

CHAIRMAN'S ADDRESS, SECTION ON THE PRACTICE OF MEDICINE.

By ARTHUR W. WHITE, B. S., M. D., OKLAHOMA CITY, OKLA.

I have chosen for discussion in this paper a condition, or rather, a class of conditions, remarkable principally for obscurity and difficulty of diagnosis, and for the meagerness of our clinical knowledge thereof. Not that I may be able to add much, if anything, in an original way to that already made known, but more that it may serve as a representative of a great many conditions to stimulate you to greater care and completeness in examinations and more strict attention to the observance of clinical symptoms and signs.

At this time, especially in Oklahoma, when fad and faddist, whose stock in trade is treatment, treatment based not on scientific principals, or on knowledge of pathology and diseased conditions or dependent upon skilful diagnosis, but based wholly upon the whims and credulity of people, is so defended and protected by law and society, it behooves us, and particularly those of us most interested in what we term internal medicine, to look to our claims as scientific men and continue in the progress that has so distinguished men in our line of work heretofore.

I believe the time has come when we must cease to be staisfied with our present knowledge of the underlying conditions of most of our chronic affections, for that knowledge, in great part, at least, is of the dead, and not of and for the living. We must develop a new pathology, one not solely of interest to the coroner and the laboratory worker, but one that will aid us in the incipiency of disease to a recognition that may be of some practical value to the individual sufferer.

How many conditions there are which we are prone to overlook, and if perchance they are discovered early, to pass over lightly, until some grave or alarming symptom develops to force our attention, and then often we are worried because the patient is beyond permanent help.

A notable example of this type is chronic disease of the myocardium, the more common types of which are often spoken of as "fatty heart." This term "fatty heart," of course, should not be limited, as it was formerly, to a mere deposit of fat beneath the epicardium and between the muscle fibers, or those disturbances of heart action which bear a direct relation to the obesity of the patient, but also those conditions developing independently.

Unfortunately, it is too often believed that when cardiac insufficiency appears in corpulent people it is due to an excessive deposit of adipose tissue or to fatty degeneration of the heart muscle, and always directly due to the obesity of the patient. Cardiac insufficiency very frequently in the obese is not due to fatty overgrowth. This has been substantiated especially by both Leyden and Romberg, that hearts loaded down with fat tissue have not always given signs of inadequacy, and on the other hand, many hearts which were insufficient in their function during life have not shown, at the post mortem, fat deposits in sufficient quantity to weaken the muscle, and it is not uncommon to see large fat men with an hypertrophy of the heart, with no evidence of a fatty affection.

Again, we find at the post mortem table hearts which do show both a fatty degeneration of the heart muscle and in infiltration between the fibers—in people who were quite slight and free from fat during life.

In anemia, for instance, the heart shows very extensive fatty changes in almost every case. It may be so flabby that if held up by the apex it will collapse. The endocardium shows a mottled yellow appearance. The papillary muscles of the left ventricle show especially marked changes. Microscopically fat drops are seen to take the place of the striae and nuclei.

In chronic pulmonary disease we find almost the same conditions. At times the heart is completely encased in a capsule of fat.

In the hypertrophied heart of chronic valvular disease, also that resulting from over-exertion, e. g., the athletic heart, as age advances, it is not uncommon to find more or less fatty changes of this kind. This latter condition is due principally to an ischaemia as a result of stenosis of the coronary arteries.

Therefore the heart difficulty in obese patients must arise from some other condition than mere general corpulence. Many corpulent individuals of indolent habits are anaemic and have a flabby musculative. In them the heart muscle, through anaemia and want of exercise, is incapable of responding adequately to the work required of it by the great exertion of moving the large corpulent body, and hence we soon find symptoms of heart weakness.

In such cases the heart is over-taxed, even when the body is in repose; consequently the condition as continually increasing instead of diminishing.

Marked symptoms, as a rule, first make their appearance after some unusual exertion or after an attack of some acute infectious disease. Occasionally the heart may rupture, or the coronary arteries be diseased, and death result from angina pectoris. But these conditions are wholly independent of general corpulence. Hence we see how one fat individual may show marked heart changes not exhibited in another of like corpulence.

Fatty infiltration when found is usually

well distributed over the organ, and the fat usually lies between the cells. It may, however, be deposited within the cells. · Fatty degeneration consists of a conversion of the proteid cell contents into fat. It may be either diffuse or circumscribed— as a rule the left ventricle is most affected. The heart is usually a distinct yellow color. The muscle is soft and flabby, and when cut imparts a cheesy feel to the fingers. In advanced stages it may be readily torn.

Microscopically we see the muscle fibers studded with **fat droplets**; these occupy the interfibrillary sarcoplasm, and are disposed in rows extending from the poles of the nuclei. In advanced stages the striae and nuclei may, however, be entirely obscured by the fat. In chronic cases the fibers are usually atrophied and pigmented and separated here and there by fibrous tissue.

There is nothing especially peculiar in the symptomatology and physical signs of fatty diseases of the heart, for the most part, further than is found in any inadequate heart, and it is not a difficult matter to diagnose cardiac inadequacy. The real problem is whether the heart is only potentially not equal to its work or is incompetent as a result of fatty infiltration or degeneration.

Among the early symptoms shortness of breath is probably the first noticed, and may exist some time before the physician is consulted in regard to it. Stooping or bending forward is apt to cause great dyspnoea, and as cardiac feebleness advances distressing shortness of breath declares itself on the slightest exertion, as that incident to the taking of food or to conversation. Another early symptom, vertigo. is noted especially on change of position. as in getting on the feet. This may amount even to a syncope, and the patient may fall and remain unconscious for several minutes. the feeble heart failing temporarily to maintain cerebral circulation.

Also the digestive system, very early in the disease, furnishes its quota of trouble for the sufferer. He finds his usually small appetite is diminishing, and so soon as he has eaten is oppressed by an uncomfortable fullness in the epigastrium and a shortness of breath. Unquenchable thirst compels him to drink large quantities of water, which but increase the oppression, and he is annoyed by frequent eructations of gas. The bowels are sluggish, the urine scanty and high colored.

Many associated conditions, as melancholia, partial loss of memory, hesitating speech, palpitation of the heart, angina pectoris, congestion of the ears and lips, sallow skin, double vision, and, late in the disease, cheyne-stokes respiration, are found in advanced cases of both fatty infiltration and degeneration.

On examining the patient we find in fatty infiltration increased cardiac dullness, both superficial and deep, a slow, full pulse, which may even be bounding; while in fatty degeneration we find no increase in the size of the heart. The impulse is weak and feeble, and the pulse is, as a rule, weak and irregular. The first sound of the heart is frequently absent, but if heard is short and feeble; the second sound likewise is short and seems far away. A soft mitral regurgitant murmur is often heard at the apex.

Thus we see that the signs and symptoms are for the most part none other than we see in a failing heart, and in summing up we might draw this conclusion: that if the pulse is normal in rate and quality and if subjective symptoms are felt only on exertion, are slight, and soon disappear with rest, the heart walls are presumably intact; especially if careful inquiry fails to bring out a history of cardiac strain, acute infectious disease, bad habits or any other influence that might serve to affect the integrity of the myocardium. On the other hand, degenerative changes are probable if the patient is past middle life. if the pulse shows marked divergence from normal in quality and rythm, and if the heart seems inadequate when the patient is at rest. If the patient be both fat and anaemic and the muscles are flabby, the incompetency is doubtless due to fat changes in the myocardium, but if symptoms of inadequacy develop in the fat and plethoric, whose body muscles are large and firm, it may be reasonably concluded that the heart is over-strained, perhaps dilated, but not hampered by fat deposit.

And finally, if symptoms of cardiac inadequacy develop in any corpulent individual, it is the part of wisdom to make a diagnosis of cardiac incompetency, and not of fatty heart, for there is as yet no positive means known of determining during life whether fat be present in the heart muscle.

Delivered at the seventeenth annual meeting of the Oklahoma State Medical Association, Oklahoma City, Okla., May 11, 12, 13, 1909.

MALINGERING.

By DR. R. E. RUNKLE, EL RENO, OKLAHOMA.

Opportunities for fraud in the domain of opthalmo-otological practice are few as compared with those of the general practice, thanks to the various diagnostic appliances which we now have at our command. Yet as it is we are frequently harassed by deceptions of a surgical nature the detection of which is not always an easy matter. In the following I will eliminate those stimulated affections of a hysterical nature and endeavor to confine my remarks to those spurious disorders which are assumed for a given purpose. To charge a fellow being with a willful misrepresentation of his physical state either for a monetary or other purpose is a serious matter and one which should neither be surmised at nor regarded lightly. The former because facts must be established,

the latter because something of material importance must be connected with the assumed condition. My experience has been that the ignorant class furnishes by far the majority of these cases, yet it occasionally occurs that we are confronted by one whose educational qualifications and knowledge as to the subject of their claims are not found wanting. The statements of the former are rarely misleading to the experienced observer but the latter class often causes considerable annoyance. Again it occurs that to our own minds we are thoroughly satisfied as to the attitude of the patient but should it become necessary for us to expose our reasons before a body of laymen we would probably find ourselves at a loss to impress them with the same views. We therefore must content ourselves with silence until such a time as we are prepared to convince the most skeptical. The happiest of families might be dissolved by hasty action, large sums of money may be lost and even our own reputation with possible financial loss may result from a mistake in such affairs. All stand innocent until proven guilty and fairmindedness and due deliberation must guide us at all times. It must be borne in mind that a successful examination depends largely upon the attitude the examiner and claimant assume toward each other, hence the former must establish a friendly relationship regardless of his personal feelings. He must show no signs of suspicion, must be pleasant and at times it may be best to be a little sympathetic.

My case records show that deafness forms the basis of the majority of allegations among this class. Why this should be I am not able to say unless it is because of a sense of safety from detection as against other parts. In many instances an actual injury does exist but the allegations are far reaching as compared with the actual conditions existing. Indeed claims are seldom made without some lesion being present to incite them such as a middle ear catarrh being the foundation for an asserted loss of hearing due to concussion as from the firing of guns or from a blow on the side of the head. These cases I have frequently met with and are not so easily detected as one might suppose. The patency of the tube, position of the drum head, and other objective signs may determine the presence of an otitis media but if we have an actual injury to the internal ear remains to be proven. In so much as nature provided such good protection for these delicate structures of which the internal ear is composed injuries to these parts are comparatively rare hence the existence of such an injury is doubtful. Such allegations are usually those of total deafness (odinarily uni-lateral) and tuning fork and other tests are generally futile, so far as the establishment of positive evidence is concerned. Certain rules for the detection of malingerers are referred to in our text books but in practice they are of but little use. Our only hopes are to catch the patient unawares determining his hearing power at this time and by the objective signs. Their personal histories are usually conflicting with the conditions assumed.

I might here mention a case which came under my observation a while ago. This patient, a man past sixty years of age, was sent me for examination as a suspected malingerer. His claims were for total deafness in both ears due to concussion. He was a bright fellow and well educated, having held responsible public positions. His stubbornness and affectation convinced me at once that he was shamming. He would respond to none of the tests either for air or bone conduction. The objective signs were those of a middle ear catarrh. I was unable to communicate with him except by writing. I was satisfied the claimant was malingering but how was I to prove it. I dismissed him with instructions to call the next day for further examination. Within half an hour after leaving my office I had the pleasure of standing beside him in a public building listening to a very quiet conversation he was engaged in with another party. You can imagine his feelings when he saw me within arm's reach of him. It is needless to say that he did not return for the "further examination." Yet this same individual was receiving pay for total deafness.

As before stated simulated affections of the eyes have not been so numerous with me as those of the ears and of this I am indeed sorry for the various aids to diagnosis such as the opthalmoscope prisms, etc., places the facts within easy reach. As in cases of alleged deafness there is usually some lesion of the ocular structures to stimulate the claims made but occasionally we find that the allegations are without any such foundation whatever, as in the following case: This was a case of alleged disability due to impairment of the vision in both eyes in which the visual defect was so great as to render the patient unable to find my office unattended. If this person had any disease or had every received any injury to the visual apparatus I failed to find any evidence of the same. I extended my sympathy mildly to him and suggested that perhaps a very strong lense would aid him. The conversation drifted toward glasses and their power and at the close of the interview I had given him vision to the extent of 20-15 with either eye with a plain lens. This person was of the very ignorant class but he had fooled others to the extent of receiving a pension on the grounds of having defective vision caused by disease contracted during the late war.

In bringing this subject before you I do not do so in the hopes of enlightening you or setting forth anything new, but purely in the expectation of bringing out a discussion. I am considerably interested in this class of cases being engaged in government and corporation service and I am sure that these patients have been rather numerous with me. Such individuals are a disgrace to modern society and unless the medical profession gives more attention toward the detection of these fakirs

their number promises to increase.

Presented at the 1910 meeting of the Oklahoma State Medical Association, Oklahoma City, Okla., May 11-13, 1909.

THE OVARY, ITS CONSERVATIVE AND RADICAL ATTENTION.

By DR. CHARLES NELSON BALLARD, OKLAHOMA CITY, FORMERLY OF CHICAGO, ILLINOIS. ASSOCIATE PROFESSOR OF GYNECOLOGY AT COLLEGE OF PHYSICIANS AND SURGEONS (MEDICAL DEPARTMENT OF THE UNIVERSITY OF ILLINOIS), SURGEON TO MARION SIM'S SANITARIUM, CHICAGO, ILL.; ATTENDING SURGEON WEST SIDE HOSPITAL, CHICAGO; ATTENDANT IN GYNECOLOGY, WEST SIDE DISPENSARY.

Only a few days ago my attention was directed to the fact that I was to prepare a paper for this most important meeting.

Realizing the fact that I must fill the place assigned to me if possible for me to do so, I made note of the subject assigned to me and wondered how I would dare present such a time worn subject to such an intelligent audience. However I was somewhat relieved when I noticed the other subjects on the programme.

This organ, though quite small, is a very important one and gives many troubles and heartaches to its possessor. Oft-times it is annoying because of its active reproductive power, again it is brought to our attention on account of its inability to produce.

Many accusations are placed upon its roll of dishonor that are not justly attributable to it primarily.

Many uncomfortable feelings are placed to its credit by its possessor, and many reflex phenomena are referred to it by the medical advisor, when if carefully studied might be more properly credited to the misconduct of some other organ whose pathology, or even whose physiology is not so familiar to us.

A complete resume of the pathological conditions to which the ovary is subject would require volumes to contain, hence I shall only touch on some of the points, discussing only that part which I consider of most value to us. We may differ as to these points and that will elicit a discussion which I consider the most interesting part of any paper.

Some of you will, no doubt, remember during the days spent within the confines of your Alma Mater, that your clinical instructors were in the habit of performing ovaryatomies very promiscuously, not considering the existing pathology as is now so closely studied.

During the present decade we do not consider that our examination of a case is complete until we have studied its pathology thoroughly. If this can be done before operative procedures then it is taken into consideration afterwards, for it is only in this way that we are able to arrive at an acurate diagnosis. You may suggest that there is but little to be gained from a post-operative diagnosis, yet can we do better than to correct by future study that which we do not already know?

Pathology is the foundation upon which all careful diagnosticions base their conclusions. Without its study all diagnoses are wanting in part.

The sway of the pendulum has had its effect in the confines of gynecology as elsewhere in the surgical field.

Since the first ovaryotomy performed, which was done by Ephraim McDowell, in 1809, we have seen the extremist venturing farther and farther with some special technique in his operation upon the ovary, until he is checked in his frantic effort to see the fullest benefit to be obtained by his work, by some more conservative surgeon, or by himself seeing the unfruitfulness of his efforts.

It is necessary for every special branch of medicine and surgery to have these extremists in order to accomplish extreme things. Following this forward movement there is always a reaction, the swing of the pendulum never stopping at the medium, but going far beyond, however usually stopping short of the old standard, hence some permanent progress is made by each effort in this direction.

These self-constituted individuals can not be ignored, for it is to their everlasting progressiveness that our greatest advances in medicine and surgery is due.

In the early months of utero-gestation, there is developed from the Wolffian body, the genital glands which later form the ovary. The ovary is the germ bearing organ of the female, the analogue of the male testicle. Normally there are two of these organs situated in the pelvis on a level with its brim, partly above and partly below the line of the brim.

It is in relation anteriorly with the anterior layer of the broad ligament and the round ligament; posteriorly with a portion of the posterior layer of the broad ligament; external and below is found the ampula of the tube as well as the mingled layers of the broad ligament forming the infundibular ligament; internally the ovarian ligament and vessels.

The axis is obliquely to the pelvis with a little inclination forward. It rests in the posterior layer of the broad ligament as if fastened, in a slit in the posterior layer, attaching itself to the edges of the slit, thus placing itself partially posterior and partially anterior to the posterior layer of the broad ligament.

The germ bearing portion of the ovary is within the peritoneal cavity, hence it is not covered with peritoneum. The anterior lower portion is practically extra-peritoneal, lying between the layers of the broad ligament, being held in position by a reflection from the inner surface of the posterior layer of the broad ligament, known as the mesovarium. That portion within the peritoneal cavity is covered by germinal epithelium.

The ovary, normally, is about the size of an almond. The thickest portion is external and the thin pointed end internal, toward the uterus to which it is attached by the ovarian ligament. This ligament is composed principally of muscle fibers and connective tissue, intermingled with ovarian stroma.

It varies in size however, becoming larger at the menstrual period and during pregnancy. It is usually at its largest about six weeks after parturition. After menapause it shrinks to more than half its original size.

The color of the organ varies with the age and activity of the woman. Its normal hue is pinkish-grey, at the time for the menstrual period it becomes darker and at menapause much lighter, if physiological. Following ovulation a dark spot occurs, due to an accumulation of blood following the rupture of a graffian follicle and the voidance of an ovum. This color changes in time: absorption takes place and at the end of a few weeks there is left only a shriveled up spot known as the Corpus luteum, which in time disappears and leaves only a ciccatrix to mark the spot and this remains permanently. This process continues, ova are voided, blood clots formed and absorbed, and ciccatrides occur until the once smooth pinkish-colored ovary now becomes irregular, lighter in color, smaller, and more firm in consistency.

If there exists any cause preventing the rupture of the Graffian follicle, then the ovary becomes larger and irregular on account of the many existing retention cysts thus produced.

Sections made from the ovary entire, show two kinds of tissue constituting its greater portion, the medulary and cortical. The latter or peripheral layer constitutes the greater portion within the peritoneal cavity; dipping deepest at about the central part of the convex surface, sometimes to the depth of three millimeters. When the central portion is incised it has a pearly glistening appearance and is soft in consistency. This substance is studded throughout with small vessicles, varying in size, sometimes as large as a pea. They can often be seen infringing upon the surface, thinning it sometimes to the point of rupture.

Ovulation effects this layer most and the scars spoken of above are found here principally.

Before puberty we find large spheroid cells, with very prominent nuclei upon the columnar or germinal epithelium. These represent young ova. The germinal epithelium grows inward here infringing upon the stroma. These ingrowths are tubular in appearance and are known as the ovarial tubes of fluger.

Immediately beneath and practically inseparably from this epithelial layer is to be found the Tunica Albuginea, a fibrous membrane, very thin in texture normally. This membrane contains muscle fibers. Until recently the ovary was not supposed to contain any muscle tissue. This latter tissue is a very important part of the ovary to us.

It is not fully developed until between the third and fourth year. It becomes quite a firm membrane when subject to any sort of inflammation. It being a very superficial part of the ovary, practically enveloping it, it is most seriously effected by infections beginning superficially. The ovaries anatomical location subjects them most intimately to such infection. Micro-organisms are usually deposited here by continuity of tissue, by way of the genital tract, through the tube, into the peritoneal cavity, in direct contact with the germinal surface of the organ, effecting almost immediately this covering. It soon becomes congested, thickened, and loses its former elasticity. It is necessary that this tissue remain elastic to allow for the physiological expansion at the menstrual period and during pregnancy. The inelasticity of this membrane is one of the most common causes of ovarian pain at the menstrual period and in early pregnancy. The reason why this pain occurs

is the pressure produced by the normal expansion of the tissue within this cavity, surrounded by this new pathological inelastic membrane.

The rupture of the ripe Graffian follicle is prevented and from it is developed a retention cyst. Each month more of these cysts are formed, sometimes remaining as individual cysts. This condition we call cystic degeneration. At other times the pressure becomes so great that the cyst walls are absorbed coalescence occurs and one common cyst is formed. Should the now general cyst wall become so diseased by pressure, that it continues to secrete the fluid thus increasing the pressure upon this confining membrane it will become thinned and much enlarged, the source of our larger ovarian cysts.

In entering into the pathological conditions in this organ we have many features to consider. Its relation anatomically and physiologically are such as to make it almost always only a part of a pathological picture. When it becomes infected there is practically always some other closely associated organ also entering into the pathology. We seldom find an infection confined to it alone, but have some complication to consider; some other kinds of tissue, acting differently under the same type of infection, and responding differently to the various remedial agencies.

A statement is made by most authors that all inflammations of the ovary, like the tube, are due to bacterial infection. This is a broad statement and will admit of some modification. It is true in the majority of cases, but we must admit that displacements, irritations, strangulations, or new growths produce hyperemias, and this, if long continued, results in change of tissue simulating very materially that caused by the continued action of the less verulent germs. Physiologic hyperemia exists at the time of menstruation, sexual excitement, and pregnancy. Pathologic hyperemia occurs when we have a displaced ovary, with a torsion of the mesovarium, interfering with the venous circulation; when there exists natural or unnatural sexual excitement, an ill-fitting pessary, or a near-by tumor. Should this blood pressure continue to increase, BY IT ALONE, transudation of the serum, and migration of the lucocytes take place, thus transforming hyperemia into a true inflamamtion. The transuded elements later become organized and a true hyperplasia is produced. During this excessive hyperemia, the tissue is over abundantly supplied with nutrition and the pre-existing histologic elements become enlarged and a true hypertrophy is the outcome. This character of hyperemia presents when examined microscopically, dilated blood vessels and thickened vessel walls, many of which are thrown into folds projecting into the lumen of the vessel. There are some reasons for considering the bacteria of the ovary on account of its differing somewhat from the other genital organs. Its anatomic structure, its periodic physiologic function, its giving birth to the ovum, lacerating tissue, exposing open vessels, congesting the veins by torsion of the pedicle, ALL are conditions making the ovary most susceptible to any bacteria.

This may explain why it is that infected Graffian follicle cysts are so frequent while abscess in a cystic ovarian tumor is exceedingly rare.

Three principal routes of invasion by the bacteria can be considered; blood vessels, lymphatics and continuity of tissue, the latter seeming to be the route of selection for the gonococci. This explains why the latter is the most frequent source of peripheral infection. Bacteria may pass through the intestinal wall into the peritoneal cavity, gravitate to the pelvis and produce inflammation in this way, or the Bacillus coli Communss may be transmitted through the degenerated walls produced by adhesions to the ovary. Strep-

tococic infection ordinarily reaches the ovary through the lymphatics or blood vessels. Milliary abscesses are formed which are so characteristic of this special form of infection. This invasion always occurs through some abrasion or trauma·in some portion of the genital tract. The bacteria may first make their presence known in the muscular wall of the uterus. They may stop in the surrounding cellular tissue, or go on their journey, and be made manifest first in the ovary. These three points may appear as so many stages of the infection, or they may occur simultaneously. The rapidity of the invasion depends upon the verulency of the micro-organism and the resisting power of the patient. The lymphatic chain distributed throughout the genital organs, with its many radiating branches, makes it possible for many points to become infected during its travel frcm the foci of infection, hence the ovarian infection, usually constitutes only a part of the clinical picture.

The peritoneum is usually implicated, adhesions form binding the surrounding organs together in a mass, the freeing of which is one of the most difficult operations allotted to the destiny of modern surgery.

In considering the infections of the ovary and their development we must not lose sight of the fact that the infectious diseases are very frequently the source of ovarian inflammation in the child. This class of diseases frequently check the development, or produce a chronic inflammation that is usually overlooked until menstruation begins to be established. I have been unable, at times, to account for the pathology found in the ovaries of young girls until a carefully taken history I could determine a relationship existing between the onset of the symptoms and some of the infectious diseases.

Taylor, in American Journal of Medical Science, 1907, describes a case of supurating cyst of the ovary occuring eight mouths after an attack of typhoid fever. A comprehensive study mas made by him of its morphologic, cultural, and serum agglutinating properties and was definitely proven to be the Bacillus Typhosus. The possibility of this metastatic transferrence of these various micro-organisms, should not be lost sight of during the progress of the different infectious diseases, because of the difficulty, sometimes, in determining the cause for the pathology found in the ovaries of young girls.

In acute ovaritis, when the cause of the inflammation is known to come from the already existing uterine septic infection, then we must treat the pathology with the general condition for it is only a complication. When it is an individual inflammation and we have such accompanying symptoms as a burning, lancinating pain in the ovarian region, radiating down the thighs, into the lumbosacral region; tenesmus of the rectum and bladder, and pain in the breast of the corresponding side, we must direct our attention to alleviating the symptoms originating from the pathology of the organ itself. Determine the cause, if possible and remove it; if not able to do so then apply measures common in such inflammations, such as absolute rest, salines, and the ice bag. I insist especially on the use of the ice bag, if early, for it relieves congestion, assists in preventing supuration, lessens the amount of exudation, and is the most effective curative agent at our disposal. If supuration can be prevented, recovery may be expected, but if not radical measures will be necessary.

There is at the present time much discussion as to the time for conservatism. When the ovarian tissue is undergoing degeneration we are too prone to attempt to save a portion of an ovary, not fully appreciating the fact that there is much pathological tissue that can not be detected microscopically.

Only too often is conservatism abused to the point of becoming radicalism. It is most perfect conservatism to do radical work on these cases, as this condition in the ovary is seldom cured unless complete extirpation is done.

It is our duty to save this most vital genital organ in the young woman during her reproductive period, but we can expect to do this only when a diagnosis is made before the trophic condition occurs. When a diagnosis of hypertrophy is made before cystic degeneration has begun, and it does not respond to palliative measures, then we are justifiable in doing a resection to relieve the pressure and establish normal circulation. This is the only stage, it seems to me, in which resection of the ovary is beneficial.

Chronic inflammation of ovarian tissue first shows itself in proliferative activity in the stroma, followed by rounded celled infiltration, and a deposit of new connective tissue. This increases the firmness of the organ, presses the blood vessels, sometimes to obliteration, cutting off the nutrition from the Graffian follicle, resulting in its destruction. Sometimes this change of tissue is most persistent at the surface of the organ, and then, even though the Graffian follicle is not destroyed, it is prevented from voiding the mature ovum, owing to the thickened cartilaginous Tunica Albuginia. When this process takes place peripherally the ovary becomes enlarged, but when it progresses throughout the stroma the reverse is the case. If it is excised in this latter condition, its appearance will be much whiter than the normal ovary owing to the greater portion of the tissue now being firm connective tissue. After all this change in tissue has taken place, not one of us would expect to be able, ever, to make of this organ a real ovary. Its normal ovarian tissue has been transformed into entirely different tissue. This now abnormal organ, composed of abnormal tissue can only produce abnormal symptoms and hence, is not only of no use to its possessor but a real injury to her. It is an incurably sick organ and must be dispensed with in order to give relief.

Though it can be said of this little portion of the female anatomy, without its presence in the early development of the female being there could not be produced, in the full sense of the word, a real female. The female reproductive power would be wanting as well as that characteristic gentleness, which belongs to this sex.

These little portions can be dispensed with after the female has become fully developed and no apparent difference as to sex can be noted, but not so if removed before all the organs, differentiating the sexes, have been developed.

So all in all this is a very useful organ, when properly developed and cared for. Its loss when normal, is deplored by all real women but when abnormal can only be fraught with danger, and the economy is better when freed from its task of supporting which has now become really foreign to its existence.

Conclusions.

(1). Use conservatism when any real normal tissue can be saved.

(2). Use radicalism when necessary to relieve the sick.

(3). Try the first, but resort to the second before it is too late to do good.

Dr. Goddard, Alderson:

I want to say that the paper was classic, and the summary that he gave here was very very excellent. Conservatism at the beginning until you see that conservatism is not going to do the work, and then radicalism. That to my mind was a splendid ending up of a very excellent paper. I wish to thank the doctor for the paper.

Dr. Kuhn, Oklahoma City:

I didn't hear Dr. Ballard's paper, but I would like to get up some interest about

the conservatism of ovarian operations. It is my rule never to sacrifice an ovary unless it be a case of malignancy of the ovary. I never sacrifice both ovaries when one can be saved.

Dr. Russell, Oklahoma City:

I see no reason for removing an organ, whether it be ovary or any other organ if you can save it. I think a good many things come up that helps to decide that question, as is brought out by this paper.

If a party has this ovarian condition and has no offspring and thinks there is no chance for it, then we should try so she can leave an offspring. Everybody wants to leave an offspring if they can. If there is only half of an ovary, save it, for pregnancy has taken place when there is less than half of an ovary. Now there should be no question about taking out the ovary when the tubes are removed. They have a close connection with the nervous organism. If these ovary tubes are entirely removed, why should we take out the ovaries? They get no pregnancy but will continue to have menstruation, which is a good thing for a woman. It is a bad thing for a woman to have to cease menstruating too early in life because from a nervous standpoint and other reasons, she doesn't seem to be quite satisfied. Leave her as near to her natural condition as possible.

Dr. Vance, Checotah:

Mr. Chairman: I want to say that I think that a most excellent paper, and I enjoyed the reading of it very much and its explanations are good. And while we are talking of conservatism, I think that this is one of the cases where we ought to exercise a great deal of conservatism. I do not believe the ovary should be removed except the case be, as my friend on the right said, unless it is of malignant character and can not be cured, although I do not believe in removing the entire ovary or both ovaries. I believe that the rule ought to be to save as much ovary as possible.

The removal of the ovary has a moral effect on a woman. A woman, as a rule, is proud of her natural condition and most all of them tell you when you go to operate when they have some suspicion that you are going to remove a uterus, they seem to have a feeling they want you to leave these parts if possible. I heard a request made to a doctor in a hospital one morning. A lady said, "Take whatever you think necessary, but don't take the ovaries, if you can help it."

———

Discussion closed by Dr. Ballard, Oklahoma City:

I thank you doctors for the discussion. There isn't much for me to say in closing. The principal point I think in our work on the ovary as far as conservatism is concerned, is to make a differentiation when we can. Now, the doctor on my right spoke of not removing an ovary unless it is malignant. It is true we want to save these if we possibly can—it is our duty—but when we have an ovary that is affected, we all know it is a difficult point for us to know just how much to take out and just how much to leave. I don't think there are any of us who will say we know just how much to leave that will not still go on and on through the process of degeneration. If we do this we will soon have the same condition we are trying to relieve, so at this point it is a difficult matter to decide. I think it would be better to sacrifice a little over and cut out all the diseased parts and save another operation. There are some patients who would rather run the risk of another operation than to be relieved of their ovaries entirely, but we take it upon ourselves and the blame of not doing what we should do. And so this is a point hard for us to decide. We have got to use our judgment and do the best we can. Try to prevent a

second operation and try to save as much as we can. There are many that are removed that are not malignant, or even approaching it.

Read before the seventeenth annual meeting of the Oklahoma State Medical Association at Oklahoma City, Oklahoma, May 11-13, 1909.

———

DRAINAGE IN BELLY SURGERY.

By CHAS. BLICKENSDERFER M. D., TECUMSEH, OKLA.

———

By drainage is meant the removal of disease and wound secretions. This may be accomplished by one of a small number of procedures. The subject may be subdivided under the heads of natural, artificial and postural drainage; any one of which may alone or in combination with the other two be employed as the exigencies of the case may require.

By natural drainage is meant the leaving open of wounds (whether accidental or otherwise) in order to facilitate the escape of retained or accumulating secretions. These openings, of course, should be left in the most dependent portion of the wound.

Artificial drainage is obtained by the use of gauze wicks, cigaretts, rubber, glass or bone tubes or, large amounts of gauze, so placed that they bring into communication the deepest recesses of infected dead spaces and pockets, and the exterior, their usefulness being enhanced by the combined forces of gravitation and capillary attraction.

By postural drainage is understood one of the positions of the patient in bed. The one being known as Fowler's, is one in which the head of the patient is raised so that the secretions of the peritoneal cavity gravitate toward the pelvis. The other known as Clark's position consists of raising the feet of the patient facilitating the gravitation of peritoneal fluids towards the diaphragm. These two positions are based upon the knowledge that absorption of peritoneal secretions is accomplished by the diaphragmatic and omental peritoneum, there being a normal steady flow of secretion from the pelvis to the diaphragm as was proved by the experiments of Muscatelle. This flow upward is accelerated or retarded as the feet of the patient are raised or lowered. The philosophy of these two positions is as follows: The periteneum under normal conditions is capable of disposing of large amounts of infectious material. This ability is lessened in direct proportion to the trauma sustained by this membrane and the diminished resistance or vitality of the individual caused by shock or disease.

In the Fowler position the head of the individual being raised lessens the rate of flow toward the diaphragm and consequently of absorbtion; the peritoneum thereby being enabled, in its crippled condition to dispose of its contained infectious bodies at a rate that will not overtax its capabilities, and in this we find a vaginal drain sometimes a most potent assistant. This position is very properly used in conjunction with artificial means that have for their object the removal of secretions from the abdominal cavity to the exterior.

In the Clark position the lower extremity of the patient being elevated the rate of flow from below the diaphragm is accelerated allowing the rapid absorbtion and disposal of contained infectious material before it can reproduce itself in quantity sufficient to make its removal impossible, without artificial means.

Abnominal drainage is often an excuse for poor surgery, yet to affirm that drainage has no place in belly surgery would be as erroneous as to proclaim its usefulness as a routine measure in all abdominal operations. As a matter of fact, however, the use of drainage in operations of selection is a practical admission of incomplete and unclean surgery. Of course drainage may be and is in a small per cent of these

cases indicated, as it more frequently is in operative procedures characterized as emergency. To drain the muscles and fatty layers here is of far greater importance than to drain the peritoneal cavity. It may be stated as axiomatic that to know when to employ artificial drainage requires a greater degree of judgment than to know when to dispense with its use. In other words, when in doubt don't drain. The condition of the operative field and the state of the patient when taken together, alone, furnish the indication for drainage or otherwise. Operations that are relatively clean, in which there remains no blood clot, no accumulation of fluid in the spaces, with a minimum amount of shock and a moderate amount of traumatism to the peritoneum require no artificial drainage. The less injury that can be inflicted upon this membrane the more competent it is to deal with septic infection to its own advantage providing the infecting agent is not encompassed by clots of blood or fibrin or other foreign body that allows of its rapid multiplication safe from the action of the phagocyte; the foreign bodies in the meantime inflicting by their presence peritoneal injury that forms new fields for the multiplication and development of the bacteria.

Drainage is very properly used in the following cases: Appendiceal abscess where limiting adhesions have been formed walling off the pus from the general cavity.

For this purpose a gauze drain wrapped in gutta-percha, and long enough to reach from the bottom of the cavity to the exterior; or the drain may only be sufficiently long to enter the cavity from without In large cavities of this kind the drain may be brought out through the incision or there may be instead, or in addition, a drain introduced through a stab wound in order to make the force of gravity available. In placing a stab drain, only the skin and fasciae should be incised, the muscle fibres separated by divulsion and the gauze wick or cigarette, be slipped into place by means of a forceps or hemostat. The gauze drain is to be preferred to the glass, bone or hard or soft rubber tubes on account of its efficiency, easy removal and for its lessened liability to cause fistula or other injury to the surrounding or underlying structure. A drain of this kind will remove large quantities of serous fluid by cappillarity while allowing pus to escape around it.

A drain is indicated in gangrene, sloughing or perforation of the appendix, where there are no limiting adhesions, and as before a small wick or cigarette of guttapercha covered gauze is sufficient. It is imperative to make our drain efficient in these cases that the peritoneum be as little injured as possible, the time of separation be short, and that artificial drainage be supplemented by the following means, as advised by Murphy, of Chicago.

Posture and the instillation of normal salt solution into the rectum drop by drop at a temperature of 100 degrees Farenheit to the amount of tolerance, usually from one to two pints twice daily or more. The position or posture keeps the accumulation below in the neighborhood of the drain making it more efficient, besides keeping the hitherto uninfected serus membrane comparatively free from agents of infection. To effectively drain there must be a medium for transportation. This is supplied by the normal saline solution taken up by the rectum, distributed by the systemic or portal circulation and supplying the peritoneum with this solution in a physiological manner diluting the toxins and hastening their removal. This is of paramount importance in thin subjects and those in whom the infection is highly virulent. Besides getting an increased effect due to the mechanical and physical action of the normal saline when thus used, the period of shock is shortened and its intensity lessened, stimulation of the circulatory apparatus ensues and all the emunctories driven to increased activity in the dilution and elimination of toxic bodies. This is particularly true of the renal secretions.

Drainage is also indicated in acute pelvic inflammation. This applies to infection following labor and abortion—puerperal sepsis—accumulations of pus from other sources following inflammation of the uterus and its adnexa.

For the proper treatment of these it is well to drain the pelvis by way of the vagina where this is at all possible. Where the inflammation is of a virulent type involving the middle or upper areas of the peritoneal surface it may be necessary to open the abdomen for additional drainage and for the removal of pus pockets that are otherwise inaccessable.

In establishing vaginal drainage the same gauze drain but of larger dimensions will give as good results as any, although a preference may be given to soft rubber tubes of a large calibre. This should be enclosed by layers of gauze which are in turn covered by layers of gutta-percha tissue.

In acute diffuse peritonitis, especially if the focus of infection can not be removed, a small gauze drain should be placed in the lower angle of the wound or in a stab wound communicating with the seat of infection. The drain should be moistened, preferably with salt solution and squeezed dry before placing.

Put the patient in the exaggerated Fowler position and introduce normal salt solution as before directed.

When these attacks of peritonitis can be treated surgically before they have had time to spread over but a small extent of peritoneal surface, the foci of infection removed, no drainage is necessary. This is true even when a small residium of sepsis remains, drainage, if any, being only supplied for the muscular and fatty tissues of the abdominal wall.

These cases in which it seems advisable to introduce into the gut solutions of Epsom salts during operation modify the manner in which the normal salt solution should be administered in order to supplement drainage. According to the studies of Hay and others all strong saline solutions of a strength of seven parts or more per thousand when brought in contact with animal tissues causes a flow from the tissues toward such solution. It will thereby be readily seen that absorbtion from the rectum will be retarded and probably interrupted and it will be advisable under such circumstances to give the saline by infusion or hypodermoclysis.

The principal subject to which we wish to draw the attention of those who practice obstertrics, is the drainage in puerperal sepsis. It may be pointed out that these are first cases of puerperal peritoneal sepsis which are soon converted by lymphatic and peritoneal absorbtion into cases of general septicamia. the mortality rate of which is such as to justify almost any means that. in the least, gives a promise of a chance of ultimate recovery.

The prompt drainage of these cases while they are yet subjects of peritoneal sepsis or before the intoxication and infection are general offers at least better results than the routine curettage, uterine irrigation and packing. or internal medication. Personally, preference is given to the method of Pryor. who opened the pelvic cavity by puncturing the posterior wall of the vagina and packed the pelvis with iodoform gauze. The opening through the vagina should be sufficiently large for the packing of gauze all around the uterus and its appendages. This drain performs a four-fold service. It lets out the infected and toxic collection of serum at once, establishes drainage into the gauze from all the surrounding structures: stimulates the formation of protective adhesions from the general cavity and mechanically obstructs the lymphatic circulation from the uterine interior into the

general circulation. In this operation the interior of the uterus should also be packed and drained and all pus pockets incised, cleaned out and drained.

The gauze should be removed from the pelvis in two days, when the cavity may be gently irrigated with saline solution and a gauze wick or a gauze covered soft rubber tube replaced to maintain an opening for the discharge of objectionable secretions.

Read before the 1909 meeting of the Oklahoma State Medical Association, Oklahoma City, May 12, 1909.

Discussion.

Dr. Jackson, Kansas City, Mo.:

I feel a little embarrassed to open the discussion on this paper which is one of the best papers I ever listened to. I think I cannot take issue with him on anything and I like to differ with a man on some things.

I believe we will all agree that the general tendancy of surgery is for less drainage than a few years ago, especially is this true in the peritoneal cavity, which has the function of absorption and secretion. The peritoneum on account of its absorptive power, can take care of a great deal of poison.

There is one type of infection in which we cannot get along without drainage. That is in cellular tissue, in which if drainage is not afforded there will be difficulty. Likewise in cases of peritoneal abscess where cellulitis and peritonitis exist, drainage is necessitated, but in ordinary cases of peritonitis, even though pus is there, if the appendix has been removed there will be no need for drainage. But in all cases where pus is brought out of the belly, you must drain down through the belly. In many of the cases where we have secondary abscess we do not have to open up the peritoneum always. but the cellular tissue must be looked after. If the entire focus is removed we close the peritoneum. but drain the cellular tissue. The doctor spoke of posture drainage. In a virulent infection posture drainage is not only of great value in allowing pus to get out but in focussing it. For the past year or two in cases of appendicitis, I have been in the habit of turning the patient over on his belly. He gets along better than when on his back. Attention to this point was called a few years ago when a patient died from paresis. If there is gas, or if you have intestinal paresis the conditions will be relieved by turning the patient over on his belly.

One other thing I would say, I agree with the doctor in the matter of the rubber drain and the cigarette drain.

Another point is that gauze drainage is contended by many not to drain. If hot salt solution packs are used there will be good drainage. Gauze, if moistened, will drain. Capillary drainage should be reserved for the drainage of fluid secretions, and in cases where we have gross tissue necrosis, then use tubular drainage.

Dr. Ross Grosshart, Tulsa, Okla.:

There is one point in regard to drainage brought out by the doctor in his paper, that is, in regard to opening through the pelvis and packing after abortion or labor. This is a neglected field in child-bed fever. The opening of the abdominal cavity and packing gauze in it will act the same as giving the patient a dose of anti-toxin, or phagacytosis. The theory is, and the microscope shows, that under these conditions you produce a leucotysosis.

Dr. J. Hutchings White, Muskogee, Okla.:

Nothing has been said of the removal of drainage. To me it is a very interesting point, because I believe the early removal of drains means a good deal to the patient. I think drains should be removed by the end of the third or at least of the fourth day.

Dr. Harry Breese. Henryetta, Okla.:

I heartily agree with Dr. Blickensderfer's paper.

Dr. A. L. Blesh, Oklahoma City, Okla.:

Closing: I would like to say that in making drainage in the peritoneal cavity I prefer cigarette drains. I roll rubber and gauze together—gauze, gutta-percha, gauze and so on. You get a nice drainage through the gauze. You remove soluble toxin through the gauze part of your drain.

I cannot take issue with the doctor as to drainage, but must say I don't like rubber tubes. I have better results from simple drainage and a very small amount of manipulation of structures.

Dr. Grosshart mentioned the action of phagocytes. I think in opening the cul de sac of Douglas, you remove a large amount of sero-serum. By the presence of gauze you have a further drainage from the surrounding structures. Instead of allowing absorption to go on you interrupt it and turn its course into the vagina.

NEW MORPHINE SUBSTITUTES.

Gelseminine is rapidly growing in favor, as presenting most of the benefits accruing from the use of morphine without any of its disadvantages. Gelseminine is a sedative; uniform in its actions, widely applicable, and safe in that when the doses are pushed beyond the remedial limit it affords unvarying indications (ptosis, etc.) of this fact long before an unsafe dose has been reached. It can be given in the usual way, or hypodermically, causing no irritation in the latter instance. It is especially applicable as a sedative, antipyretic and relaxant in cases of children, as well as in those of adults.

The Abbott Alkaloidal Co., presents gelseminine in granules containing 1-250 of a grain (per 100, 26c; 500, $1.15; 1,000, $2.25), and hypodermic tablets containing 1-50 of a grain (per tube of 25, 35c; 100, $1.30).

This remedy combines beautifully with solanine, the "vegetable bromide," one grain of which is equivalent, as a sedative, to 150 of K. Br.

This is furnished in granules of gr. 1-67 as follows: 100, 24c; 500, $1.28; 1,000, $2.50. This combination is especially in-dicated in "tic." in all facial-nerve affections, as a general sedative and a hypnotic where cerebral congestion predominates.

EDITORIAL

SOME PROPOSED FREAK LEGISLATION.

New York, Pennsylvania, New Jersey, Massachusetts and Illinois respectively have had their turn of bills proposing to regulate vivisection, none of which have been near passage, but as it is well to notice and regulate the small infection before it spreads into something of a graver type it will be well for Oklahoma to be prepared to meet just such freak propositions as that of vivisection regulation.

England has had a restrictive Act for thirty-two years, that is a regulation calling for registered buildings, inspections, licenses, etc., yet it is pointed out that that country is most active in its unwarranted and dangerous tampering with the medical profession, through the various anti-vivisection societies and that their object is not to restrict experimentation to proper channels, but to totally abolish it. One eminent English medical authority has stated that "England offers in this respect at least an example to be shunned alike by her offspring and by her fellows."

The proposals of these cranks are answered by the Council on Defense of Medical Research of the American Medical Association about as follows:

That restriction is impracticable in cases of the country practitioner.

That reports of experimentation are necessarily highly technical and that they would only serve to bring about unnecessary and futile prosecutions by persons incapable of appreciating, through their ignorance and prejudice, the true trend of such reports.

That premature publication to the public of experiments might work great harm to a community.

That it would lack wisdom to appoint Inspectors to report on such matters whose qualifications are not known and that gross errors of judgment from every standpoint are likely to occur from the acts of such unqualified persons.

The general objections to such legislation are that it is unnecessary as nearly all the demands made by such proposed legislation are already carried out and observed as far as possible in all laboratories. That it is class legislation. The function of the state is to enact general legislation prohibiting cruelty to animals and that so far as this part is concerned all states now have statutes governing cruelty to animals, through which anyone may be prosecuted.

W. W. Keen several years ago ably pointed out in a letter to some leader of the vivisectionists creed the utter absurdity of the legislation and the great harm that would be done to mankind in general by the passage of such laws.

When one considers the rapid strides made in surgery in Europe and America in the last twenty years and places the credit duly for it; to vivisection, one wonders why an organization can so far forget itself as to propose to stop all the good that may be done in the future by restriction of animal experimentation. Not alone has surgical work been advanced to a wonderful degree, but internal medication has advanced with it. Under their regulations all future experiments where it is necessary to use any of the lower animals would be hampered and interfered with to such a length that eventually they would become things of the past.

Let each medical man look well to these matters and be forewarned by the history of our sister states.

AN ADDITIONAL DELEGATE FOR OKLAHOMA.

At the Atlantic City meeting the Committee on Reapportionment allotted two members of the House of Delegates to Oklahoma.

This apportionment holds good for the years 1910-11-12. At the end of this period we must be clamoring for another delegate, which is only in keeping with the growth of the state in all other lines.

THE PRIVATE DRINKING CUP.

It is gratifying to note that there is an extended effort on the part of State Boards of Health and medical organizations to induce public utility corporations to use intelligent means to prevent the spread of disease in the matter of using the ordinary drinking cup as is seen at public fountains, hotels and on railway cars.

This is one of the most potent sources undoubtedly in carrying infection and the medical press will welcome the day when universal regulations are ordained which will remedy to the fullest extent these sources of trouble.

Several states have already taken up the matter of requiring transportation companies to provide for a separate bowl to be used for dental purposes in sleeping cars. As the condition now usually prevails one goes into the smoking room, washes his teeth and expectorates during the performance into the bowl used by the passengers in common for face and hands. Some roads have already provided, of their own volition, bowls for such uses, but it will probably require a law to force most of them to provide these ordinary needs.

THE PRESIDENT'S ADDRESS.

As many enquiries have reached the Secretary's office with reference to the address of the retiring President, Dr. B. J. Vance, not having appeared in the June issue of the Journal as it should have done, we have this explanation to make and make it so that all may be informed:

One of the first acts of the incoming Secretary was to write Dr. Vance and request that he send the copy of his address to this office as it was not left with the reporter of the meeting as it should have been.

Not having a reply to this communication and having occasion to write Dr. Vance later on other matters the request was renewed and the information was returned that he did not turn the address over to the reporter as he wanted to revise it somewhat and that after reaching home he was called away and did not have an opportunity to attend to it and that he would send it to the Journal soon.

As no communication has since been received from him we conclude that it is still in preparation and promise to publish it in the first issue after it is received.

In this connection it is not out of place to remind all those contributors to the Oklahoma City meeting who failed to transmit their papers to the reporter that their so doing now will save considerable correspondence and delay. If the Editor desired ever so much to publish the transactions of the Oklahoma City meeting it would be a physical impossibility to do so until these papers are all in our hands.

It should also be remembered that these papers are the property of the State Association and should be transmitted to this office.

THE FIFTH COUNCILLOR DISTRICT

Letters having reached the Secretary's office with reference to the Fifth Councillor

District, an explanation of the situation in that district will probably not be out of place.

Dr. T. A. Rhodes, of Goltrie, was elected Councillor at the Oklahoma City meeting and resigned. An attempt was made then to elect some other person to represent the district, but as it was late in the meeting no selection was made, leaving the district without a Councillor.

Dr. Bradford, the President, takes the position that he has not the power to appoint anyone to fill the vacancy, but will designate some one to act in that capacity from time to time and as occasion arises demanding a Councillor in the district.

COUNTY SOCIETIES

ADAIR COUNTY.

A meeting of the Adair County Medical Society is called for July 27, 1909, at Stilwell, Oklahoma.

The program:

"Gastro Enteric Diseases of Children," Dr. C. C. Barnes, Westville.

"Typhoid Fever," Dr. Lane, Westville

"Report of Case, Puerperal Eclampsia," Dr. P. C. Woodruff, Stilwell.

"Malarial Fever," Dr. Jas. A. Robinson, Dutch Mills, Ark.

"Sanitation and Prophylaxis," Dr. Jos. A. Patton, Stilwell.

The latter paper, "Prophylaxis and Sanitation," is an address to which the public has been invited and is delivered by the County Superintendent of Public Health. This occurs to us as a step in the right direction for just so long as the people look with indifference on their unsanitary surroundings or are uninformed as to how they should be remedied, just so long will many of our preventable diseases run rampant and remain uncontrollable. There is no reason why an intelligent public should not co-operate in the eradication and prevention of disease.

President. T. S. Williams, M. D., Stilwell.

Vice President, C. C. Barnes, M. D., Westville.

Secretary-Treasurer, C. M. Robinson, M. D., Stilwell.

ELLIS COUNTY.

The Ellis County Medical Society was organized April 26th with the following officers in charge:

President, Dr. H. W. Hubbell, Grand.

Vice President, Dr. J. O. Ralston, Arnette.

Treasurer, Dr. L. T. Green, Shattuck.

Secretary, Dr. John F. Sturdivant, Arnette.

DELAWARE COUNTY.

Physicians composing the proposed Delaware County Medical Society have determined, for the present, to postpone organization until some time in the future.

This is a matter of regret to the State Association for Delaware county contains many good men who want an organization and the State Association wants them.

We trust the matter will be concluded at an early date.

HUGHES COUNTY.

The next meeting of the Hughes County Medical Society will be held in Holdenville July 29, 1909, with the following program:

"Malaria," Dr. Floyd E. Waterfield.

"Fads and Fancies in Gynecology," Dr. Z. C. Denney.

"Quinine," Dr. J. T. Drake.

"The Reason Why All Doctors Should belong to the County Society," Dr. W. D. Atkins.

"Clinic," Dr. J. D. Scott.

"Thirty Minutes Quiz: Anatomy of the Shoulder," Dr. F. B. Hicks.

"Illustrated Lines on a Skeleton," Miss Jessie Butts.

"Social and Professional Courtesy, What It Is and What It Should Be," Dr. W. C. Bradford, of Shawnee.

"What Constitutes a Successful Doctor?" Dr. A. M. Butts.

This program, especially of the evening, is liberally interspersed with musical selections from the young ladies of Holdenville.

LE FLORE COUNTY.

The LeFlore County Medical Society convened in Poteau July 1st. No special program was rendered, but case reports and discussion thereon was had and the question of refilling prescriptions was fully discussed, resulting in an arrangement by which the druggists of LeFlore county will participate in the next meeting and a full understanding of the question will be reached.

A winter course of study has also been agreed upon.

The following resolution was unanimously adopted:

"Whereas, In the furtherance of his plans for life Dr. John B. Wear has seen fit to retire from the active life of a busy physician; and

"Whereas, Since its organization the doctor has been an honored member of the LeFlore County Medical Society, one whose council and advice has always been timely and of inestimable value to its members, his departure from us will be felt in the workings of the Society, his friendly greetings will be missed and his opinions on the subjects under discussion will be wanting. Now therefore, be it

"Resolved by the said LeFlore County Medical Society in session, That in the loss of Dr. J. B. Wear from our membership, we give expression to the hope that in his new home his life will be replete with the good things that fall to good men,

"That we commend he and his good wife to the people with whom they may come in contact as people well worthy their unlimited confidence, whom to know is a pleasure.

"That our Society loses one of its most valued members and that the medical profession of LeFlore county loses one of its shining lights, a leader and a professional gentleman in every sense of the word.

"B. D. WOODSON, M. D.,
"President.
"R. L. MORRISON, M. D.,
"Secretary."

PERSONAL MENTION.

Dr. J. W. Kerley, of Cordell, is taking a post-graduate course in New York.

Dr. K. D. Gossam, of Custer City, is taking post-graduate work in New York.

Dr. W. O. Weiskotten, of Uitca, New York, has located in Morris, Oklahoma.

Dr. Walter Hardy, of Ardmore, is doing post-graduate work in Europe during the summer.

Dr. J. O. Callahan, of Muskogee, who has been seriously ill for some time, is slowly improving.

Dr. S. A. Ambroswef, of Muskogee, will visit Seattle during the Exposition, taking in Yellowstone Park and points of interest on the Pacific slope.

Dr. R. M. Anderson, of Shawnee, spent part of June visiting in Tennessee and attending the meeting of the American Medical Association in Atlantic City.

Dr. D. H. Patton, of Woodward, President of the Woodward County Medical Society, is taking a vacation of several weeks duration in the East.

Dr. H. D. Shankle, of Morris, Oklahoma, has removed to Muskogee, Oklahoma. Okmulgee county loses an active practitioner and the County Society one of its most useful members, Dr. Shankle being the President of the County Society.

EXCHANGES

HEMORRHAGE IN CHILDBIRTH.

The frequency, causes, and treatment of hemorrhage from the parturient canal in childbirth are discussed by J. F. Moran, Washington, D. C. (Journal A. M. A., June 12). These, he says, may occur before, during or after labor, and those occurring before or during labor are either accidental or unavoidable. The accidental are due to partial separation of the placenta from its normal situation, while the unavoidable type is caused by vicious implantation of the same structure. Hemorrhage occurring after delivery may originate from any part of the parturient canal, but postpartum hemorrhage properly speaking is only from the placental site. Accidental hemorrhage from premature separation is not of common occurrence, but it probably passes often unrecognized. Placenta praevia, or abnormally low implantation of the placenta, occurs in from 1 in 300 to 1 in 1,000 pregnancies. The causes are not definitely known, but multiparity and endometritris may be regarded as predisposing factors. Other abnormal conditions probably have influence and each case must be judged by itself. We are powerless to prevent accidental or unavoidable hemorrhages, but postpartum hemorrhage can be prevented usually by proper management and can usually be controlled by measures at our command. The vaginal tampon, which is so effectual in placenta praevia, Moran says, has no place in the management of accidental hemorrhage because of the danger of concealed hemorrhage. In marginal and lateral placenta praevia, rupture of the membrane usually admits of a normal labor by compressing the structures. But in central implantation, bipolar version, perforation, or separation by the fingers are the usual methods of treatment. It has reduced the maternal mortality, but the child's life is usually sacrificed, and to avoid this abdominal Cesarean section has been more or less occasionally resorted to. Moran considers that it has a limited but clearly defined field, in complete placenta praevia in primiparae with undilated cervix. Miller has practiced and recommended ligation of the uterine arteries to avoid hemorrhage in central implantation, and claims that maternal mortality can be eliminated, except by infection, though the fetal mortality might be slightly increased. The objection to this is that, as in the older methods, the chances of the child are too much neglected. The most frequent cause of postpartum hemorrhage is improper management of the third stage of labor, and every nurse should be instructed in the Crede method of placental expression, should not be attempted, however, too soon. While the mortality, in accidental and un-avoidable hemorrhage, is high, even in the practice of skilled obstetricians, post-partum hemorrhage and that from lacera-tions, are most amenable to treatment, but require an intimate knowledge of the cor-rect procedures under such conditions. His reasons, therefore, for calling attention to so familiar a subject is not its frequency, but the emergency of the situation, which requires prompt and correct management.

The Newfoundland Society for the Pre-vention of Tuberculosis is carrying on a vigorous and necessary campaign this year in the island. The death rate from the dis-ease in Newfoundland is very large. About one in every five of the total population dies of it, and, what is worse, in the last six years the death rate, which is station-ary or decreasing elsewhere, has increased about 50 per cent. Such a state of affairs calls loudly for a remedy, and the Society for the Prevention of Tuberculosis has call-ed the forces of society against the common enemy. As in too many places in Canada, fresh air seems to be dreaded in Newfound-land, and the people spend the long winter closely housed without oxygen. The gov-ernment of Newfoundland has given the campaign a splendid start. It has made a grant of money sufficient to bring to St. Johns all the teachers of the island to at-tend a teachers tuberculosis convention, so that every teacher in the colony will be a leader in the educational campaign.—Medi-cal Brief.

CHLOROFORM IN HEMOPTYSIS.

Joseph B. Fish, Edgewater, Colo., (Journal A. M. A., June 12), after refer-ring to a previous paper on the successful use of chloroform in pulmonary hemorrhage (Journal A. M. A., March 13, 1909, page 883), says that he has continued his experi-ments and now practices this treatment alone in such cases. The effect of chloro-form on the circulation is chiefly to decom-press the vasomotor system, causing an extraordinary fall of blood pressure. Com-plete vascular relaxation follows and the patient, so to speak, is bled into his own vessels. There is also some cardiac enfee-blement and dilatation, which also contrib-ute to lowering the blood pressure. Chlo-roform has also a depressant effect on the respiration, and, as it produces the coagula-tion of the blood in vitro, it is possible that some direct contact with the bleeding point by the vapor may also have some effect. He describes his mode of administration of from 2 to 4 c.c. of chloroform on an or-dinary inhaler or wad of cotton held near the nostrils of the patient. The hemor-rhage will cease within five to ten minutes, and during the following twenty-four or forty-eight hours the patient will be bring-ing up blood clots. The inhalation of from fifteen to twenty drops every hour is con-tinued for a few days and ammonium chlo-ride, with small doses of codein, is given internally every four hours to expel the re-tained secretions and prevent excessive coughing. It is a good plan, he says, also to give a teaspoonful of magnesium sul-phate to keep the bowels free. In the lim-ited number of cases in which he has used this treatment the results have been all that could be desired, and he recommends it to further trial by others.

THE TREATMENT OF BURNS IN THE BERLIN CHARITE.

Pels-Leusden describes the method of handling burns in this noted institution. Extent of surface involved has much to do with the prognosis. The patient almost always succumbs if more than one-half of the surface of the body is involved. One-third of the cutaneous surface involved is frequently followed by death. The determination of the degree of the burns is next in importance. Burns may appear to be of the first degree and later show the formation of blisters or scabs. The third point of importance is the time which has elapsed between the time of the burn and the examination. Hemoglobinemia and hemoglobinuria are seen in many cases, the temperature sinks and other symptoms indicate an intense toxic action. It is therefore necessary to administer digitalis and large quantities of fluids. As the patients are usually thirsty there is no difficulty in getting them to swallow large quantities of strong coffee and tea, brandy and champagne. Repeated enemata of physilogical salt solution, 100 c.c. each, or if the blood pressure is sinking, intravenous injections of the same, often do good. This treatment will not always save, but acts well in many cases of doubtful prognosis. Morphine must be given to allay pain and to quiet the patient. The general symptoms must always be treated first, and it must be remembered that the treatment of the local condition may increase the shock. As a rule general symptoms pass off in from five to six days, but death has been seen after eight even ten days without sepsis or duodenal ulcer being present. Local treatment of burns of the first degree he considers unimportant, but this is not so in burns of second degree. Avoid infection of the wound by first thoroughly disinfecting the burned area. This is extremely painful and can not be properly done without some form of anesthesia. Non-extensive burns may be disinfected by local anesthesia, in other cases a conduction anesthesia or a lumbar anesthesia. In extensive burns of the head or body a general anesthesia may be resorted to. The vesicles are well opened and the whole surface well washed with soap and water and a brush for ten minutes. Alcohol and perchloride of mercury solution are then applied for two minutes, and lastly the wound is covered with gauze dressing, with a thick layer of absorbent wool and another of nonabsorbent wool. Exclusion of air relieves pain. If the secretions of the wound are free it may become necessary to change the wool but not the gauze. In ten or fourteen days the whole dressing is spontaneously cast off. The wound is then found to be epidermizing well and the scars are usually satisfactory. Splints may be necessary in the process of healing to prevent contraction of joints. Early injection of thiosaminine of frobrolysine are usual to obviate contracting scars in the skin.

SOME POINTS OF INTEREST IN TUBERCULOSIS OF THE LARYNX.

By Charles Graef, M. D., of New York, instructor in Throat Department, New York Post-Graduate Medical School and Hospital.

There is probably no pathological condition in any part of the body which presents a more diversified picture than may be seen in a series of cases of tuberculosis of the larynx. Diagnosis is not made especially difficult by this fact, but treatment and prognosis are necessarily modified and many of the "suspiciously long lists" of curative agents which one may find named as successful by various writers on the subject, owe their reputation to the same fact.

In this short contribution I purpose limiting myself to those phases of the disease which are most likely to come under the observation of the practitioner and shall, therefore, limit myself to the consideration of some points in diagnosis, treatment, and prognosis.

Tuberculosis of the larynx is seldom, if ever, a primary matter. Some pulmonary lesion is commonly in evidence when the throat trouble is noted, and in such event diagnosis is comparatively easy. In other cases, however, the first signs of tubercular invasion present here, and these instances are sufficiently numerous to make early recognition a matter of much consequence.

Aside from a suggestive family history, perhaps no single early sign is of such importance as loss of voice. A patient who becomes husky at frequent intervals, with perhaps imperfect restoration of tone between the attacks, should be regarded as a likely subject and kept under careful observation. Miliary tubercle is the form in which the disease presents in the larynx, and frequently large numbers of small seed-like tubercles can be seen through the mucous membrane. As they increase in number, cell proliferation proceeds to the point of death from blocked nutrition, and softening, with spreading ulceration, ensues. Pallor of the mucous membranes is accordingly another very suggestive early stage. The grayish-yellow color of these tissues is very striking, and once observed is likely to be recognized in future cases. This pallor is seen not only in the lower throat but in the pharynx, and especially on the soft palate. In syphilis, malignant disease, and lupus, with which active tuberculosis of the larynx is most likely to be confounded, the membranes are injected and hyperemic.

Pain is rarely complained of until the disease is well advanced. In the early stages a dry, burning feeling in the throat is more often spoken of by the patient, and this may be accompanied by an irritable, tickling cough, particularly troublesome at night when the patient is recumbent, or cause him periods of wakeful discomfort towards morning. The affection is more common in men than in women, and most of the cases occur between the ages of twenty and thirty-five years. To the early signs, in insidious cases, which I have mentioned, must be added the loss of appetite and energy, so familiar in many tuberculous cases, and nowadays, the result of one or more of the tuberculin tests must also be given due weight. Later, as the disease advances and ulceration is progressing, the pain and

cough become severe from erosion of the nerve elements, or pressure from tubercle formation and swelling. Loss of function is also more marked and voice defects, depending on the location and extent of the changes in the larynx, vary from a degree of huskiness to complete aphonia. The lesions are most common on the back parts of the larynx, thickening of the arytenoids, which assume a characteristic "club-shape," being perhaps oftenest seen as the first sign. Ulceration of the epiglottis is also common and destruction of this part of the larynx has been, in my experience, a strong indication that the case would prove one of poor resistance and rapid progress to the end. Cases in which the cords are chiefly involved, especially if this is unilateral, the cord being affected on the side corresponding to the lung in which an area of disease is located, are more likely to respond to treatment. Examination of the sputum is not of much help except in the way of determining, by thus finding the bacillus, that disease is present in the lung. In laryngeal tuberculosis the bacilli are rarely located in the sputum. A brief resume of the chief points by which tuberculosis of the larynx is characterized, and through which it may, in most instances, be distinguished from other diseases, is as follows:

The mucous membranes are pale. Health is generally impaired for some time before attention is drawn to the throat and in most cases there is previous or coincident pulmonary trouble. Its early appearance is most often on or between the atyrenoids where the occurrence of small spots of induration is rapidly followed by marked edema. Ulcers are not deep but spread widely and are accompanied by pain in speaking, coughing and swallowing. Stenosis of the larynx is seldom seen and treatment with iodides is either without effect, or, by increasing the edema, may aggravate the symptoms.

Prognosis: This has become distinctly

better of recent years as the understanding and management of tuberculosis in general has improved. Only a few years ago a prominent writer on the subject felt justified in saying: "As a rule the prognosis can be given only on the basis of the weeks or months of life yet before the patient. The prognosis is most unfavorable." Such a dictum cannot be accepted today. Well-known workers in this field report that they have raised their percentage of cures from two to twenty, by modern methods. These consist chiefly in general hygienic measures, fresh air, nourishment, etc., and, locally, the clearing away of the diseased tissue by curettage, followed by local applications, of which the best is probably lactic acid, or by galvanocautery and subsequent healing applications. Recently some considerable success has been reported by those who have used tuberculin in suitable dosage, and I have personally had some promising progress in a few cases in which I have added a spray of the culture of lactic acid-producing bacilli, to the local treatment of tuberculosis of the larynx. It is, of course, too early to do more than mention it as a possibly useful material in this connection.

A difficulty in treatment of these cases is that the patient can, himself, do little toward effective medication of the part. Sprays and gargles practically have no more useful function than that of cleansing the pharynx, though with practice a patient may learn to reach the laryngeal disease with a good atomizer. He can aid the cure much by giving the larynx complete rest, and this is a point that should be strongly urged.

Pain is sometimes difficult to control, no single drug being effective in all cases. The juice of the ordinary pineapple is sometimes helpful and can be safely recommended for use by the patient. Of drugs, probably orthoform, either as insufflation or in ten grain doses in emulsion, is as effective as any if not quite the best. Cocaine, in 5 to 10 per cent strength, sprayed into the larynx, gives ease but requires repeating at frequent intervals. Later in the disease, where treatment becomes largely palliative, morphine must be used. For the burning feeling already spoken of, a gargle or spray of equal parts of peroxid of hydrogen, extract hydrastis (colorless), and cinnamon or chloroform water, is very soothing. If dryness is a marked feature, an oil spray, of which benzoinol is a good example, should be prescribed.

1076 Boston Road, New York.

References:

Kyle. Diseases of the Throat.

Herzog. Tuberculosis of Upper Air Passages.

—Interstate Medical Journal.

THERAPEUTIC NOTES.

Gargle For Quinsy.

According to Journal de Medicine de Paris for June 27, 1908, Guisez uses the following gargle in the treatment of amygdalitis:

R Carbolic acid ....m xv;
  Glycerine .... ʒiss;
  Menthol .... gr. v.;
  Cherry laurel water .... ʒv.

M.

Sig.: A tablespoonful to be dissolved in a glassful of hot water and used as a gargle morning and evening.

Headache of Neurasthenia.

Bingl prescribes the following pill to be taken at bed-time:

R Quinine sulphate .... gr. xv
  Arsenic troxide .... gr. j
  Extract of cannabis indica .... gr. vij
  Pulverized valerian root,
  Extract of valerian, each q. s.

Mix and divide into thirty pills.

Hemorrhoids.

R Extracti belladonnae fol ....
  Extract opii .... aa, gr. xv;
  Antipyrinae .... gr. xlv;

Cerati plumbi subacetatis _____ ʒiiss;
Unguenti _____ ʒi.
M. et Sig.: Use externally as directed.

Pyelitis.

In cases of chronic pyelitis the following is recommended internally:

R   Quininae tannatis _____ gr. xv
    Sacchari albi _____ gr. xxx
M. Ft. cap. No. vj.
Sig.: One capsule three times a day.

In calculous pyelitis due to lime or uric acid deposits the following may be used:

R   Sodii phosphatis _____ ʒj
    Sodii bicarbonatis _____ ʒij
    Lithii carbonatis _____ ʒiiss
M. Ft. pulvis.
Sig.: One teaspoonful in a pint of water t.i.d.

In the treatment of uric acid calculi Yeo states that excellent results have been obtained by the administration of large doses of glycerine by the mouth. the good effects being due to changes produced in the urine.

The amount given is 1 to 4 ounces dissolved in an equal quantity of water taken between meals every two or three days for a period of several days. Some authors state that it renders the specific gravity such as to produce a change in the urine.

EPIDIDYMITIS.

Ichthyoli _____ fl. ʒvj.
Ungt. hydrargyria _____
Ungt. belladonnae _____ aa ʒiv
Cerati plumbi subacetatis _____ q. s. and ʒii
M. Sig.: Apply to scrotum freely twice or thrice daily. and support with large suspensory bandage.—Merck's Archieves.

BOOK REVIEWS.

The Principles of Pharmacy.

By Henry V. Arny, Ph. G., Ph. D., Professor of Pharmacy at the Cleveland School of Pharmacy. Pharmacy Department of the Western Reserve University. Octavo of 1,175 pages. with 246 illustrations. mostly original. Philadelphia and London. W. B. Saunders Company, 1909. Cloth, $5.00 net: half Morocco, $6.50 net.

Professor Arny in this excellent work divides his subject into the following seven parts:

I—Deals with pharmaceutical processes;

II—With the galenical prepartions of the Pharmacopeia and many unofficial preparations of value;

III—Deals with the inorganic chemicals used in pharmacy, also containing a chapter on chemical theories:

IV—Deals with the organic substances of pharmacy from a practical as well as theoretical standpoint;

V—Is devoted to tests of pharmacy and has them systematically grouped, a decided innovation in such works:

VI—Is the most thorough discussion of prescription writing and compounding so far given by any work and should be closely observed by every student of medicine:

VII—Is devoted exclusively to laboratory work and especially to the work as taught by Professor Arny in the Cleveland School of Pharmacy.

Treatment of the Diseases of Children.

By Charles Gilmore Kerley. M. D.. Professor of Diseases of Children in the New York Polyclinic School and Hospital. attending physician to the New York Infant Asylum and Maternity, assistant attending physician to the Babies Hospital. consulting physician to the Savilla Home for Girls and to the New York Home for Destitute and Crippled Children. consulting pediatrist to the Greenwich (Connecticutt) Hospital.

Second edition revised.

W. B. Saunders Company. Philadelphia and London.

Professor Kerley in this work has given the profession an improvement on what was already the most thorough work from the American press on the "Treatment of the Diseases of Children" and one which should be in the library of every general practitioner of medicine.

It is exhaustive and minute with reference to the care of the infant from birth, leaving no subject untouched, the chapters on infant feeding are perfect and the section devoted to drug dosage is one that we believe is not found in any other work, especially in the convenient and accessible form here given.

The chapters on general hygeine and gymnastic treatment of various affections of childhood are also extremely thorough.

It should command the attention of every general practitioner.

———

Bier's Hyperemic Treatment.

By Willy Meyer, M. D., and Professor Victor Schmieden. The new (2nd) edition enlarged.

"Bier's Hyperemic Treatment in Surgery. Medicine and all the Specialties: a Manual of Its Practical Application," by Willy Meyer, M. D., professor of Surgery at the New York Post-Graduate Medical School and Hospital, and Professor Dr. Victor Schmieden, assistant to Professor Bier, at Berlin University, Germany. Second revised edition. Octavo of 280 pages, illustrated. Philadelphia and London. W. B. Saunders Company, 1909. Cloth, $3.00 net.

While this work is comparatively speaking new to many of the Oklahoma profession a close study of it will be of lasting benefit.

The first edition was rapidly exhausted and enthusiastically received by the profession generally.

The work considers the treatment from the hyperemic view point of practically all inflammatory conditions, being every complete as to tubercular affections of joints and bones.

MISCELLANEOUS

THE UNIVERSITY OF KANSAS.

———

Announcement is made by a committee of the faculty of the University of Kansas that a review week will be held September 13, 14, 15, 16, 17 and 18, complimentary to the graduates of the medical department and of the several colleges which were consolidated when the clinical department was founded.

The general plan is to review for the practitioner the recent progress and current status of some of the more important subjects of medicine and to this end several lectures, demonstrations and some clinical work will be had with hospital visits; provision is also made for laboratory work and there will be some operative clinics during the time.

College reunions, a banquet and theatre parties are arranged for the evenings and all alumnae of the merged colleges are requested to attend.

———————

THE WYNNE EYE, EAR
AND THROAT HOSPITAL.

———

Dr. H. H. Wynne announces to the profession that The Wynne Eye, Ear and Throat Hospital, 107 North Broadway and Park Place, Oklahoma City, is open for their consideration and support.

The hospital contains twenty-two rooms, is of modern construction and a considerable sum of money has been expended in making it all that is desirable in such an institution.

NEW MEMBERS OKLAHOMA STATE MEDICAL ASSOCIATION.

E. A. Jones, Sweetwater.
H. H. Gipson, Erick.
G. W. Henry, Carter.
H. P. Hampton, Rhea.
D. C. Adams, Taloga.
E. E. Lawson, Seiling.
A. H. Atkins, Aledo.
A. L. Hotcher, Texola.
G. Pinnel, Erick.
G. A. Share, Seiling.
J. G. Marshall, Fountain.
J. B. Leake, Taloga.
W. T. Royce, Cestos.
R. E. Leathercock, Putnam.
Changes in address:
J. S. Meradith from Coralea to Russell.
J. W. McQuaid from Friendship to Korn.
G. M. Clifton from Denver to Norman.

C. A. THOMPSON,
Secretary-Treasurer.

THE ARLINGTON HEIGHTS SANITARIUM.

Announcement is made that Dr. John S. Turner, of Fort Worth, Texas, formerly connected with the Arlington Heights Sanitarium, has removed to Dallas, Texas, where he will devote his time exclusively to the practice of his specialty, mental and nervous diseases.

Arlington Heights Sanitarium will hereafter be under the management of Drs. William L. and Bruce Allison, who have heretofore been connected with this well known institution.

OKLAHOMA PUBLIC HEALTH.

During the five months ending May 31st, 1909, there were 218 deaths from tuberculosis in the state, the rate of mortality from this disease being higher than from any other cause.

During the above period nineteen physicians died from various causes.

On August 1st a rule will be promulgated by the Oklahoma State Board of Health requiring that all tubercular cases be reported to the County Superintendents of Public Health and that all typhoid fever cases be reported to the same officers.

The necessary blanks for these reports will be furnished the profession at an early date and the laboratories of the State University will be called into use in assisting the diagnosis in cases of doubt.

Muskogee and its dirt has been receiving due attention from both Dr. J. C. Mahr, Superintendent of Public Health, and Dr. W. T. Tilly, President of the Board of Examiners. The city was required to abate many nuisances of a small character and to remedy defective sewerage conditions in its septic tank system.

OKLAHOMA STATE BOARD OF HEALTH.

Grosshart vs. Means, case continued until October meeting.

Brown vs. Randle, case continued to October meeting.

Thrailkill vs. Peters, under advice of the Attorney General's office a license was issued to Dr. Peters in this case, on purely technical and legal grounds, Dr. Thrailkill, on the same advice and the advice of his attorneys, withdrawing the charges. New charges were immediately filed covering the same facts and this case will come up for final hearing during the October meeting of the Board

Board vs. Woody and others, licensed by the Peters Board, temporary license was granted Dr. Woody and others until October when they are to show cause why their license should not be permanently revoked.

The Board decided that hereafter any-one wishing to obtain temporary license until the following meeting of the Board must pay a fee of five dollars, not return-able, and take the examination at the next succeeding meeting. This action is caused by the habit of some men obtaining tem-porary license, practicing until the Board met and then removing to some other state.

Next meeting, Credentials Committee to pass on the credentials of applicants and the reciprocity features of the various ap-plicants will meet Monday, October 11. Court day for trials and hearings Tuesday, October 12. Examination days October 13, 14 and 15.

CASES TO BE INVESTIGATED BY THE STATE BOARD OF EXAMINERS

Grosshart vs. Means, action to revoke license, abortion.

Board vs. Lee.
Board vs. Norvall.
Board vs. Lindsay.
Board vs. Harrell.
Board vs. Green.
Board vs. Jameson.
Board vs. Clark.
Board vs. Wilson.
Board vs. Weiser.
Board vs. Davis.
Board vs. Beasley.
Brown vs. Randel.
Thrailkill vs. Peters.
Durham vs. Board, demand for certificate.
Floyd vs. Board, demand for certificate.

The most important of these cases is that of Thrailkill vs. Peters. This case is well known to many of the profession of the state as being one in which it is alleged that as a member of one of the old Indian Territory Board of Examiners, Dr. Peters illegally registered many physicians, who under the terms of the Act of Congress could not be registered. The final out-come of this case will be watched with great interest as the Board of Examiners of Oklahoma have so far refused to regis-ter many of the men so registered by Dr. Peters and the gist of the charges against Peters is that he should not be registered on account of his acts as a member of the Indian Territory Board. His registration would probably encourage those applicants already denied registration to renewed ef-forts along that line.

AS TO WATER AND SEWER SYSTEMS.

A. M. Alden, Assistant State Bacteriol-ogist, of Norman, Oklahoma, State Uni-versity, sends out the following questions to health officers:

1. What kind of water supply has your town? a. Where does the water come from? b. What kind of reservoir have they? c. Is there any chance for con-tamination?

2. Has your town a sewer system and if so what disposition is made of the sew-age?

3. How many cases of typhoid have you in your town at present?

If you suspect that there is any chance for contamination in the public water send a sample for analysis. All public work is done gratis and for private work, such cases as the physician may suspect of con-tamination, a fee of $5.00 is charged, this fee being paid by the parties owning the well or reservoir."

The new Washington state law providing that applicants for marriage licenses must undergo medical examination went into ef-fect on June 10th. Ten couples appeared at the license clerk's office without phy-sicians' certificates, and two couples, when informed of the new law, said they would go to British Columbia to marry. County officials say the new law will result in many Americans marrying in Canada.—Medical Fortnightly.

OFFICERS OF THE OKLAHOMA STATE MEDICAL ASSOCIATION.

President, Dr. Walter C. Bradford, Shawnee.

First Vice President, Dr. C. L. Reeder, Tulsa.

Second Vice President, Dr. D. A. Myers, Lawton.

Third Vice President, Dr. J. W. Duke, Guthrie.

Secretary, Dr. Claude Thompson, Muskogee.

LIST OF COUNCILLORS WITH THEIR RESPECTIVE COUNTIES.

First District, Dr. J. A. Walker, Shawnee. Canadian, Cleveland, Grady, Lincoln, Oklahoma, Pottawatomie and Seminole.

Second District, Dr. John W. Duke, Guthrie. Grant, Kay, Osage, Noble, Pawnee, Kingfisher, Logan and Payne.

Third District, Dr. Charles R. Hume, Anadarko. Roger Mills, Custer, Dewey, Blaine, Beckham, Washita and Caddo.

Fourth District, Dr. A. B. Fair, Frederick. Greer, Kiowa, Jackson, Comanche, Tillman, Stephens and Jefferson.

Fifth District, _____, _____. Cimarron, Texas, Beaver, Harper, Woodward, Alfalfa, Ellis, Woods, Major and Garfield.

Sixth District, Dr. F. R. Sutton, Bartlesville. Washington, Nowata, Ottawa, Rogers, Mayes, Delaware, Tulsa and Craig.

Seventh District, Dr. W. G. Blake, Tahlequah. Muskogee, Creek, Wagoner, Cherokee, Adair, Okmulgee, Okfuskee and McIntosh.

Eighth District, Dr. I. W. Robertson, Dustin. Sequoyah, LeFlore, Haskell, Hughes, Pittsburg and Latimer.

Ninth District, Dr. H. P. Wilson, Wynnewood. McClain, Garvin, Carter, Love, Murray, Pontotoc, Johnston and Marshall.

Tenth District, Dr. J. S. Fulton, Atoka. Coal, Atoka, Bryan, Pushmataha, Choctaw and McCurtain.

Delegates to American Medical Association, Dr. C. S. Bobo, Norman; Dr. L. A. Hahn, Guthrie.

Alternates, Dr. C. L. Reeder, Tulsa; Dr. J. A. Walker, Shawnee.

EPSOM SALTS MADE PALATABLE.

A very fine preparation of epsom salts, according to Burnett Physicians Drug News, October, 1908, is made by taking two pounds of the salts, one ounce of the tincture of cardamon, twenty grains of vanilla, three drachms of saccharin, two ounces of alcohol, two ounces of glycerine, two ounces of coffee (roasted and ground) and water to make a half gallon. Stir the coffee in the half gallon of hot water and let it stand for fifteen minutes and let it draw, then add the salts, vanilla and tinct. of cardamon to the alcohol and shake; then add the glycerine and the saccharin, and when coffee mixture is cold enough, mix all together and filter. A half ounce of the salts is contained in each ounce of the mixture. It keeps well, acts well, tastes well, and children cry for it.

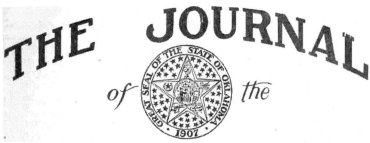

THE JOURNAL of the
Oklahoma State Medical Association.

VOL. 2.   MUSKOGEE, OKLAHOMA, AUGUST, 1909.   No. 3.

CLAUDE A. THOMPSON, Editor-In-Chief.

ASSOCIATE EDITORS AND COUNCILLORS.

DR. J. A. WALKER, Shawnee.   DR. JOHN W. DUKE, Guthrie.
DR. CHARLES R. HUME, Anadarko.   DR. A. B. FAIR, Frederick.
DR. F. R. SUTTON, Bartlesville.   DR. W. G. BLAKE, Tahlequah.
DR. G. W. ROBERTSON, Dustin.   DR. H. P. WILSON, Wynnewood.
DR. J. S. FULTON, Atoka.

Entered at the Postoffice at Muskogee, Oklahoma, as second class mail matter, June, 1909.

This is the Official Journal of the Oklahoma State Medical Association and every member of that organization is entitled to a copy and if, through accident or oversight, you fail to receive a copy notification of that fact to this office will receive prompt attention. All communications should be addressed to the Journal of the Oklahoma State Medical Association, English Block, Muskogee, Oklahoma.

THE DIAGNOSIS AND TREATMENT OF MALARIA IN DIFFERENT LOCALITIES

DR. F. B. ERWIN, WELLSTON, OKLAHOMA

Read before the Seventeenth Annual meeting of the Oklahoma State Medical Association, Oklahoma City, May, 1909.

This is one of the most common diseases which the general practitioner has to treat in this section of the country. This being the case, it would seem useless to attempt to offer a few thoughts along the diagnosis and treatment of this disease. Yet we profit by the exchange of ideas though no new ones be offered. I desire to handle this subject, as nearly as possible, from the standpoint of a country practitioner.

When we speak of malaria we frequently think of it in a great deal the same way as we think of hysteria. There is not very much the matter and does not need much

treatment. Just a little quinine and calomel and everything will come all right. While it is true that many cases are easily controlled, yet it is also quite true that there are a large number of cases which are very difficult to treat, successfully.

Malaria is a disease, which is acquired in the summer months, from about May or June till cold weather. It is an endemic disease which is characterized by a destruction of red blood corpuscles, enlargement of the liver, enlargement and in chronic cases hyperplasia with pigmentation of the spleen. It is due to a germ, known as the Plasmodium Malaria, which is found in the spleen and blood. In all cases of malaria there is passive congestion of the liver and spleen. It has marked effect on the vaso-motor system producing a partial or complete paralysis of the coats of the blood vessels. Hence the great tendency to local and general congestion.

The Plasmodium Malaria which produces or is the causative factor of malaria is found in three forms, namely: Tertian, Quartan and Aestivo-autumnal.

The tertian parasite is characterized in the earlier stages by small hyaline bodies and possessed of amoeboid movements. As they increase in size they become surrounded by pigmented granules.

As they enlarge the granules collect toward the center and the amoeboid movements cease. Segmentation then begins and the parasite divides into from fifteen to twenty-five parts. Then the blood cell bursts throwing them into the system. This produces the chill. It requires about forty-eight hours to complete this cycle so that a single group of the cells produce a paroxysm every other day. A double infection would produce a paraoxysm every day, quotidian fever.

The quartan parasite has less pigment, of a more coarse type, less spores and segmentation requires seventy-two hours. So that the chill would come every third day.

The aestivo-autumnal type is smaller, being about one-half the size of a red blood cell and contains less pigment than the preceding. It appears in the blood cells as small hyaline bodies and causes the corpuscles containing it to assume a shrunken, crenated appearance. After a week or more large ovoid bodies, crescentic in shape, appear in the corpuscles. Segmentation occurs only in the spleen and other internal organs. The cycle of this parasite covers a period of forty-eight hours.

If all cases of malaria had the characteristic objective and subjective symptoms in all localities then the diagnosis of this disease would be practically easy without the use of the microscope. But many are the cases which we meet that have symptoms simulating other diseases so closely that it requires very close differentiation to be absolutely sure that it is only a case of malaria.

Malaria manifests itself in two general forms of fever: Intermittent and remittent. And we have three distinct stages in the fevers: The cold stage or rigor, the fever and the sweating stage. The cold stage lasts from five minutes to one hour; the fever lasts from one to ten hours; and sweating stage lasts from one to five hours.

For the typical intermittent or remittent type in adults we have the following characteristic symptoms: The cold stage begins with lassitude, yawning, headache, nausea, skin becomes pale and wrinkled, nails and lips are blue, features pinched. Temperature begins to rise.

The hot stage begins as the cold one ceases and temperature continues to rise. The surface of the body becomes flushed, the pulse rapid and full. Headache, backache, nausea and great thirst. Urine scanty and high colored and increased specific gravity.

The sweating stage begins gradually, appearing first on the forehead and extending over the entire body. All other symptoms subside as perspiration becomes free. In children these stages are not so well marked. Sometimes they begin abruptly with vomiting or convulsions. Malaria chills in children under five years of age are rare. They have cold hands and feet, blue lips and nails, sometimes slight cyanosis, pallor, drowsiness and prostration. Headache is very common usually frontal and may simulate tubercular meningitis.

The aestivo-autumnal form presents the following types: Gastro-enteric, Thoracic, Cerebral, Hemorrhagic and Algid.

The symptoms of the Gastro-enteric are: Nausea, vomiting, purging, thin discharge from the bowels, burning sensation in the stomach, intense thirst, weak pulse, cold hands and feet, cramps, marked depression. Lasts from one to several hours.

Thoracic type: Usually combined with the preceding, attended by dyspnoea, oppressed cough with some blood streaked sputum, frequent weak pulse, cold surface, terror stricken features.

Cerebral type is marked by violent delirium, followed by stupor and full, slow pulse. Flushed or livid surface due to congestion of the brain.

The Algid type is that in which the body surface is intensely cold, rectal temperature frequently 104 to 107, cold sweat covers body, pulse slow, feeble and often absent at wrist. The mind is clear, but the countenance is death like.

The differential diagnosis should be made from cerebral apoplexy, meningitis, uremia, yellow fever and cholera.

In the foregoing we have noted some of the subjective and objective symptoms of the typical types of malaria. Now let us notice some of the symptoms of the atypical types of which we see so much, indeed, we see them so frequently that we think sometimes they are in the majority.

Some cases come in our office in which we can find no history of chill or chills, or no sweating stage. We find the history of fever every third day or every other day or maybe a little fever continuously. If the fever has continued for any length of time, probably about the first thing we notice is a cachectic look and an emaciated appearance. They complain of a loss of appetite, headache, nausea or vomiting, probably constipation. pain in one or both sides and general weakness.

Upon a physical examination the liver or spleen or both may be found moderately or considerably enlarged. The digestive organs will generally be found to be deranged. The abdomen may be enlarged with considerable tympany or it may be emaciated. The urine will generally be found to be dark in color, decreased in quantity and increased in specific gravity. The sclera of the eyes may be slightly jaundiced. Upon examination of the blood quite a decrease in the number of red blood cells and the Plasmodium Malaria will be found in quantities proportional to the advancement of the disease.

In some cases the symptoms very much simulate typhoid fever. The temperature has the characteristic morning and evening rise and fall of typhoid. The dry brown coated tongue, the enlarged spleen, the tympanitic condition of the bowels and sometimes the delirium. As a rule there is constipation but sometimes diarrhoea. There is sometimes a rash similar to typhoid rash.

In parturient cases malarial fever develops a few days after the delivery. Several cases have come under my notice. One which I desire to call attention to was a case of a lady about forty years of age. Before parturition considerable swelling of the limbs and a little irritation of the bladder was all that seemed to bother her. She gave birth to twins and got along nicely for three or four days. Then suddenly a high fever developed. The attending physician had been very careful in the delivery to prevent sepsis, as we always are or should be, and thought it almost impossible that it was a septic condition. The third day of the fever, to be absolutely sure that he was right in his diagnosis, he thought best that a microscopical examination be made, and asked me to see the case. After carefully examining for the Streptococci I failed to find any. Upon examination of the blood I found quite a number of the Plasmodium Malaria. The patient was placed upon a rigid malarial treatment and soon made a nice recovery. This case very much simulated a case of septic infection but proved not to be.

The treatment of malaria resolves itself

into the preventive and curative.

The preventive consists in keeping all the emunctory organs in good condition, that is, the use of purgatives to keep the bowels active and from two to four grains of quinine three times daily, at intervals, to keep the resistive power of the blood such as to overcome the Plasmodium Malaria as fast as they develop in the system.

In the curative treatment there are about three methods as regards the administration of quinine. First, give large doses of quinine a few hours before the expected paroxysm to destroy the parasite before maturity. Then small doses during the interval. Second, give large doses of quinine during the sweating stage to destroy the young spores which are floating around in the blood. Then give small doses in the interval. Third, give continuously to destroy both the parasite and spores.

In the treatment of malaria quinine is the chief drug to use, as it is the one that acts directly against the Plasmodium Malaria. However, adjuvants are needful in the treatment as well: such as iron, arsenic, and strychnine. Experience has proven that the hepatic gland must be aroused and made active before the quinine will have its proper effect.

Hydrargyri cloridum mite is denied by some as having any specific action upon the hepatic gland. However, some authorities claim that there is a possibility of the mild cloride being acted upon in the intestines by the alkaline ferments and changing part of it into the corrosive cloride which does have a specific action upon the liver. While authorities claim and many physicians practice the use of small doses of calomel, Hare says "that large doses of calomel in warm climates produce a large flow of bile" which small ones will not do. It seems that the warm climate produces an inactivity of the liver which calomel will overcome. Experience has proven that it is necessary that large quantities of bile be

thrown off for the other medicines to have their best effect.

There is a difference among physicians as to the amount of calomel to be given. However, nearly all are agreed that it is better to give it in broken doses. Some say to give small doses about one-tenth to one-half grain every thirty minutes till eight to ten doses are given. Others give one-half to one grain every thirty minutes till four to six doses are given. Always follow with a saline or if not well borne by the stomach use an enema.

In some localities the first and second methods seem to prove very successful but in our locality the third method has proven the most effective treatment.

When the patient is first seen begin with one grain of calomel every thirty minutes till three to five grains are given; follow with a saline or enema. Then begin the administration of quinine, two or three grains every two hours till four to six doses are given. Then continue the use of it every three hours till the fever has subsided. After that give three or four doses daily for several days. As an adjuvant use some form of iron, as the corbonate one grain with the quinine. Also give about one-twentieth of arsenious acid three or four times daily. If the secretions are stubborn and inactive give one-half grain of calomel every three hours till six or eight doses are given. Follow with a saline or an enema. If necessary use tonics for the stomach as indicated. The use of one-fourth to one-half grain of capsicum with the quinine sometimes proves beneficial.

In obstinate cases of chills the use of opium combined in the quinine for a few doses has given good results in our section of the country. Just before or during a chill if a hypodermic of one-fourth of morphine with one-hundredth and fiftieth of atropine be given the chill will be averted or checked.

A case of the cerebral type of the Aestivo-autumnal form came to my notice. A lady about thirty years of age. While in a store she suddenly fell to the floor in a convulsion, something of the Hystero-epileptic form. She was unconscious from the beginning. Face flushed, stertorous breathing, frothing at mouth, pupils widely dilated at first, reflexes diminished. Convulsions were controlled with bromides and chloroform. After convulsions were controlled she was unconscious for about thirty-six hours. Pupils continued to be dilated, reflexes somewhat diminished deglutition poor, fever high, breathing slow, pulse rapid and weak, bowels constipated and retention of urine.

After eliminating the conditions which might cause this comatose state, such as uremia, cerebral hemorrhages, etc., a microscopical examination of the blood was made and the Plasmodium Malaria was found in great numbers.

She was given strychnine to support the heart, and was forced to resort to croton oil to move the bowels. The bladder was emptied with catheter. Then about twenty grains of the bisulfate of quinine was given hypodermically and was repeated in twelve hours. At the end of thirty-six hours she regained consciousness and was then placed upon rigid malarial treatment as indicated above by the mouth and in about ten days she was able to be around again.

Having noted the different forms of malaria or the different ways in which it manifests itself we see that the locality has considerable to do with the diagnosis and treatment of this disease.

DISCUSSION.

Discussion opened by Dr. Burch, Norman:

In regard to malaria, the best way to give quinine is to give all you are going to give in one dose. I think you will find that one large dose is better than several two or three hours apart. A patient I had not long ago came into my office, his lips were as blue as they could be and he was shaking, and I gave him one big dose of quinine, and he was soon all right.

Dr. Harper, Afton:

I wish to call your attention to the part mentioned in the paper on preventative treatment, especially after an individual in the family has developed a case, he is a source of infection to the remaining members of the family, and the malaria carrying mosquito. I think one of the most essential measures of treatment is to explain this to the patient or to the family; have the proverbial rain barrel about the house cleaned or emptied. Enough mosquitoes can be raised in an oyster can full of water to spread malaria over a neighborhood and will do it provided the water stands out a few days. In a case of acute malaria, the patient should be screened with mosquito netting and should be saturated with quinine. After a few doses of quinine the parasites in the blood are destroyed. I think the best way of destroying the mosquitoes about the place is in preventive treatment.

Dr. Adams, Chandler:

I beg to differ with the gentleman over here in regard to single large doses of quinine. I have known people to thoroughly try quinine in large doses before they came to a doctor. I have had them come to me after they had taken a teaspoonful of quinine at a time, and the chills would keep on just the same. You have got to have some calomel, and you have got to have some strychnine, a little arsenic and a little iron in there to break up chills, and rather than take one large dose of quinine, I believe in giving three grains every few hours.

Dr. Landram, Olustee:

I liked the paper. but it didn't begin far enough back. There are a great many mosquitoes, but there is only one kind that cause malaria, and it is not a difficult matter, but a very interesting study and a very pleasant pastime, to take a little net and go out along the river and catch these mosquitoes. I think it is very important that we should become familiar with these mosquitoes, and any physician would find it very profitable to study them. I have done it a few times and I found it very interesting, and I surely think the mosquitoes around the house in an oyster can are harmless. If you are close enough down by the river you are liable to be affected, but if you are up on the hill, the mosquitoes up there are harmless.

Dr. H. M. Williams, Wellston:

Mr. Chairman: I wish to speak of the paper as a whole in very complimentary terms. It seems to me that the doctor had carefully studied the subject. As to the mosquito being the only cause of malaria; why is it we find malaria where there is no mosquito to be found? In my section of the country we meet with malaria in the winter season as well as in the summer, and I wish to emphasize the fact as to diagnosis of malaria. So frequently we have complication diseases and we go on and treat our case for malaria only when there may be some other disease that has undermined our case. Especially this is true in malarial districts, and I believe it is the duty of every one when he has a case that he make a thorough diagnosis of the case, and the best thing is the use of the microscope.

Dr. Burch, Norman:

I came from down in the swamps near Norman and I have seen the most malignant cases of malaria, and I have seen it down in Texas, and I believe in heroic doses of quinine, but as the gentleman over here said, quinine is not the only thing; now it is a foregone conclusion that you give quinine and calomel both. I think the best method of administering quinine for ma-

laria is to give all you can give. The gentleman alluded to the type of malaria where the fever will never go down. Now, you will find physicians not familiar with that class of disease, and many doctors have got the idea, that you mustn't give quinine while fever is on; but you can reduce any kind of fever if you give enough of it. You can start in about 2 o'clock in the morning if your patient has a high fever and give heroic doses of quinine and by day the fever will be down. If you give small doses of quinine, you will find that you will probably have a case that will run three or four weeks, when it might as well only have been two or three days.

Dr. Bailey, Carmen, Okla:

In regard to this disease, it is one that has interested me greatly for the last nine years, since the opening of this country. At the opening of this country, I came in contact with people that said they had "slow fever," and I was just out of college at that time and had rather a scientific idea in my mind that if we had a microscope and we would puncture about and examine a drop of blood, and whether it was due to our inability to make the examination or not, at any rate we could not locate the malaria plasmodium, we could not find them in the blood. Many of these cases would drift away and when they would get back to the states, quinine wouldn't break this up. I came to believe in the meantime that we had very little malaria, and unless a case came to me with a plain history of the chills and fever and the day of feeling pretty well with no fever, I hardly knew what to call it. Recently I have had a number of cases of the malarial fever of the tertian type, I would call it, where the chills occur every other day, and the gentleman who has just left the floor has outlined my treatment exactly, and if they give the exact history of the case and the exact hour of the day they had the chill, I didn't have to make the second call on the case. I frequently give about a quarter grain of colomel about six hours apart. I have done that on their well day, or in the evening and then if the chill came on about 10 o'clock the next morning, I would give ten grains of quinine at one dose. There is no use to sit up in the night to give quinine, but I just write the prescription for quinine in capsules and if they gave me the history correctly they will not have the chill; but there is a symptom they often overlook, they skip one chill, and then they sometimes overlook the directions.

Dr. C. S. Bobo, Norman:

I was very much interested in that paper, it was not only interesting, but I think it was one of the most scientific papers on the subject that I have heard for sometime, and the manner in which he took up the different phases of malaria. The doctor is certainly to be complimented and congratulated upon his most excellent paper.

As for the treatment of malaria, I would rather hear from some Arkansas doctor, if we want to get a wholesome, successful treatment of malaria, than from most any man that practices medicine in the country. I am not from Arkansas I want to tell you, but some years ago I had a partner just from the swamps of Arkansas, and he gave me more valuable information in regard to the treatment of malaria than I ever learned from the colleges and practical bedside experience. He had been up against every kind and he had it down pretty pat as we call it; in other words, he was successful and treated his cases successfully. I think that a good brisk calomel purge is very necessary before your anti-malaria remedies, to prepare the system and then give the quinine. There is only one sure method of administering quinine and that is hypodermically. That is the only mode of administration that the doctor can absolutely swear by. He will get the effect of his

quinine when he gives it hypodermically. It has been my experience that my patients stood large doses of quinine by the stomach in order to interrupt the next paroxysm of malaria. As a rule the stomach is a little brackish and you give that stomach twenty or twenty-five grains of quinine poured into it at once and my experience is that it rebels against the dose.

Dr. Fisk, Kingfisher:

I have seen patients that could take a teaspoonful of quinine and would not get any affect from it; you take the same amount of quinine and put it into a capsule, it will be absorbed shortly. They will absorb any portion of quinine that is given. The same rule will apply to some of the coco-quinine preparations.

Dr. Rector, Hennessy:

After thirty-five years practice. I want to endorse the doctor's paper thoroughly. There isn't anything any better in my judgment. I am an Arkansas man and believe in taking a teaspoonful of quinine every two hours for six or eight days.

Dr. Medaris, Helena:

I am not from Arkansas, but I have been practicing medicine in Indiana in a malarial district, and I think I have had my part of experience. Now, gentlemen, I notice some of you don't get the affect of quinine. I know this, when you give quinine on a dry tongue, it will not be absorbed; quinine given on a moist tongue will be absorbed and you can get the affect. I have not had the experience with large doses, because large doses were not given in that day. We begin with small doses from two to three hours apart until we get the affect.

Dr. Duke, Guthrie:

I am not from Arkansas, but I am from the east side of the river and people living in that section suffered very greatly from malaria. And the doctors practicing medicine in my part of the country give large doses of calomel to raise the action of the liver and these physicians give their quinine hypodermically, bi-sulphate, believing it would be impossible to get sufficient absorption to relieve the malaria in that region. The article on malaria just read is a very scientific article and deals with it very clearly and plainly, but the doctor failed to mention one type of malaria which is very common which is the hemorrhagic type. No physician would ever administer quinine by the mouth for this type of malaria; they always resort to the hypodermic instead and usually use bi-sulphate or something that would dissolve the quinine. I also believe that a great many cases of continued fever are diagnosed malaria that are not malaria. I think we have many types of a low grade of continued fever in this country, and especially among the young which is simply auto-intoxication the circulating fluids of the body infecting it with a substance that poisons the system causing this fever, and if the microscope was used more than it is I think we would find much less malaria in Oklahoma than we now seem to have. The mosquito, I believe, is the one source of conveying malaria, but he is not so common in the high hills; I think the majority of cases of so-called malaria in these regions are due to something else.

———

Discussion Closed by Dr. Erwin, Wellston:

Mr. Chairman, Ladies and Gentlemen: I appreciate the high compliments which have been paid to the paper, and also I have profited by the discussion, though they weren't all in favor of my idea of treatment. I noticed that possibly a few of the doctors didn't take into consideration that that paper didn't deal with treatment alone, but diagnosis and treatment. And then there was another idea brought out that possibly some of the cases might be typhoid, but after several examination of the blood are made for the typhoid and also for the malaria, you will either find the plasmodium or you will find typhoid. They spoke a great many times of not giving large doses of quinine by the mouth or not having any taken by the mouth. The idea has also been brought out that the secretions should be brought out by the stomach. If the secretions are not roused there would be no effect of the quinine, therefore, we give calomel and other things that the quinine may be absorbed. The doctor asked the question as to why give quinine; the only reason we should give it is because it is the specific for plasmodium malaria.

ABDOMINAL MYOMECTOMY FOR LARGE UTERINE FIBROIDS

W. J. FRICK, M. D., AND H. P. KUHN, M. D.--READ BY DR. W. J. FRICK AT THE MEETING OF THE OKLAHOMA STATE MEDICAL ASSOCIATION, MAY 11, 12, AND 13, 1909

The treatment of fibroid tumors of the uterus resolves itself into either a radical procedure involving the sacrifice of that organ or in some form of extripation of the myoma, leaving the organ intact.

Other methods of treatment including the medical, electrical, etc., have been discarded either for failure to cure or danger to the patient. At the present time, the consensus of opinion for the treatment of fibroids is about two to one in favor of some form of hysterectomy. (1)

In review of the recent literature and from personal experience, we are convinced that simple extripation or myomectomy should take a wider field.

Myomectomy is to be contrasted with hysterectomy not only in that it leaves the uterus intact and capable of pregnancy, but conserves important rectal and bladder supports. Hysterectomy at its best sacrifices all chances of maternity and unless some of the modified methods of high amputation are undertaken leaving an ovary, the climacteric is precipitated. We believe that an artificial menopause is no more troublesome than a normal one, yet it is a condition to say the least, unnatural.

It is unfortunate that in dealing with fibroid, we have a disease for which we do not know the cause. Whether a fibroid is to be regarded as a fibrosis similar to the change in the prostate in the male (2) whether it is a developed Cohnheim area (3) or whether it bears the same relation to a terminal blood vessel as neuromata to epineurium (4) would to some extent determine radical or conservative treatment. Herein will lie the great objction to myomectomy, for not knowing the etiology, we do not know the chances of recurrence.

An average of statistics show that 21 per cent of all women have fibroid (5). This pronounced tendency to fibrosis might remain after enucleation of all growths. It is difficult to draw conclusions from postoperative statistics as there are so few reports. A. Martin had two cases recur out of ninety-six (6). The German authorities give 6.4 per cent of recurrence (7). C. P. Noble had no recurrence in sixty-six cases (7). The fact there are so few reports would argue in favor of non-recurrence. It would appear that this danger of recurrence is relatively slight since the growth of these tumors is slow, these cases would tend to reach the menopause and the fibroids retrogress before they were large enough to give symptoms (8).

Other advantages aside, that of pregnancy is the most important: Following myomectomy, we have Winter and Noble's statistics. Winter's series comprised twenty-eight cases of sub-serous, sub-mucous and interstitial fibroids of which six became pregnant (7). C. P. Noble had in forty-four vaginal myomectomies, one pregnancy in twenty-two abdominal, two pregnancies. Taking Winter's high percentage and Noble's low in ninety-four myomectomies we have nine pregnancies or 2 per cent. This rather low per cent is worthy of consideration with the other factors in favor of myomectomy.

The post-operative sequellae of myomectomy are of no small import. There is no prolapse of the bladder and resulting cystitis as in hysterectomy. The most important anterior supports of the rectum and sigmoid are not disturbed and rectal prolapse is not so likely (10). Vaginal hernia and general visceral prolapse into the empty pelvis as well as secondary atresia of the vagina are prevented (11). Myomectomy is a rapid operation with a trivial loss of blood, no shock and an easy convalescence.

The danger of overlooking malignant disease of the body of the uterus is an important desiderum. There is no doubt that carcinoma of the body of the uterus and fibroid have some intimate relationship since 5 per cent of all cases of fibroid have accompanying carcinoma of the body or have it develop later in the cervical stump. (12) Noble states that carcinoma of the body is increased twenty-six times in the presence of fibroid. (12) There appears to be no relationship between carcinoma of the cervix and fibroid.

Even though carcinoma be not present in the body or cervix we are confronted with the fact that in patients where supra-vaginal hysterectomy has been done, they have died later of a malignant disease of the cervical stump. (13) Winter, Manton and Noble report cases of malignant disease of the cervix as common after supra-vaginal hysterectomy (14). Pichelot reports three cases of cancer of the cervix occuring in fifteen cases where he had done supra-vaginal hysterectomy. (15) Lisobre' states that it is an unquestioned fact that the cervical stump is prone to degenerate (16). If these cervical stumps are so frequently the seat of degeneration we must question the value of supra-vaginal hysterectomy. There remains then but the two extremes of uterine surgery, pan hysterectomy and myomectomy. By assuring ourselves that there is no accompanying malignant disease, myomectomy must be considered more often.

The so-called degenerations of fibroids into sarcoma are rare. Von Franque found it to occur in from 1 to 3 per cent of his cases; Fehling in 2 per cent, and Noble in 2,274 cases only 1.4 per cent. The clinical significance is of no great importance only in that it offers for removal of the fibroid wherever it is discovered. (17).

TECHNIQUE.

The technique of myomectomy is simple but should be carefully carried out in its steps. With the patient in the Trendelenberg position, the abdomen is opened in the median line with an incision long enough to deliver the uterus. The intestines are walled off and the uterus surrounded with gauze pads secured with a tape and haemostat. The assistant grasps the cervical portion with the gloved hand and by compression controls the blood supply. If this method is not possible especially where the uterus cannot be delivered, Moynihan clamps after the method of Hertzler (18) are applied. Sometimes the hemorrhage can be controlled by a gauze pad rolled in the form of a rope and tightly compressed about the neck after the fashion of a tourniquet. In fibroids of the sub-mucous variety, or where they are situated well beneath the surface of the uterus, the incision is made over the most prominent part of the tumor. In the pedunculated growths, the incision is carried in an oval about the base. The tumor being exposed, blunt dissection with the knife handle or with Kelly's crenated myomectomy enucleator readily lifts the growth from its bed. This is easily accomplished. Should there be any efferent vessels running into the tumor, they are ligated. The control of the blood supply is now loosened so that any free bleeding from the cavity can be stopped. The surplus uterine tissue is trimmed down to obliterate the cavity. It will be noticed that the uterus contracts after enucleation of the deeper seated myoma and care must be taken not to trim off too much tissue else the edges will not approximate nicely. If the endometrium is torn, it is repaired with a running suture of No. o iodized cat-gut. The cavity is again inspected for free bleeding and the interrupted figure of eight haemostatic suture of No. 1 iodized cat gut is placed about one-half to one-quarter inch from the margin of the incision deep into the tissues of the uterus. With this method the edges usually approximate cleanly. To further close the incision, running suture of No. o cat gut is placed in the peritoneal coat. After we are satisfied that no more myoma exist, the uterus is dropped back into the pelvis.

Occasionally it is necessary to plicate the broad and round ligaments to take up slack in these supports (19.) The abdomen is closed in layers with No. o and No. 1 cat gut.

CASE HISTORIES.

Mrs. R. Mc. A. Aet. 29. No children. There was no typical history of fibroid. Patient herself noticed a gradual enlargement of the abdomen. Rather profuse menstral periods.

Operation: Uterus found to be symmetrically enlarged. A fibroid five inches in diameter was enucleated from the fundus, of the sub-mucous variety. A considerable amount of thinned out uterine tissue was resected to close the cavity left by the fibroid. The uterus was closed in the usual manner and the abdomen without drain.

Post operative: Patient left the hospital in two weeks with an uneventful recovery.

Twenty-two months later she has gained twenty-five pounds and is in good health with normal menstrual periods.

Mrs. D. S. Aet. 31. No children. Patient has had hemorrhages lasting for fifteen days at each menstrual period. Lost considerable weight.

Operation: Uterus was found to be covered with small fibroids. These were subserous and inter-mural and readily enucleated. One large fibroid the size of a grape fruit was enucleated from the fundus of the sub-mucous variety. The uterine incisions were closed in the usual manner and the abdomen without drainage.

Post-operative: Recovery was uneventful, patient leaving the hospital in two weeks. Twenty-four months later she has gained twenty pounds and her menstrual periods are normal.

Mrs. W. Aet. 40. No children. Patient has had a uterine tumor for fifteen years with recent pressure symptoms. She is in critical condition at time of operation from vomiting and pressure sumptoms.

Operation: Abdomen rapidly opened from ensiform to pubes. A large pedunculated fibroid filled the entire abdominal cavity. This was delivered from the abdomen and a wedge-shaped incision involving its base made in the fundus. The patient was in extreme condition. The uterine incision was rapidly closed and the abdomen with through and through suture. She rallied and made a rapid convalescence.

Post-operative: Twenty-eight months later she has gained forty-three pounds and has no symptoms referable to the pelvis.

Mrs. H. S. Aet. 45. One child. Menstral periods have been two weeks apart for three years. Nodular mass palpated in pelvis.

Operation: One sub-serous fibroid size of a billiard ball and a sub-mucous fibroid size of a walnut enucleated at the fundus. Uterus and adbomen closed in the usual

Post-operative: Sixteen months later

patient has gained weight and has normal menstral periods. Approaching the climactory.

Miss M. S. Aet. 25. No children. Rather profuse menstral periods with considerable dysmenorrhoea. Fibroid discovered at operation for acute appendicitis three months before.

Operation: Uterus was found to be symmetrically enlarged. A fibroid of the sub-mucous variety size of a billiard ball enucleated from the fundus. The tumor was solitary. The uterus was closed in the usual manner and the abdomen without drainage.

Post-operative: She left the hospital in ten days with no complications. Nine months later she is having no hemorrhages, no dysmenorrhoea and is gaining weight.

Mrs. A. D. Eat. 39. No children. Patient has had hemorrhages for two years with an increasing tumor in the pelvis.

Operation: One fibroid size of a billiard ball at level of the internal os, posterior of sub-serous variety readily enucleated. Another the same size at the fundus of the sub-mucous type was removed with some of the endometrium. This was repaired with No. o cat gut and the uterine incisions and the abdomen closed in the usual manner.

Post-operative: She made a rapid convalescence, leaving the hospital on the tenth day. One year later she has no symptom referable to the pelvic cavity.

Mrs. A. G. M. Aet. 49. No children. Patient came in for operation for chronic appendicitis. No history of fibroid.

Operation: Adherent appendix removed. Uterus was symmetrically enlarged. Fibroid size of an orange enucleated from the body of the uterus. Usual uterine closure and abdomen without drain.

Post-operative: Convalescence uninterrupted. leaving hospital at end of second week. Patient has been lost sight of.

Mrs. G. Aet. 43. No children. Severe

hemorrhages for six months. No evidences of carcinoma from uterine scrapings.

Operation: A sub-mucous fibroid five inches in diameter removed from a uterus symmetrically enlarged.

Post-operative: Patient left the hospital in two weeks. Ten months later she is having no hemorrhages and is gaining weight.

Mrs. P. Aet. 40. No children. Patient gives a history of pain and hemorrhages for six months.

Operation: One sub-serous fibroid and two sub-mucous fibroids averaging two inches in diameter removed from fundus and cornua of uterus. The uterine incisions were closed in the usual manner and abdomen without drain.

Post-operative: Patient left hospital in two weeks and one year later she has gained weight and has no symptoms referable to the pelvic cavity.

Mrs. A. L. K. Aet. 40. Two children. Patient has never been well after second baby ten years ago. Severe hemorrhages for two years.

Operation: Six small fibroids enucleated averaging one inch in diameter. Three of these were sub-mucous and the others subserous· and pedunculated. Uterus looked like a honey-comb before suturing incisions.

Post-operative: Patient made an uninterrupted recovery and left the hospital in two weeks. Three months later she is having a normal menstral period and has no symptom referable to the pelvis.

Summing up these reports, we find there was a wide selection of cases both as regards age as well as type of fibroid and complications. In every case the operation was entirely successful in relieving the symptoms and the treatment seemed to have resulted in a cure. In some of the cases, the operation was practically a Cassarean section while in others it was more simple. In either type of operation, the result was good and the convalescence as prompt. We

have in no case any cause to regret the procedure.

The literature gives such widely divergent views as to the curative value of myomectomy that perfection of technique must enter into the estimate. Winter cures 73 per cent of his cases (9). Noble has a higher percentage (20). Sutton and Giles hold that the after effects of myomectomy are admirable (21). Howard Kelly has good results and considers supra-vaginal hysterectomy in women under forty too radical a procedure if it can be avoided.

In a recent compilation by J. H. Carstens of fibroids complicating pregnancy of 498 cures in the literature up to January 1st, 1908, gives a percentage of recovery of .8 per cent favorable to myomectomy over some form of hysterectomy.

The older literature as a rule give a rather unfavorable mortality as compared to hysterectomy. J. N. West holds that it is a more dangerous operation than hysterectomy. (23) J. M. Baldy has had no deaths. (24) The Johns Hopkin's reports up to 1908 have a mortality of 4.5 per cent as compared to 3.1 per cent for hysterectomy. (10) These percentages only show that the personal factor in selection of cases and perfection of technique determines the mortality.

Authorities differ somewhat on the selection of cases suitable for myomectomy but that of Howard Kelly includes those most generally embodied (25).

Myomectomy should be prefered to hysterectomy in women under forty where there are no complication septic tubes or pelvic disease. In women over forty where the tumor is not enlarging and the menopause is distant myomectomy is the operation of choice. If the fibromata continue to grow after the climacteric, hysterectomy is indicated for it is in these cases that we have the highest percentage of carcinomatous degeneration. 64.9 per cent (28).

CONCLUSIONS.

Myomectomy is especially indicated in women under forty where the genital tract can be left intact.

The limits of myomectomy should be extended under proper technique to cover part of the field of supra-vaginal hysterectomy.

Myomectomy is the operation of choice for fibroids of the lower uterine segment in pregnancy.

REFERENCES TO THE LITERATURE.

(1) Howard Kelley, Text Book—"Operative Gyne.," Vol. II, p. 359.
(2) Crossen, Text Book—"Diseases of Women," p. 625.
(3) Kieffer, Bulletin d.Acad.—"Royal de Med. de Belgique."
(4) Bland Sutton, Text Book—"Tumors In. & Malig," 1903, p. 186.
(5) J. F. Jordan, Brit. Med. Jour., Jan. 26, 1907.
  S. S. Bishop, Text Book—"Fibromata of Uterus," 1901. (Boyle 20 per cent. Klob. 40 per cent).
(Boyle 20 per cent. Klob. 40 per cent).
  J. N. West, Amer. Jour. Obst., Vol. 56, p. 700, (12 per cent).
(14 per cent Ellice Mc. Donald).
  R. Williams, Brit. Med. Jour, 1904, p. 461, (20 per cent after 35 years).
(6) Weill, Ann. de Gyne., Paris, July, 1889.
(7) C. P. Noble, N. Y. Med. Jour., Vol. 83, p. 1012.
(8) W. P. Manton, Amer. Jour. Obst., Vol. 53, p. 73.
(9) G. Winter, Zeitschrift fut Geb. et. Gyne., Vol. LV., p. 49.
(10) L. J. Hirschman, Jour. A. M. A., Oct. 31, 1908.
(11) M. F. Porter, Amer. Jour. Obst., Vol. 52, 744.
  Sutton & Giles, Text Book—"Dis. of Women," 1897, p. 209.
(12) J. W. Bovee, Surg. Gyne. & Obst., Vol. IV, No. 3, p. 209.
  J. W. Williams, Bost. Med. Jour., Oct. 3, 1908.
  ...lice McDonald, Jour. A. M. A., Vol. 52, p. 952.
  Picquard, Ann. de Gyne., July, Aug., 1905.
  C. P. Noble, Jour. A. M. A., Vol. 47, 1906.
  Iisobre, These, Paris.
  J. ... Bovee, Amer. Jour. Obst., Vol. 152, p. 203.
  H. F. Lewis, Amer. Jour. Obst., Vol 152, p. 481.
(13) Crossen, Text Book—"Dis. of Women." p. 625.
(14) J. W. Bovee, Surg. Gyne. & Obst., Vol. IV, No. 3.
(15) Pichelot, Ann de Gyne. et Obst., Paris, Vol. 54, 1900.
(16) Lisobre, Thes., Paris, 1907.
(17) E. A. Schumann, Amer. Jour. Obst., Vol. 59, N., p. 375.
(18) A. E. Hertzler, Jour. A. M. A., Vol. 53, p. 869.
(19) R. C. Coffee, Surg. Gyne. & Obst., Vol. 7, No. 4, p. 383.
(20) C. P. Noble, N. Y. Med. Jour., Vol. 83, p. 1012.
(21) Sutton & Giles, Text Book—"Dis. of Women," 1897, p. 415.
(22) J. H. Carstens, Amer. Jour. Obst., Vol. 59, No. 375, p. 451.
(23) J. N. West, Amer. Jour. Obst., Vol. 56, p. 705.
(24) J. M. Baldy, Amer. Jour. Obst., Vol. 52, p. 771.
(25) Howard Kelly, Text Book—"Operative Gyne.,"
(26) J. B. Sutton, Surg. Gyne. & Obst., July, 1905, p. 88. Vol. II.

DISCUSSION.

Dr. Leroy Long, McAlester, Oklahoma:

I was much interested in this excellent paper by Dr. Frick. In the surgical world there is no difference of opinion as to what should be done with fibroids of the uterus. The only question is "How shall they be removed with the greatest safety to the patient?"

One of the greatest advantages by doing a myomectomy—the doctor points out—is that we do not leave a woman in a condition in which she cannot bear children. This should have great weight in deciding which operation should be done. Another thing we do not run the risk of having abdominal collapse.

Another advantage that he points out is doing a supra-vaginal hysterectomy of the uterus. We run the risk of malignant degeneration of the stomach which seems to be a condition so frequent as to require our attention.

The objections that may be offered to myomectomy are, that sometimes the tumors return, but this is, as statistics show, only about 2 or 3 per cent. I mean a myomectomy of the interstitial tumors that involve the entire wall of the uterus, in which it is necessary to go down and have—whether we want it or not—a rupture of endometrium amounting to Caesarian Section. Hemorrhage and sepsis are the principal dangers. However, in the hands of a man who is expert I believe he has taken ground that is tenable. For the average man, not expert in this work, a hystorectomy may be safer than a myomectomy.

Dr. A. L. Blesh, Oklahoma City:

I am sorry that I did not get to hear all of Dr. Frick's paper.

The question is sometimes raised whether a fibroid uterus is ever worth saving, for many of these cases return, but even after a myomectomy a woman may have borne children and for that reason it was well worth saving.

I believe where we have a well defined myoma and where important structures ar not destroyed—where the fibroid is single and not multiple—that the field is one for a myomectomy; but I don't believe that in cases of multiple fibroma that myomectomy should be considered.

I heard the conclusions of the doctor's paper and am in harmony with them.

———

Dr. U. L. Russell, Oklahoma City:

The speaker has voiced my sentiments in regard to fibroids. Fibroids are recognized largely between the ages of thirty and forty-five. At the age of thirty the chances of maturity are less; the chances of having a child are less. In the fibroids I have removed I have seldom found a single fibroid, I find quite a number. I think that where there is a single fibroid a myomectomy should be performed, and in women in whom pregnancy may occur or is present, myomectomy can be performed without producing aboreion.

In hysterectomy you have the chances of carcinoma already removed.

In the _____ hospital it is the rule to go low down and take out all the mucous membrane and all round the external os, leave enough of the cervical tissue and take the stump of the round ligament and so maintain the support of the cervix, and this tends to prevent the bladder from falling back so much. You will have few chances of malignancy.

I think a large fibroid, single, should be removed by myomectomy.

Dr. Frick, closing:

In the last two years I have done a number of myomectomies for fibroids. Previous to that time I had done hysterectomies for such cases. I believe myomectomy is the operation of choice where it can be performed. Myomectomy for large tumors and for small tumors. Hysterectomy should be, in my opinion, the exception and not the rule.

The danger of hemorrhage is slight, according to my notion. I don't remember of ever ligating a blood vessel. In this operation the uterus is brought out of the abdominal cavity and surrounded by gauze.

In regard to the recurrence of fibroids after a myomectomy, the records show only a few recurrences. Where a hysterectomy is indicated it should be a complete hysterectomy and not take any chances.

USE AND ABUSE OF THE CURETTE

BY DR. T. J. DODSON, MANGUM, OKLAHOMA

The subject of the use and abuse of the curette is one which is naturally divided into two classes: One in which the proper use of the curette is indicated; the other where it is improperly used if indicated at all.

I am a strong believer in the proper use of the curette but confess that I have been guilty of its improper use myself, and be-

lieve others have been more guilty, while some have been most guilty.

The gynecologist often meets with a class of patients, which might be called neurasthenics, who come to the office for treatment, accompanied by their mother, aunt, or some old lady friend, who have come for the special purpose of informing the doctor that the patient has "female trouble" and has been treated by certain doctors, for so long, and you are expected to know the doctors personally and thoroughly understand their methods of treatment.

These patients have come for local treatment and will not be satisfied without it. Some of them need curetting from a scientific standpoint; some for the purpose of relieving the mind; while others would be benefited most if you could convince them that they had no such thing as a uterus. The unfortunate patients are often the victims of the doctor who is anxious for the fee, in the first place and is also anxious to advertise himself as a specialist in this class of work.

The principal class of cases in which the curette is used is in the different forms of endometritis, which includes the simple, acute, chronic, and septic or specific endometritis.

In considering the anatomy of the endometrium, we find that the internal os divides the lining membrane of the uterus into two different portions. The endometrium begins here and lines the whole inside of the body of the uterus, and extends, modified, into the openings of the fallopian tubes. Its characteristic features are these: It is firmly attached to the muscular tissue by connective tissue in which is found lymphoid structures only. The mucous membrane of the cervix is dense, hard, free from lymphoid elements, and is a true mucous membrane.

In acute metritis the whole organ-body, neck, and mucous membrane is implicated; in endometritis the mucous membrane alone is involved; in parenchymatous metritis the muscular tissue is added, and in perimetritis, that of the peritoneal covering is also involved. To these cases we might add, acute septic metritis and chronic septic metritis. The curette may be properly used in all of the above cases if a correct diagnosis is made of each individual case. It is not so

much a question of whether the curette should or should not be used, as it is, what form of endometritis have we to deal with, and how the curette should be manipulated.

In simple endometritis, the membrane may be hypertrophied or atrophied. In the first condition the vessels are enlarged and increased in number; the lymph-spaces are increased in size and the muscular walls much thickened. If the membrane be atrophied the follicles with their epithelial linings are decreased in size, the lymphoid tissue is not rich in cells, and the whole membrane is below the normal in thickness. There is an abrupt demarcation between the mucosa and the muscular structures, therefore, in curetting an hypertrophied membrane we should be very careful to use no more force than is absolutely necessary to remove the membrane, and not interfere with the muscular structure of the uterus.

We do not have here, as in cancer, to remove a hard resisting tissue, but to simply scrape over a muscular wall covered by soft investment, which is still further softened by inflammation. All that is necessary is to remove the endometrium.

Acute and chronic septic endometritis also calls for the use of the curette, but should be used with great care and used early, before the staphylococci have penetrated the muscular wall.

I have seen the curette used in infecte' cases, after labor, where the muscular wall was being scraped off; the operator claiming that it was parts of retanied placenta when, in fact, it was the muscular tissue. Therefore, it is as important to know where to stop as it is to know when to begin.

If portions of the placenta or membranes remain attached to the uterine walls, after labor at full term, and uterine contraction fail to separate them entirely from their attachments, a blunt curette may be employed. If septic symptoms have appeared, the cavity should be explored with the utmost care as the uterine walls are thin and softened and there is always danger of perforating them.

If the infection has extended to any great degree, and we have a parenchymatous metritis, the uterus would be in a subinvoluted condition, with the endometrium lying in folds in a traverse way all through the entire length of the uterus. It would be impossible to thoroughly disinfect such a uterus, and it would be folly to attempt to do so with a sharp curette for you would only gouge along the walls of the uterus, over the folds of the endometrium, and open up new avenues for further infection; and such a uterus would have been in a better condition if the sharp curette had never been invented.

Yet much good may be accomplished with a large, blunt, irrigating curette; the larger the better. This is introduced up to the fundus of the uterus, and with a hot antiseptic solution. The irrigator is gently swept all around the entire body, being very careful not to make any fresh abrasions, but going into all the folds of the endometrium, giving it a thorough irrigation, then packing the uterus with gauze establishing free drainage. This I consider much better treatment than any effort at currettment. I believe that the curette is more often abused in this class of cases than in any other.

While the operation of dilatation and curettage is usually considered a safe procedure and is followed by little or no mortality, it may have decided dangers which must be considered. The uterine secretions contain germs of no kind, while germs are constantly present in the cervix; therefore, any operation upon or through the cervix should be conducted under the strictest antiseptic and antiseptic precautions. A failure to do this might lead to serious pelvic inflammation and even death.

Another point worthy of note is the method of dilatation of the cervix. After the perineal retractor is introduced the anterior lip of the cervix should be caught with a double tenaculum and the cervix drawn well down to the vulva. A sound should be introduced to determine the direction and depth of the canal. If the uterus is in a normal position we have but little trouble in passing the smallest size dilator; but if we have an antiflexed uterus and use much force there is danger of piercing the posterior wall at the cervical junction.

With the blades of the instrument well introduced dilate the canal first in one direction then relax the pressure, the blades closed, rotate the dilator a little, gently dilate another portion, and so on, continuing all around the circle back to the first point. Such a method of dilating by repeated pressure on the cervical canal from all directions is far better than the common method of opening the dilator, controlled by a screw, and expending all the force in one direction, until the fibers split and a tear is produced. By observing these precautions we avoid the danger of sceptic infection; the scar left when the rent heals, and the possibility of the development of carcinoma.

When the dilatation is completed the uterine cavity should be irrigated with creolin or lysol solution. The curette is introduced to the fundus and the scraping begun at some easily recognizable point— for instance at on e cornu—letting each stroke extend from the fundus to external os, or as nearly so as possible. One can always pass over the same place twice with safety, provided, the force used is not too great and is always directed obliquely to prevent perforating the walls of the uterus. The fundus should be scraped separately by moving the curette along its surface from side to side.

Normally the uterine wall is firm and resistant. And even marked pressure made upon it by the sharp curette would not be sufficient to perforate its walls. Occasionally the muscular tissue is thin and friable and even the slightest pressure is sufficient to cause a rupture. This is especially liable to occur in curetting septic cases after abortion.

In one case of this kind where there was great infection of three or four days duration, and the patient almost in a dying condition, I think I made a perforation myself, because of the great depth to which my curette suddenly passed in the direction of the umbilicus, and the great pain produced at the time; although, I was very careful and made no more pressure, as I thought, than to determine the depth of the uterus. Yet without any resistance the curette plunged into the abdominal cavity. I afterwards learned that the woman had been wearing a stem pessory, or some such instrument, for the purpose of producing an abortion. And it may have been that the stem pessory produced the perforation and my curette found the opening. This is more probable from the fact that the patient already had diffuse peritonitis.

When the canal is large enough, as is usually the case in a miscarriage, after the third month of pregnancy, the index finger, well sterilized, is by far the best curette that can be used. Pieces of tissue will often be found clinging to the placental area, which can be freed by the finger; and with the external hand making firm pressure through the abdominal wall the uterine wall can be felt distinctly and will sometimes feel almost as thin as paper.

In a case seen by Dr. M. D. Mann, of Buffalo, New York, a young practitioner forcibly dilated the cervix in order to remove the ovum in an early abortion, which the patient had induced by means of a catheter. In using a sharp curette and his finger, after cleaning out the ovum, he caught hold of and tore a loop in the intestine. Dr. Mann was called, opened the abdomen and found a hole in the fundus large enough to admit the finger.

Dr. J. B. Harvie, of Troy, New York, reports a case in which after dilating the uterus a young practitioner passed a pair of forceps to catch the ovum and drew out and cut off six feet of bowel without realizing what he had done. Hence the necessity of being very careful with the curette.

Read before meeting of the Oklahoma State Medical Association, May 11, 12 and 13, 1909.

DISCUSSION.

Dr. Hulen, Pond Creek:

Gentlemen of the Association: I am not sure that I understand that proposition. Shall I go back and take up the discussion of Dr. Dodson's paper, or shall I pass on to the paper just read? Not that I expect to make a systematic lengthy address at all, what few remarks I make shall be of a rambling character.

The paper on "Puerperal Infection" is one that is of interest to every practitioner. There is a point or two I want to touch on.

First, treatment. The other parts of the paper have been thoroughly discussed, but I desire to lay a little stress on it. In thirty years' experience with over a thousand confinements, without the loss of a mother, I believe that you will either have to say that I have been extremely lucky in getting the right cases, or I have been lucky in striking out on the right line in treatment of the case. In puerperal infection, or if there ever was a fever or dangerous case of placenta, provided I believe it is infection, a physician should be there at all times. I am not in a hurry to say we ought to cure that, but I am here to say we should differentiate the cure. It is a very easy matter to do that without the curette. A little cotton and disinfectant will tell you whether you have anything in that uterus that ought to be curetted. I am not here to tell you what you should do, but I will tell you what I do, and you will think less of your treatment, or more of it, just as you please. After you have sterilized the uterus, saturate to what I have been disposed to call dry saturation, not thorough saturation, a quantity of gauze in 95 per cent carbolic acid, and carry that to the fundus of the uterus and oscillate until you are as sure as possible, allowing it to remain from three to five minutes, and place nothing more or less in its place than plain gauze. If the temperature of this patient is 104 when you begin, by the time you are through it will have reduced two degrees, or perhaps more, and in two hours or two and a half hours you will find it is reduced to almost normal.

Now to the curette. If you will pardon me for digressing a little bit, I want to touch on a point that the paper didn't touch on. That is, what is the good effect of the curette, how is it brought about? In order to illustrate it, we want to get clear away from the profession of medicine. Many times when we meet a friend with a smile, they uncover gums bulging and swollen. If struck by a tooth brush would produce hemorrage. If, in that case, you take a little scalpel and make two strokes around that tooth, and instruct that patient to use any simple antisceptic solution, in two weeks you will find that the little gum vessels have contracted and that the gum has taken on a healthy appearance. When you made that little stroke with the scalpel, you cut many blood vessels. The walls contract the other blood vessels and obliterate a large share of the other blood vessels. The same thing will follow the operation with the curette, but we ought to be careful in distinguishing which cases should, and which should not, be curetted. I recall a case not a great while ago in which a patient had been taken to a hospital, having been curetted because of menorrhea. She was put to bed a few days and given the rest cure. When she left

the bed, the hemorrage returned. It is a difficult matter to diagnose whether you have only one or both ovaries are involved. In these cases you should be able to find or differentiate whether the case demands curetting or whether it demands the removal of an ovary. If you close the little urinal cavity and then place in a little cotton you will be able to tell whether you have a straight path or not. Again there is danger in curetting a case that has just passed through a miscarriage. If you are not extremely careful, as was brought out in the paper, you puncture the uterine wall with the curette, as happened in my own case on one occasion. There was a case brought to me to make an operation for retained placenta. This case had suffered a miscarriage something like three days before. As was customary then, we curetted for the sake of cleanliness. The wall of the uterus was so softened and in attempting to reach it, we did not find it and having attached to the hollow tube a funnel containing 1-2,000 of bi-chloride of mercury, the curette plunged through the wall carrying with it 1-2,000th bi-chloride of mercury. I speak of this for in many cases we are extremely liable to do this when we least expect it. There are many things that could be said along this line, but I fear I have already taken up more time than I should have been allowed.

———

Dr. Gillis, Frederick:

I took a few notes, but I see you have quite a number of others present and I have been discussing all the papers heretofore because there didn't seem to be enough to go round hardly. As I said once before this afternoon in speaking of the curette, my experience has been that whatever curette a person is in the habit of using, that is the one for them to use. Personally, I have always used a sharp curette and couldn't do anything with a dull curette. I have seen other people who always use a dull curette, and I think they were in my condition only the reverse, they couldn't do anything with a sharp curette. Wherever a curette is indicated I think the person that is curetting, if they understand what condition they want to get and they use the curette they are in the habit of, will get the result, it doesn't make any difference about what kind they use. Now, I think Dr. Dodson said in his paper that the finger was the best curette; probably so, if you could reach the infected side or the side wanted with the finger, but now I think it is almost impossible to use the finger as a curette in almost any kind of a case; I don't think you can get to the site of infection or whatever you are trying to get at in the uterus, if your hands are as big as mine, you can't get at it with the fingers. I think it is a mistaken idea to try to use the fingers.

Now as far as happening to perforate the uterus, gentlemen, that occurs among surgeons. That doesn't occur among us country practitioners. I never saw anything of the kind, and I never hesitate to use the curette. I think it is just among surgeons that that happens. The more work a man does on a given line, and the more he knows about the case, the more negligent, I believe, he will become. I think it altogether happens among the people who have too much to do.

Dr. Thrailkill, Chickasha:

I wanted to rise to answer one point that the gentleman brought out. He said he didn't believe the uterus was ever perforated except by surgeons. I want to tell you of one instance when the uterus was perforated eighteen inches and the the rectum was brought down through the uterus and the woman died. I believe

that the uterus is perforated more by the general practitioner than by the surgeon. I believe that the uterus is sometimes perforated by ulcerations and not by the curette. If perforated by ulcerations, it would be easy for either the surgeon or the general practitioner. I would advise any physician who own any of the instruments I speak of to throw them in the well or do something with them so he wouldn't ever be attempting to use them.

Dr. Russell, Oklahoma City:

I want to say a word, but I didn't get in in time to hear the paper. Of course, the curette ought to be used in such a manner as he feels it should be. Now the curette should be used cautiously. Don't jam the curette through the fundus, but pass it up carefully and bring it down until you get the uterus clean. Now in general cases, it is not much necessary to use it, but when it is used pass it gently through the fundus and not carelessly down on all sides.

Dr. Dodson, Mangum, closes discussion:

I haven't much to say in closing. I thank you for the discussion. As I said in reading, I always think there is more learned from the discussion than from the paper.

In reference to the finger being a good curette, I simply said that in abortion after about three months, that the finger was better than the curette, because you can feel very well, and if there is anything to be removed, I don't believe it would be so firm but what it could be removed without any difficulty. I think that a dull curette should be used in any case of that kind.

There was another point I tried to lay stress on in the paper, and that was, where the curette was used to try to make a diagnosis, and then be careful with the curette to handle it in the proper way. Insofar as perforating the wall of the uterus, or the walls are perforated after the curette has been used, we don't know what has taken place. It may be that the walls of the uterus are perforated oftener than we think for. I had that happen once and one gentleman who discussed the paper said that fell to his hands once. I don't see why it should fall in the hands of the surgeon any oftener than any one else.

EDITORIAL

THE COUNTY SECRETARY.

"Section 4. The Secretary shall record the minutes of the meeting and receive and care for all records and papers belonging to the Society, including its charter. He shall notify each member of the Society as ciety which may come into his hands. He shall keep an account of and properly turn over to the Treasurer all funds of the Society which may come into his hands. He shall make and keep a list of the members of this Society in good standing, noting of each his correct name, address, place and date of graduation, and the date of the certificate entitling him to practice medicine in this state; and in a separate list he shall note the same facts in regard to each legally qualified physician in this county not a member of this Society. It shall be his duty to send a copy of such lists, on blank forms furnished him for that purpose, to the Secretary of the State Association at such a time as may be designated by the State Association.

"In making such lists he shall endeavor to account for each physician who has moved into or out of the county during the year, stating, when possible, both his present and past address. At the same time, and with his report of such lists of physicians and members, he shall transmit to the State Association his order on the Treasurer for the annual dues of the Society."

Now, Brother Secretary, you can greatly aid the cause and further the interests of the Association by complying with the above, which is an extract from the By-Laws of your County Society. It is not the intention of the writer to chide you in any manner for not having done this before; many of you have sent prompt reports and gone even further than that by sending in the happenings of your locality for publication from time to time and the object of this is to stimulate each of you to renewed efforts in that direction.

The Secretary of the American Medical Association requires a monthly report from your State Secretary of new members, removals, deaths changes of address, resignations, etc., and without your prompt compliance with this section of your laws the work necessarily lags.

You are earnestly requested to carry out these provisions and do everything in addition that occurs to you will be beneficial to the organization.

If any of you are out of the necessary blanks or need any information in the possession of the State Secretary you will be promptly supplied upon request.

Suppose you try to help in this matter? It will be to the mutual interest of every physician in the state that you do so; it will go far in making our state body second to none and in making your Journal one of interest to all its readers.

AFTER THE CHIEF CRIMINAL.

The Tulsa City Physician, Dr. W. E. Wright, is making a very sane campaign for the extermination of the active housefly, and has taken most effective means to call the attention of the laity to its dangers.

A large card was printed, the center showing just how the sources of infection were carried from place to place and interesting data is given concerning the breeding and propogation of this common nuisance and universal danger to human health and comfort.

Terse directions are given for their extermination and one is struck with the thoroughness of the advice, nothing being left to the imagination as to their destruction.

The margin of the placard on the left is given up to pictures or etchings of a consumptive spittoon, garbage can, dirty dairy, dead animals and open outhouses; these are accompanied on the opposite or right hand side by the pictures of an infant's nursing bottle, fruit, cake, dining table and a case of typhoid fever.

The doctor admits at the bottom of the forceful creation that it is a disgusting picture, revolting to the stomach, but says the end justifies the means and that disgust created by the eye is as nothing compared to the benefit to be derived from taking warning from the picture.

Every Health Officer, Board of Health, City Physician and Sanitary Officer in the state should have a copy of this placard and the good done by a common display of it in every neighborhood in the state from April to October cannot be even estimated.

COUNTY SOCIETIES

COUNTY SOCIETIES.

The Secretary of each County Society is earnestly requested to keep this office advised of deaths, marriages, removals, changes of address, new comers in the profession, etc., in their respective counties, this being the only method by which items of interest to the Journal's readers can be had without entailing an enormous amount of unnecessary correspondence.

You are especially requested to forward promptly, the transactions of your County Society.—Ed.

TILLMAN COUNTY.

The Tillman County Medical Society was scheduled to meet July 27th at Frederick, with the following program announced:

"Erysipelas," Dr. A. B. Fair, Frederick.

"Intestinal Antiseptics," Dr. J. H. Hansen, Grandfield.

"Malaria," Dr. J. P. Van Allen, Frederick.

Subject announced later, Dr. G. A. Camp.

HUGHES COUNTY.

The Hughes County Medical Society will hold no meetings during the summer months, resuming their program October 28, 1909.

TULSA COUNTY.

Tulsa county will hold no meetings during the summer months, resuming their work October 2nd.

LINCOLN COUNTY.

Program of Lincoln County Medical Society, Wellston, Oklahoma, August 11th.

1909, beginning at 10 o'clock a. m.:

"Importance of Early Diagnosis of Tuberculosis," Dr. J. O. Glen, Sparks.

Discussion opened, Dr. A. H. Taylor, Wellston.

"Treatment of Incipient Pulmonary Tuberculosis," Dr. F. C. Brown, Sparks.

Discussion opened, Dr. W. A. Pendergraft, Carney; Dr. J. W. McIntosh, Sparks.

"Treatment of Tuberculosis in General," Dr. E. E. Lumm, Stroud.

Discussion opened, Dr. C. M. Morgan, Chandler.

"Tuberculosis Sinuses," Dr. A. A. West, Guthrie.

Discussion opened, Dr. J. J. Evans, Stroud.

"Pathology of Tuberculosis," Dr. J. M. Postelle, Oklahoma City.

Discussion opened, Dr. A. M. Marshall, Chandler.

"Duty of Community to Tubercular Patients," Dr. F. H. Norwood, Prague.

Discussion of topics open to public:

"Necessity of Organization Against White Plague," Mrs. Ed O. Johns, Chickasha.

Discussion opened, Prof. O. F. Hayes Chandler.

"Necessity of a State Sanitarium," Dr. C. W. Bradford. Shawnee.

MARSHALL COUNTY.

Program of the Marshall County Medical Society held at Madill July 6, 1909:

"Etiology and Treatment of Puerperal Eclampsia During Labor," Dr. S. P. Winston, McMillan.

"Why Physicians Should Attend Their County Medical Society," Dr. T. A. Blaylock, Madill.

"Gastro-Intestinal Toxemia, Etiology," Dr. J. Erwin Gaston, Kingston.

"Symptoms and Treatment of Renal and Vesical Calculi," Dr. E. F. Lewis, Kingston.

"The Uterine Curette, Its Indication and Contra-indication," Dr. F. A. White, Madill.

"Summer Diarrhoea in Children," Dr. J. Gumm, McMillan.

The above is said to have been the best attended meeting ever held by the Marshall County Society; the Secretary says—it is due to a very intimate letter sent each member urging him to be present. The letter strongly called the attention of the members of their Society, its importance to them from every standpoint; incidentally touching on the amount of work necessary to arrange a meeting and program. It is gratifying to know that the letter produced good results.

BLAINE COUNTY.

The Blaine County Medical Society met at Geary, Oklahoma, July 21st. Dr. Charles R. Hume, Councillor for the Third District, attending the meeting.

Dr. J. A. Hatchett, El Reno, read an interesting paper on the "Relation of the Surgeon to the Interne."

Dr. J. M. Campbell, Watonga, read a paper on the "Summer Diseases of Children."

These papers were fully and ably discussed by the members present.

President, Dr. J. W. Browning, Geary; Secretary, Dr. J. M. Campbell, Watonga, Oklahoma.

MEDICAL ASSOCIATION OF THE SOUTHWEST.

Dr. F. H. Clark, Secretary, El Reno, Oklahoma, sends out the following letter with reference to the meeting which we publish in full as we wish to assist in every way in making the meeting a success:

Dear Doctor:

The coming meeting of the Medical Association of the Southwest which is to be held at San Antonio, Tex., Nov. 9-11, 1909, should be a matter of the greatest interest to every member of the profession in the five states making up this Association for many reasons.

First—It is to be held in the largest state in the Union, and while it is not the oldest by any means it is one of the best organized so far as the profession are concerned of any one of the states.

Secondly—The meeting is to be held in one of the oldest historic cities of this country. It is a city of more than 100,000 inhabitants with beautiful buildings, points of historic interest, principal among which might be mentioned the Alomo.

Thirdly—The splendid meeting of last year at Kansas City, and the royal entertainment accorded all who attended are still fresh in the minds of those who were fortunate enough to be there and it is no idle boast that those who have the planning of this meeting in charge have set their stakes to surpass even the splendid meeting of last year.

Fourthly—We have a conditional promise that we are to have with us as our guest of honor at this meeting Dr. Welch, of Baltimore, the honored President of our parent Association, the A. M. A., and Dr. W. L. Rodman, of Philadelphia, who will deliver the oration on "Surgery."

Fiftly—The profession of San Antonio are expecting you and are making great plans for your comfort and entertainment and you ought not to disappoint them.

Sixthly—Because after the meeting is over an opportunity will be given you by means of an excursion, the itinerary of which is enclosed, to visit at a very nominal expense the beautiful country and city of Old Mexico. You can't afford to miss this.

Lastly—Don't be selfish and leave your wife at home, to look after the business, but lock up the office, take the wife with you and make up your mind you are both going to have the time of your life and will not be disappointed for the meeting will furnish a "feast of reason" as well as great social pleasures and the ladies will be royally entertained every minute of the time.

NEW MEMBERS.

J. W. Tucker, Purdy.
P. S. Johnson, Indianola.
G. C. Mullins, Kiowa.
W. E. Sanderson, Altus.

CHANGES OF ADDRESS.

Dr. T. W. Hartman, from Woodville to Ada, Oklahoma.

Dr. M. D. Belt, from Madill to Woodville, Oklahoma.

Dr. McLain Rogers, from Geary to Clinton, Oklahoma.

Dr. N. P. H. White, from Geary to Clinton, Oklahoma.

Dr. Allen Bell, from Maude to Geary, Oklahoma.

Dr. A. P. Grayson, from Shawnee to Huntsville, Ala., Route 3.

Dr. Jas. W. Scarborough, from Russell to Mangum, Oklahoma.

Dr. T. E. Evans, from Shawnee to Amarillo, Texas.

PERSONAL MENTION

Dr. G. H. Funk, of Madill, has located in Geary, Oklahoma.

Dr. Allen Bell, formerly of Maude, has located in Geary, Oklahoma.

Dr. H. L. Wright, of Hugo, is doing post-graduate work in Chicago.

Dr. D. F. Stough, formerly of Parsons, Kansas, has located in Geary, Oklahoma.

Dr. J. B. Murphy, Stillwater, spent the month of July in California.

Dr. Robert C. Robe, of Pueblo, Colorado, visited relatives in Muskogee in July.

Dr. J. L. Blakemore, of Muskogee, spent the month of July visiting in Emory, Virginia.

Dr. J. O. Callahan, Muskogee, will spend August and September in Manitou, Colorado.

Dr. W. H. Vann, of Claremore, has sold his practice and will locate elsewhere in Oklahoma.

Dr. J. C. Ambrister, of Chickasha, has been taking a vacation of several weeks duration.

Dr. E. E. Rice, of Shawnee, is spending several weeks with the Mayo Brothers in Rochester, Minn.

Dr. P. P. Nesbitt, of Muskogee, spent part of July in the White river region of Southern Missouri, fishing and hunting.

Dr. H. A. Wagoner, of Shawnee, who has been sick for several weeks, is convalescing at Eureka Springs, Ark.

Dr. Bruce Younger, of Whitesboro, Texas, is now associated in the practice of medicine with Dr. J. C. Mahr at Shawnee.

Dr. L. Haynes Buxton, Oklahoma City, is spending his vacation in the Rocky Mountains at Grand Lake, Colorado, where he will remain until September.

Dr. F. S. King, of Pryor, is spending his vacation at the Alaska-Yukon Exposition and in visiting points of interest in the Northwest.

Dr. Louis A. Turley, State Bacteriologist is spending the summer months at Harvard doing special work in his field. During his absence the laboratory is in charge of A. M. Alden.

Drs. McLean Rogers and N. P. H. White, of Geary, have sold their partnership practice to Dr. D. F. Stough, of Parsons, Kansas, and have removed to Clinton, Oklahoma.

EXCHANGES

THE PHYSICIAN AND PUBLIC HEALTH.

Walter Wyman, Washington (Journal A. M. A., June 12), discusses the duties of the physician engaged in private practice in his relations to public health and emphasizes the fact that no physician can separate himself from his fellows and their general interests. A most natural sequence of a doctor's practice is an interest in general sanitation and hygiene, and he illustrates his ideas by the modern movements against epidemic diseases which are now so prominently to the fore. He gives particulars to to what the government is doing by regulations for its own employes, for emigrants, seamen, etc., and dwells on the need for instruction of the tuberculous in hygienic rules to be observed by them for the welfare of their fellow citizens. The responsibility of the general practitioner in this matter is not a small one. Wyman goes at some length into the history and functions of the Public Health and Marine Hospital service, its importance to the country's welfare, its relations to local state governments, etc. In conclusion, in addressing those who are just starting into professional life, he urges them not to be delinquent in observing and attending to the general physical welfare of the communities in which their lot may be cast.

GALLSTONES AND HEART DISEASE.

R. H. Babcock, Chicago (Journal A. M. A., June 12), calls attention to the gastric and digestive tract symptoms of gallstone disease and their association with cardiac derangements, which often overshadow those pointing directly to the hepatic disorder. This last was the case in eleven of the thirteen cases he reports. The symptoms referable to the heart predominate, the gall bladder becomnig an object of suspicion either on account of digestive troubles or something in the history of the case. In each of the cases, however, careful palpation detected a swelling over the gall bladder which in most cases was shown by operation to be a Riedel's lobe. He divides the cases into four groups: 1. Five cases of pronounced cardiac incompetence showing considerable dilatation with arrhythmia and feebleness of heart's action with murmurs. 2. In two cases there had been attacks of pain, of anginoid character followed by evidences of cardiac muscular inadequacy, and one case in which there was dull infracardiac pain together with irregular pulse and a moderate degree of dyspnea on exertion, both dependent on recognizable, though not great, cardiac dilation. 3. In this group were three cases of intermittent pulse of long standing and very intractable, but without dyspnea or other marked subjective symptom of myocardial inadequacy. Patients in this group were greatly benefited by operation, more so than by any other line of treatment. 4. This group includes two cases of valvular disease in which cardiac competence was destroyed, either by evident attacks of hepatic colic, or by distressing symptoms attributed to the stomach, at first, but later referred to the gall bladder, because of the recognition of a Riedel's lobe. The cases are reported in detail, and the question arises how to explain the effects of gall-bladder disease on the heart and why all persons with chronic gall-bladder disease do not develop cardiac symptoms. Babcock admits his inability to answer the first of these questions, but suggests a pre-existing myocardial condition as accounting for the occurrence of the symptoms in some and not in other cases. Several theories may be advanced for the bad effects of gall-bladder disease on an already predisposed cardiac muscle; such as (1) the circulation in the blood of bacteria or their toxins; (2) the depressing influence of bile constituents on the heart muscles; (3) disturbances of the splanchnic circulation, and secondarily of the systemic circulation, of the heart; (4) reflex inhibition through the vagus. Each of these are taken up separately and their probability or possibility shown. Babcock closes with a discussion of the literature of the subject.

MEDICAL PSYCHOLOGY.

E. J. A. Rogers, Denver (Journal A. M. A., June 12), argues that physicians have neglected too much the study of the mind and its functions, and asks if really psychology is not as essential a study for a physician as anatomy and physiology. He refers to the addresses at the last meeting of the British Medical Association by Haldane and Francis Darwin, especially the discussion by the latter of qualities in plants which we usually classify as characteristic of intelligence. He says if vegetable cells manifest such qualities it is not difficult for us to surmise that individual cells of the animal body may possess, to a certain extent, similar characteristics, though always under the control of cells higher up in the functional scale. Thus step by step we go upward until an ultimate central and always active control is reached. There must be zone beyond zone of directing intelligence, each in its sphere guiding all above it, until the whole is brought into perfect unity. We must realize that while every cell in the body is, in a degree, an individual, still every cell is under the controlling influence of the higher cells until the highest physiologic center in the brain is reached. When we reach the high controlling centers we are very near to consciousness, though the ordinary acts of this control, as shown in physiologic processes, are habitually involuntary. Now we come to the all-important question, can acts habitually involuntary be in any way controlled by the conscious mind or will? The importance of such control of cell functions by the will is self-evident, if it exists. Professor William James, who, as we know, is a graduate in medicine as well as a psychologist, comes as near, Rogers says, to an affirmative answer to the above question as any one he has seen in a short article, in his presidential address to the American Philosophical Association in 1906. Rogers quotes from this several passages, showing that, in every one there are latent powers over the body through the mind when aroused by extraordinary stimuli, which enable one to do and suffer what might have been deemed impossible. All so-called faith healing, if we accept this view to its fullest extent, comes to be simply a volitional act, and he thus explains all the phenomena of suggestion, some forms of which we are using in every phase of everyday life. There is of course a wonderful difference in the facility with which this is done by different individuals, and we have not been able to give the process or any guide by which susceptibility may be determined, except by individual experience. Every-

thing being equal, however, the higher the scale of intelligence, the more easily can concentration and the action of the will be aroused. The power of self-control can, by direct suggestion, be developed more than is possible by any other means, and it is in this way that the mind exercises its influence on the body even to the controlling, it may be, of the primary tissue cells.

ECTROPION AND ENTROPION.

S. L. Ziegler, Philadelphia, (Journal A. M. A., July 17), recommends and describes a method which he has employed for many years with success in entropion and ectropion and some other conditions of the lids. It requires but two instruments which are figured, a short galvanocautery point and a lid clamp. He usually employs local anesthesia with 4 per cent cocain on the conjunctival surface, but in nervous sensitive patients it is necessary to employ nitrous oxid, bromid of ethyl, chloroform or ether. If ether is used it must be removed before the approach of the hot cautery point. The lid clamp is adjusted with its straight bar 6 mm. from the lid margin. The galvanocautery point is applied to the surface with considerable pressure. The button on the handle is pressed down to turn on the current, while the point is quickly pushed through the cartilage and as quickly withdrawn. The punctures are made 4 mm. from the lid margin and separated from each other by an equal interval of 4 mm. These should be made on the side on which we wish the contraction to take place, namely, the conjunctival surface in ectropia and the skin surface in entropion. If necessary we can repeat in a few weeks. From one to three sittings will accomplish as much as would a plastic operation. He has seldom seen any reaction follow, but if there is a little cellulitis and puffing of the lid, the use of continuous ice-pads for a day or two will control it. Two or three repetitions are generally required, at intervals of from two to four weeks, according to the case. The procedure is perfectly under control. In repeating the operation it is well to alternate the punctures locating the second series between the first. The eschar of the cautery causes no disturbance and usually clears off in about a week. Fourteen cases are briefly reported, showing the effects of the procedure in the class of cases for which it is adapted. The article is illustrated.

MISCELLANEOUS

THE DOCTOR'S TELEPHONE.

Read before the Ladies' Auxiliary of the Oklahoma State Medical Association by Mrs. Buchanan, May, 1909.

The telephones met in convention one day,
And each told his story of work or play;
They told of the service they were to man,
And from these tales a discussion began
As to which telephone in his office or store
Was of the most use to mankind the world o'er.

The grocery man's phone was the first one to speak,
And said without him man could not live a week;
That while one woman was on her way to the store,
He could deliver the orders for a dozen or more.
It was plain to him that no other phone
Could be of as much service in business or home.

The phone whose home was the dry goods store
Felt put out and a little sore
That the others so very important should feel.
'For he clothed man from his head to his heel.
And since Eve ate the apple from the tree of knowledge,

An education in dress is more important than college.

The tale the lovers told
Was one of romance, gay and bold.
Through him true lovers find a way
Of meeting each other day by day.
And though all the world should object to the match,
Love laughs at locks and breaks the latch.

The minister's telephone told a story
Of sorrow and happiness, shame and glory.
"Never a day but I must bring
To the minister a tale of sorrow and sin.
One of the fallen ones needs his care,
And he must go any and every where.

"At the marriage feast he participates,
He joins their lives and seals their fates.
From there he is called to the bed of a friend
Whose life is probably nearing its end.
And there he must comfort with prayer and song
That dying friend until the soul is gone."

Last but not least in this strange convention
Rose the doctor's phone, and demanded attention.
He said, "I'm afraid this silly discussion
Is likely to give my brain a concussion.
Men eat and dress and love and pray,
But these things happen every day.

"But when a man is really sick,
I'll tell you he needs a doctor quick.
'Tis then I prove to you, my brothers,
That I'm of more importance than you
    to others.
For I slip 'twixt life and death
And call the doctor while yet there's
    breath.

"I bring the man that carries the dope
That scatters sunshine and raises hope.
I call him out on cold winter nights
When the fires are out and also the lights,
And send him out on missions of love,
Where his pay he will probably get from
.   above.

"And when a new little life appears,
Through me they can banish their doubts
    and fears
As to what makes the poor little baby cry,
And what shall they feed it, and how, and
    why.
And when it cries all night wrapt warm in
    its blanket.
Is it really sick or shall they spank it?

"And thus, my friends, you can easily see
All important messages a r e carried
    through me.
Men suffer from Gastro-Anastomosis,
Ataxia, Bacteria, or Osteo-Necrosis,
But no matter what their trouble may be,
They find their family physician through
    me.

"They love him mightily when they are
    sick,
But when they are well they forget him
    quick;
And when the statement the doctor sends,
They swear that now all friendship ends.
'It is an insult to receive such bills
And they never again will take his pills.'

"But the doctor knows human nature well,
And he says to me. 'You never can tell,
Old friend. what a day or two will bring,

By tomorrow these very same people may
    ring,
One of them with an accident has met,
And they know my ability and they will
    not forget.' "

These phones are like the men they repre-
    sent
Each thinks his profession is heaven sent.
That without his services to the human
    race
This world would be a different place.
But though each himself is a very small
    man,
It requires the whole to complete God's
    plan.

MIND VERSUS MATTER.

Dr. Dudley, of Chicago, who attended
the Oklahoma City meeting, told the following story relative to this question:

A couple living in the neighborhood
constantly entertained their neighbors with
their family rows, quarrelling night and
day and constantly causing every one in
the vicinity to wonder what the next outbreak would be like. There was no peace
in that family, the God of War seemed to be
constantly on the job until they were finally
induced to join the Christian Science organization when a remarkable change occurred; their bickerings and black eyes
ceased, they were as lovely as two doves
in a cote, cooing to each other and lovey
doveying everything about them and declaring that there was no such thing as
fighting, etc., that it was all due to and
purely imagination.

About this time the family dog had the
misfortune to sustain a broken leg; the
small boy of the family had not yet reached
the ecstatic stage of his superiors, he had
no imaginary foolishness bothering him,
he could see that dog's broken leg and he
wanted it fixed right away for the dog was

the prize fighter of the block, evidently having absorbed some of the former frame of mind and idiosyncrasies of his master and mistress. The boy carried the dog to the ex-family physician, who was not feeling very good toward that family on account of their defection from his clientele.

"I am not a veterinary," said the doctor, "you take that dog to your Christian Science doctor, your parents have her to do the work when they 'imagine' they are sick, what do you come fooling around me with your dog for?" The boy pondered a moment only and then said: "Doctor, what are you trying to give me? I want you to fix that dog, do you think I want to take my good fighting dog to that Christian Science woman; that's a good dog, doctor. I don't want all the fight taken out of that dog."

PA AS A PATIENT.

Pa, he's become a patient, the doctor told
  us so;
He caught the influenza about a month
  ago.
He stays home from the office about three
  days a week
And seems to want to show us that he ain t
  mild and meek;
He scolds us and he grumbles and rips and
  tears around;
He grits his teeth and mumbles and jum.
  at every sound;
He tells us that he wishes he was drowned
  in the sea—
Pa's a blamed impatient patient, so at
  least he seems to me.

Ma begs him every morning to stay at
  home in bed,
Then he rages and he scolds her and our
  hearts get full of dread;
The doctor comes to see him every other
  day or two,

And he s takin' twenty-seven kinds of stuff
  to pull him through;
But he don't seem to be gettin' any better
  very quick,
And he keeps on sadly frettin' and he's
  made ma nearly sick,
To catch him here the doctor has to track
  him like a sleuth—
Pa's a blamed impatient patient, if you
  want to know the truth.

He thinks the world is goin' to the dickens
  right away,
And we almost think so with him when he
  stays at home a day;
Last night he kicked a panel nearly from
  the bathroom door
And got wild because the baby left his
  toothbrush on the floor;
He seems to think he's dyin' every time he
  has an ache,
And he wastes his money buyin' all the
  stuff he's told to take;
It seems to make him nervous if we even
  dare to wink;
Pa's a blamed impatient patient if you
  ask me what I think.

This morning when the doctor came before
  pa could escape,
He asked: "Well, how's our patient? Is
  he rounding into shape?"
Gee, you out 'a' hear pa roast him!
  "Why, you darned old quack," he said,
"With the treatment that you gave me it's
  a wonder I'm not dead!
You get out of here and stay out, I've got
  through with you for good!"
So the dcotor found his way out, and I
  guess he understood;
But ma couldn't keep from cryin' as she
  stood and watched him go—
Pa's a blamed impatient patient, but we
  dasn't tell him so.
          —Medical Brief.

OFFICERS OF THE OKLAHOMA STATE MEDICAL ASSOCIATION.

President, Dr. Walter C. Bradford, Shawnee.

First Vice President, Dr. C. L. Reeder, Tulsa.

Second Vice President, Dr. D. A. Myers, Lawton.

Third Vice President, Dr. J. W. Duke, Guthrie.

Secretary, Dr. Claude Thompson, Muskogee.

LIST OF COUNCILLORS WITH THEIR RESPECTIVE COUNTIES.

First District, Dr. J. A. Walker, Shawnee. Canadian, Cleveland, Grady, Lincoln, Oklahoma, Pottawatomie and Seminole.

Second District, Dr. John W. Duke, Guthrie. Grant, Kay, Osage, Noble, Pawnee, Kingfisher, Logan and Payne.

Third District, Dr. Charles R. Hume, Anadarko. Roger Mills, Custer, Dewey, Blaine, Beckham, Washita and Caddo.

Fourth District, Dr. A. B. Fair, Frederick. Greer, Kiowa, Jackson, Comanche, Tillman, Stephens and Jefferson.

Fifth District, _____. Cimarron, Texas, Beaver, Harper, Woodward, Alfalfa, Ellis, Woods, Major and Garfield.

Sixth District, Dr. F. R. Sutton, Bartlesville. Washington, Nowata, Ottawa, Rogers, Mayes, Delaware, Tulsa and Craig.

Seventh District, Dr. W. G. Blake, Tahlequah. Muskogee, Creek, Wagoner, Cherokee, Adair, Okmulgee, Okfuskee and McIntosh.

Eighth District, Dr. I. W. Robertson, Dustin. Sequoyah, LeFlore, Haskell, Hughes, Pittsburg and Latimer.

Ninth District, Dr. H. P. Wilson, Wynnewood. McClain, Garvin, Carter, Love, Murray, Pontotoc, Johnston and Marshall.

Tenth District, Dr. J. S. Fulton, Atoka. Coal, Atoka, Bryan, Pushmataha, Choctaw and McCurtain.

Delegates to American Medical Association, Dr. C. S. Bobo, Norman; Dr. L. A. Hahn, Guthrie.

Alternates, Dr. C. L. Reeder, Tulsa; Dr. J. A. Walker, Shawnee.

OKLAHOMA PUBLIC HEALTH.

BIRTHS.

During the month of June, 1909, there were 2,054 births reported in Oklahoma, with the following special information:

Couplets 57
Three per cent "still born" 68
Unnatural labor 124
Difficult labor (same as above) 124
Abnormal presentation:

Breech 15
Abnormal 2
Foot pres. 4
Faulty 2

Shoulder 4
Transverse 1
Mal Position 3
Placenta Praevia 7
Premature Labor 31
Deformed pelvis:

Deformed pelvis 2
Justo-Minor 2
Contracted 21
Small pelvis 3
Flattened 1
Mothers age 2
Uterine inertia 19
Accidents with cord 3
Cause not assigned 4

DEATHS.

Deaths from typhoid fever 23
Deaths from tuberculosis 52
Deaths under five years of age................338

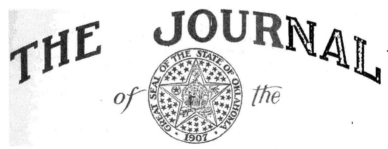

Oklahoma State Medical Association.

VOL. 2.   MUSKOGEE, OKLAHOMA, SEPTEMBER, 1909.   No. 4.

CLAUDE A. THOMPSON, Editor-in-Chief.

ASSOCIATE EDITORS AND COUNCILLORS.

DR. J. A. WALKER, Shawnee.   DR. JOHN W. DUKE, Guthrie.

DR. CHARLES R. HUME, Anadarko.   DR. A. B. FAIR, Frederick.

DR. F. R. SUTTON, Bartlesville.   DR. W. G. BLAKE, Tahlequah.

DR. G. W. ROBERTSON, Dustin.   DR. H. P. WILSON, Wynnewood.

DR. J. S. FULTON, Atoka.

Entered at the Postoffice at Muskogee, Oklahoma, as second class mail matter, June, 1909.

This is the Official Journal of the Oklahoma State Medical Association and every member of that organization is entitled to a copy and if, through accident or oversight, you fail to receive a copy notification of that fact to this office will receive prompt attention. All communications should be addressed to the Journal of the Oklahoma State Medical Association, English Block, Muskogee, Oklahoma.

TUBERCULOSIS IN INFANCY AND CHILDHOOD

DR. W. M. TAYLOR, OKLAHOMA CITY, OKLAHOMA

Read before the 1909 meeting of the Oklahoma State Medical Association, Oklahoma City, May 11, 12 and 13, 1909.

Tuberculosis is a very frequent disease of early childhood. The importance of this fact becomes more evident the more one studies the subject of pulmonary tuberculosis in children. Holt says, "the frequency of tuberculosis in infants and children has not been appreciated, because we have not been accustomed to looking for it with sufficient thoroughness."

More careful application of our means of diagnosis has made possible the recognition of tuberculosis in very many cases where otherwise it is likely to be overlooked. Therefore there is no better place to begin the study of tuberculosis, than in young children.

With the understanding we have today of this condition—it is believed there are five portals of entry to the tubercular-bacillus:

1st. By the placental circulation, heriditary tuberculosis.

2nd. By contact with eye. ear and skin.

3rd. By the respiratory tract.

4th. By the digestive tract.

5th. By the genito urnery tract, which is very rare.

The two courses which concern us most are the respiratory and digestive tracts; the former source constituting 90 per cent of all cases of this malady in children.

Schlossman says, "infantile tuberculosis deserves especial consideration—because it differs generally in pathology, clinical course and prognosis. It is characterized by a rapid generalization of the disease—it is not localized in one organ—it is nearly always of the acute miliary form—does not become circumscribed or calcified. The tissue of infants seems to form an excellent culture medium for the bacilli.

I shall report a case in a breast fed infant, of five months, in which the source of infection was doubtless respiratory. The baby was born here in Oklahoma City, healthy and well nourished at time of birth. When two months of age was taken by mother to visit family in Missouri, staying one month, and when mother returned baby was coughing, and she thought it had taken cold while traveling on the Pullman. Cough remained persistend of a dry harsh nature. Physical signs at this time showed only roughened breathing and some mucous rales. Cough continued and I was called two weeks later to explain high temperature that had developed—I first excluded middle ear disease and malaria. I found temperature ranging from 100 to 104 and at times baby was slightly cyanotic—slight intestinal disturbance but nursed well and remained in remarkably well nourished condition—spleen began to enlarge extending over the umbilicus—liver also enlarged but not so marked.

There was a constant rolling of head from side to side.

The probable diagnosis of tuberculosis was made from the above group of symptoms. During the third week the temperature became very high—ranging from 102 to 104—cyanosis marked at times. Blood examination for malarial plasmodia negative.

Drs. Jolly and A. D. Young saw case with me at this time and concurred in the probable diagnosis of tuberculosis—thought I had made repeated efforts to get a specimen of sputum for examination by swabbing throat after coughing spells I had failed. While Dr. Young and I were examining baby at this time she coughed and vomited immediately afterwards and from the vomitus I secured a specimen for the microsopical examination which I was sure had come from the lungs—this we found under the microssope to be loadad with tubercular-bacilli. Of course only till then was the diagnosis of tubercular infection positive. When told that recovery was impossible and that it was only a question of a week or so the family called in an osteopath, and he finished up the case—the baby died four days later.

From family history I found that while on a visit at home—a sister of the mother had taken care of the baby and at the time of baby's death had been sent to Colorado for a chronic bronchitis of probably tubercular origin. This was proven later by her death from pulmonary tuberculosis—and here we find the source of infection almost beyond question. This single case brings out several points worthy of consideration. This case was beyond one of acute miliary tuberculosis—involving the spleen, which we found much enlarged—involving the meninges as evidenced by the cerebral irritation present and involving the lungs which the physical and microscopical examinations showed. Another feature especially interesting to me, was the fact that the baby became more cyanotic in certain positions and it occurred to me that enlarged bronchial lymphnodes by pressure at this time was the cause of the increased cyanosis.

For miliary tuberculosis of infants there is no remedy; we can use only prophlyactic measures. Tuberculosis in childhood or in school children offers a contrast to the symptoms and course in infancy. A large percentage of the cases seen in school children—do not complain of illness until the disease has reached an advanced stage—

therefore thorough examinations of school children should be made at regular intervals, and our school teachers should be on the look out for any children who develop the persistent winter cough, not only for the protection of that particular child but for the welfare and protection of their schoolmates. Tuberculosis is the most dangerous disease for children between the age of 5 to 15 years.

The family physician has other duties than simply prescribing for these patients, and when he knows there is a predisposition or a family history which directs his suspicious to tubercular trouble, it is little less than criminal for him not to teach the parents or rest of family all the prophylactic measures at our command, such as attention to enlarged tonsils and adenoids, with their attendant catarrhal conditions; prohibit the pernicious habit of kissing babies—warn them against coming in contact with people having a chronic cough, not forgetting that tubercular infection very frequently follows measles and one should be careful in following up those cases of bronchitis which often date from an attack of measles.

Teach cleanly habits as washing hands before eating, for the finger nails are a favorite site for the deposit of dirt and bacteria.

The campaign against tuberculosis can be waged only if we prevent infection during childhood—for it is during this period in a great many cases that the infection takes place, although the disease may not become manifest until later in life. Someone has said that tuberculosis is simply the last act of a drama begun in childhood. I believe this would be more fully appreciated if we were more vigilant in our search whenever symptoms develop which should make one suspicious. And these symptoms are always evidenced in some way if we rightly interpret them and appreciate their significance.

We know that incipient tuberculosis is a curable disease in childhood—therefore the necessity for being ever on guard for the first symptoms, and once our suspicion is aroused keep an ever constant watch over the patient—never forgetting to insist on all prophylactic measures at our command. All we may hope to accomplish depends on an early diagnosis.

So much time and research has been given this subject I feel that it might be of interest to add here a brief report as offered by Dr. Woods Hutchinson, our American delegate to the International Congress, for study of Tuberculosis—but only where it has a special bearing from a pediatric standpoint.

Prof. Koch still maintained that—notwithstanding all that had been said to the contrary, there was practically no authentic case on record of the undisputed transmission of bovine tuberculosis to a human being, and that he felt justified in saying that it played but a small part in the reproduction of the disease—and Dr. Hutchinson further adds that if it were decided by the impression made the palm of battle remained with Koch.

Incidentally, another side of the question of the spread of disease was a very remarkable series of papers on the incidences in children of tubercular parents reported by Bowditch and Floyd, of Boston, and Miller, of New York. As soon as a case is reported at the dispensaries, a nurse follows the case into his or her home and gives the patients instructions, as to how to fight the disease first; second all the children in that household are brought to the clinic for examination. The result was appalling. From 25 per cent to 50 per cent of these were found to be tuberculosis.

Another feature was that many of the children showed no signs of impairment of the general health, but appeared to be in fair condition, until the examination and reaction test was made, emphasizing what we have long believed, that most of the so-called pretubercular symptoms are really early signs of the disease itself.

Finally we find from these reports that 80 per cent of tuberculosis can be traced to some previous human case, and the inference is clear that by stopping this we shall be able to stamp out from 80 per cent to 90 per cent of tuberculosis.

DISCUSSION.

Dr. Charles R. Hume, Anadarko:

The paper is of such vital interest to all of us that I would emphasize everything the doctor has brought out in his paper. It becomes every one of us to watch for the Great White Plague. The report of the State Board of Health shows that deaths from tuberculosis numbered more than all other causes. (Year 1908).

Children do not develop pulmonary tuberculosis so much as lypmhatic tuberculosis. The avenue by which the tubercular bacillus enters the system is often through the alimentary tract, this in spite of the theory so long held that human beings are not infected by bovine tuberculosis. I think we should educate the people concerning tuberculosis and show them it can be treated at home as well as away. I think that as physicians we should educate our patients to understand they can be treated at home as well as away, especially is this true in the cases requiring enforced feeding. A patient of mine told me that it was pitiable to see how many cases were in New Mexico seeking health and who had no way of living except at restaurants and who were forced to depend upon poorly cooked food and food that would not nourish.

Dr. Fair, Frederick, Oklahoma:

It seems to me very important that the disease should be diagnosed in its incipiency. One case, a boy three years old, the son of my partner, Dr. G., of Frederick. In some manner the disease found entrance.

we are inclined to think that its point of entrance was through the nose, for the boy had had ulcers of the nose. He had had indigestion and complained of pain in the stomach and bowels. We were not able to make a perfect diagnosis of the disease. The father took his boy to Chicago and there the trouble was diagnosed as Potts disease. There was nothing to show he had an abscess at that time. It is important to discover the incipiency of the disease. The case above referred to is now better and runs around much like the other children, but he has a knuckle on the spine.

Dr. Harper, Afton:

I had the pleasure and privilege of attending the Tuberculosis Congress in Washington last year. Dr. Koch was, of course, the center of attraction, if not the center of authority. Eminent men from several foreign countries were there. Koch is a forceful man. He announced several years ago that he had never seen a case derived from bovine tuberculosis. There was a secret session of the leading lights on this subject of tuberculosis and he was urged to recede from his position, but he did not do so.

There was an interesting and extensive display at this Congress of exhibits from animals used in research work. There were rabbits, guinea pigs, rats and mice.

I firmly believe that many children die from what is diagnosed as diarrhoea when really there is tuberculosis of the bowels, and the intestinal tract is unable to digest the food and there is ilio-colitis.

The cases of tuberculosis in children are much more acute than in adults. Of course there is little doubt but that most of our cases of human tuberculosis are derived from previous cases of human origin. Taking it for granted that 80 per cent of the cases of tuberculosis are from human origin then there are 20 per cent that could be prevented by taking care of the milk supply. Even from an apparently healthy cow we may get tubercular milk. We ought to use our means to have the state establish means to educate the people on this subject. The milk supply ought to be tested for tubercular bacilli.

Dr. Day:

There is one thing that should be mentioned in connection with tuberculosis of children. It is one often neglected at early stages. Until the medical profession took an interest in the origin and source of tuberculosis, little was known as to the origin of lupus vulgaris, a skin disease. And the individual with his face disfigured with scars lived out his life in that way. This has been found to be a localized tuberculosis. It is a tubercular condition which when properly recognized can be treated successfully. And the patient can be restored to a normal condition. Too much stress cannot be laid upon the subject merely from this fact. And whenever we find a skin trouble of a chronic nature with pus exuding at times we are not excusable unless we make care-

ful examination for tuberculosis bacillus. The use of the X Ray works like magic in these cases.

Dr. Tralle, Purcell:

I am not prepared to go into à scientific discussion of the case, but I have to say a few words from eleven years' practice which may be of interest.

The beginning of tuberculosis in children nearly always starts with the digestive organs. When you find a child cranky as to when it eats and what it eats—then is the time to start treatment. When you have a mother possessed of good common sense there is no trouble in beginning, but when you have a mother that insists upon giving the child everything it wants, then you may look for loss of child in a few years at latest. I believe that we as general practitioners should pay a little closer attention to peevish and fretful children, those that are cranky about their eating. Many children will not take milk but they can be taught to do so if they are under the right management.

THE TREATMENT OF PURULENT CONJUNCTIVITIS

BY DR. W. ALBERT COOK, TULSA, OKLAHOMA

Read at the Oklahoma City meeting of the Oklahoma State Medical Association, May, 1909.

The first step in the treatment of every case of purulent conjuctivitis should be the microscopical examination of the pus, so as to ascertain the variety of the microorganism present. Treatment need not, and should not, be delayed on this account, as in many instances every hour is of moment; but certainly no case can be intelligently treated without this information.

In cases that have the clinical appearance

of gonorrhoea strong germicides should be at once applied, while in cases of less severity, and presumably caused by less virulent pus germs, it would certainly be a mistake to make the same application. In fact, the selection of the germicide is a matter of no little tact. Many effective germicides cause a certain amount of traumatism to the conjunctiva, although in some recent preparations this is reduced to a minimum, and we must consider carefully whether the effect we wish to gain is worth this disadvantage.

The gonococcus is the most virulent germ we have to deal with in the eye, leaving aside the rarely occurring diphtheria bacillus, and the clinical picture is apt to be suggestive. Almost every one is familiar with the brawny, swollen lids, the chemosis, the profuse, thick discharge of creamy pus—all coming on with great rapidity after infection, whether occurring in the adult form, or in the modified form in the newly-born infant. The disease varies somewhat, but in the great majority of cases is considerably more severe than the worst cases caused by other infections. In fact, I have come to doubt the existence of the so-called "mild cases" of gonorrhoeal conjunctivitis.

It is reasoned by many that we should find mild infections in the eye as well as in the genital tract, but the clinical fact remains that in mild cases of conjunctivitis we do not find the gonococcus. Such cases are often called gonorrhoeal on insufficient evidence. Indeed, it is too often supposed that the eye condition is gonorrhoeal without any examination of the pus. In gonorrhoeal cases the treatment should be first of all directed to the destruction of the gonococcus, and our best means to this end is by the application of nitrate of silver. None of the new germicides seems capable of replacing silver entirely, and they are of use chiefly in cases in which silver is not well borne. It is imperative in adult cases that the application should be made at the earliest possible period after the infection. As soon as we see a case, a microscopical examination should be made and silver applied, as on this point often depends the success or failure of the case. If the gonococci once have a chance to penetrate the conjunctival tissue thoroughly, the eye will probably be lost, as it is impossible to reach them by germicides, and the process goes on until the cornea ulcerates. In babies, the results of delay are not apt to be so serious, as the cases are more manageable, but in every case the silver should be applied as early as possible.

When we see the case before the lids are much swollen—a period of a few hours in adult cases—it is sufficient to apply a two-per-cent solution. This should be done by a swab of cotton on applicator. The eye should be cleansed, and the applicator carried entirely through the cul-de-sac under the upper lid; then the lower cul-de-sac is to be swabbed out in the same way, so that the silver is applied to every part of the conjunctiva. This, of course, cannot be done with children. We have to be satisfied with a less thorough application, which, however, will usually be sufficient. A certain amount of reaction invariably follows, but this can easily be controlled by iced cloths, and the irritation is of small importance compared with the seriousness of allowing the gonococci to penetrate the conjunctival tissue, which they always do with great rapidity. No other germicide is so much to be depended upon in this connection as silver. If the gonococci have penetrated, the swelling will have begun and the discharge will be profuse, and stronger solutions of silver may be necessary. When the disease is well developed, as it is apt to be by the third or fourth day after infection, the two-per-cent solution gives the best results; but before that time stronger solutions may abort the process.

It is impossible to lay down any rule as to the limits of the time when the abortive plan of treatment may be used, but my own practice is always to attempt it whenever there is any prospect of success. If I see a case two days after infection, and the swelling or discharge seems not to be at the greatest height, I apply a three-per-cent or a four-per-cent solution of nitrate of silver as thoroughly as possible, and then meet the further indications as they arise, using two-per-cent as a daily application. It is best in using a stronger solution than two-per-cent to neutralize with salt-solution on account of the danger of staining the cornea, or even to lay a pledget of cotton soaked in salt-solution upon the cornea while making the application.

Where silver irritates, as shown by the increased discharge of serum, and a tendency of the conjunctiva to bleed readily when handled, a six-per-cent solution of protargol may be used. It has been claimed for this germicide that it is without irritating properties, but this is certainly not so. It is, however, very much less irritating than silver, and many persons do not feel the application of a six-per-cent solution at all. Stronger solutions are of no particular advantage—the irritation is more marked and the germicidal properties seem to be not appreciably greater. Protargol is a valuable drug in Ophthalmia neonatorum—in cases in which the conjunctival thickening is not great enough to support applications of nitrate of silver. It may be dropped into the eyes twice daily.

In other forms of purulent discharge, that is, those caused by the pneumococcus, or other pus organisms, silver is not to be used, but protargol in six-per-cent solution. applied once a day, is a most efficient germicide, and will often limit an attack of "pink eye" to a few days, which otherwise would last two or three weeks. Protargol has the further advantage of not staining the tissues as readily as silver nitrate; and it is good practice to flood the corneal ulcer occurring in the course of a gonorrhoeal conjunctivitis, with a six-per-cent solution once a day. It has been claimed that protargol will not stain the conjunctiva, but cases have been reported in which its prolonged use has led to a slight stain. The claim at first made for it that it will penetrate the tissues and destroy germs more deeply than silver, seems not to be borne out by clinical experience. In severe cases of gonorrhoeal conjunctivitis with

papillary hypertrophy the astringent action of the silver is to be desired, and the discharge subsides less readily under protargol than under silver. Argyrol, 25 per cent, or silver vitelline, fulfils all the above indications for protargol, and is absolutely non-irritating. It also is less effective than silver when an astringent is required; but when a non-irritating germicide is required, it is certainly ideal. I have seen it injected into the anterior chamber of an infected eye with remarkable checking of the process, and without any irritation of the iris whatever.

The other indications for treatment in purulent conjunctivitis are best met on the old-fashioned lines. Constant cleansing with saturated boracic-acid solution resists the development of corneal ulcers and keeps down a number of germs. Boracic acid is merely a non-irritating wash, and has no germicidal value. If we use plain water on the conjunctiva, or any other mucous membrane, there is a tendency to exosmosis set up at once in the blood vessels, which dilate —a phenomenon frequently observed when the eyes become red after being filled with tears in weeping. The least irritating solution, therefore, is one which has nearly the same specific gravity as the blood. The cleansing should be done often enough to keep the eye clean, even if that is every ten minutes day and night.

For the swelling of the lids, iced cloths, applied constantly, are best, and these have another very important action, as has already been pointed out, in reducing the temperature of the conjunctival cul-de-sac below the point at which pus organism grow best. It is possible to reduce the temperature several degrees, while heat can not be applied constantly, and most pus germs bear slight degrees of increased temperature better than diminished temperature.

Corneal complications are to be met on

the usual lines, the only advance in recent times being the use of protargol or argyrol, either of which will destroy the germs in corneal ulcers as well as in the conjunctiva, and that without irritation and danger of staining which makes the use of silver in this connection impossible. In a certain small proportion of cases, when the chemosis is severe and the discharge not free scarification of the chemosis is of value, notwithstanding the fact that it has fallen into disrepute of late years, the reasons for this latter fact being that its advocates at first claimed a much wider field for its application than was justifiable as is so commonly the case with methods and remedies in this disease. Scarification will not reduce every case of chemosis, by any means; but in certain cases when the discharge is scanty and the chemosis is of a boardy character, scarification will relax the chemosis in a way that no other means will accomplish.

Cauterization of the cornea, in cases in which the chemosis is not severe, is a most valuable means of combating corneal ulceration, and is particularly useful in ophthalmia neonatorum. Pure carbolic acid is the best cauterizing agent to use. It need hardly be said that we should be reasonably certain that the tissues will react well to the cautery, which will not be the case if the chemosis is very severe, or if the patient's general condition is much reduced. When corneal infection appears, hot water applications are to be used for the purpose of stimulating the corneal tissues.

ECTOPIC GESTATION

DR. FRED H. CLARK, SURGEON EL RENO SANITARIUM, EL RENO, OKLA

Ectopic Gestation or "Extra Uterine Pregnancy" may be defined as that condition brought about by the Spermatozoae of the male and the ovum of the female coming in contact and fertilization taking place while the ovum is in transit somewhere between the fimbriated extremity of the fallopian tube and the opening of the tube into the cornu of the uterus.

This may occur: first, in the tube itself; second, in either ovary; third, as stated by some authorities between the folds of the broad ligament or "intra ligamentous;" fourth and lastly, in the free abdominal cavity.

The form most frequently seen is that occurring in the tube itself the mass forming usually in the central portion of the tube. While authors of good standing present authenticated case reports of these other forms many equally good men consider that these forms are the outcome of a pregnancy first started in the tube and then either because of a rupture of the tube during which the foetus has escaped through the rent, while the placenta was not detached from the lining of the tube thus furnishing support to the foetus which has continued to grow while within the free abdominal cavity until it came to full term, or because of the unusual size of the fimbriated extremity of the tube the fertilized ovum has slipped through without detaching the placenta and it by this means has been enabled to go on to full term.

It is not quite so easy to account for the gestation which takes place in the ovary, and yet while the reality of this condition taking place is questioned I will report briefly at the close of this paper a case of this character.

I have not been fortunate enough to have seen a case known as the "intra ligamentous" and so will refrain from a discussion of this form.

A glance at the history of Ectopic Gestation would lead one to believe that like appendicitis it must have gone undiscovered for a considerable period of time as Parry in 1876 was only able to find 500 cases reported: but in 1892 the increase was very apparent as Schrenk collected reports of 610 cases occuring in the five years just previous to that time. This increase was, however, without question more apparent than real and was undoubtedly due to a better ability to make a correct diagnosis, for as late as 1883 this condition was said to be of interest chiefly from its pathological standpoint and few, if any, cases were recognized clinically.

DIAGNOSIS.

Probably no single pathological condition is so frequently overlooked in proportion to the number of times it occurs as Ectopic Gestation. This is not hard to understand if we stop to think that in a large number of cases the early days of the Gestation do not differ materially from those of a normal case, and secondly the ordinary general practitioner does not have many cases of this kind even in a number of years practice and consequently is not so keen to notice the peculiarities in the case as he does for instance in a suspected case of appendicitis or of some form of obstruction of the bowels.

Let me say in all seriousness that no more grave condition confronts a patient than an undiscovered extra-uterine pregnancy, especially after rupture has occurred.

I am reminded just now of a case seen in the early years of my practice, which occurred in the clientile of a prominent and splendid practitioner of the city in which I resided and which was unrecognized until some little time after rupture had taken place, when she was hurried to the hospital, prepared for operation as quickly as possible and the abdomen opened; it was found filled with clotted blood which was literally scooped out by the hands full, the ruptured tube was hurriedly ligated and the abdomen closed, but the patient died a little later from shock though everything possible was done to overcome it.

Without doubt instances of this kind could be multiplied for I presume no one present who has been in practice any great length of time but who has had one or more such cases.

How then shall a case of Ectopic Gestation be recognized and diagnosed before rupture, and what are some of the conditions for which it might be taken? Perhaps the most common symptom which brings the patient to the physician is a continuous menstrual flow; not of a severe or flooding type but simply a steady flow sufficient to cause more or less annoyance.

A careful history should always be secured and it will usually reveal the fact that the woman has been having her usual normal monthly menstrual periods until possibly the second month preceeding her visit to the physician when she did not "come around" as usual and since that time has been annoyed by an almost constant dribbling which has caused her to wear a napkin all the time.

This is practically all the history one will be able to get in the ordinary unruptured case if seen early.

If it is, say one month later or in the neighborhood of the tenth week, we will have a patient complaining of more or less pain which may be on either side or in the back. Practically all writers agree that few cases of Ectopic Gestation go beyond the twelfth week unruptured so we may expect if our case is approaching the middle or latter part of her third month to have a considerable pain.

With this history before us what may we expect to find on examination per vagina, and what other conditions might be present which would require a differential diagnosis. First, we must exclude a normal pregnancy; if we have a normal pregnancy which has reached this stage we should find, first, a uterus somewhat enlarged and inclined to the right: the cervix may be slightly enlarged and soft and as we have a continuous flow we will not find the os closed; these with the blue color of the vaginal wall, might be stated as the more common symptoms to be found on examination of the pregnant woman. Failure to find these symptoms present should lead us to a further examination and in which we will presume we found an abnormal mass in the left side of the pelvis. We are now called upon to differentiate between the conditions which might cause this mass. We note first the character of the mass; is it round, oval or oblong or sausage shaped? Is it firm and tense or soft and yielding and boggy to the touch? If it is the former shape and consistency we would be justified in assuming that it was of cystic origin probably of the ovary. If it was oblong or sausage shaped we would undoubtedly be dealing with either a hydro- or a pyo salpinx. If we find the mass nearly round, and of the soft boggy feeling with the history already given we may safely conclude we are dealing with an Ectopic Gestation.

An excellent gynecoligist said in my hearing once that a man might consider himself a good diagnostician if he diagnosed this condition before rupture while any one could make the diagnosis after rupture had occurred.

One other condition might be mentioned which I have had the misfortune to come in contact with, and not correctly diagnose, is a retroverted uterus fixed in its position. I will cite very briefly a case to illustrate this.

In the latter part of December, 1908, I was called to see a lady suffering with severe pain in the lower right side. It was one of the families at Fort Reno where I was contract surgeon and as the case was not a severe one I left her in the care of a member of the Hospital Corps with instructions to report daily and I would call when necessary.

Twenty-four hours later I was informed that she was threatened with an abortion as I had already learned that she was pregnant and in her third month. Some two years before I had examined her at the request of one of the physicians of our city and had found a retroverted uterus and a mass in the left side of the pelvis. She was making the usual convalesence from the appendicitis when she began to complain of a severe backache which I ascribed to the retroverted uterus. She was waiting for the acute symptoms of the appendicitis to subside when I was to operate upon her and while calling upon her during this time, I examined her and finding what I took to be the retroverted uterus pressing down into the Cul-de-sac and the old mass in the left side I attempted to return the fundus to its proper place. This I thought I did and the patient said she had not been as free from pain in weeks as she was after doing this.

You can imagine my surprise then when on opening the abdomen forty-eight hours later as I incised the peritoneum to have come welling up large quantities of dark colored blood and to find a ruptured Ectopic Gestation on the left side, originating in the left ovary which is the case mentioned earlier in this essay.

This shows how easily one can make a mistake in the diagnosis of pelvic conditions.

Thus far we have been dealing with a class of cases which have no alarming symptoms; but of the cases in which rupture has taken place this is not true.

Many of these cases are in extremis when reached by the family physician who is called to the case first in nearly every instance. Many of the patients will state that they had started the menstrual flow when they were suddenly seized with a severe pain in the lower bowels; thinking they had caught cold they tried simple home remedies for relief but to no avail, then they called the physician.

On his arrival he finds often times a patient whose very face tells the story. Exsanguinated from internal hemorrhage, pulse feeble and rapid, covered with a cold clammy perspiration and often times in a condition of profound shock due to the excessive hemorrhage. A hurried examination and history brings to light the fact that the patient has missed two monthly periods and is in her third month. She has been wasting for some little time oftentimes sufficient to cause her to wear a napkin; she has felt some unusual fullness in one side of the pelvis; but having many of the ordinary symptoms of pregnancy and supposing herself to be in that condition she has only been afraid she was threatened with abortion and had simply been attempting to avoid that when she was suddenly seized with an almost unbearable pain in the pelvis after which she soon grew sick and faint and had been steadily getting worse until her present condition was reached.

These are the typical symptoms of a ruptured Ectopic Gestation and which I confess cause me great alarm when they confront me.

TREATMENT.

Here is where there is great diversity of opinion. My own experience has been so limited in comparison with that of many who have written upon this subject that I prefer to draw from their experiences and quote them rather than my own.

First. The treatment of an unruptured Ectopic is purely surgical and there should be no delay for but few will be fortunate

enough to see this condition and if they are they certainly should profit by it.

I shall not take time to more than mention the other forms of treatment suggested and formerly practiced, namely the use of electricity and injections of poisons for the destruction of the foetus for they are practically things of the past and are only mentioned by the better men of today to be condemned.

Regarding the diagnosis of these cases Dr. Herman J. Boldt, of New York, said recently, after having seen upwards of 300 cases that extra-uterine pregnancy is but rarely recognized before rupture and then by accident.

Dr. McCalla also said in a recent article, "The importance of immediate operation in all cases after the diagnosis is made and prior to the rupture can not be over estimated." Whatever the condition it is a surgical one. The origin of this operation is credited to Dr. Tait in 1883.

Quoting Dr. P. A. Harris, who cites more than 130 cases of his own, he says; "That 90 per cent of these should have been correctly diagnosed though they were not, and that the common error is made of calling them miscarriages."

I will cite but one other writer, Dr. Grandin, of New York, in a recent article after going over the different methods of treatment sums it all up when he says "From my own personal experience I maintain that prompt surgery should convert this malignant disease into one carrying the certitude of recovery, other things of course being equal. I shall also maintain that the ideal surgery is to operate before rupture. To go further I shall maintain that operation should be resorted to upon presemptive evidence, it being my preference to be proved wrong in diagnosis rather than to sit on the fence awaiting the diagnosis made at the time or rupture."

The cases, however, which will tax the

skill of all in whose hands they may fall, and often times cause him to wish he had done the other thing, are those severe cases following rupture when the patient is already in a state of collapse and shock.

There is a wide difference of opinion on the plan to be followed here among all operators, one side maintaining less mortality when a reasonable time is allowed to lapse before operation and citing a large number of cases to prove their point, claiming that the natural pressure formed by the clot checks the hemorrhage. On the opposite are an equally large number of good men who quote as many cases also and who insist upon immediate operation.

Which of these shall we take? My own belief is that early operation presents the most hopeful outlook for I can not make myself believe that one can be at all safe with as much surface bleeding as there is with a .rupture of the tube and absolutely out of reach except by the surgeon.

Of course the question of what route should be taken for operation must of necessity be left to the individual preference of each operator, my own preference being for the abdominal route.

I shall present briefly one further case report which shows another condition which might readily be mistaken for Ectopic but which is not. Miss C., age about 22— this was a patient belonging to my associate, Dr. Hatchett, but which I was first called to wait upon during his absence from the city. I was called one Saturday afternoon to see her and to relieve her from a severe pain in the pelvis supposed to be caused by her menstrual period though she had not gone the ordinary length of time since her last period. I found her in bed but not apparently in very great pain and only flowing moderately and leaving an anodyne to relieve her and requesting her to report her condition the next day I left her. She did not report, however, but I learned incident-

ally that she was up and had attended church, so did not think anything further about the matter. On the Friday morning preceding my first visit I afterward learned she was on her way to school, as she was a teacher, and there was a very strong wind blowing at the time and she was carrying a rather large umbrella to protect herself from the rain, and it was about all she could possibly do to walk against the wind and when she reached the school room she was suffering some pain in the pelvic region which she supposed was due to the strain of walking and holding the umbrella. She began to flow very freely about this same time, so much so that the other lady teachers tried to persuade her to go home for the rest of the day but she did not do so, but remained until the close of the day. The next day I saw her; a little more than a year before we had operated upon her for a case of suppurating appendicitis draining a large abscess from which she seemed to have fully recovered but on taking her history at this time we found that prior to this attack she had a considerable trouble in the right side of the pelvis supposed to be some sort of an inflammation; she ran along for several days after I first saw her without reporting to me and about this time Dr. Hatchett returned home and she began to get worse and he was called to see her when upon examination he found a large mass in the right pelvis which he diagnosed as a pelvic abscess and had her removed to the hospital and made a vaginal incision and drained and was very much surprised to secure nothing but blood from the mass and no pus; I was absent from the city that day but returned home during the night and early the next morning we examined her made a blood count and found the count of reds exceedingly low and at once opened the abdomen and tied off the right tube which we found ruptured near the fimbriated extremity and tried our best to save the life of our patient but we could not and she died as the result of the shock caused by the hemorrhage although we did everything we could possibly do to save her. She was a single woman of good character and nothing present to suggest. anything except the rupture of a tube which had probably been included in a mass of adhesions and which could not withstand, the strain caused by the struggle against the wind that morning going to school, after which she began to flow. Under the conditions this would probably not be correctly diagnosed by any one before the time of the vaginal incision.

SYPHILIS OF THE CENTRAL NERVOUS SYSTEM

ANTONIO D. YOUNG, M. D., PROFESSOR OF NERVOUS AND MENTAL DISEASE, EPWORTH COLLEGE OF MEDICINE
NEUROLOGIST TO ST. ANTHONY HOSPITAL, OKLAHOMA CITY, OKLAHOMA

Syphilis produces pathological changes in the central nervous system in two ways: first, by the direct action of the etiological micro-organism or its toxines upon the histological structures of the brain and cord; second, by so affecting the nervous elements that degenerative changes will eventually ensue. Loco-motor ataxia and paresis are the only known examples of the latter variety and will not here be considered.

The neurone theory, which seems to fit most of the known facts of neurology, assumes that the true nervous element is the neurone which is composed of the cell body and processes called dendrites and neuraxones. In the central nervous system these neurones are arranged in groups and cables and are known as tracts and columns. Each neurone has no relation with its lateral neighbor and joins the next neurone in line not by continuity but by contiguity. The cell body is the center for nutrition. The dendrites transmit incoming impressions and the neuraxone, the centrifugal ones.

Neurones are: motor, sensory, trophic, etc., and the only histological difference among them is in their terminations called end-organs. Most of the neurones are medulated and are surrounded by a membrane, the neurilema. Degeneration is the only pathological change to which the neurone itself is subject. When a nerve process is separated from the cell body, its nutrition is cut off and it degenerates. This degeneration is a peculiar process and occurs somewhat as follows: the myelin sheath, first breaks into fragments each containing a small portion of axis cylinder. This is eventually absorbed leaving a cavity surrounded by the neurilema which if the process goes on to complete destruction is replaced by connective tissue (sclreosis). There is a similar result if the cell body dies from any cause.

Frequently the degenerative process is arrested and the neurone regenerates. This rejuvenating process is induced by small bodies called the nuclei of the neurilema. The medullary sheath and the axis-cylinder are reproduced and its function restored.

In addition to the neurones the brain and cord are composed of: meninges, blood vessels, connective tissue, lymphatics and neuroglia.

Whatever the ultimate pathological result in nervous syphilis the initial lesion is in the blood vessel and is a specific arteritis. There is a thickening of the vessel wall and a round cell proliferation may occur in its immediate vicinity. The changes in the artery may induce a thrombus causing occlusion and softening of the parts supplied by the vessel or a rupture may occur with consequent hemorrhage. The exudate about the vessels sometimes spreads over the neighboring parts in a membrane like fashion. This is what usually occurs in syphilitic meningitis and frequently is limited to the base of the brain. At other times the exudate is formed into more or less spherical nodules called gummata. A guma consists of a mass of granulation tissue with areas of caseation.

Syphilitic pathological process may be confined to one branch of a blood vessel and in this way only one of the cranial nerves may be involved. At other times a group of blood vessels may be affected producing a localized meningitis or a localized softening as the case may be. Again one hemisphere alone may be the seat of syphilitic changes or the gummata may be irregularly distributed throughout the brain and cord. While the changes that occur are constant it can readily be seen how the symptomatology may vary according to the seat of the lesion.

The exudation and proliferation may be so slight that no remnant of it remains and the resulting change is a degeneration seemingly without a previous inflammation. However this is only apparently true as the degeneration must have been preceded by inflammatory process.

After a gumma develops it becomes a source of irritation leading to obliteration or rupture of the blood vessel producing a hemorrhage or softening respectively. Gummata developed primarily in the brain are rare but by spreading from the meninges may infiltrate the cerebral tissue to a greater or less extent producing a meningo-encephalitis. A round cell proliferation may occur in the epineurium independent of any change in the blood vessels with a resulting interstitial neuritis.

In this condition processes are projected among the bundles of nerve fibers destroying them by pressure atrophy. The chiasma, optic nerve and motor-occuli are usually affected by this type of nervous syphilis.

Brain syphilis or spinal syphilis existing alone is a rarity, but is theoretically possible. Usually both are simultaneously affected. It is very doubtful if there exist a "functional" syphilitic disease of the nervous system. They are called "functional" because of the inability of our present methods to discover the histological changes.

A hereditary nervous weakness is the prime factor in causing syphilis to attack the nervous system: but the immediate production of the outbreak is brought about by excesses of any kind. It is believed that those cases exhibiting mild, secondary symptoms are more likely to be followed by an invasion of the cerebro-spinal axis. Men are more frequently victims of syphilitic nervous disorder, than are women on account of the greater preponderance in their lives of the exciting causes.

Sometimes during the course of cerebro-spinal syphilis the symptoms are so markedly intra-cranial, intra-spinal, or neural that for the sake of convenience we speak of brain syphilis, spinal syphilis, and nerve syphilis. However it should not for a moment be forgotten that the disease is an invasion of the entire nervous system as the subsequent history will reveal if the case is sufficiently prolonged.

One of the peculiar features of the disease is the changeableness of its clinical manifestations. Symptoms appear and disappear; appear in one locality today and in another tomorrow; become better and worse at frequent intervals. Symptoms of brain and cord syphilis are in no way distinctive. They are essentially the same as those of tumor, or meningitis or occlusion of blood vessels from other cause.

Headache is very common and its special

characteristic is, the exacerbations usually are accompanied by vertigo and occur each night. It seldom disappears entirely but is much less severe during the day. Sooner or later after the appearance of the headache the patient becomes mentally dull and apathetic: is given to periods of somnolence, loses his appetite and his weight is decreased. He may have attacks of "cerebral" vomiting at which time his vertigo is increased. After these clinical signs have become established nerve palsies develop. The disease process may involve any of the cranial nerves but more often the third nerve is attacked producing ptosis and strabismus. Next in frequency comes the seventh (facial) and then the optic with resulting hemianopsia or blindness. The olfactory and the fifth nerve may share in the trouble producing disturbance of their functions.

In untreated cases next comes attacks of hemiplegia which in no external way differs from the hemiplegia of other origin. A hemiplegia in a person under forty, when not due to cardiac embolism, is almost conclusive evidence of cerebral syphilis. Prior to the hemiplegia, general or local epileptiform convulsions may occur perhaps followed by coma. This condition in a person under thirty when not due to uremia or alcoholism is always caused by syphilis.

If the disease is acute and of rapid development these symptoms may be absent and be replaced by a deep coma coming on early and followed by death.

As will be seen the symptoms in brain syphilis are caused by a meningitis or a meningo-encephalitis usually of the base but also of the Rolandic area and elsewhere.

The symptoms of spinal syphilis are those of transverse myelitis but the initial changes occur in the meninges, blood vessels and nerve roots and are the same as those occuring within the cranium. There may be a specific meningitis of any of the layers,

with or without gummata, endartertis and thrombosis with consequent softening.

The usual type clinically is a progressive paraplegia known as syphilitic spinal paralysis and comes on gradually with spasticity and considerable pain. In cases with numerous spots of softening the clinical signs are those of disseminated sclerosis. A striking feature of spinal syphilis is a changeableness of its symptoms. When the disease begins as a meningitis and extends to the substance of the cord, the outward manifestations are continually changing as the disease progresses. With the formation of gummata comes the signs of tumor of the cord.

When the disease is meningial, the earliest symptoms are pain, paraestheia, spasm and paresis, caused by irritation of the roots of the spinal nerves. Of course the patient refers the pain to the peripheral terminations of the affected nerves. The tendon reflexes are exaggerated. The girdle sensation is present when the dorsal or lumbar region is affected.

The motor symptoms are: rigidity of neck and limbs, tremor and exaggerations of reflexes terminating in complete paralysis. In the end the sphincters are involved.

The diagnosis of spinal syphilis is best made by exclusion. A history of syphilitic infection is of great aid but many cases subsequently found to be luetic, earnestly and perhaps honestly, deny knowledge of having contracted the disease. The prognosis depends so much on a proper diagnosis that a physician should use every available means to discover the nature of the infection. The unequal distribution, the instability, the disappearance and reappearance of the symptoms, their prompt amelioration when under treatment, finally their disseminated character are sufficiently typical in the majority of cases to make a diagnosis. (Alfred Gordon). Many cases of spinal syphilis may be practically cured while the degenerations, though in a large measure the counterpart symptomatically are beyond therapeutic aid. It is equally important to make the diagnosis early. After the disease has passed the inflammatory stage and degeneration of the true nervous structure has occurred the damage is irreparable. Nothing can restore life to a dead tissue; but by prompt and vigorous treatment the disease may be stopped short of this destructive change. Close investigation usually shows an involvment of both the cerebrum and spinal cord although the predominant symptoms are referable to one or the other.

Aside from the root neuritis of the spinal nerves in specific meningitis the peripheral nerves usually escape syphilitic invasion. There is some evidence however to support the view of a special form of neuritis due to syphilis but most observers doubt its existence. Isolated syphilitic exudates may occur along the course of nerves producing the usual signs of irritation and compression. This seldom occurs.

Inherited syphilis produces the same changes seen in the acquired form, the pathological findings are identical and the diagnosis is made from the same signs.

Persons infected by syphilis should be warned to live a regular life free from excesses of all kinds, especially alcoholic. When stimulants are used to assist a worn out body to carry an excessive load, the danger of invasion of the nervous system is undoubtedly increased.

Mercury and potassium iodide are the sheet anchors of treatment. Persons who are properly treated from the beginning long before the nervous system is affected stand a much better chance of escape.

If the poison is already at work on the brain and cord the treatment must be promptly and vigorously pushed. Mercury, the main reliance, should be given hypodermically, in the form of the cyanide, 1-10 grain every second day, gradually increased to 1-5 grain.

The iodide should be started in a week and pushed to the point of intoleration. One of my patients according to his own statement, increased his dose to nine hundred grains daily but only for two days when I advised him to begin decreasing it. In addition to the regulation of the patient's habits and the administration of these drugs other hygenic measures tending to maintain the resistance at the maximum. will suggest themselves from time to time. Mercury and the iodide should be repeated at intervals of six months throughout the life of the patient.

During the preparation of this article it has been my pleasure and profit to consult the following references: Organic and Functional Nervous Diseases, by M. Allen Starr; Text Book of Nervous Diseases and Psychiatry, by Charles L. Dana; A Treatise on Diseases of the Nervous System, by L. Harrison Mettler; Nervous and Mental Diseases, by Archibald Church and Frederick Peterson; Diseases of the Nervous System, by Alfred Gordon, and numerous articles appearing in current medical literature.
634 Security Bldg.

LOCAL ANESTHESIA

BY JOHN A. WYETH, M. D., L. L. D., SENIOR PROFESSOR OF SURGERY IN THE NEW YORK POLYCLINIC MEDICAL SCHOOL AND HOSPITAL

Of the many great advances in modern surgery it may be said that none in general usefulness surpasses local anesthesia.

The very natural dread of the surrender of consciousness and the number of distressing after-effects of a general anesthetic, deters many a human being from seeking early relief from physical distress, causing them to be robbed of health and life by that "thief of time," procrastination.

Probably one-half of all surgical lesions which become formidable enough to demand a major operation under full narcosis are susceptible of cure by a minor procedure under local anesthesia if taken in their incipiency. One of the great duties of the profession is to educate the people in this direction.

Realizing the importance of this fact, it has been one of the chief objects of surgical research and practice 'at the Polyclinic for nearly a quarter of a century, during which period operation under local anesthesia has made such tremendous strides that not only has the field of minor surgery been gleaned but the domain of the major procedures well invaded.

In my clinic within the last few months. Dr. Charles R. Hancock, my assistant, has done five appendectomies (one child of seven and four adults) with cocaine infiltration alone—one-fourth on one-per-cent solution. The demonstration of the practical insensibility of the intestines was complete, the adult patients asserting this during the manipulation of the caecum and appendix outside the peritoneal cavity.

The number of herniotomies by Professors Bodine, Lyle and Robertson and others of the staff in this institution has nearly reached the two thousand mark while the list of more formidable and serious procedures without general narcosis is rapidly lengthening.

In the satisfactory employment of this form of anesthesia not only is a thorough acquaintance with the technic essential, but there must be added the subtle influence

of suggestion and insistence upon the fact that no pain will be felt. This is where the personal factor counts.

The operator by his manner and method must impress the patient with the confidence of success, and that he is at home and perfect master of the situation. He must also omit no effort to distract the mind and attention of the patient from the field of operation. For this reason conversation is constant and general and no instrument desired is called for. The assistant should know what is needed and should hand it unobserved to the surgeon. Even the scissors must move so smoothly that the blades do not "clip" or make a "cutting noise." Traction, if employed, should be light and care taken not to invade the sensitive area beyond the anesthetic zone.

The method of infiltration is now so well known that it need not be here repeated. Chiefly the weaker cocain solutions have been employed, viz: one grain of cocaine hydrochlorate to two, three or four ounces of distilled water.

The stronger solutions are employed only in extremely sensitive areas and in the minutest possible quantities.

Lately Professor L. L. McArthur has recommended novocain as less toxic and somewhat superior to cocain in local anesthesia but as yet we have not fully tried this agent. We have in no instance observed any annoying symptoms to follow the use of the weaker cocain solutions.

THE UTERINE TAMPON IN POSTPARTUM HEMORRHAGE

BY T. J. CROWE, M. D., DALLAS, TEXAS. IN AMERICAN JOURNAL OF OBSTETRICS

Several years ago I read in one of the representative journals a paper, from the pen of a professor of obstetrics, condemning the uterine tampon as worse than useless, often positively injurious in the treatment of postpartum hemorrhage.

Had this paper been contributed by a recent graduate, it might have passed unnoticed, but coming, as it did, from a man whose teaching and writing carry conviction to hundreds of students and young physicians without experience sufficient to disprove his assertions, it should not have been allowed to go so long unanswered, because, when properly applied, the tampon is both effective and safe.

Fortunately, postpartum hemorrhage is not of frequent occurrence. Many a physician has gone through a lifetime service without witnessing a genuine case. Many of the reported cases have been little more than hemorrhage from vaginal and cervical lacerations. I have witnessed rather troublesome bleeding from tears in the anterior commissure on either side of the urinary meatus, also from a badly lacerated cervix; but these, while troublesome, are neither as alarming or dangerous as real postpartum hemorrhage, which, when it does occur, places the physician face to face with a very alarming and dangerous condition, and one that will tax his skill and ingenuity, if life is to be saved.

This is one of the conditions in which a few minutes will determine the result— whether life is to be saved or lost, and where a cool head, a clear brain and a ready hand may snatch from the grave, as it were, a human life. It behooves us, therefore, to hold fast to that which is effective, notwithstanding the condemnations of a few.

That the tampon has failed and that it has been the carrier of infection, I do not question, but that is the fault of the man who applied it, and not of the tampon.

Because some bungling farm-hand misapplies the forceps and destroys a woman's life, must we abandon the forceps? The forceps or any other instrument is dangerous in the hands of a man who does not understand the nature of the condition with which he is dealing nor the scientific use of the instrument with which he is trying to meet it.

That we may know how to control postpartum hemorrhage it is necessary that we should understand the conditions under which it occurs. What is that condition? There is but one answer: Uterine relaxation. How is the presence of relaxation determined? By palpatation through the abdominal walls.

When the uterus can be found as a solid, pear-shaped tumor, about the size of the closed first, midway between the umbilicus and pubes, it is firmly contracted, and hemorrhage, if present, must be sought for elsewhere than from the cavity of that organ. When it cannot be definitely located or made to contract, by kneading, manipulation, etc., so that it can be distinctly outlined, it is quite likely that the flow, if any, is coming from the open sinuses in the cavity of the relaxed uterus, and then, if resort to the usual measures fail to cause contraction and stop the bleeding, the tampon is a last resort and, properly applied, a veritable life-saver.

I say this without fear of successful contradiction, and that, too, in the face of the fact that I have heard learned professors say that the womb would on such occasions swallow up a hatful of gauze without appreciable result.

To effectually apply the uterine tampon, it is necessary that the obstetrician should know how hemorrhage from other parts of the body, as the nose, an alveolar cavity, or even a limb, is stopped by tampons and pads. We know that we can stop such hemorrhages only by compressing the walls of the bleeding vessels between a pad and a bone or some other resisting substance with sufficient force to obliterate their lumen. Why, then, should we expect to check the rush of blood from the uterus, in a case of postpartum hemorrhage, by simply stuffing its cavity full of gauze, applying pressure to the vessels on one side only?

If the muscular tone of the uterus is

sufficient to furnish its own resistance, as is the case in miscarriage during the early months of pregnancy, firm pressure from the inside by a tampon will be sufficient to control any hemorrhage that may occur, but, unfortunately, this muscular tone is the very thing that is lacking when we have hemorrhage following labor at full term.

The manipulation incident to packing a relaxed and bleeing womb may cause the organ to contract upon the tampon and, for a time, check the flow of blood, but its overdistended, semi-paralyzed walls will again relax after the packing is placed and bleed as violently as before. This is why the tampon has been considered ineffectual and why it has been so bitterly condemned.

The failure of the tampon in such cases is due to the mistaken idea that filling the cavity of the womb with gauze should stop the flow of blood without counterpressure other than that furnished by its muscular walls.

That the proper application of the tampon will stop hemorrhage from the womb as elsewhere in the body is proven by the following report of a case which will sufficiently describe what I consider the proper method of applying counterpressure to the bleeding vessels and amply demonstrate the value of the procedure.

Several years ago I was engaged to attend Mrs. A., the wife of a division commander in the Salvation Army, during her confinement. She was then the mother of two children whose entrance to the world had occurred without untoward incident. She was healthy and robust; family and previous personal history negative.

I made the usual urinary and preliminary vaginal examination: the urine was negative, presentation and position normal.

About a week before the expected time I was called to see her. When I arrived at the house I found her suffering severe pain in the right side, just above and to the

left of the anterior iliac spine. There was no tenderness to touch or pressure. She had been suffering for nearly twenty-four hours when I saw her, but said nothing about it until she noticed a slight flow of blood from the vagina which led her to believe that labor was coming on and that I should be called.

The discharge was so slight that I gave it little attention further than to ascertain whether or not labor had commenced. Failing to find any evidence of uterine contractions or cervical dilatation, I left her a prescription for the pain with instructions to call me if she had any further trouble.

Six days later I was again called, and when I reached my patient, at 2 o'clock a. m., found her squatting in the middle of the bed in an agony of pain, which did not cease until, twenty minutes later, the baby and after-birth together were violently expelled, and following them came a torrential rush of blood. I at once realized that I had a desperate condition to deal with and promptly resorted to the usual methods for controlling it, but, in spite of my kneading, clearing out of clots, hot douching, etc., the flow continued unabated until, by introducing my right hand into the vagina and seizing the cervix and with my left grasping the fundus, I succeeded in doubling the uterus upon itself and applying pressure, when I had the hemorrhage temporarily under control. In the meantime the woman was nearly exhausted, complaining that she could not see and struggling for air.

Thus I held the womb for twenty minutes, during which time I got a breathing spell and a chance to decide what I should do if the hemorrhage reappeared when I released it. After twenty minutes I relaxed without removing my hands; immediately the flow was resumed as violently as before. I then instructed the husband to hastily call Dr. C., who resided but two blocks away. The doctor responded promptly, and I requested him to prepare for packing while I maintained pressure, and thus avoid any further loss of blood while gauze, instruments, etc., were being sterilized. When all was ready I withdrew my hand from the vagina and the doctor commenced packing the uterus while I continued to hold the fundus so that the organ might be steadied and kept contracted. The uterus and vagina firmly packed. I released the fundus and waited to see if our efforts had been successful. I did not have long to wait, for in less time than it takes to tell it the packing was saturated and a steady stream of blood flowing from the vaginal orifice.

Realizing that we had failed, I again grasped the fundus and forced it down against the packing, at the same time instructing the doctor to secure three towels and a sheet; each towel to be folded and rolled into a solid cylinder three inches long and two and a half in diameter; the sheet to be folded so that it could be used as a binder. Having been secured and prepared, I placed one of the towels above the fundus and one on either side of the uterus, extending from the transverse pad to the pubes, and fixed them with the binder drawn as tight as possible. This held the womb in a solid box, as it were, with the spinal column behind, a solid pad on either side and above and the binder in front.

Having thus forestalled any possible relaxation beyond the space within my splints, I hastily withdrew the vaginal packing and added the length of two sterile gauze bandages, one inch wide to the packing already in the uterine cavity and repacked the vagina. This effectually stopped the hemorrhage, and so completely that the new vaginal packing was not even soiled when removed.

The hemorrhage stopped, I turned my attention to the baby and after-birth; on inspection of the latter I found what appeared to be the cause of all of my trouble. In the center of the placental mass, on the maternal side, I found a firm blood-clot, about the size of a fetal head, thoroughly adherent and apparently several days old. This it was that caused the pain in the side and the slight discharge of blood which made its appearance several days before labor commenced and continued until the baby was born.

This enormous clot had so distended the segment of uterus above it that it was paralyzed and incapable of contraction, as is the overdistended bladder after prolonged retention, consequently the sinuses remained open and poured out a torrent of blood that nothing but properly applied pressure could stop. The increasing tension over the steadily growing clot probably accounts for the pain in the side, complained of during my first visit.

That the reader may have a better conception of the position and size of the clot I shall describe the combined mass as hat-shaped: the clot corresponding to the crown and the free margins of the placenta to the rim of a hat. The remarkable thing about it is that enough of the placenta remained attached to save the child, which was born alive.

I have never heard of another case of postpartum hemorrhage where splints were used, as in this case, to secure counter pressure for a tampon. If any have been reported I have overlooked them. I have treated several cases by the same method, but all of the others were slight hemorrhages which could have been controlled, no doubt, without the outside padding.

Aside from neuralgic pains which lasted for two days and at one time or another involved almost every portion of the body, even the fingers, this woman's convalescence was uninterrupted, notwithstanding the fact that, in his haste, the doctor forced the steel rib from the Cook packer into the womb, from which it was removed with the gauze thirty-six hours later.

The after-treatment consisted of a pint of saline solution hypodermically immediately following the final packing, and high elevation of the foot of the bed, which I had resorted to before assistance was called. I had to keep this woman in the inverted position for more than a week, dropping the foot of the bed a little each day until the horizontal was reached. Because of the sliding toward the head of the bed and other discomforts complained of by the patient, I made several earlier attempts to drop the foot of the bed all the way down, but in each instance she became dizzy and faint, and it had to be returned.

Those of my readers who have had a simliar experience can appreciate something of the trials of that dreadful night which, fortunately for the patient and myself, terminated more happily than I, at one time, thought it would. Until Dr. C. came I had no help except what I got from the husband, who was so badly frightened that he was worse than useless.

While I do not presume to question the opinions of physicians of mature judgment and large experience, I consider one well demonstrated fact of more practical value than a volume of theoretical speculation. I contend, therefore, that the uterine tampon with properly applied counterpressure is a successful method of controlling postpartum hemorrhage, and when due precautions to secure asepsis are taken, there is little danger of infection. In any event, the hemorrhage must be controlled, and the risk of infection, which is of secondary importance, must be taken.

Before concluding this paper, I wish to say that I have always made it a practice to go to every case of labor prepared for any emergency, always anticipating hemorrhage, and I shall continue to do so. My obstetrical bag is unnecessarily heavy and cumbersome forty-nine out of the fifty times I carry it, but I prefer the load to parting with the sense of security it gives me.

252 Browder Street.

EDITORIAL

THE EVANS' PLAN FOR THE SELECTION OF REGENTS FOR THE STATE UNIVERSITY.

President A. Grant Evans, of the State University, is considering the advancement of a proposition looking toward a change in the system now in vogue for the selection of Regents of the State University.

The proposition in the main requires that the Regents be nominated by various representative bodies now a power in Oklahoma rather than that the appointive power be vested in one person.

President Evans thinks that the Educational interests will be better served if Regents were nominated and appointed on the recommendation of the Alumnae Association of the University, Trades Unions, Governor, State Medical Association, Bar Association and the State Commercial bodies, each to select one member and the entire membership to be so appointed that some of the older ones would hold over, giving the body the necessary experience for the management of the institution's affairs.

Theoretically the plan appears to be excellent. It is not new by any means, so far as its application to other appointive bodies goes. Many of the states, especially in the South, have recently adopted laws by which the Governor was required to appoint various boards on the recommendation of those people more likely to be advised of the fitness of the prospective members.

South Carolina and Texas have this plan in execution so far as the appointment of a State Board of Medical Examiners is concerned. but the law has not been in force long enough to judge its merits.

However, scattering the appointive is not likely to be harmful and we wish President Evans success.

THE SHAWNEE WAY OF DOING THINGS.

Ten months ago the Pottawatomie County Medical Society concluded to have a city hospital and a contagious and infectious hospital together with an up-to-date ordinance calling for a city Health Department.

Solely on account of their superb medical organization all of these benefits are to-day assured. This condition was brought about by a united medical profession who placed the matter in the hands of an active committee, and Drs. Sanders and Byrum, respectively City Superintendent of Public Health and County Superintendent of Public Health.

This committee and the gentlemen named together with the profession generally overcome a great many obstacles which at first seemed unsurmountable and the success of their efforts is now testified to by a bond issue of twenty thousand dollars to make the necessary improvements.

The city of Shawnee has in like manner created a City Health Department whose duty it shall be to enforce needed health regulations according to the requirements of the Oklahoma public health laws and the rules of the Board of Health of Oklahoma.

Too much praise cannot be given those concerned in bringing about this successful termination of the struggle. Hospitals as a rule are not money making institutions and it is no more than fair that all the people be concerned in their buildings and maintenance and this plan which is being executed by Shawnee occurs to us as being very feasible as it places the burden on all the people and not the small minority of managers and enthusiasts as is usually the rule.

It is to be hoped that other cities in Oklahoma will follow this plan and give themselves what they need more than any other municipal improvement; a modern hospital.

THE MEDICAL ASSOCIATION OF THE SOUTHWEST.

This organization which is a comparatively new one is making every effort to make their meeting at San Antonio, Texas, in November, a success from a scientific and also social standpoint. In addition to a program which promises to be replete with excellent productions and the assured presence of many men famous in the medical and surgical history of our country, a trip is being planned after the meeting, to take in Mexico and its capital.

Many men are unable to attend the meetings of the American Medical Association for various reasons and this Association, comprising the states of Oklahoma, Kansas Missouri, Texas and Arkansas gives them a large and fruitful meeting at their doors, which can be reached with little loss of time and comparatively small expense.

The American Medical Association has become. according to the views of many men a complex machine, the understanding of which requires much time and work and participation in its affairs is necessarily confined to few men when the total membership is taken into consideration.

This Association of the above named states gives the profession in them an opportunity to meet many new and prominent men and at the same time to participate more or less according to their wishes in the transactions of the body.

In our opinion its membership will grow and prosper as time goes on until it will become secondary only to the parent body —the American Medical Association.

CHANGE IN MANAGEMENT OF SANITARIUM.

It is announced that the responsibility for the management and control of the Duke and Rucks Sanitarium, Guthrie, Oklahoma, will in the future be assumed by Dr. John W. Duke. The location remaining as heretofore, 310 North Broad street.

Dr. W. W. Rucks will assume the general practice of medicine. The ability of Dr. Duke to conduct this institution in a successful manner is too well known to require comment here.

FULL TERM BABY AND FOETUS AT SAME CONFINEMENT.

May 10th, 1909, call to see Mrs. R. in first confinement. Age 22, family history good, labor normal in every respect.

Third stage progressed till placenta was practically out of vagina when suddenly it stopped, after a few minutes I made some traction and found it was fast; I twisted or turned the placenta over in order to rope the membranes and made a little more traction, thinking the membrane was detached and simply stuck in the vagina. I then pressed two fingers into the vagina under the placenta, by this time pains had come on and I could feel a mass protruding through the os and in another moment the entire mass was expelled.

The placenta was apparently normal except a white fibrous mass of membranes or sack attached to the border; on opening the sack I found a fairly well developed foetus, four and one-half or five inches long, there was a trace of cord attached to foetus but I could not make out where the other end had been attached. The membranes and sack about the foetus were white and of a fibrous character.

IRA W. ROBERTSON, M. D.,
Dustin, Oklahoma.

Dr. C. A. Thompson,
Muskogee, Oklahoma.

Dear Doctor: As I am reported as stating that quinine will be rendered quickly soluble if placed in a capsule, it may be well to rise and explain what was said. It is like the play of Hamlet with Hamlet left out. The procedure mentioned is really worth while and it may not be taking too much of your valuable space to explain it. As a prescription it will look like this:

Quinine Sulphate................Drachm 1
Acid Sulphuric Aromatic............q. s.
Glycerite of Starch................q. s.
Mix and dispense in twelve capsules.

The acid is dropped onto the quinine until it is reduced to a thin paste and it is then made into pill mass with the glycerite of starch. When made right it is easy to shape the material and slip it into capsule. The powdered liquorice can be used in making the mass of proper consistence, but it dries out rapidly and is not so suitable as the starch.

C. W. FISK.

PERSONAL MENTION.

Dr. F. B. Fite, of Muskogee, is spending his vacation in North Carolina.

Dr. J. E. Hillis, Pryor, had the misfortune to lose his office equipment in the recent disastrous fire in that city.

Dr. V. M. Gore, of Kingfisher, was operated on for appendicitis in St. Louis, Mo., August 21. At last report he was doing nicely.

Dr. Milton K. Thompson, Muskogee, will make a trip around the world in 1910, stopping in Europe for some time for postgraduate work.

Dr. Harry McQuown, of Fallis, has bought out Dr. S. M. Barnes, of Stillwater, and has removed to 'that place where he will make his future home.

Dr. Sydney Hagood, Durant, Oklahoma, spent a few of the hot days in Sulphur Springs, Ark., visiting his professional friends in Muskogee on his return.

Dr. W. G. Brymer, of Comanche, Oklahoma, is offering his home and fixtures for sale with the intention of taking post-graduate work in New Orleans and New York and later locating in some city.

· Dr. J. B. Smith, of Durant, has returned from his California trip. While absent Dr. Smith attended the Elks Convention in Los Angeles. He was accompanied home by Mrs. Smith and their daughter.

Dr. J. H. Adcock, formerly located in Morris, Oklahoma, but who has been spending some time in the New York Polyclinic Medical School and at present an interne in Bellevue Hospital, visited Oklahoma recently. Doctor Adcock will return to Oklahoma eventually.

FOR SALE.

The Journal has tuition to the amount of forty-four dollars in the New York Polyclinic School and Hospital which will be sold at a reduction from the usual rates. Address The Journal.

A GOOD LOCATION FOR SALE.

I will sell for cash my home, consisting of five-room house, one acre of land, concrete storm house 6x8x9, and buggy and team of three horses, with about one hundred dollars worth of drugs, for $800.00.

This includes my practice of about eight miles square in a prairie agricultural country, twelve miles southwest of Duncan and twelve miles northwest of Comanche, Oklahoma. There is no competition, the nearest physician being twelve miles distant. The practice amounts to $2,000 annually, collections good, being 95 per cent. Good schools and lodge, with all churches represented with organization.

Will sell for cash only and will introduce buyer. Am going to take post-graduate work and move to city. If you mean business, write or come, but don't bother if you do not want a good village and country practice. Address Dr. W. G. Brymer, Fair, Route 4, Comanche, Oklahoma.

NEW MEMBERS.

F. M. Edwards, Fairland.

T. J. Bond, Miama.

Lester H. Murdoch, Okeene.

Ira F. Smith, Fay.

Dr. J. Scott Lindley, Fairview, Major County.

Dr. Wiley Brown, Cleo, Major County.

CHANGES OF ADDRESSES.

E. D. Ebright, from Carmen to Enid, Oklahoma.

J. W. Childs, from Noble to Carmen, Oklahoma.

M. L. Gorton, from Pawnee to Lindsay, California.

M. A. Warhurst, from Remus to Maud, Oklahoma.

M. H. Levi, from Elk City to Oklahoma City, Oklahoma.

Harry McQuown, from Fallis to Stillwater.

J. J. Hardy, from McCurtain to Poteau.

EXCHANGES

HYDROCEPHALIC MONSTROSITY.

Dr. W. H. Davis, Castle, Oklahoma.

On April 25th I was called to attend Mrs. G. in confinement. She was 24 years of age, and had had four previous confinements; all preceding labors had been natural, but at each time she had had a spell of sickness either before or just after. the last time being measles. When her husband called me, he said he feared we would be too late, though they lived only two blocks from my office; he said the "waters (liquor amnii) had already broke before he left home." When I made examination I found the womb high up in the abdomen, and the cervix dilated to about the size of a dime. I also found a sac extending above the pubis which appeared to be more a "gob of .fat" than anything else; this could be noticed externally. The mother said the fetus had been moving every half hour. After my arrival pains almost ceased, and I told them we would have to wait several hours before delivery. The mother complained that she could not bear the pains when they did come because they seemed to press upon the bladder, and gave her great pain, however, I knew that she was mistaken, because she would urinate every fifteen minutes. After waiting about eight hours for pains to become good, I gave a dose of ergot—this I would not have done had she not been two weeks over the nine months. At the same time I gave one-eighth grain of morphine, in order to stop what as I thought were hysterical pains. The medicines did not seem to have any effect upon her, so about twelve hours after being called, I administered hypodermically twenty-five drops of fluid extract of ergot. After ergot was absorbed, pains became good, when I noticed there seemed to be something abnormal about the head of the child, at which I ordered my wife, who was assisting me, to administer chloroform and I would use the forceps. Pains became very good, and I succeeded in delivering a dead "something" weighing about seven pounds, which was hideous to look upon. The head of the fetus appeared to have no bones in it and was as big as the head of an adult, and as large as all the rest of the body. Its features were more those of a human than anything else, but greatly distorted; but the thing that attracted my attention most was the cord—where it left the abdomen of the child it was at least an inch in diameter, and eight inches from the abdominal attachment was a large pouch looking something like a bladder and which I found contained a fluid of the color of urine, and also a full set of intestines.

This pouch was as large as a man's closed fist. But the cord then became contracted and was about eight inches longer and attached to the placenta, which was normal. The abdomen of the fetus appeared to be natural, and was filled with the viscera. The mystery in this case to me is, how were those intestines formed in that umbilical cord, as the cord contained the vein and artery to supply the fetus with circulation, and I know these were intestines from the fact that they were divided into cecum, colon and rectum, and became lost in some other material at the beginning of the cecum. The mother is making an uneventful recovery. Now, my reason for writing this is that some brother practician may tell me what caused this. I have delivered several monstrosities, including a frog, a rabbit. pups, etc., in my seventeen years practice, but never saw anything like this umbilical cord. What do the others think of this?

CALCIUM SALTS IN EPILEPSY.

A. P. Ohlmacher, Detroit (Journal A. M. A., August 14), has hitherto refrained from publishing his remarkable success following his first trial of the calcium salts in epilepsy, but now since Littlejohn (Lancet, May 15, 1909, p. 1382) has reported results with the same agent, he wishes to supplement it with his case. It was a child four years and four months old, with no heredity of epilepsy, in whom the disease had begun and continued from a month after his third birthday. When first seen he was having from 34 to 73 attacks a month and his mental growth had apparently stopped. The grand mal attacks as seen by Ohlmacher were very severe but never became the typical full status epilepticus. The child had frequent nosebleed following these attacks and its nurse asserted that she could detect the odor of

blood on the breath during convulsions and prior to the appearance of actual hemorrhage. At the time Ohlmacher had been working on therapeutic immunization where the problem of blood coagulability presented itself, and he had employed Wright's method of measuring the time of blood coagulation and of using calcium salts to fortify a defective coagulability. Accordingly, when his attention was called to the hemorrhages, he made a blood clotting test and finding that it was slow in clotting, he began giving calcium lactate in doses of seven to ten grains dissolved in hot water and added to the milk three times a day. This medication has been continued from the first beginning, on June 2, 1907, with no change, except occasionally reducing to one or two doses daily, to the present time. The coagulation time was soon reduced to normal and since the cessation of the epilepsy, three months after commencing the calcium lactate, the child has had occasionally nasal hemorrhages apparently related to periods of lowered coagulability. At the time he began the medicine McCallum's observation on calcium metabolism as related by parathyroid intoxication and to tetany had not been published nor had Carle's paper on calcium chlorid in therapeutics appeared. Incomplete observations on several additional cases similarly treated tend to confirm the favorable results with the first case.

INFANTILE DIARRHOEA.

First noticing the findings of other authorities of the Bacillus dysentericus as the cause of the summer diarrhoea of infants, C. G. Grulee, Chicago (Journal A. M. A., August 14), mentions the investigations of J. S. Welch and himself, with failure to find the above organism and their conclusion that true dysentery in infants must be relatively rare in Chicago. He says there are many reasons for believing that the B. dysentericus is not etiologically connected with a large percentage of the diarrhoeas in infants. In the first place, the cases showing this organism in the stools showed no clinical differences from those in which it was absent. In the second place, the dysentery bacilli were usually few and hard to find, and, in the third place, agglutinins were by no means constantly present, as far as could be learned, and the antidysenteric serum seemed to have no effect. The dysentery bacillus has never been cultivated from the blood of these infants nor has it ever been found outside the human body, except in the laboratory animals. He therefore regards the connection of the dysentery bacillus with the summer diarrhea still, at least, an open question, with the burden of proof on those who assert its etiologic relationship. Since the infectious nature of the disorder has not been proved, we must seek elsewhere for its causes. Within the past year Finkelstein has described a disorder of nutrition which he calls metabolic intoxication. The symptoms are the same as those of summer diarrhea as we encounter it. He has proved that this disorder is caused primarily by the inability of the organisms to properly assimilate sugar, a condition to which too much fat in the food predisposes. Czerny and Keller, while agreeing with Finkelstein, to a certain extent, suggest that we may have a toxicosis due to the decomposition of the food by bacteria, either before ingestion or in the gastrointestinal tract. Grulee, after discussing the condition and pathologic findings, comes to the conclusion that while infection in the intestinal wall probably occurs in some cases it is not the usual cause of a summer diarrhea in infants, but that this infection is, as a rule, due to disturbance of metabolism or to decomposition of the food. As regards. treatment it is evident that, if this is the case, the first in-

dication is to stop the food and put the child on a low diet. This is not all. There must still be a supply of fluid for the system and this we accomplish by giving barley water or weak tea. It is occasionally impossible to give this by the mouth, and it is well to resort to a continuous enema or even to a subcutaneous administration of normal salt solution. After ten to forty-eight hours of the starvation treatment it is time to give the patient food, the symptoms having usually disappeared. For the past two years he has usually employed skim milk as the first food for these children. He has, as a rule, had this boiled, which kills the bacteria and seems to be more readily digested. This skim milk is given in the amount of one and a quarter to one and a half ounces to the pound weight of the child, each twenty-four hours, and diluted sufficiently to afford the proper quantity at each feeding. This is a temporary measure and, as soon as possible, milk sugar must be added and whole milk substituted for the skim milk. The condition of the child must be the guide. The greatest trouble with this method is the tendency to constipate when the skim milk is being replaced by whole milk, and the addition of malt may be useful. The vomiting may continue and require stomach washing and bismuth in extreme cases. Reduction of temperature can be accomplished usually by the measures already suggested, but hydrotherapy is often useful. The distention which occurs only in the more protracted cases can be temporarily relieved by the introduction of a tube into the rectum, the other end of which is placed in a vessel containing hot water. We may also use colonic flushings and hot external applications to the abdomen. Collapse can best be met by mustard packs followed by saline infusion and continuous saline enema. Grulee does not favor the use of calomel in these cases and he believes it has been much abused. As for intestinal antiseptics generally, he sees no indications for them in these cases.

THE COLON TUBE AND THE HIGH ENEMA.

The question of how far the soft rubber colon tube can be inserted into the bowel to administer an effective high injection, is taken up by H. W. Soper, St. Louis (Journal A. M. A., August 7), who describes experiments performed by him in which the position of the tube was verified by the X-Ray. Sixty cases were examined where it was attempted to pass long blunt end soft rubber tubes, with side openings, into the rectum, the patient being in the knee chest and side positions. The only case in which he succeeded in passing the tube above the dome of the rectum was one of Hirschsprung's disease or congenital idiopathic dilation and hypertrophy of the colon, end even here it was necessary to use the sigmoidoscope to introduce the tube. He thinks it is only in cases of abnormal development of the sigmoid that it is possible to introduce a soft rubber tube higher than six or seven inches in the rectum. A short tube six inches in length is therefore best for all sorts of enemata when using water for fecal evacuation, and it is possible, as he has frequently demonstrated, to thoroughly cleanse the entire colon by using a large caliber (one-half inch) short tube. It is also best when retention of liquid is desired.

SKULL FRACTURE.

C. R. C. Borden, Boston (Journal A. M. A., August 7), points out the ways in which basal fractures of the skull are of interest to the aurist and rhinologist because of their contiguity to the organs of special sense and to the regions affected by ear and nose disease. The extent of basal injuries is rather remarkable and certain parts, such as the petrous portion of the temporal, the greater wing of the sphenoid, an the orbital plates of the frontal, are specially liable to be involved. Hemorrhage from the ear is a common symptom and Borden considers it as not necessarily due to contrecoup. The temporal bone is situated practically in the center of the skull, and when autopsy records tell us of fractures eight and nine inches long, the contrecoup theory is not necessary to account for them Hemorrhages from the ears are not, so far as he can determine, especially important as prognostic indications. He has analyzed 400 cases and a little more of fracture of the skull taken from the records of the Boston City Hospital. As regards sensory symptoms, there were 307 cases recorded; 168 patients were unconscious, and 58 conscious, the remainder being in the intermediate stage of confused or dazed mentality. Of those patients conscious on admission 13 per cent di d and 87 per cent were discharged relieved. On the other hand, of those unconscious on admission 51 per cent died, while of 9 admitted in a comatose state 66 per cent died, and where the mental condition was intermediate, the mortality was comparable to that of the unconscious patients. As regards pupillary reaction there was a wide range of conditions, the greater number were normal, and next in frequency were those in which one pupil was dilated, usually on the side of the injury. Of those with normal reaction, 24 per cent died and of those with unequal pupils, two-thirds recovered. Of 8 individuals with equally dilated pupils seven died. and contraction of pupils is more serious than dilatation, about 50 per cent of deaths occuring in this class. The worst pupillary condition appears to be wide dilatation of one with pin-point contraction of the other, all the eight recorded cases being fatal. Contrary to his expectations a slow pulse was not the rule. In only 14 out of over 400 cases was there below 60. It seems to him that the reason for this is that pressure is more evenly distributed over the surface of the brain than in tumors or abscess where slow pulse is usually met with. Slow pulse may develop later and then indicates either incipient meningitis or extension of hemorrhage or increase of cerebral spinal fluid. On the other hand a rising pulse is a distinctly bad symptom. In the majortiy of cases death is caused by failure of the respiration. Temperature ranged from 95.1 to 110.8 F. In 5 cases it was subnormal and the patient died in a few hours. Respiration therefore is the most important symptom to be considered. The records give it as stertorous in 41 cases, rapid and labored in 7, slow and labored in 5, slow in 5, irregular in 4, Cheyne-Stokes in 3, blowing in 1, infrequent in 1, and gasping in 1. Vomiting was not specially prominent, though it was noted in 55 cases, but only in 5 was it persistent or considerable. Convulsions were noted 25 times and facial paralysis 24. Delirium is common. Age is of no special importance except in young children who survive spectacular tumbles, etc., though they occasionally succumb. Such patients however should be kept quiet and under observation after these injuries. Any other course is risky. Borden notes the fact that hemorrhage from skull fracture does not cause such definite symptoms as tumor or abscess, and he accounts for this by the softer nature of the blood or clot pressing on the brain. Contusions are more or less common and infected areas are occasionally found at autopsy, both these and contusions occurring chiefly in the sphenoidal and frontal lobes. The nervous symptoms from skull fracture in this series of cases have already been analyzed by Thomas (Journal A. M. A., July, 1908, p. 271). The treatment of the cases at present is surgical. Many of the patients recover in 15 or 25 days and while the mortality from fractures of the vault is comparatively small, in that of the base it is high.

NITROUS OXIDE AND OXYGEN ANESTHESIA.

C. K. Teter, Cleveland, Ohio (Journal A. M. A., August 7), gives his experience with nitrous oxid and oxygen anesthesia. He first gives a sketch of the history of this method, crediting the first reported cases in which it was used to Dr. E. Andrews, of Chicago, who, however, did not use it to any great extent. It was studied by Paul Bert but its extended use is more due to Dr. F. W. Hewitt, of London. Warming the gas improves its effects and safeguards best against post-operative bronchitis or pneumonia, besides requiring a much less volume of gas to produce the narcosis. The elimination takes place principally through the respiratory tract and a patient with good circulation will come out of the anesthesia very quickly. It has been advised against in brain surgery but with the proper addition of oxygen he has never had any difficulty with it. If air is used instead of oxygen there is less asphyxia but the anesthetic effect is diminished. He reports cases in which the effect on the brain was directly observed, showing, in his opinion, that the discoloration and dilatation were not due to the anesthetic but were purely asphyxial manifestations. The asphyxia, moreover, is not dangerous as compared with that from ether or chloroform. Several cases are reported also, illustrating points of special interest, such as strength of narcosis, the effects of age of patient, physical condition, primary shock, etc. He has kept a patient under this anesthetic for several hours, and considers it safer in this respect than any other of the general anesthetics, without exception. The aged as a rule are good su but in children it is best to watch the symptoms closely, as the effects are very rapid. It is not always best to continue with nitrous oxid and oxygen under all circumstances, for, in some cases, it may be impossible to retain the desired depth of anesthesia. In some cases it may be better to change to a more stimulating or tolerable anesthetic, either in combination or sequence. He has had a few cases showing shock, probably more than would be noticed with other agents, owing to the fact that the nitrous oxid was selected on account of abnormal conditions present. He has had but one fatality which he reports and that was due to shock and primary cardiac failure. He emphasizes the importance of continuous auscultation and describes his method of performing it during an operation with an improved Kehler stethoscope, which is especially adapted for the purpose. One of the main objections to nitrous oxid is the rigidity encountered in about 10 per cent of cases and his best results in meeting this difficulty were obtained with an injection of from 1-4 to 1-8 grain of morphin sulphate and from 1-100 to 1-150 grain of atropin, injected half an hour before the operation. He does not advise the use of morphine as a preliminary, however, to any one not experienced in this method of anesthesia. The apparatus and the technic for this operation are described, together with the variations required when operating on the mouth and throat. The dangers are enumerated in some detail. The principal one is asphyxia. But he believes that nitrous oxid can produce death without the asphyxial element coming into it at all. Ordinarily, the cyanosis is not so severe as to be very objectionable, the principal result being a post-operative headache. Another undesirable symptom is tetanic cramps in the arms, hands, feet, and legs, but in every case in which this was observed the patient's physical condition was either bad or he was of a neurasthenic temperament, or both. Blood pressure is slightly raised during nitrous-oxid anesthesia and this point and other effects on the blood have been brought out by Hamburger and Ewing. Their experiments, the author thinks, prove that nitrous-oxid anesthesia does not reduce hemoglobin and thereby cause anemia; that it does not increase hemolysis, and that what apparent change it does produce, is transient and of no clinical significance, and that nitrous oxid causes no permanent effect of any significance from the standpoint of blood changes. The advantages are the freedom from nausea and vomiting, the better after-effects, and fewer complications retarding recovery.

PRURITUS REMEDIES THAT WORK.

Pruritus of the skin, anus or vulva, especially when attended by scaling of the skin of the hands or feet, may be invariably set down as due to autotoxemia from fecal absorption. This condition is admirably met by the following combination:

Juglandin gr. 1-6, to stimulate secretion, relieve costiveness, and favor the loosening of fecal matter adherent to the coats of the bowels; physostigmine gr. 1-250, to stimulate peristalsis and the ejection of fecal matter; berberine gr. 1-6. to induce contraction of the relaxed and dilated bowel. This dose should be given from three to seven times a day (with the morning Salithia flush) and continued as long as the necessity exists.

Much better results will be obtained from such application of exact remedies to meet the conditions they exactly remedy than from the ignorant combination of cathartics without regard to the specific action of each, and the administration of such remedies in very large doses which soon exhaust the irritability of the intestines and require constantly increasing doses with constantly decreasing effects.

THE MODERN TREATMENT OF HAY FEVER.

Whatever be the accepted views as to the pathology and etiology of hay fever, there is little difference of opinion concerning its importance and the severity of its symptoms. An agent that is capable of controlling the catarrhal inflammation, allaying the violent paroxysms of sneezing and the abundant lacrimation, cutting short the asthatic attack when it becomes a part of the clinical ensemble, and, finally, sustaining the heart and thus preventing the great depression that usually accompanies or follows the attack—in short, an agent that is capable of meeting the principal indications—must prove invaluable in the treatment of this by no means tractable disease.

In the opinion of many physicians, the most serviceable agent is Adrenalin. While not a specific in the strict meaning of the word, Adrenalin meets the condition very effectually and secures for the patient a positive degree of comfort. It controls catarrhal inflammations as perhaps no other astringent can. It allays violent paroxysms of sneezing and profuse lacrimation by blanching the turbinal tissues and soothing the irritation of the nasal mucosa which gives rise to those symptoms. It reduces the severity of the asthmatic seizure, in many instances affording complete and lasting relief.

There are four forms in which Adrenalin is very successfully used in the treatment of hay fever: Solution Adrenalin Chloride, Adrenalin Inhalent, Adrenalin Ointment, and Adrenalin and Chloretone Ointment. The first solution, first mentioned, should be diluted with four to ten times its volume of physiological salt solution and sprayed into the nares and pharynx. The inhalent is used in the same manner, except that it requires no dilution. The ointments are supplied in collapsible tubes with elongated nozzles, which render administration very simple and easy.

It is perhaps pertinent to mention in this connection that Messrs. Parke, Davis & Co. have issued a very useful booklet on the subject of hay fever, containing practical chapters on the disease, indications for treatment, preventive measures, etc. Physicians will do well to write for this pamphlet, addressing the company at its home offices in Detroit or any of its numerous branches.

OFFICERS OF THE OKLAHOMA STATE MEDICAL ASSOCIATION.

President, Dr. Walter C. Bradford, Shawnee.
First Vice President, Dr. C. L. Reeder, Tulsa.
Second Vice President, Dr. D. A. Myers, Lawton.
Third Vice President, Dr. J. W. Duke, Guthrie.
Secretary, Dr. Claude Thompson, Muskogee.

LIST OF COUNCILLORS WITH THEIR RESPECTIVE COUNTIES

First District, Dr. J. A. Walker, Shawnee. Canadian, Cleveland, Grady, Lincoln, Oklahoma, Pottawatomie and Seminole.

Second District, Dr. John W. Duke, Guthrie. Grant, Kay, Osage, Noble, Pawnee, Kingfisher, Logan and Payne.

Third District, Dr. Charles R. Hume, Anadarko. Roger Mills, Custer, Dewey, Blaine, Beckham, Washita and Caddo.

Fourth District, Dr. A. B. Fair, Frederick. Greer, Kiowa, Jackson, Comanche, Tillman, Stephens and Jefferson.

Fifth District, ..., ... Cimarron, Texas, Beaver, Harper, Woodward, Alfalfa, Ellis, Woods, Major and Garfield.

Sixth District, Dr. F. R. Sutton, Bartlesville. Washington, Nowata, Ottawa, Rogers, Mayes, Delaware, Tulsa and Craig

Seventh District, Dr. W. G. Blake, Tahlequah. Muskogee, Creek, Wagoner, Cherokee, Adair, Okmulgee, Okfuskee and McIntosh.

Eighth District, Dr. I. W. Robertson, Dustin. Sequoyah, LeFlore, Haskell, Hughes, Pittsburg and Latimer.

Ninth District, Dr. H. P. Wilson, Wynnewood. McClain, Garvin, Carter, Love, Murray, Pontotoc, Johnston and Marshall.

Tenth District, Dr. J. S. Fulton, Atoka. Coal, Atoka, Bryan, Pushmataha, Choctaw and McCurtain.

Delegates to American Medical Association, Dr. C. S. Bobo, Norman; Dr. L. A. Hahn, Guthrie.

Alternates, Dr. C. L. Reeder, Tulsa; Dr. J. A. Walker, Shawnee.

CHAIRMEN OF SECTIONS.

Section on Obstetrics and Gynecology, Chairman, Dr. G. H. Thrailkill, Chickasha.

Section on Pediatrics, Chairman, Dr. H. M. Williams, Wellston.

Section on the Practice of Medicine, Chairman, Dr. R. H. Harper, Afton.

BANDAGING THE EYES AFTER GENERAL ANESTHESIA.

By J. Allen Jackson, M. D., Pathologist, Central Indiana Hospital for the Insane.

The bandaging of the eyes after general anesthesia is so very simple and the results obtained therefrom so gratifying as to warrant the bringing of the subject before the medical profession, with the idea in view that it may be further studied and at the same time act as a preventive against the most exhausting and deleterious effect of post operative vomiting.

Post operative vomiting may be divided into what may be called the essential vomiting and the vomiting due to other causes not well understood. By essential vomiting is meant the stomach emptying itself of the excess of mucus which accumulates there during the time of anesthesia. The cases of the second group are those in which, even though the stomach has been thoroughly emptied either with natural resources or artificial means, such as a stomach pump, vomiting still continues.

If, at the time the surgeon says "no more ether" you will carefully bandage the eyes, with small pieces of gauze over them to protect them (if irritated from ether, saturate pieces of boric acid solution) and allow the bandage to remain until the patient asks for it to be removed, you will find it very beneficial. How it acts is not understood.

During my service as surgical interne at the Philadelphia Hospital all of the cases under my care were subjected to this simple procedure. The summary of the results is as follows:

1. In all cases patients rested more quietly until consciousness was restored.

2. Vomiting only occurred in very few cases, and if it occurred the patient usually spat up a small amount of mucus and was not nauseated further.

3. Post operative vomiting in its truest sense was not encountered.

These few remarks and results are offered to those who are in a position to study the effects more fully with the hope of preventing this most disagreeable sensation as well as detrimental complication.
—Indianapolis Medical Journal.

OKLAHOMA PUBLIC HEALTH

The following resolution was adopted at the Kansas City meeting of the Medical Association of the Southwest with the request that State Secretaries give the matter wide publicity:

Whereas, The tendency of physicians and charitable organizations over the country is even now to send advanced, indigent consumptives from their homes to climatic resorts, notably parts of Texas, Colorado and the Southwest, and

Whereas, The consensus of opinion among the best authorities is that climate alone can not cure tuberculosis, and

Whereas, The boarding houses and hotels in many resorts no longer open their doors to this class of people, thereby depriving them of any chance of securing proper accommodation, and

Whereas, The sanitariums and eleemosynary institutions of the Southwest are already over burdened with such cases and the people are called upon to do double duty in that they must take care of others besides their own consumptives:

Therefore, Be It Resolved, That all states and territories throughout the country and all physicians and charitable organizations be urged to discourage the aimless drifting of the average consumptive, and that all advanced consumptives be kept within the confines of their own city, county, or state and the legislatures of the several states be urged to pass such laws as will insure the building and maintenance of sanitariums for curable cases and hospitals for advanced and incurable cases.

SUBSTITUTIONS AND ADULTERATIONS.

An extract from the report of State Drug Inspector, Mr. C. B. Bellamy, to Dr. J. C. Mahr, Commissioner of Health for Oklahoma, shows the following common substitutions to be practiced:

Salt Petre, adulterated with rock salt.

Olive oil, wholly without any trace of olive, artificially colored, adulterated with cotton seed oil.

Spices, practically every character, adulterated with wood and sand.

Turpentine is being shipped into Oklahoma, containing 40 per cent coal oil adulteration.

Linseed oil, without a trace of linseed, made from a rape seed.

Especial attention is called to the use of cheap imitation flavoring extracts being used by practically all bottling works in the state. These flavors are known to be injurious to health. These extracts are largely made from ether, chloroform and such injurious drugs.

The use of wood alcohol in the manufacture of iodine and bay rum by retail druggists is quite different in some of the smaller towns. Several confiscations have been made where the druggists professed ignorance of the pure food and drug act.

One of the most general abuses to be found is the disregard of the rule governing the mislabeling and branding of goods. Considerable difficulty has been experienced in impressing upon the minds of the druggists the absolute necessity of proper labeling the use of the word "Imitation" in plain letters on every label used on a substitute, being demanded in all cases.

OBITUARY.

DR. MASON F. WILLIAMS

Dr. Mason F. Williams was born in Louisville, Ky., February 18, 1851, and died in the Muskogee Hospital a few hours after operation for peritonitis following rupture of the gall bladder August 15, 1909.

Dr. Williams received the A. B. and A. M. degrees from Princeton, class of 1871, and graduated in medicine from the University of Louisville March 4th, 1876, spending most of his life after that time in the Indian Territory during which time he held many positions of trust and honor.

For several years he was pastor of the Presbyterian church in Muskogee and relinquished that position on account of his manifold duties in his professional field.

During his thirty years of active life in Muskogee he endeared himself to many people and his loss will be distinctly felt by the people, especially in the humbler walks of life to whom he was always a friend in need.

At various times he held the position of United States Pension Examiner, Physician to the United States jail, Physician to Henry Kendall College and was Secretary of the first United States Examining Board for the Western District of Indian Territory, which position he held until the advent of statehood. He was a member of the Muskogee City, Muskogee County, Oklahoma State and American Medical Associations.

A wife and one son, now a professor in Princeton, survive him to whom the sympathy of the medical profession of the state will be sincerely extended.

DR. ANTONIO D. YOUNG
Disease of the Mind and Nervous System
Security Building

Long Distance 'Phone 384-X.   OKLAHOMA CITY, OKLA.

J. M. TRIGG, M. D.
Surgery and Diseases of Women
Main and Bell Streets

Phone 194   SHAWNEE, OKLA.

DR. S. R. CUNNINGHAM
Practice Limited to
Surgery and Diseases of Women

Phone 158.   Main and Harvey.   OKLAHOMA CITY, OKLA.

OKLAHOMA PASTEUR INSTITUTE
Oklahoma City, Oklahoma
For the
Preventative Treatment of Hydrophobia
S. L. MORGAN, M. D., Director

1025 West Reno Ave.   L. D. Phone 3311

DR. E. S. LAIN
Practice Limited to Diseases of
Skin, X-Ray and Electro-Therapy

Indiana Building   Phones—Office 619, Residence 2828
Cor. First and Robinson Sts.   OKLAHOMA CITY

A. K. WEST, Internist   S. R. CUNNINGHAM, Surgeon
DRS. WEST & CUNNINGHAM
Consultants in
Internal Medicine and Surgery

Main and Harvey   Phone 158   OKLAHOMA CITY, OKLA.

DR. H. H. WYNNE
Oklahoma City, Okla.
EYE, EAR, NOSE AND THROAT
The Wynne Eye, Ear, Nose and Throat Hospital

Corner N. Broadway and Park Place—Take University' or N. Broadway Car Going
North.   Phone 2316
Down Town Office, 208 1-2 W. Main St.   Up Town Office, 107 W. Park
Opposite Scotts' Drug Store,   Place (just east of Broad-
Phone 3054   Circle).   Phone Black 2316

DR. RALPH V. SMITH

Surgeon

Phone No. 237   GUTHRIE, OKLAHOMA

Office Phone 8   Residence Phone 3
W. ALBERT COOK, M. D.
Practice Limited to
Eye, Ear, Nose and Throat
Glasses Fitted
308 and 309 First Natl. Bldg.

Hours 9 to 12—1:30 to 5   TULSA, OKLA.

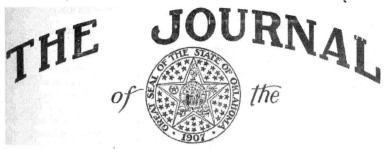

Oklahoma State Medical Association.

VOL. 2.   MUSKOGEE, OKLAHOMA, OCTOBER, 1909.   No. 5.

CLAUDE A. THOMPSON, Editor-in-Chief.

ASSOCIATE EDITORS AND COUNCILLORS.

DR. J. A. WALKER, Shawnee.   DR. JOHN W. DUKE, Guthrie.

DR. CHARLES R. HUME, Anadarko.   DR. A. B. FAIR, Frederick.

DR. F. R. SUTTON, Bartlesville.   DR. W. G. BLAKE, Tahlequah.

DR. G. W. ROBERTSON, Dustin.   DR. H. P. WILSON, Wynnewood.

DR. J. S. FULTON, Atoka.

Entered at the Postoffice at Muskogee, Oklahoma, as second class mail matter, June, 1909.

This is the Official Journal of the Oklahoma State Medical Association. All communications should be addressed to the Journal of the Oklahoma State Medical Association, English Block, Muskogee, Oklahoma.

DIFFUSE SUPPURATIVE PERITONITIS

BY A. L. BLESH. HORACE REED AND G. E. LEE, OKLAHOMA CITY, OKLAHOMA. MAY 14. 1909.

This disease existed and was recognized at a time far more remote than written records reach, evidences of it being found in mummies of a period antedating the Christian era by four thousand years. In all these ages, so remote that they can be grasped by the human mind only as shadow pictures, doubtless it presented the same deadly characteristics. The evolution of our understanding of it has progressed just in proportion as our minds have grasped its pathology and etiology and as it has been lifted from the realms of conjecture and mystery. With the banishing of the mystery of "idiopathic peritonitis" has come a clearer conception of the history and course of the disease and a more hopeful and justifiably optimistic view of the results of the rational application to it of surgical principles. We have, somewhat to our surprise, found that the peritoneal cavity might be considered. when infected with pus-forming organisms, as a large abscess and that it is amenable to treatment as such along well-recognized surgical lines; and that simplicity here, as everywhere else. is the key to progress. But, notwithstanding a clearer conception of the true pathogenesis of the disease. a bitter warfare of words has waged about its nomenclature. In this sense, perhaps. the use of the term "general peritonitis" to designate or describe the disease, in contra-distinction to localized or circumscribed peritonitis, has been unfortunate. There are those who sincerely believe that a case of "general peritonitis" is doomed and can never recover. If by this term it is understood that the entire surface of the peritoneum is involved, they are doubtless quite right, for this is most surely a terminal condition; it is end-pathology. Considering the enormous expanse of this membrane and its important functionating capacity, it might be as reasonable to suppose that a patient could recover whose entire cutaneous surface is thrown out of commission by a burn.

Then, there are those who believe just as sincerely that many, in fact, *most* of the cases of "general peritonitis" should recover, and do so, if proper surgical treatment is instituted. The misunderstanding seems to arise from a difference in definition, so it becomes necessary for us to define what we mean by "Diffuse Suppurative Peritonitis" before we proceed further. By diffuse suppurative peritonitis we shall be understood to mean that form of the disease against the advances of which Nature has placed no protecting barriers of adhesions, let the extent of the involvement of the peritoneum at the time of the operation, be large or small. This in contra-distinction to "circumscribed" or "localized" peritonitis in which such protecting barriers have been set up against the advancement of the disease, whether the area so involved is large or small. To illustrate: The writers have seen a "diffuse peritonitis" that involved as yet but a very small portion of the peritoneum, but it was truly of the "spreading" type, in that there were no protecting adhesions thrown about it. While, on the other hand, we have operated cases of "circumscribed peritonitis" that involved considerably over one-half of the abdominal cavity as a cavity, but which

were most truly "circumscribed" in that such protecting walls had been thrown about it. To the experienced surgeon it is no open question as to which of these two examples is the most dangerous to life and requires the greater skill and judgment on the part of the surgeon.

Again: A case which is at one time "diffuse" may in its progress become "circumscribed," just as a case which has been "circumscribed" may become "diffuse" by breaking through the barriers, and this process may go on through several repetitions, involving an ever-widening area. As a matter of fact, every case in its beginning is most likely "diffuse." Whether a case is to become circumscribed or not depends upon several factors which will be considered later.

CAUSES OF PERITONITIS.

As to the causes of peritonitis, we may consider that, speaking in a broad way, they are always infective, but with the so-called chemical variety we, as surgeons, have little to do.

The sources of infection are:

(a)   From some hiatus in the gastro-intestinal tube;

(b)   Hematogenous;

(c)   A breaking down of suppurating mesenteric glands fed from some extra abdominal source, as, for instance, suppurating inguinal glands;

(d)   In the female, through the genital tract.

Where the infection arises through or from the gastro-intestinal tract, the appendix is to blame in perhaps something over sixty (60) per cent. of the cases, so that the mortality of peritonitis must be reckoned largely as an appendicitis mortality —a sad reflection to those who deny timely surgical relief to those suffering from this disease. It has been demonstrated over and over again that the most virulent forms of infection of the peritoneum arise from the appendix perforations. This is in perfect harmony with the fact that the ilio-cecal region teems the most plentifully with pathogenic bacteria, and that they diminish both in virulence and numbers as we ascend or descend from this point. This is because of the stagnation of the fecal current at this point. Moving fluids do not offer as favorable conditions for the multiplication and growth of bacteria as do still pools. The fecal stream is here checked by the ilio-cecal valve and the sharp angulation between the ilium and colon.

Perforation of the stomach, duodeum and gall bladder in the normal state would not give rise to an infective peritonitis. But in all pathological perforations of these organs (those due to ulcers of the stomach and duodenum and to gall stones), they are not in a normal state and are themselves the seat of infected processes although of a less virulent nature than those of the appendiceal region. In those cases where, upon operation, the atrium of infection cannot be demonstrated, it is not fair to assume that such an atrium does not exist, for, if the perforation be due to tubercular ulceration, it may be so minute as to escape detection. Also, the destruction of the epithelial lining will act, so far as the transmission of germs is concerned, as would an opening through all the coats. Perforating typhoid ulcers come in for a fair share of the blame and owing to the typhoid state are frequently undiagnosed, or, diagnosed too late to be of surgical value.

The female genital tract offers an open doorway to the peritoneal cavity, which is responsible for a percentage (rather small) of the cases. That this percentage is small is due to the fact that absorption from this region is not active and that it is favorably situated for localization. So, while

circumscribed peritonitis is very common from this source, the diffuse form is rather exceptional.

It would be impossible to estimate correctly the number of cases for which infected mesenteric glands might be justly held responsible, or for those of hematogenous origin. However, as compared to the total number, they are probably inconsiderable.

The special infections, as the pneumococcus* and the gono-coccus, it will not be within the sphere of this paper to elaborately discuss. Suffice it to say that so far as the pneumo-coccus type of peritonitis is concerned, it is extremely probable that the route of infection may be either by the blood stream, or locally, through the primae viae, but that it is most frequently the latter; that it occurs most often in children; that its most probable source, especially in children, is locally through the gastro-intestinal tract and at its greatest point of vulnerability—the appendix region. This is true in our opinion and is also in accordance with the results of our observation, because of the fact that a child rarely ever expectorates material from the respiratory tract, whether normal or pathologic. Very often, central pneumonias are not diagnosed in the beginning of the attack, and if the consolidation does not approach the lung surface, not at all.

Again, this type of pneumonia not infrequently involves the diaphragm before it does the parietal pleura, hence it is possible to have extension to the peritoneum by continuity. What secretion is raised by the child is immediately swallowed, mixed with a mucuous secretion. This substance coats the stomach and bowels with its tenacious substance and is passed along, alive

---

*The pneumo-coccus plays so varied a pathological role in the surgical sense that it is our purpose later to prepare a special paper on this subject.

as it is with pneumo-cocci, until some vulnerable point is reached, where it takes hold.

A case illustrating this method of infection with operative and bacteriologic findings is here appended.

CASE: A. A., male child, aged 7. Family history negative; personal history: When a little child had "bowel complaint" of a chronic nature; has had several attacks of bronchitis.

Present attack began one week ago with vomiting and looseness of the bowels of a diarrhoeaic nature, and pain in the abdomen. This pain in the course of a few days localized itself quite definitely over the appendix. Temperature ranged from 99 degrees to 102 degrees; pulse from 100 to 120; nausea and vomiting continuous. Physical examination revealed nothing definite in chest. Operated December 24th, 1907, through a one-inch grid-iron incision. Appendix deeply injected and inflamed, but, upon section, showed no pus. Microscope showed pneumo-cocci in abundance with a few colon bacilli. Twenty-four hours after operation a frank pneumonia of the left lung was manifest. This appeared so suddenly and was so extensive as to preclude the supposition that it had developed within the preceding twenty-four hours. It probably existed as a central pneumonia at the time of the operation and for several days before, for the patient began within a few days after the operation to expectorate pus in large quantities. This case illustrates the route of infection. Query: Are not many of our cases of so-called pneumonia really a localized pneumo-coccic peritonitis. Pneumo-coccic peritonitis may also be either diffuse or localized in type.

The gonorrhoeal form may also be carried locally or through the blood, probably most often by the former. It more often gives rise to localized forms because of the slowness and semi-chronicity of its progress. It is rarely fatal in prognosis.

PHYSIOLOGY OF THE PERITONEUM.

The physiology of the peritoneum, so far as it relates to absorption, has a great deal to do with the treatment of peritonitis, and should be briefly considered in order to comprehend the value of the mechanics involved, for to the writers' minds this resolves itself largely into a problem of physics. This problem is surprising in its simplicity. The idea that the peritoneum is supplied with so-called inter-cellular stomata, through which and by which absorption occurs, has been disproved by Muscatello and others, and they have further demonstrated that this absorptive surface consists of a net-work of lymphatics which underlie the peritoneum, and that this network is, for all practical purposes, limited to the diaphragmatic peritoneum. The rapidity with which absorption occurs is surprising and there are other, perhaps several, factors, concerned in it which are not as yet fully understood, but into which phagocytosis enters as an important element. As to time, it has been demonstrated that particles of carmine may be recovered from the thoracic duct seven minutes after injection into the free peritoneal cavity.

The physiological scheme of absorption holds true and dominant sway only for the normal peritoneum, but we have this factor plus another—the blood vessels in the abraded peritoneum. Every inflamed peritoneum is in a positive sense an abraded peritoneum in that its natural defense, the endothelial cells, are put out of commission, i. e., there is a break in the continuity of the protecting endothelial lining.

The physiological absorptive areas of the peritoneal cavity are principally the diaphragm and the mesentery. The lymphatic net-work which lies beneath the peritoneum sends its projections from behind forward into the mesenteric folds. The diaphragm, from the moment of birth to that of death, is never at rest. This muscular activity has much to do with the circulation, especially, in the passive vessels, such as lymphatics and veins. This enters as an important factor in peritoneal absorption of pathologic elements, and in peritonitis it is important to bear in mind constantly that in peritonitis it is absorption (of toxins and bacteria—toxemia and bacteremia) that destroys life. The mechanical principle is the same, whether this absorption occurs through stomata, in accordance with the views of Von Recklinghausen, or by phagocytosis, which is more in harmony with the views of Muscatello, or the still later investigations of McCallum, who believes that the permeation may be intercellular. The factor in absorption that we as surgeons are mostly concerned with is, that, however it takes place, it is in and through the upper zone. Absorption is favored by:

(1) Position (gravity);

(2) Peristalsis;

(3) Muscular activity, especially of the diaphragm, and intestinal peristalsis.

(4) Mechanical and chemical insult; prolonged operative interference involving much exposure and manipulation;

(5) Peritoneal abrasion (operative—accidental or incidental);

(6) Pressure (as of contained fluids);

(7) The removal (operative) of protecting fibrin.

It follows naturally that the converse holds true in preventing or limiting absorption, and this knowledge is the key to successful operative interference. The application of these principles will be considered in the treatment. Alonzo Clark had more than a modicum of truth in his "opium treatment," and if the patient survived the first period of toxemia, recoveries were not infrequent.

Great as is the name of Lawson Tait, it is our most sincere conviction that the dogma of the "saline treatment," which by his powerful personality and genius he so deeply impressed upon the professional mind of his time, has been the means of retarding the rational evolution in the treatment of this disease at least fifteen years. So mighty has been the influence of his name that even now men depart from his teachings with fear and trembling. When the medical history of this generation is finally written the names of Murphy, Ochsner, Fowler and Clark will occupy a high position.

DIAGNOSIS.

At the outset let us understand that to wait for the classical clinical picture is to await terminal conditions and an endpathology, death having already set his seal upon the patient. Indeed the old book picture of peritonitis is but that of lethal toxemia. The symptoms in order of importance are:

First—*Pain.* This is at first, as a rule, diffuse, later localized about the point of attack, to become again diffuse later in the course of the disease. It is sharp and lancinating, especially in the beginning, when it reaches its acme with the peristaltic wave.

Second—*Increase in pulse rate.* With change in the character of the pulse. Pulse becomes more tense and wiry.

Third—*Nausea and vomiting.* This appears, as a rule, early. At first, the vomitus is stomach content; later, bilious, and finally, may be stercoraceous.

Fourth—*Muscular rigidity.* This is characteristic and in a fairly reliable manner maps out the area involved.

Fifth—*Intestinal paresis.* This manifests itself by a practically absolute colpo-stasis and is at times difficult to differentiate from mechanical obstruction, for which it is not seldom mistaken.

Sixth—*Tympanitis.* This is dependent upon intestinal paresis and is more or less late in appearing in the sequence. For the early diagnosis an increasing leucocytosis with an ascending pulse rate and the local syndrome more or less present should be accepted as the most reliable indication.

ATYPICAL CASES.

Practically all the cases in this class have to do with a visceral peritonitis in which the parietal peritoneum is not involved. Those cases in which the parietal peritoneum is not involved are characterized by the absence of the severe type of pain and muscular rigidity. The remaining portion of the syndrome is the same.

TREATMENT.

Death in peritonitis, as indicated above, is due to toxemia, and the mortality bears a direct ratio to absorption. On this hypothesis the treatment, to be effective, must be based. It has been conclusively demonstrated that the upper or diaphragmatic peritoneum absorbs very rapidly. Even bacteria placed in the region of the diaphragm are soon found in the circulation. Also, it is known that the absorption from the lower, particularly the pelvic peritoneum, is slow. Then it naturally follows that we should bend our efforts toward keeping the toxic material away as far as possible from the region of the diaphragm, and pay little attention to those parts where its presence does little harm. In the so-called Fowler position this end is accomplished. It is not sufficient that the shoulders alone be propped up, but the whole trunk should be elevated to an angle of at least 45 degrees. It has been shown that unless at least this angle is reached that the lumbar spaces will not be drained into the pelvis and the absorbing surface will be thereby increased.

The time to begin the use of Fowler's position is immediately, that is, as soon as the diagnosis is made. We will go further and suggest that it should be used in anticipation of spreading peritonitis. To this end we now advise that the patients having localized infections of the peritoneal cavity should be placed in a chair; a cab as a conveyance from station to hospital is preferable to the ambulance stretcher. Bearing in mind that every moments delay in instituting an upright position means an increased supply of toxins in the circulation, action must be prompt and continuous. It is not enough that the patient sit up twenty-three out of the twenty-four hours, for in a few moments time, with the diaphragm bathed in bacterial toxins, sufficient poison may be absorbed to turn the tide against the patient. This point is vividly illustrated in the following case:

L. I., aged 60, while lifting a large stone into a wagon box, allowed it to slip. Falling, it struck him on the abdomen. Pain was immediate and terrific and the shock so great he could not walk. He was found some two hours later by some neighbors. He was pale, was bathed with cold perspiration, and vomiting. Was seen three days later by surgeon in consultation with attending physician. The entire abdomen was rigid and distended. There was apparent fluctuation in the left lower quadrant. Vomiting has been persistent, but was now under control by large doses of morphine. Tongue dry and brown; pulse wiry at 120; temperature 98 degrees.

Under primary ether anaesthetization two rubber tube drains were inserted; one in the pelvis, the other in the left lumbar space. Pus of a foul odor and under such great tension that it spurted at least eighteen inches above the patient, was found when the peritoneum was incised. Operation consumed not to exceed five minutes.

Patient was returned to bed and placed in Fowler position, pulse 118. Within six hours pulse dropped to 100 and never went above that for over forty-eight hours. The hypocratic facies was supplemented by a bright, cheerful expression. About two days following operation, in spite of positive instructions of the surgeon to the contrary, the nurse allowed the patient to lie down. And according to the chart, which the nurse herself kept, the patient became immediately worse and died in two days more—toxaemia—from simple failure of the nurse to maintain the Fowler position.

There are indeed difficulties in the way of maintaining the sitting posture. This is particularly so in bed. The patient will grumble and unless closely watched will slip down, leaving only the shoulders elevated. Special contrivances for avoiding this difficulty have been described, but we cannot always have one at hand when most needed. As a makeshift, we have found the old-fashioned high-backed rockers answer well. The chair can be well padded and blocks placed under the rockers to prevent rocking. This contrivance has the distinct advantage that is found in almost every home.

The sitting posture should be maintained until the septic material becomes localized and sufficient adhesions have formed to prevent its escape. Just how long in any individual case this will require it is impossible to say. We have found that in the average case it will take from five to seven days. It may, however, require a much longer time, and rarely, a shorter.

Next to position in limiting absorption, comes rest. It would be useless to set the patient up, endeavoring to protect the upper zone of the peritoneum, if the bowels were in a continuous state of peristalsis. Peristalsis must be controlled. To this end, food and drink must be prohibited. To allay the intense thirst sips of hot water only are allowable.

How long must food be withheld? What has been said as to the time the sitting posture should be maintained is equally true in answer to this question? We have had patients that went from seven to ten (7 to 10) days without food of any description by mouth.

When should the bowels be opened? Not until the patient has recovered. In this respect practice Ochsner's dictum—"Masterly Inactivity." This is a hard concession for some physicians to make, and particularly so for the patient's friends, but a mistake is always made when a physic is given during an active peritoneal involvement, either local or diffuse.

As a further control of peristalsis we do not hesitate to use morphine. Restlessness—a tossing patient—is not conducive to localization of free septic material within the peritoneal cavity, and we have found it a universal necessity to use morphine.

Contrary to the statements of others, we have not been misled by the freedom from pain experienced by the patient, and the apparent improvement in the general condition, and the mild cardiac stimulation produced, giving a false sense of security leading to "dangerous" delay, by the judicious use of opium. The intelligent physician understands the action of opium and should not let a fear of his memory lapsing stand in the way of his administering to his patient a drug the indication of which is so apparent as in peritonitis.

PROCTOCLYSIS.

The process of absorption having been checked so far as it is within our power to do so, we now direct our attention to measures producing elimination of toxins already accumulated. This is accomplished by virtually washing the blood stream. To Murphy of Chicago belongs the credit of having popularized the method termed "proctoclysis." The modus operandi by which it accomplishes such marked results is now definitely known. Large quantities of salines will be absorbed by the colon and in a remarkably short time. Murphy reports a case of a child eleven years of age who retained thirty pints in twenty-four hours. It is contended and easily demonstrated that the average adult will absorb through the colon during the first twenty-four hours an average of one pint per hour. This fluid is not all stored up in the lymphatics and blood vessels without taking the place of something else. The fact is that within a few hours after the flow of the saline begins, all the avenues of elimination are opened up: The skin is bathed in perspiration; the kidneys act freely: the dry, brown tongue becomes moist and the pinched expression gives way to one of brightness and relief.

DESCRIPTION OF METHOD.

"The best plan is to place a pint and a half of the saline solution in the container every two hours. The container should be elevated sufficiently to allow all this to flow into the rectum in forty to sixty minutes, giving the rectum a period of rest from the income of fresh fluids approximately an hour before it flows again."

The best device thus far described for this purpose is a fountain syringe, the nozzle being the ordinary vaginal type which has been bent upon itself so that the angle formed is not greater than 130 degrees. The greatest difficulty we have encountered in administration is the tendency in attendants to raise the syringe too high. With the great pressure the fluid rushes into the bowel and by over-extension peristalsis is stimulated, with the result—expulsion of the fluid, soiled linen, and disgusted patient. There never should be

more than fifteen inches hydro-static pressure, and more often four to six inches is the amount used. The tube leading from the container should not be constricted but free and open. In case of over-distention or irritation which would cause the patient to strain the fluid should be free to pass back into the container.

The tube should be strapped to the patient's buttocks or thigh and not removed unless it should become obstructed. The fluid may be kept warm by placing water bottles around it. Proctoclysis should be kept up from two to four days. The solution used is plain salt—one (1) dram to one pint of water; or, salt and calcium chloride of each one dram to the pint. Gastric lavage is of value in the cases of persistent vomiting and should be practiced. Such patients experience a sense of relief following stomach washing.

OPERATION.

Diffuse suppurative peritonitis is essentially a surgical disease. There are, however, difficulties to be met requiring rare judgment and skill. When to operate is the first question. For this there can be no hard and fast rule. Murphy operates as soon as he sees the patient. All his reported cases were seen rather early. When closely questioned as to what he would do in cases seen at a later stage of the disease, he replied: "It is useless to operate on those already dead." We believe in early operations under certain conditions, that is, in all cases of known perforations in which the opening would likely be so large as to allow the escape of faeces into the abdominal cavity, also in cases in which the clinical picture and the differential blood count indicates sufficient resistance in the patient to withstand the additional toxemia and shock incident to the operation. The latter class could be treated tentatively but their convalescence will be more sure and they will be less liable to have post-operative obstructions if the abdomen is drained before multiple dense adhesions are formed. We do not believe in immediately operating these cases who have all but the lethal dose of toxins. This class is usually seen late and have not, as a rule, had treatment as suggested under the first part of this heading. The abdomen is usually greatly distended and the muscles boardlike in their hardness. Tenderness on pressure is universal, in fact, these cases are approaching the end and correspond to the classical clinical picture of peritonitis as described in antedated clinical text books. To operate these cases in this condition means to hasten death. The blood count may or may not be of assistance in this class. If the toxemia of the patient, as indicated by the clinical picture, is profound, and the differential is not correspondingly high, it usually indicates that the resisting quality of the blood is paralyzed or at least greatly reduced. The operation, however, skilfully done, means an additional raw surface through which it may be only a small amount of toxins will be absorbed yet in sufficient quantity to turn the tide against the patient. For such conditions the treatment has been described under the head of elimination. In our report of cases, which follows, may be seen what results followed this line of treatment. We have seen the lower two-thirds of the abdominal cavity converted into an abscess sac which had the appearance before operation of a marked case of ascites. Then it follows there are two classes of cases in a surgical sense:

First: Those operated when first seen.

Second: Those operated after the toxemia has been reduced and the general process converted by the treatment into a local one.

To operate, the patient must be retained in the sitting or reclining posture. When operating the first class a general anaesthetic is required. Rigidity of abdominal muscles is not conducive to rapidity of technic in operating. Under local anaesthesia rigidity is always present. In no other field of surgery can the operator do too much so easily. He must be quick and must not do more than absolutely necessary. Newly formed adhesions should be respected. The operation simply consists in opening the abdomen, closing the perforation, putting in rubber tube drainage, either single or multiple, one of which should always drain the pelvis. As Murphy says: "Get in quick and get out quicker."

In the second class are those in which the process has been localized, single or multiple drains may be inserted through incisions made under local anaesthesia without moving the patient from his bed or chair. The after treatment differs in no way from the pre-operative, that is, salines are continued and food withheld until the process has sufficiently subsided and the abdomen becomes flat and soft.

Finally, there are cases which completely recover without operation. We believe these to be exceptional.

Further than this we have no remarks.

PATHOLOGY OF PERITONITIS.

Foreword: After the surgical principles of the present treatment of peritonitis had become well mastered there arose quite a question as regards the value of the laboratory findings in this class of cases as an aid to the knowledge of when would be the most opportune time to operate. At first those who laid most stress upon the value of laboratory findings and depended less upon their clinical judgment, finally began to condemn the laboratory findings. This state of affairs has existed is nearly all else that has had any laboratory connections.

Formerly, when the presence of a leucocytosis was found quite high and there was coupled with it the clinical phases and symptoms of a diffuse peritonitis, then much stress was laid upon the presence of a marked leucocytosis, as regards prognosis. When the leucocyte count was found quite high—20,000 to 30,000—some claimed that the operation should not be delayed except when there was a rapidly ascending leucocytosis, then it was thought best to wait until the leucocytes became stationary or falling. This state of affairs soon became unpopular, as is quite obvious from observing its incompleteness. The most important factor, namely, percentage of polynuclears, not having been as yet taken into consideration. Later, some few very able men called attention to this important fact, and since that time the value of the finding of the absolute and relative leucocytosis has become an important factor in the complete intelligent diagnosis and treatment of diffuse peritonitis.

Technic: So very few men have worked along this line, that, without apology, we shall give a few words as regards the method of procedure. When we are shown the patient, he is propped up, or being brought to the hospital in a sitting posture. After the cleansing of the lobe of the ear, a short deep incision is made, one that will flow freely without having to be expressed. Then the "white" pipette is filled with blood to the .5 mark then with a diluting fluid (3 per cent acetic in distilled water, with a sufficient quantity of pyoktannin to stain the nuclei of the corpuscles), and is drawn up to the 11. mark. When the laboratory is reached, the counting

chamber (Tuerk's) is prepared and, first, the total of all leucocytes is obtained, then the same fields are again gone over carefully, but only the polynuclears are counted this second time. These, divided by the total number, gives the percentage of polynuclears in the external circulation. This method, as to obtaining the percentage, has carefully been checked against the counting on the stained slide for the percentage, for over a year, with the result that this has been adopted as the most accurate method. This method also corresponds most closely with the clinical phases and symptoms and is more reliable for prognosis.

LABORATORY FINDINGS AND PROGNOSIS.

If we find a markedly increasing leucocytosis, 18,000 to 25,000, and 89 per cent to 93 per cent polynuclears, he is not operated until such time as the absolute leucocytosis has increased and the relative leucocytosis has diminished, or both. But should the patient have a comparatively highly absolute and a low relative, or equal leucocytosis, he is safely considered as being:

(a) One who has built up a resistance; or,

(b) One whose infection is not of such a virulent type but that he can endure a rapid operation for drainage and yet recover.

This is a safe rule and there are but few exceptions when he has a fibrinous fibro-purulent or purulent process. Should he have, however, septic peritonitis, neither the leucocyte estimation nor much else will avail. Then one's clinical judgment is depended on quite heavily in order to save the patient in any instance.

The above refers to the cases in particular that are pneumococcic or streptococcic in origin, and strictly to septic peritonitis

Absolute   Relative

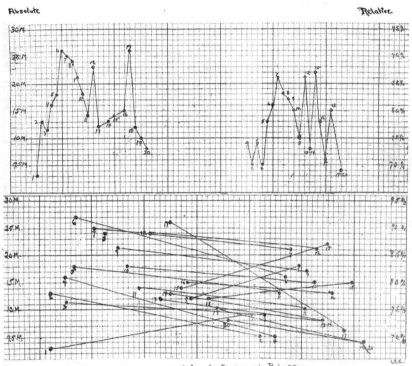

Upper chart compares variation in Absolute and Relative.
Lower chart compares Absolute Leucocytosis with corresponding Relative Leucocyte count.

Case No. 828   Class No. I

CLASSIFICATION OF CASES.

In the following classification we have attempted to keep as much as possible all similar cases under one heading.

Class 1. Diffuse, purulent plastic peritonitis. The chart (Class No. 1) selected to represent this class of cases shows on the first count (1) a rising line that is

terial. The cases selected to represent this class are:

(a) Streptococic.

(b) Pneumococcic.

There is little of importance in this class of cases except to note that we have a rapidly progressive process that terminates fatally in the majority of instances. Those working for statistics alone leave out this

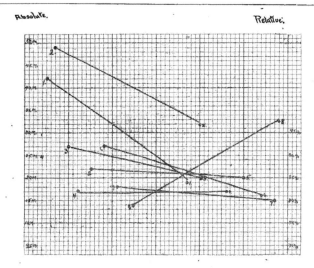

Absolute.   Relative.

Case No. 1108   Class No. II

a higher relative than absolute leucocytosis, hence pre-operative treatment was continued for twenty-four hours, when No. 2 revealed the opposite to the preceding.

Allow us here to digress enough to state that the clinical chart did not show this gain in increased resistance until later. It is noticed that in this group of cases we have, except rarely, a higher absolute leucocytosis than relative.

Class 2. Virulent septic peritonitis without appreciable plastic or purulent ma-

group entirely. It is to be hoped that in the future we will have success in dealing with this class of cases when we make an anti-serum from the patient's own particular srtain of coccidial infection. The worst feature, however, in these foudroyant cases is the lamentable lack of time to institute and carry out any line of treatment.

Class 3. Gangrenous appendix with early peritonitis and tubercular peritonitis. In this group the classification is given, not because of any similarity in either the bacteriological or pathological findings, but because of the striking similarity of the range of leucocytosis, both absolute and relative, when the charts of these two conditions are compared. In this group we have a comparative straight or falling line as regards the relative compared with the absolute leucocytosis.

This refers only to conditions recognized as such and operated early.*

abdominal cavity. The visceral is that part which is reflected over nearly all of the abdominal organs as well as the uppermost portions of the pelvic organs, except in the female, the fimbrae of the fallopian tubes. The peritoneum externally contains small branches of lymphatics, nerves and minute blood capillaries within loose, areolar white fibrous connective tissue. Overlaying this are endothelial cells. Given, an insult such

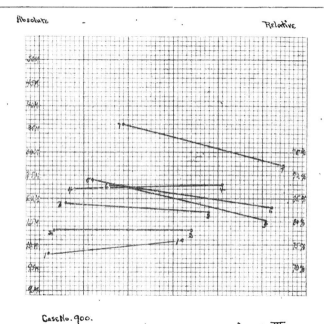

Absolute   Relative

Case No. 900.   Class No III.

HISTO-PATHOLOGY OF THE PERITONEUM.

The peritoneum is a closed sac. The parietal portion of which walls the entire

*The charts that we use are taken as an arbitrary standard and were decided on as a working basis, first by Charles L. Gibson of New York. The figures, however, were all supplies by our own findings, also the classification is entirely our own and is so arranged for brevity only.

as microbic invasion, or trauma; the well-known processes of inflammation become established. There is first a stasis of the blood capillaries, causing the dark bluish condition seen on opening the abdomen. This causes an exudation and invasion of lymph and microbes and their toxins, either or both, into the peritoneal cavity. There is also squeezed out from the blood capillaries themselves an immense number of polynuclears. The more of these phagocytic elements the better is the prognosis, provided that trypsin or some other chemically inhibiting material is not present; because of the fact that when we have a thick viscid process of sufficient specific gravity the largest amount of the toxic material can be carried mechanically (position and drainage) to the lower portion of the abdomen where there is far less danger of rapid absorption.

BACTERIOLOGIC FINDINGS.

When the peritonitis is caused from a gangrenous process or from intestinal perforation or both, the principal factors we have to deal with, are—B. Col. Communis,' and B. Pyocyaneous, unless we have a perforation from' B. Entericus. In the event of such a process, should the patient, either during or later, have an added infection from Staphylococcus albus, his chances for recovery will be greatly enhanced because of the fact, first, increased presence of polynuclears and the large amount of pus cells subsequently formed.

Should the patient have a peritonitis caused from pneumococcus or streptococus there is a marked lack of plastic or fibrous exudation. The serum normally formed in the peritoneum, together with the amount added because of the presence of these germs, is a most favorable inducement for the rapid proliferation and spreading of these most virulent types of infection.

Tubercular peritonitis is of no great interest here, but is most markedly deserving of mention. The etiologic factors here as well as the subsequent pathologic changes are quite similar to those of the pathology of tuberculosis elsewhere.

We often find on opening the abdomen no discernible cause for the peritonitis that is so manifestly present; this, formerly, was termed *idiopathic peritonitis.* Very rarely we have been able to find minute ulcerative patches which have eroded from some portion of the bowel through the parietal peritoneum.

ANIMAL EXPERIMENTS.

Our older writers have carried out some very interesting experiments as regards the induction in animals artificially of peritonitis by using different chemical and microbic cultures. The most important of these that can be mentioned is trypsin. Pawlowsky introduced trypsin in varying quantities, together with bacteria of different degrees of virulence, through a series of forty-one animals, with the result that when trypsin was added in any considerable amount the virulence of bacteria and its toxins was not inhibited, but that all efforts on the part of Nature to wall off by fibrinous exudates, or to otherwise inhibit the progressive process, signally failed. Other experiments more or less interesting have been carried out by very able men. One bacteriologic experiment that is worthy of mention is, that on injecting Staphylococcus albus, an appreciable exudate occurs that is markedly tinged with Hemoglobin as well as the red blood corpuscles themselves.

It has been considered by very able authorities that when we have a mixed infection the presence of staphylococcus albus tends to enhance the chances for recovery. The theory for this contention is that there is an increased stimulus to phagyocytosis. Streptococcic infection is highly virulent in peritonitis, while gonococcic infection is not. One very able English authority contends that we need in all cases a polyvalent anti-baccillus coli serum. The most important questions as to the harmlessness of drainage is—have you left raw surfaces around the exit or have you injured important tissues or vessels within the abdomen?

Peritonitis (septic) may be caused by pathogenic microbes which, at present at least, are not classified as such.

Peritonitis (suppurative) cannot exist, however, without at least an infection mixed with pyogenic bacteria. In most cases of septic peritonitis pyogenic bacteria can be demonstrated.

CASE REPORT.

Case 1. E. B., merchant, aged 36. Was taken Saturday night at ten o'clock with intense abdominal pain, soon followed by nausea and vomiting. The following morning pain was localized at McB.'s point and patient had fever. About 3 P. M. Monday pain became suddenly severe and diffuse At 7 P. M. same day patient was found tossing on his bed. He had a pinched expression, abdomen very rigid and tender. Temperature 100 degrees; pulse 90 and wiry. Morphine, 1-4 gr. hypo, had failed to control pain and restlessness.

Treatment: Patient placed in barber's chair. Salines by bowel. Morphine qs. to control pain and restlessness. One week later was brought to hospital, sitting in barber's chair from which he had not been removed from the first. Eight days from time treatment was instituted operation was performed; it consisted in evacuation of the abscess which filled the pelvis. Convalescence from this time rapid. Discharged from hospital in three weeks, well.

Case 2. C. B. W., hotel keeper, aged 37. Attack began April 30 at 8:00 P. M., with pain in abdomen so intense in character it required morphine, hypo, for relief. Nauseau was present and at 11 P. M. had fever. May 1, fever continues and pain localized at McB.'s point; refused to enter hospital at this time. May 2d, pain again became diffuse, followed in rapid succession by vomiting, abdominal distention and hiccough. In this condition was taken to hospital; pulse 118, temperature

96. Pinched expression. Treatment as above. May 12th, under local anaesthesia, large amount of foul smelling fluid and pus evacuated. For this operation patient was not removed from his position in bed. Subsequently, at intervals of from one to three weeks, localized abscesses were evacuated in like manner. During this time patient developed fecal fistulas. These eventually closed spontaneously within six months. Since which time there has been no further trouble.

This case was very interesting and the blood count, as shown in the pathological part of this paper, was very interesting and instructive.

Case 3. H. G., aged 21, grocery clerk. Eight months previous had abdominal abscess, which being opened through left flank, drained for six weeks. August 14th pain began in abdomen; diffuse; nauseated; abdomen rigid; pulse 110; temperature 99 degrees; treatment as above.

Operation on the following day, evacuation of large quantity of sero-purulent matter; tube drain in right flank and pelvis. Was able to be out of room in four weeks; returned to hospital October 12th and had stump of appendix removed, since which time he has been free from trouble.

Case 4. A. V., aged 14; entered hospital August 3rd with ——— sysmptoms of peritonitis acute. Four days previous began with pain in right side, followed in rapid succession by vomiting and fever. Pain spreading and in twenty-four hours was diffuse. Patient cyanotic and pulse bad, abdomen greatly distended. Under regular treatment had improved and the operation was performed August 6th. Pelvis and right flank drained with separate tube drains. Three days later, August 9th, abdomen was soft and flat; patient feeling good, when he suffered a severe hemorrhage through one of the drainage tracts, a recurrence of same, August 11th, resulted in death.

Case 5. F. F. F. Entered hospital with symptoms of bowel obstruction of three days' standing; pain from the beginning paroxysmal in character. Temperature ranged from normal to 99. On entering hospital it was 99 and pulse 78. Abdomen greatly distended and sensitive to pressure over entire area. Greatest distension on the right side. Free fluid could be demonstrated. Operated immediately, incision through right rectus. Large quantity of sero-purulent fluid escaped. Adhesions throughout general cavity undisturbed; greatest trouble apparently in appendiceal region; its removal could not be accomplished without too great a disturbance of the numerous adhesions and it was let alone. Two drains, one in right flank, and the other in pelvis completed the operation. Patient was discharged in three weeks, drainage tracts all but closed.

Case 6. L. I. Reported in body of paper illustrating effects of treatment.

Case 7. F. M. G., aged 55, carpenter. Had trouble in region of appendix for twelve or fifteen years. Two days previous to entering hospital was taken with colicky pains in right side. In addition to these symptoms had had fever; rigid, retracted abdomen and general tenderness over entire area, with exception of small part of upper left zone. Operated immediately. Appendix found perforated in middle portion and large quantity of pus free in abdominal cavity. Peritoneum injected. Appendix removed; two drains, region of appendix and pelvis. Patient discharged in 24 days.

Case 8. William J. M., aged 16; farmer boy. Trouble began July 2nd, with pain in abdomen; nausea and diarrhoea. Family physician called two days later and found patient with temperature of 101 degrees.

pulse 120; distended abdomen. Tenderness diffuse; dry, brown tongue; occasional vomiting, fecal in character. Brought to hospital in sitting posture.

Treatment: Fowler's position; starvation; salines by bowel and morphine for pain; gastric lavage. July 14th, three large abscesses evacuated and drained, one drain in flank, and the other in the pelvis; discharged August 31st, wound still slightly discharged; patient in good condition.

Case 9. A. D., aged 17, farmer. Was injured over abdomen by fall on pommel of saddle, and for several days following had diffuse abdominal pain, but not severe. After one week suddenly became worse; abdomen tender and hard. Large amount of morphine required for relief of pain. Pulse 108, temperature 101; pinched expression, tongue dry, brown, and breath foul. Operated immediately. Incision through rectus; large amount of sero-purulent fluid escaped when perineum was opened. Peritoneum injected. No points of rupture discernible; pelvic drain. Patient returned to bed and regular treatment begun. Improvement steady, discharged in three weeks.

Case 10. G. G., aged 11, school girl. Had more or less abdominal pain for one week; pain finally settled in region of appendix; on the train coming to hospital, pain became more severe; on entering hospital patient very much exhausted; abdomen greatly distended, diffuse tenderness. Temperature 102 degrees, pulse 130; usual treatment in Fowler position; improvement prompt. Two days later, drainage instituted. On opening perineal cavity pus gushed out, escaping from free cavity. Usual pelvic and flank drainage.

Condition improved for two days when pericarditis suddenly developed and the patient died the following day.*

*This was a case of pure pneumo-coccic peritonitis.

Case 11. F. B. T., aged 27. Began 48 hours ago with severe, diffuse, abdominal pain and vomiting, some fever. At present abdomen is distended, tenderness diffuse; pulse 74; temperature 98 degrees; operated immediately. Free pus in cavity. Pelvic and flank drainage. Regular treatment began after the operation. Recovery prompt. Discharged in two weeks—wound still draining.

Case 12. School girl, aged 8. Was seen in home in consultation with attending physician. Five days before patient seized with severe pain at McB.'s point, followed by the usual appendicitis syndrome. Within 48 hours this pain had subsided, with evidence of localization. Twenty-four hours later she was again attacked with severe abdominal pain, diffuse in character, with general rigidity and tenderness; an increasing pulse frequency; temperature ranging from 99 to 101. This was followed by progressive tympanitis and coprostasis. When seen by the consultant, pulse was 105, temperature 99 degrees and the facies indicative of peritonitis. Abdomen very much distended. General rigidity; sensitive all over, in short, a typical case of peritonitis, involving a large area, evidently arising from a rupture of appendiceal abscess which had been clearly defined by attending physician previous to second attack of pain.

No operation. Regular treatment instituted, resulting in complete disappearance of all symptoms in two weeks.

Case 13. F. C. H., aged 39, druggist. Had had five previous attacks, diagnosed appendicitis. Present attack began in typical manner. At the end of three days, while being given an enema was suddenly seized with severe pain in the region of McB.'s point which rapidly became diffuse. Circulation somewhat embarrassed and respiration reached 40 and was shallow. Twen-

ty-four hours later was seen by consultant who found conditions as follows:

Abdomen presented general rigidity. Considerable tympanitis, most marked over right side; pulse 92; temperature 99 degrees.

Treatment: Fowler's position, salines by bowel, morphine. Seven days later was brought to hospital in sitting posture; condition at entrance, process well localized in lower abdomen. Operation. Drainage. Appendix not removed. Recovery uneventful. Discharged in 12 days. Drainage tract not quite closed.

Case 15. Mrs. R., aged 38. Began with intense abdominal pain. Vomiting; sub-normal temperature; rapid pulse. Entered hospital three days later in what appeared to be hopeless condition. Temperature, sub-normal; pulse rapid; skin cold; abdomen greatly distended; rigid; patient stupid. Operation advised against.

Treatment: Postural; no food or drink. Morphine for restlessness and pain; strychnine for the heart. Conditions remained practically unchanged for three days longer, when patient began to show signs of improvement. At the end of one week free fluid could be demonstrated in the abdomen. Operation advised at this time, but refused. Improvement continued, all the symptoms gradually abating until at the end of three weeks they had all disappeared and patient was discharged.

RESUME.

1. Peritonitis of the diffuse suppurating type has from time immemorial been recognized as one of the most fatal diseases, and treatment, before, and for many years after, the dawning of the surgical era had little, if any, effect upon its frightful mortality.

2. The use of the term "general peritonitis" to designate the disease in question has given rise to misunderstanding and

controversy because it does not convey a true clinical conception. The idea conveyed by this term is that the whole of the peritoneal surface is involved in the process—a condition almost, if not quite, impossible in a living subject. Hence it is that many brilliant surgeons deny the possibility of recovery, a view which from such a standpoint is eminently correct. The term "general peritonitis" (suppurating) should, therefore, give way to a nomenclature more nearly adapting itself to the clinical picture as found by the operating surgeon. Such a term is found, we believe, in the title of this paper. The term "general peritonitis" owes its existence to dead-house pathology and is, therefore, expressive of terminal conditions necessarily fatal.

3. The etiology of peritonitis from the surgeon's standpoint may, for all practical purposes, be summed up in a leakage from the visceral content of the abdominal cavity. This leakage is most frequent about the appendix. The next in vulnerability is the right upper abdominal quadrant including the gall bladder and ducts and the pylorus and deodenum. In the female the genitalia are sometimes the source.

4. The demonstration that the upper or diaphragmatic zone is the area which has the most to do with absorption has an immensely practical bearing in treatment.

5. The bacillus pyocyaneous plays a part in the early processes of the disease, but just what that part is our studies have not fully determined. We have found it to be present invariably in the early hours of attack in every case operated sufficiently early. The most common bacillary agent present has been the colis communis.

6. To Alonzo Clark came the happy fortune of catching the first glimmer of light in the treatment of this disease. By his opium treatment he accomplished a limi-

tation in the dissemination of the infection by quieting intestinal peristalsis. Next came Ochsner with his "starvation" plan, which still more effectually quieted peristalsis. A little later Fowler added the postural treatment, now known as the "Fowler position," and last of all, Murphy with his "get in quick and get out quicker" axiom.

7. The application of the general principles noted in conclusion six (6) has transformed the mortality tables in this heretofore appalling disease until, at the present time, it has been removed from the hopeless to the hopeful class.

8. The disease is strictly surgical and its treatment surgical, and every case of even probably beginning peritonitis, whether appendicular or otherwise, should be at once subjected to the postural and starvation treatment, with or without operation according to the indications in the given case. After the diagnosis is made morphine sufficient to relieve the pain should not be withheld.

Posture should be *continuous* and maintained until localization is accomplished, and normal saline by the rectum by the drop method given to the limit of toleration.

9. Patients with peritonitis do not die from the disease per se, but from toxemia, the limitation and elimination of which are the fundamental facts of the treatment outlined above.

10. The pain of peritonitis is occasioned by the involvement of the parietal peritoneum. A patient may have visceral peritonitis with but little pain history, and since the muscular rigidity is due to the same cause, with but little rigidity.

11. The differential blood count is of value in deciding the time for operation. In cases where a favorable prognosis can be given there is either a high absolute with a low relative leucocytosis, or a compara-

tively high absolute with a correspondingly level or falling relative.

12. Cases that are inoperable clinically show a very high relative leucocytosis and a very low or very high absolute leucocyte count.

13. The comparison of the relative with the absolute leucocytosis is of the most importance before the operation and subsequent counts are of value in determining the efficiency of drainage.

DISCUSSION.

Dr. J. H. White, Muskogee:

In reference to the paper, I don't understand how the peritoneal cavity can be opened while patient is in sitting posture. Should think it would be a difficult problem.

Dr. Cunningham, Oklahoma City:

As to the symptoms I can say nothing. As to the treatment, however, I would like to make a few remarks. I would like to call it Ochner's treatment for Murphy stole it from Ochner.

I use and am using now a very simple apparatus for proctoclysis. I take an ordinary steamer chair, costing only about a dollar and a half, a canvas chair. In this chair I make a hole—rather large—and put the chair in bed.—Illustrating at blackboard.

The doctor speaks of rest, but you cannot get much rest sitting in an arm chair. But in this position (aided by the use of pillows and cushions for the arms and hands), the patient can have complete muscular relaxation of the entire anatomy. That you must have if you get the patient to retain properly the salt solution.

Some of our men say they have complete failure in using this treatment. I think the reason is that the tube used irritates the rectum. I take a glass tube with aluminum ————, heat one end of it

until it closes, then I blow into it until it becomes bulbous, then I perforate it three or four times. Then I bend it into proper shape. It does not irritate the bowel and thereby does not cause action.

Dr. D. A. Myers, Lawton:

I have nothing to say in criticism of the paper, but when a man or a body of men can conquer such a disease as peritonitis they have done great good. Some time back I was unfortunate enough to lose some cases of that character. I am going to try to save the next one.

Dr. Grossheart, Tulsa:

I would like Dr. Reed in closing to discuss his method of operation and his drainage. He spoke of drainage in the abdominal and pelvic region. Is the tube well in the peritoneal cavity or just so it can go into the pelvis, or so it will go through the omentum. These are points that I should like explained.

Discussion of A. L. Blesh:

In closing the discussion of this paper, I will state that it is the joint product of all three of us working together to try to evolve a method whereby we could save those hitherto hopeless cases. Many of them we could not see in time for the Ochsner treatment to be of avail in localizing within small limits and most of them were seen after the time that Murphy characterizes as hopeless. Our claim is that we have been successful in saving a large percentage of these cases that all of you have looked upon as beyond salvation.

As regards the inquiry as to how the abdomen can be opened with the patient in the sitting posture, I will merely say that it is not a difficult feat. All of the cases reported were operated in this position and one of them was so weak that we feared removing him to the operating room and the drainage was made under local anesthesia while in the Fowler position in bed.

This patient developed several abscesses subsequently which were operated and drained as they appeared. The diagnosis of them was easy and was made by the physical signs, and the blood count. Invariably the leucocytosis would ascend and we noted this before even the clinical chart would show any change, that is to say, before the physical signs were manifest. In this particular case the abscess covered more than half of the abdominal cavity, but we succeeded in truly localizing it. Before the localization so far as we or any one else could see, the whole abdominal cavity was involved in the inflammatory process. The whole abdominal wall was rigid. Paresis with distension was present and a toxemia so profound that the patient actually seemed in extremis. Position by gravity favored the localization in the lower regions where absorption was sluggish, thus limiting the absorption of the poisonous products and the patient rallied sufficiently to permit of the drainage at the opportune time.

Now a word in closing as to the value from a clinical standpoint, of the blood count. We have always found that the differential is the most important feature of it. A high differential indicates a most dangerous time for operative interference. The reason is simple. When we find the polynuclears in the blood stream in a plus quantity, it is a fair assumption that they are not out on the firing line where the battle is raging. The added insult of operation at this time will completely overwhelm them, perhaps, and turn an orderly retreat into a veritable rout and panic. A little help by way of lessening the absorption of toxins will enable them to rally and again assume the offensive and we will now find the differential will be relatively low. This always happens when localization is accomplished. Finally we wish to thank the Association for the cordial reception of the paper and the frank discussion that followed its presentation.

PREVENTIVE PUERPERAL SEPTISEMIA

DR. JAMES W. SCARBOROUGH, RUSSEL, OKLAHOMA.

Mr. President, Ladies and Gentlemen of the Association: First in introducing for your consideration this always interesting subject, I do so with no hope of presenting anything new, but for the simple purpose of getting this ever important question before these able representatives of our profession with hopes that something may be brought out in the open discussion whereby the suffering humanity from this malady may in the future be benefited.

I repeat the importance of this subject and will say that it should receive more attention from the medical profession than it ordinarily does. There are few things in our professional lives which make a deeper or more lasting impression upon our memory than the death-bed scenes of patients dying from any cause, but more especially if the objects of our solicitude happens to be an ideal young woman in the bloom of existence, battling for life within the poisonous clutches of peurperal infection. This can be worse and is why we believe that it has been through neg, gence on our part for not having used all the preventive methods.

Experience has confirmed the theory

that this disease is one of the most dreaded in the long list of maladies known in connection with childbirth. Peurperal fever may be infectious or non-infectious; the infectious variety are usually due to bacteria or ptomains which finds it way into the genital tract which may effect the uterus, tubes, pelvic tissues, peritoneum, bladder, ureters, kidneys or rectum.

Non-infectious puerperal fevers occur in malaria constipation, exposure to cold and reflex irritation, etc.

As we are all truly familiar with the oncoming symptoms of this subject under consideration we will be brief in mentioning same, notwithstanding they vary some according to the type with which we have to deal with, but the usual cases are as follows: Patient has chill on third or fourth day following confinement, followed by high fever, severe headache, thirst, anorexia and insomnia, pain in hypogastric region which later becomes general. Respiration accelerated, pulse, first full and bounding, later, rapid and weak. Temperature 105 to 106 degrees F.; tongue coated, brownish fur—bowels constipated first, later may become loose—abdomen bloated and tympanitic, urine scanty, uterus large and tender—milk secretions if begun usually cease—skin hot and dry at first, later begins perspiring when it becomes cool and clammy.

The above symptoms we should be ever mindful of when in our obstetrical work, remembering the Noah adage, "that an ounce of preventative is worth a pound of cure." True to this fact we should confine ourselves more closely to the aseptic technic in our general practice, but more especially to our gynecological duties—to this we should be as careful, disinfecting gloves and hands as if we were going to do a major operation of some nature. On our past conduct we may see the error of our way and should we not for the sake

of humanity take advantage of same?—we should always avoid all unnecessary preliminaries, more especially the frequent examinations for as a rule one or two vaginal examinations are sufficient. Well, yes, often times we find a patient or a midwife, who is present and thinks we are not doing our duty if we don't stand in line (equal to that of a soldier boy) trying to help her have a baby when she is only having dilating pains. These opposing facts can be easier and more satisfactorily explained than can a case of sepsis be cured. Plans are very numerous that we might mention aiding us in the preventive treatment such as educating the people to general invironments, hygene, cleanliness, dieting, the lying-in-room, etc., etc., all of which we are very familiar with and which are essential to the successful treatment of gynecological work. There are few things we should emphasize more thoroughly, however, we do not to the extent of our privilege and duty, sometimes due to negligence and oftener, perhaps, afraid that we might effect the feelings of this or that particular family, owing to their habits of living. In my practice I have given primiparas more attention, possibly due to my having been taught in school that they are more susceptible to infection owing to their protracted labor, the birth canal being narrower and its parts being softer, *but* in my practice I have never had a primipara but they have all been multipara: This may be explained by my having believed the above and have been especially particular with my primipara. In normal labor I never allow my patient to use the douche for fear an inexperienced nurse may infect the patient. Aside from this fact, why are we not satisfied when we have seen nature do her work with such perfectness?

Should I deem it necessary to use a douche I am the individual to use it, taking all responsibility myself. An experience recently converted me to this plan. Patient sick for more than three weeks and, after having visited her daily (you all know how tiresome this gets to be, especially in a case of puerperal septicemia, even though the money is cash, as this one truly was) I thought as her temperature was normal and she doing nicely otherwise, that I'd turn the patient over to the husband as he had carefully assisted me each day and after I had fully explained the usual aseptic technique I turned the case to him to douche daily and phone me each day. Agreeable to our wishes she improved nicely until the fifth day when I had a phone message stating that Mary was worse, her temperature having reached 105 degrees F., and just crazy with the headache. It is useless to tell you how I received this word after having worked so long and faithful only now to bow to my negligence. Notwithstanding my disappointment, I made the visit and when I next dismissed this patient she was well. Experience has proven to me that you cannot depend upon hardly anyone save they be a trained nurse, the malady being one that is too treacherous.

Again, we should consider the forceps more conservatively and use it a great deal less in our obstetrical practice. God, the greatest physician known to the world, has so arranged nature that we should not attempt to take His ever willing duty from Him and apply these instruments, which, no doubt, is the originating cause of more homeless and motherless children than any other complication known in child bearing. Certainly there are some exceptions to the rule, for instance, the only case I have lost in my six years of practice was an instrumental delivery, which was inevitable. Another doctor's case was called in and found she was in labor, but was too weak to produce pains, she having the typhoid fever, and was reported to have been dying for many days. This woman was a primipara with no life scarcely, so I 'phoned to Dr. D. He came and we delivered her with instruments, she being completely exhausted. In this case the instrument was as inevitable as was her death. Yet we do not attribute this death to the forceps, but to her low vitality.

It is a very unusual thing in which the infection is present in the uterus before labor comes on, which will be followed by septicemia. One case has come under my practice. A lady, nineteen, first child. When born it was dead and all appearances indicated that it had been dead for some time, it having turned dark and the skin cleaving from the flesh. After cleaning up I announced that we could expect some septic trouble. However, I began with my douches and illiminating treatment and she recovered with but little trouble. In this and like cases I believe in douches.

Next which we may consider is lacerations. It is a very wise man who looks after his slightest perineal lacerations which may prove in the end a preventive and should repair and look after same with aseptic precaution, for a woman will suffer much with pelvic ptosis which accompanies lacerations of the perineum, and may effect the bladder, causing cystisis, and suppurative changes distributing the infection possibly throughout the entire genital tract.

Since my paper is long enough I shall only mention the treatment in brief for touching the most common and favorite treatment. First, we all realize that in the treatment of aseptic fevers there should be no one rule of treatment, but should vary according to the etiology, duration and severity of the disease, also to the resistance of the patient.

The first important step to take into consideration is to remove all predisposing causes. This can only be done by the irrigation of the uterus. A uterus in peurperal fevers needs to be flushed out, relieving all abnormal conditions therein. Some use the sharp curette. I never have had cause to use one, but instead I use the blunt. Not to curett but only to take antiseptic wash into all parts of the uterus, relieving all pus formations by washing all shreds or sloughs that may be the seat of all evil. Just here I want to say the more water you use the better results you may expect. Some use normal salt solutions, others alcohol solutions, others bichloride, etc., etc., but personally, I prefer the carbolic wash with from three to six per cent with water as hot as patient can stand same. In severe cases I mop out uterus with carbolic followed in three to five minutes with alcohol mop, realizing the importance of killing all germs as quickly as possible, carbolic being one of the best agents for germicidal purposes, and, too, in like cases renders one of the best preventatives for relieving the disagreeable odor which arises from sepsis. After this has been done we recommend the packing of the uterus wtih gauze.

The general treatment consists of rest, stimulents and light nourishing food.

The medical treatment for the severe types of infections should consist of medicinal properties that will promote phagocytosis. I never lose sight of the importance of eliminating the system; for the bowels I give principally the mild chloride, may follow with the saline laxatives, but repeat my mild chloride every few days. For the kidneys I advise the drinking of much water and if this does not flush the kidneys sufficiently I put patient on potassium ac., buchu and juniper comp., or any other mild diruretic. Much depends on the condition of patient's stomach. Never use the cathether as long as can avoid same owing to the after results arising therefrom. Reduce temperature with compound of aconite, digitaline, veratrine as often as indi-

cated to reduce fever and control the severe headache.

To restore strength to the patient I recommend "egg nogg," broths, beef tea and other light diets as conditions may admit. I never fail to tonic patients in convalescence stage, producing strength and appetite.

In conclusion, since these fevers are a bacterial disease, there is no stereotyped method of treating same. However, there is a set method of the preventive treatment and if we can apply these rules to our gynecological, practice which are simple and inexpensive rules that will render our work successful, warding off this disease, why not use them to the interest of our patients? Now, many may say, Oh, we do all this, but we do not, I am negligent and so are you. In the world wide field of medicine and surgery today there is nothing more interesting than the problem of preventative of all diseases.

DISCUSSION.

Dr. Robinson, Dustin:

It is a nice paper, practical, but I can't agree with the Doctor's treatment. I don't think that a douche for puerperal sepsis is a good treatment. I believe if the uterus is infected we are apt to carry the infection further. I believe that the first thing to be done in fever after labor is to clean out the uterus with the fingers, pack it with a sterile gauze. Of course, there are cases where it might be necessary to put in drains through the vaginal route. I have seen the like done in this class of cases, and it is a practice that I have never done, but it is one that I would not hesitate to do in the case of fever after labor where I thought it was in the last stages and it looked like the patient was going to die. But this thing of douching from day to day and fever going up, is a mighty poor practice and it is carried out too much. I believe in thoroughly cleaning out at the first visit after the baby is born. Get that clean then and you are done forever. When you get it clean, pack it, and remove the packing after six to twelve hours.

Dr. Gillis, Frederick:

I think that was a fine paper and I think we ought to discuss these papers, too. The only reason I was going to say something on every paper is because there wasn't very many here and I appreciate it is something I haven't been able to do for quite a while for our society in our country is very small. In that way we get along better as I think we learn and get more out of the discussion of every-day papers than we can get out of our books, or almost any other way.

I have only one objection to the Doctor's paper and that was he said that the proper thing was to use every precaution in the first place and not get sepsis, and let the patient become affected. I think in the paper it would have been well if he had gone over his routine. I haven't had so many cases of sepsis in my own practice. I can truthfully say that I never had but one case and that was one that had a small laceration and there was a small blood clot and the next day that patient had a temperature of 106, and the next day I found in this patient's fourchette a torn blood clot, and I used the douche and the patient got along all right. I believe in using the douche if you have to. I don't think there is anything that will beat water; I don't think we can find anything that will beat water. Now, I use a sharp curette; that is simply a matter of habit. I think whatever the Doctor is in the habit of using that he can do better with. I can't use a dull curette. I have tried, but I knew before I would do anything I wasn't giving myself satisfaction, so I always use a sharp curette in any and all cases. I couldn't give

up water in these cases any more than I could quinine in malaria; I think it is just as essential. I think the principal thing for us to watch out for is to educate the family and educate the patient as much as we possibly can along lines of cleanliness, and get everything ready. Have everything ready in a case of confinement. Take things that you are liable to need up to the house and leave it there. I think that is the best way where you can. Of course, we country Doctors can't do that always, but where we can, if it is understood that we do these things, and always get ready for these cases before hand, I think it will eventually make us money, and I know it will make us better success.

As I said before, I am very glad to have heard the paper. I think the papers that are heard here this afternoon, we couldn't have papers of any more interest to the general practitioner.

Dr. Lef, Henry:

If I understood the Doctor correctly he has charged sepsis up to the use of the forceps. If that was his statement I want to correct that. I misunderstood you, then. There is no reason why the forceps should affect the patient any more than anything else if you understand the use of it. There is no use to let a woman lay and suffer for hours when she can be relieved in a few minutes if you understand the use of it.

Dr. Doudin, Coyle:

I want to refer to one remark in the paper that I heard made. I only heard about half of the paper on the subject. Don't make too frequent examination, one or two in the course of labor is enough. Now, I have been practicing about thirty years and I believe that the Doctor ought to know what is going on in that vagina and he is a fool to sit around and not know what is going on. Wash your hands and go ahead and examine often enough to know. If the pain is accomplishing anything, you want to know it. I see no reason why the forceps should produce sepsis. Have the forceps clean. There is a placenta forceps, one spoon always fits another spoon. I think that is a good curette. There is an inch and a half of surface and you are not going to go through that uterus while it will produce pressure on it and if there is anything left on there and you haven't scraped off any living tissue.

———

Dr. Charles Nelson Ballard, Oklahoma City:

I did not hear the paper, so can not discuss it, but I note the subject, puerperal sepsis, to be one of greatest importance to us all. I do not know whether the essayist discussed the different kinds of infection or not.

The paramount principle in this complication is to make a diagnosis. Locate the point of primary invasion. Determine the nature of the offending material. By the symptoms we will be able to distinguish the character of the infection. By a careful consideration of the symptoms and physical signs we can usually divide the condition into two distinct classes, sapremia and septicemia.

Sapremic infection we understand to be that produced by the actions of the saprophites on retained material such as, blood clot or placenta. The action of this microorganism is to produce decomposition of the retained material, liquefaction takes place and this is followed by rapid absorption. The decomposed material is a point of easy entrance and a fertile soil for the rapid multiplication of the streptococci, and in this way a mixed infection may be produced. Septicemia, however, is usually a primary affection induced by the introduction of pathogenic germs through some abrasion of the mucus membrane in the genital tract. These organisms, which are always present in the vagina, may be stimulated to renewed activity and be the first cause, but usually they are introduced from without, through the failure of the nurse or physician to observe proper antiseptic precautions.

A differential diagnosis can usually be made by close observance of the symptoms.

In sapremia, the onset occurs from three to five days after delivery. Normal convalescence is interrupted by the sudden onset of the symptoms. The lochial discharge has a very offensive odor. On examination retained material, with offensive odor, is found and when removed the symptoms suddenly subside. In septicemia, the onset is slow, but may begin within twenty-four hours after delivery. A gradual rise in temperature with chilly sensations are characteristics. Sapremia is excluded when no retained material exists. Septicemia must be carefully diagnosed from malaria and typhoid fever by exclusion.

Prognosis in sapremia is favorable, while that in septicemia is exceedingly unfavorable.

A diagnosis of sapremia being determined—make use of a dull curette, removing the offending material from the uterine cavity and cauterize the point where absorption was taking place. I advise iodized-phenol for this purpose, 50 per cent.

If a diagnosis of septicemia is made, then be sure that you do not use the curette, but locate the foci of infection being some abrasion or laceration and cauterize this and keep it well cleansed from all contaminating secretions.

However, the all important point is a differential diagnosis and a treatment will suggest itself.

———

Dr. Fowler, Pittsburg County:

I want to thank the Doctor for his very excellent paper. I want to thank him for the stress he put on the fact that nature and nature's God is the best physician in this and every case, and also for the stress he put upon the care we should use in using the forceps. Nature usually will do the work if we are able to control ourselves and the patient and the patient's family. When we do get an infection, whether it comes from the uterus itself or whether it comes from the vagina, as it sometimes does, the thing to do is to do the same as when you want to wash your hands. Infection comes from dirt and until we get some form of dry process cleaning, I believe that water is the thing to use and lots of it. There is no particular need of using anything in the water if we will use sterile water and use it hot. Hot water always cleanses better than cold water. I will never forget my talking at one time with a gentleman considerably older than myself, a man with very large experience, a close observer and splendid student. I was telling him that a man used a vaginal douche in these infections, and he says in his way: "Yes, very good, Doctor, splendid, but," he says, "it has just taken me about twenty years to find out that sterile water does better." I have never forgotten that, and I believe that that is all that is necessary to use. After the womb is thoroughly cleaned then use the water with alcohol, but what I like better is iodized phenol.

As to the use of the curette, I do not see the need of using the sharp curette in these cases. We must remember that it has only been a few days since this uterus was large, containing the foetus, and I think the curette that is best in these cases is a piece of gauze on the end of a forcep. The idea is to cleanse the uterus of little blood clots that are there, and there is no need to use a sharp or any kind of a curette.

Dr. Jas. W. Scarborough, Russell, closes discussion:

I wish to say the main idea in presenting this paper was for prevention in this trouble. As I said in the close of my paper, it is the greatest problem now known to the medical profession. As to douching, I believe in washing out because as the old adage says, "cleanliness is Godliness," and if we want to keep our sores and our infections clean, there is no other way to keep them clean other than using good sterile water and plenty of it.

Now as to the use of the forceps. I believe in them, but I don't believe in them to the extent they are sometimes used, for when we do use them we are assisting in forcing nature and it is bound to bruise.

As to frequent examinations, I don't see any cause why a physician should be making these examinations every few minutes. He finds out the condition of the lady and her general condition, and I see no reason why he should make frequent examinations; but instead, he should wait, and at the proper time he will be notified when to work.

I thank you, one and all, for your discussions. I feel that I have been benefited by the discussion.

EDITORIAL

MEDICAL ASSOCIATION OF THE SOUTHWEST.

The annual meeting of the Medical Association of the Southwest promises to be one of the great medical gatherings of the year.

A partial promise from the President of

the American Medical Association to attend has been received. Doctor W. L. Rodman of Philadelphia has promised an oration on surgery.

San Antonio is planning a royal entertainment and after the meeting special cars will take a party to the City of Mexico. It is desirable to run a special sleeper from the East and one from the West side of the state, these meeting other sleepers at Fort Worth for a joint trip to San Antonio.

It is especially desired that those wishing to take advantage of this opportunity to attend the meeting and at the same time visit Mexico, write Dr. F. H. Clark, Secretary, El Reno, Oklahoma.

THE TUBERCULAR EXHIBIT.

Wellston, Okla., Sept. 11, 1909.

Dear Doctor: The committee that was named at the State Society in May to devise a plan to eradicate tuberculosis from the state, met at Oklahoma City yesterday together with Dr. J. C. Mahr, State Superintendent of Board of Health. It was decided that this committee and the State Board, jointly, should place a tubercular exhibit at the State Fair at Oklahoma City, which begins on September 28th and continues for a period of ten days. The State Fair Association has donated this space that probably could have been sold for $200 or $300 which obligates us to put on an exhibit creditable to our state. The committee deemed it wise that there should be present each day a physician who is able to explain the display to the public. It was agreed to select ten men, three of whom should represent the State Board, the remainder the State Medical Association. The following are the names which have been chosen to represent the Association: Dr. A. K. West, Oklahoma City; Dr. Le-Roy Long, South McAlester; Dr. R. H. Harper, Afton; Dr. K. F. Camp, Oklahoma

City; Dr. A. A. West, Guthrie; Dr. F. H. Clark, El Reno; Dr. C. W. Bradford, Shawnee.

You will see that your name is included in the above list. Will you kindly notify Dr. H. M. Williams, Wellston, whether you can be present either in person or by representative and what day you would prefer, if any.

H. M. WILLIAMS, Wellston,
J. M. POSTELLE, Oklahoma City,
R. H. HARPER, Afton,
                    Committee.

THE CHIROPRACTOR AGAIN.

Dr. A. C. McCall, a chiropractor, was arrested Friday morning on the charge of practicing medicine without a license from the state board. The complaint was made by Dr. A. G. Wall.

The case will be carried to the last ditch. Its outcome will determine whether or not chiropractors shall continue to practice in this state.

Dr. McCall and Dr. Wall agree that the whole question resolves itself into the query, does a chiropractor practice medicine?

The former takes the negative, and the latter the affirmative. Dr. McCall says that the treatment he gives is purely mechanical, and no medicine is administered, therefore, he does not practice medicine.

Dr. Wall takes the position that anyone who treats diseases is practicing medicine, even if no medicine is actually administered.

Dr. McCall is alleged to have treated a typhoid fever patient. The chiropractors treat their patient by treating the spinal column by mechanical methods.

There are many chiropractors in Oklahoma, and the settlement of the matter will be eagerly awaited. The first promises to engage the attention of the entire body of "regular" physicians on the one hand and the chiropractors on the other.

Dr. Wall said: "I filed the complaint in the interest of the profession, in part, but mainly in the interest of the public, which is being gulled more and more every day by chiropractors."

Dr. McCall said: "I am glad they picked on me, because I have the means to fight the case through, and many chiropractors have not."—From the Daily Oklahoman.

SUPPRESSION OF OBNOXIOUS NEWSPAPER ADVERTISING.

The Minnesota Medical Associations have in the last few months achieved no small degree of success along the line of suppression of advertising in the daily press by the various fake medical institutes, cancer hospitals and other such institutions.

Their plan, which is the only possible one to accomplish good in that field consisted in moral suasion alone.

The matter was systematically agitated throughout the state at the same time, resolutions calling attention of the people to the danger and damage done and the general bad effect on the moral tone of the community were passed and given wide publicity.

Most of the papers of the state at once closed their advertising contracts; one of the first being the St. Paul Pioneer Press, one of the largest papers in the Northwest and the largest in Minnesota. Great pressure was brought to bear on the owners of these papers to reconsider their resolution barring them from advertising; wealthy and influential concerns sent representatives to argue the matter. To the owners it meant loss of thousands of dollars in patronage, but their moral ideas were stronger than their financial needs and today the

"Abortion Hospital," and the "Institution for the Reinvigorating of Man" flaunts not its brazen countenance to the thousands of readers of the Minnesota daily papers.

THE GRADUATE NURSE.

The Oklahoma State Association of Graduate Nurses will hold their first annual convention in Guthrie on the 5th and 6th of October. This Association has been favored with the endorsement of the Medical profession of Oklahoma and should continue to have every help the organized profession can give them. An intelligent nurse is the doctor's most faithful ally and in furthering the interest of this profession the Medical Association is only raising the standard of nursing in the state. The Oklahoma State Medical Association and its members will continue to give the Graduate Nurses' Association their support.

DOCTOR COOK THE DISCOVERER

Frederick A. Cook, discoverer of the North Pole, is a graduate physician, lately residing in Brooklyn and not a "Doctor" simply by the courtesy of our flexible language.

Whether Cook or Peary discovered the pole first is a matter yet to be determined but the profession will look with pride on the dignified attitude of Dr. Cook in contrast with the puerile action of Peary in his attempt to discredit the work of another explorer.

Dr. Cook has made thousands of friends and admirers by his manly silence and brevity of speech when he did speak and the denial of his laurels by Peary has only made the public more ready to believe that of the two Cook is decidedly superior.

A Polar expedition is fraught with innumerable hardships and those men going through one deserve great credit and one regrets the smallness displayed by Peary in coming out of the North and crying that Cook is an imposter.

The medical profession must have more proof from Peary before accepting his view of the matter and even if his contention is true he still shows up in a most unenviable light.

EXCHANGES

INFANTILE ECZEMA.

I. A. Abt, Chicago (Journal A. M. A., September 11), says that the etiology and pathology of infantile eczema are but little understood and that we should be careful not to confuse it with other skin eruptions due to irritation. The most rational view, he says, based on clinical observaifestation of some internal disorder. Constitutional conditions are the underlying cause and the presence of bacteria in the external lesions may result from secondary infection and not hold any causal relationship. The various views held by authorities—that it is due to underfeeding or overfeeding, metabolic disturbances, etc.— are stated. The French authors lay considerable stress on hereditary influences and that parental arthritis, gout, obesity, asthma, and various neuropathic conditions tend tion, is to consider eczema an external manto favor eczema in the offspring. That this view is based on facts, Abt says, is corroborated by every observer's clinical experience. Gaucher finds an inhibition of metabolism in every case and regards eczema as an autointoxication, the poisons being eliminated through the skin. The symptoms, according to the classification of Marfan, are described. In the first form there is the wet or crusty eruption on the scalp, cheeks or ears which has been known as milk scab, the limbs and trunk usually being free. If neglected, it may extend, however, over the whole body. This form is most often of the seborrheic type and, while treatment is difficult, spontaneous cure may occur at the end of the first year when the quantity of milk of the artificially fed infant is reduced. The second form is described by Marfan under the name of disseminated dry eczema, and the history obtained is usually that of an over-fed infant who is thin and delicate, suffering from chronic intestinal and nutritive disturbances. There are dry, scaly, infiltrated islands of crust with popular and pustular lesions, and sometimes moist areas. The face is most involved, the scalp only slightly. Unlike the other form there is usually itching, which is very refractory to treatment. It has been suggested that this is the gouty form. Among the complications of infantile eczema is albuminuria, with or without kidney involvement. These are undoubtedly due to toxic absorption and more attention to the heart complications has been advised by many writers. The clinical symptoms rarely indicate a fatal ending and post-mortem may not reveal the cause of death. It has been held by some that a myo-cardinal degeneration may exist, and others hold that it may be due to the status lymphaticus. An etiologic relationship between eczema and asthma has been strongly indicated in several reported cases. The treatment is given in some detail by Abt. Locally the crusts can be removed by softening with ointment but in the scalp it should be gradual to prevent serious results. Powders and pastes of zinc oxid and, in severe dry cases, some tar ointment are useful. Sulphur baths are sometimes useful. The constitutional treatment consists, in the main, in the regulation of the diet and attention to the intestinal disturbances and digestion. Good results have been reported from what is known as Finkelstein's soup, which is made of coagulated milk and oatmeal water, but Abt does not recommend it. Czerny emphasizes the need of treating any underlying hereditary factor. On the whole, it may be said that a milk-poor restricted diet with addition of cereal, and the exclusion of eggs and meat broths, as a rule, yields good results in a short time. Older infants should be also given fruits and vegetables.

THE FLEXNER SERUM IN MENINGITIS.

F. S. Churchill, Chicago (Journal A. M. A., September 11), shows how the use of the Flexner serum has reversed the proportions of death and recoveries and greatly reduced the unpleasant sequelae of the disease. He also gives his own observations of forty-one cases, of which twenty-nine were demonstrated as beyond question due to the meningococcus. In these twenty-nine, thirteen, or 44 per cent, died, but closer analysis shows that lateness of beginning of the treatment in the disease and lack of proper dosage accounts for the mortality. Hospital patients do better than those treated at home. They can be watched more closely, the serum can be given more persistently and thoroughly and more exhaustive laboratory investigations as to the blood, etc., can be carried out to guide the treatment. The most striking thing in the cases treated early in the hospital is the high per centage of perfect recoveries without sequelae and the especially low rate of mortality, it being sometimes as low as 10 per cent. in cases treated within the first three or four days. The course of the disease is materially shortened and the patient is much more comfortable. The increased phagocytosis can be observed with the successive injections. He describes the technic of the method. The injection must be made at the pathologic seat of the disease by lumbar puncture. Evacuate 30 to 45 c. c. of the spinal fluid if possible, and, if it is at all turbid, inject an equal quantity of the serum at once without waiting for an examination. If the bacteriologic examination shows the presence of the meningogoccus, subsequent injections of the serum should be given. It is better to repeat the dose daily for three or four successive days before stopping the injections, and as a rule it will then be found that the patient is decidedly improving. If the conditions do not improve, repeat the process and so on until bacteria have disappeared, giving occasional injections until no organisms are found in either smears or cultures. Five cases are reported, two of them illustrated by charts.

MERCURIAL TREATMENT OF SYPHILIS.

Recognizing that mercury is the chief available remedy for syphilis. F. C. Hay, Hot Springs, Ark. (Journal A. M. A., August 28), discusses the merits of each method of its administration, the internal, the inunction, and the injection methods respectively. The ingestion method, or mercury administered by the mouth, is one of the oldest and the one that has been most in favor, but he is opposed to depending on this alone as it is so feeble and slow in its action on the disease, disappointing and discouraging to the patient, irritating to the gums and the digestive tract when given in any adequate dose, and in any case uncertain in its action. He would depend on it only when the patient is free from all manifestations of the disease and it is only desired to keep him slightly under the influence of mercury as a matter of precaution when he is being allowed to rest in the intervals between the more active treatments. When giving mercury by the mouth he prefers a pill containing biniodid of mercury, arsenic and gold; it is non-irritating and has been productive of good results. Another favorite pill is metallic mercury combined with lanolin and purified ox gall, one-half grain each, which produces less gastrointestinal disturbance than any other he has used. The inunction method is also one of the oldest methods. It is not painful and is free from danger and is quick and potent in its action, but it is often objected to by patients because it is apparently dirty and sometimes irritating to the skin. It is, therefore, often left to institutional treatment or treatment at resorts with thermal springs, etc. At Aix la Chapelle the mercury cycle is used; that is, the mercury is rubbed on different portions of the body successively, while at Hot Springs it is confined to the back, hips, and sometimes outer surfaces of the thigh with just as good results, besides being cleaner and pleasanter. The injection method, he thinks, has really no advantage over the inunction at least when the soluble preparations are used. The insoluble preparations are the most potent drugs we have when given this way, but it is admitted by the majority of writers that their use is very painful besides being the most dangerous. He believes in the combination of all three-methods, and the important points which he wishes to emphasize are given as follows: "When first instituting treatment after infection, either inunctions or injections should be employed. followed by internal medication, instead of treatment with pills first, followed by more heroic methods, as advised by most of the leading writers. The inunctions, from my experience and observation. on an average. are superior to the soluble injec-

tions, and more lasting in their effects. The insoluble salts are too intense and profound to be employed in routine, and should be held in reserve for rebellious cases in which rapid and pronounced mercurization is desired. Finally, the long course of treatment I have advised should be pursued in all cases. The six cardinal points in the therapeutics of syphilis are to keep a close observation of the weight, kidneys, bowels, stomach, gums and nervous system; especially the latter, as some patients will never manifest any evidence of mercury in the form of stomatitis, and the first evidence you have is a profound and acute nervous prostration. The prolonged course of treatment mentioned covers five years in which the periods of treatment, mainly by inunctions or injections. alternated by periods of rest. are gradually reduced from eight months in the first to four or six weeks in the fifth year.

MEDICAL EXPERT TESTIMONY.

Much has been said and written on the subject of the medical expert in court, especially from the standpoint of the physician, but the lay and judicial opinions have not as a rule, been based on facts and firsthand knowledge. It is, therefore, with great gratification that one reads in the June North American Review a concise statement of the matter from the pen of Supreme Justice Clearwater, Chairman of the Committee of the New York State Bar Association, appointed to consider the regulation and introduction of medical expert testimony. Judge Clearwater's high standing as a jurist gives to his words the full weight of authority, while his responsible position as chairman of the committee above mentioned certainly puts him in immediate command of the facts. All efforts to remedy the present unsatisfactory status of the medical expert have failed, up to the time of the appointment of the commission, because many, both lawyers and physicians, have fought against any change.

One of the existing evils, and the first one named in Judge Clearwater's paper, is the lack of standard as to expertness. This was well exemplified in a recent notorious trial in which one of the medical witnesses proved his incompetence by foolish and ignorant answers to the simplest questions. Still he went on the stand as an expert. Other evils of the present system as named in the Judge's essay are the giving of partisan evidence; contradictory testimony from physicians in equally good standing; unprincipaled self-styled experts; trial judges who are incompetent to pass on the ability of experts or validity of their opinions; payment of witnesses by the litigant, and, consequently, the employment of the best experts by the litigant with the longest purse; the contemptuous treatment some experts have received at the hands of rude and unscrupulous lawyers and, most of all, trial judges who have sought to draw attention to themselves by their manner of admitting evidence of bad quality. In order that the ends of justice and truth may prevail, "the expert witness should be free from embarrassment, should have no clients to save and no partisan opinion or interests." He should speak judicially as an exponent of the science of medicine, with full knowledge of the highest authorities and of the most recent investigations dealing with his subject. Cross-examination plays havoc with the expert because of his personal embarrassment when he is called as one high in authority, and because of unfair attempts of the opposing lawyer to "rattle" him. Says Judge Clearwater: "Scientific opinion, to be of controlling value, can be given only under conditions of mental repose," which is seldom possible, we may add, in the witness box.

Some newspaper writers have promulgated false views of the expert's position because of their unacquaintance with judicial proceedings, and first of these is the erroneous statement that the calling of expert witnesses is of recent origin. As far back as 1532, Henry VIII., of England, in his published Code, gave power to appoint expert physicians and surgeons for the examination of injured patients before the court. And this is probably not the first instance. Then, too, the ordinary witness and his function is mistaken for that of the expert. "The ordinary witness testifies to facts; the expert witness to opinions." The expert should not form his judgment from the evidence of witnesses, and should not draws inferences from their statements. "The only legal method is to frame a question upon assumption that certain facts are true, and then to ask the witness, assuming they are true, his opinions concerning them. While the hypothetical question seems involved, the method pursued is scientific and calculated to eliminate the element of error so far as it is possible to do so."

Direct examination of the accused and the passing up by the expert of an opinion in writing is not either desirable or tenable. The sixth amendment to the Federal Constitution granting to the accused the right to be confronted by the witness against him makes any such provision unconstitutional and would lead to a mistrial. Every party has a right to call witnesses desired and to cross-examine them as seems necessary. In civil actions the deposition of a witness whose attendance in court is impossible may be taken by commission, and on application of the accused may be so taken in criminal actions, but the right to cross-examine remains. The hope is expressed in conclusion that the present efforts of the committee appointed by the Bar Association may prove fruitful. "Medical expert testimony long has been a necessary and always will be an important factor in the administration of justice. It will require time and effort to restore its sullied luster. but the aim justifies the struggle." We commend the reading of

Judge Clearwater's paper by all physicians who are interested in the problems of medical jurisprudence.—Medical Record, June 26, 1909.

COUNTY SOCIETIES

COUNTY SOCIETIES.

All county Secretaries who have not been supplied with the card index system for their counties or who have not received them from their predecessors in office should at once write the State Secretary for the system and it will be supplied them immediately and in case they have not been turned over to you with the papers belonging to the Secretary's office you should call on your predecessor for the system.

They are extremely convenient and simple and when put in operation render the keeping of the records of your county society a matter of simplicity.

Many of the newer counties in the Eastern portion of the state have never been furnished the system, while some of the older counties have had them for a long time.

JEFFERSON COUNTY.

The Jefferson County Medical Association had a well attended and enthusiastic meeting in Waurika, Tuesday, September 7.

Several scientific matters of importance to the profession were discussed.

Several matters of business were brought before the society, among which was the following resolution which was unanimously adopted:

Whereas. There are in Jefferson County twenty-one regular practicing physicians, of which number eighteen are members in good standing of "The Jefferson County Medical Association;" and,

Whereas, It has come to the knowledge of this society, that there has recently been appointed as Superintendent of the County Board of Health of Jefferson County a man who is not a member of this society; and,

Whereas, In the membership of "The Jefferson County Medical Association" there are men who are qualified to fill the office of Superintendent of the County Board of Health, in a capable and efficient manner and who are in sympathy with a large majority of the members of the profession of the county; therefore, be it

Resolved, That the membership of "The Jefferson County Medical Association" make their reports direct to the office of the Superintendent of the State Board of Health, until such a time as a man may be appointed from this body.

Be It Further Resolved, That a copy of this resolution be furnished the State Journal. the county papers and the Superintendent of the State Board of Health.

F. W. EWING.
Sec'y.

J. M. STEVENS, V.-P.,
Acting Chairman.

MARSHAL-BRYAN.

Joint meeting of the Marshall and Bryan County Medical Societies held at Aylesworth, Oklahoma, September 9th, 1909.

Welcome Address—Hon. J. Frank Adams, Aylesworth.

Surgical Aspects of the Pneumococcus Germ—Dr. A. L. Blesh, Oklahoma City.

Subject to be selected—Dr. J. S. Fulton, Councillor Tenth Councillor District, Atoka, Oklahoma.

Diagnosis and Treatment of Typhoid Fever—Dr. T. A. Blaylock, Madill.

Medical Ethics—Dr. L. S. Willour. Atoka.

Cholera Infantum—Dr. J. I. Gaston, Kingston.

Professional Ethics—Dr. G. M. Rushing, Durant.

Relapsing Fever—Dr. W. H. Yates, Bokochito.

Malaria and Its Complications—Dr. A. S. Haygood, Durant.

This program contains some of the best talent in the Southwest and the meeting was one of the best ever held in Southern Oklahoma. One of the novel features arranged for this meeting was that it was held on the banks of one of the beautiful lakes of Aylesworth where nature smiles upon her creatures. A splendid lunch was prepared and served under the shade of trees and another feature of the occasion was the presence of many of the physicians' wives. Meetings of this character should be emulated by other county societies as they cannot fail to bring the profession to a closer and friendlier acquaintance.

HUGHES COUNTY.

Program for October 28, 1909.
Morning Session, 10 o'clock.
Call to order by the President.
Prayer by Rev. Goddard.
Short talk by Judge P. W. Gardner.
Reading minutes of last meeting.
Reading communications.
Voting on resolutions and amendments.
Balloting on applications.

Unfinished and new business.
Afternoon Session.
Gunshot Wounds—Dr. J. W. Love.
Discussion—Dr. J. A. Hemphill.
Typhoid Fever—Dr. E. T. Trebble.
Discussion—Dr. C. E. Parker.
Measles—Dr. W. G. Evans.
Discussion—Dr. J. J. Edwards.
Morphine Poison—Dr. A. J. Williams.
Discussion—Dr. N. J. Johnson.
Clinic—Dr. T. J. Cagle.
Thirty Minutes' Quiz: "Anatomy, Liver and Gall Bladder"—Dr. F. E. Warterfield.

OKMULGEE COUNTY.

The above society met in joint session with the Woman's Auxiliary in Okmulgee August 22.

The ladies took up the matter of giving aid to the hospital which has recently been opened in Okmulgee and the county society outlined the work for the coming year.

A banquet had been prepared for the occasion and the affair was very successful from a social standpoint.

PERSONAL MENTION.

Dr. J. H. Proffitt, Oklahoma City, had a narrow escape September 3rd from an automobile in which he and some of his friends were riding, coming in collision with an interurban car. The car was demolished and the chauffeur was severely injured. Dr. Proffitt escaped without serious injuries.

Dr. J. Hutchings White, Muskogee, spent his vacation in Wisconsin.

Dr. J. C. Miller, who recently moved from Indiana and located at Weeleetka, was shot and killed August 25th near that town; specific details of the tragedy are not obtainable as the affair is surrounded somewhat by mystery. Dr. Miller was a young man, being twenty-nine years old at the time of his death.

———

Dr. Hubbard, City Physician of Oklahoma City, has sold his office fixtures and appliances to Dr. R. L. McMahan, who has located in that city. Dr. Hubbard will be away from the state for some time, but will return at some future date.

———

Dr. Jas. L. Shuler, Durant, is attending the New York Polyclinic. He is accompanied by Mrs. Shuler and his son.

———

Dr. F. B. Fite of Muskogee is attending the New York Polyclinic.

———

Dr. F. R. Sutton, Bartlesville, suffered the loss of his home by fire September 8th.

MARRIED.

———

Dr. J. A. Adams and Mrs. Lena Virginia Satterfield were married Thursday, September 9th, 1909, at 8:30 P. M., at the home of the bride in West Sulphur, Oklahoma, Rev. G. H. Clymer officiating.

CHANGES OF ADDRESS.

Dr. S. H. Landrum from Olustee to Altus, Oklahoma.

Dr. G. O. Hall from Chickasha to Carnegie, Okla.

Dr. S. N. Stone from Calumet to Edmund.

NEW MEMBERS.

G. O. Hall, Carnegie.
William H. Cook. Chickasha.

R. I. Bond, Hartshorne.
W. D. Baird, Davenport.

———

THE SIGN.

Ira W. Robertson, Dustin, Oklahoma.

There is an old tradition or superstitious idea among the laymen that there is something in the sign for castrating pigs, calves, etc. Not long ago I was called in consultation with Dr. Pope of Hanna to see a young married lady who was suffering from appendicitis and had been for twenty days. There was a very large appendiceal abscess. The family objected to operation, especially her father; the case lingered for twenty days longer. When I was called again I explained the matter, telling him the danger she was in and had been all the time and insisted on operation, stating that there was practically no danger. The old gentleman hunted up the almanac and after looking through said the sign would be right the following Tuesday. On that day I evacuated the largest appendiceal abscess I ever saw in private or hospital practice. The patient made a good recovery and the old gentleman attributes the success to the sign being right when the patient was operated on.

———

AN IMPORTANT LITTLE WORK ON BIOLOGICAL THERAPEUUTICS.

———

In view of the near approach of the season when biological therapeutics will claim a considerable share of the attention of practitioners, reference may pertinently be made at this time to a unique and valuable contribution to the subject which has recently issued from the press of Messrs. Parke, Davis & Co. The publication consists of 52 pages, exclusive of the cover, and appears in brochure form. It is handsomely printed on white enamel paper of first quality and bears in colors a profusion of halftone illustrations. The title is

"Serums and Vaccines." A brief chapter on the origin and development of biological therapeutics, with an injected hint as to what the opsonins may have in store for us, constitutes the introduction. Then follow chapters on serums—anti-diphtheric, antitetanic, antistreptococcic, antigonococcic, antitubercle and antivenomous; on tuberculins; on vaccines, including the new bacterial vaccines which are exacting so much attention from the medical world; on organo-therapy, its development, and some of the important products that are associated with it—"a tabulation," in the language of the brochure itself, "of such creations of biologic pharmacy as are really utilizable in medicine." There are striking pictures of the Company's home laboratories at Detroit, with numerous interior views: the research laboratory: the operating house and biological stables at Parkedale Farm (where the animals are cared for), with accompanying landscapes in nature's colors.

This little book "Serums and Vaccines," is distinctly "worth while." If you haven't seen a copy, drop Parke, Davis & Co., a postal card at their home offices in Detroit, mentioning this Journal, and get one. It is a safe guess that any physician who receives the brochure will read it admiringly and with interest, filing it away thereafter for future reference.

OUT OF THE ORDINARY.

Abbott's Saline Laxative has two features which distinguish it from the common run of saline cathartics: First, when taken in cool (not cold) water immediately on rising, it acts *once*, in an hour or two (a clean, satisfying flush), and usually no more; whereas, ordinary salines keep the patient busy all day long. The annoyance of this when one is away from home or busy in business is great. Besides, there does not seem to be any failure in the action of this saline when used continuously for long periods—no habit forming necessitating increase of dose, but rather the reverse.

In one case a physician reports that he has taken a single teaspoonful of it every morning for 12 years, and still finds that dose amply sufficient to maintain regularity in his bowels.

In the trade everywhere. Samples sent to interested physicians by The Abbott Alkaloidal Co., Chicago, on request.

EVERY PHYSICIAN IN OKLAHOMA should have on his desk a copy of our New Illustrated Catalogue—now ready for mailing, and will be sent to any physician upon request. The most complete catalogue ever issued by a Western house for the Dispensing and Prescribing Doctor.

THE MOORE DRUG CO.,
Exclusive Physicians Supplies,
Wichita, Kansas.

PROGRAMME

First Annual Convention Oklahoma State Association of Graduate Nurses—October 5-6, 1909, Guthrie.

First Annual Convention Oklahoma State Association Graduate Nurses.

Tuesday, October 5th, 1909, 10 A. M.
1—Registration of delegates and visitors.
2—Credentials and dues.
3—Committee meetings.
4—Reports of Standing Committees.
Afternoon Session, 2 P. M.
1—Call to order by the President.
2—Invocation, Rev. Wm. H. Rose.
3—Address of Welcome—Mayor A. O. Farquharson.
4—Roll call.
5—Reading of minutes.
6—Treasurer's report.
7—Business.
8—Communications.
9—Address by the President, Miss Rae L. Dessell, R. N., Oklahoma City.
10—Paper, "The Need of Special Training in Children's Diseases in Modern Training

Schools," Dr. Lelia Andrews, Oklahoma City.

11—Discussion, Miss Blanche Dreisbach, Guthrie.

12—Paper, "The Nurse's Part in the Tuberculosis Campaign," Miss Elizabeth C. O'Donnell, City Tuberculosis Nurse, Oklahoma City.

13—Open discussion.

14—Announcements, Mrs. Margie Morrison, Chairman.

Reception, 8 P. M., Ione Hotel.

Wednesday, October 6th, 10 A. M.

1—Call to order by the President.

2—Reports of committees.

3—Unfinished business.

4—Paper, "A Point in Ethics," Miss Olive Salmon, Oklahoma City.

5—Discussion, Miss Edna Holland, Oklahoma City.

Afternoon Session, 2 P. M.

1—Call to order by the President.

2—Address, Dr. John W. Duke, Guthrie.

3—Report of Convention of United States Alumnae Association at Minneapolis. Martha Randall, R. N., Oklahoma City.

4—Incidents of the Trip, Miss Mabel Garrison, Oklahoma City.

5—Paper, "Trained Nursing, Retrospect and Prospect," Mrs. (Idora Rose) Scroggs, Kingfisher, Okla.

6—Discussion, Mrs. J. W. Riley, Oklahoma City.

7—Paper, "Registration, Its Aims and Its Hopes," Mrs. Cecelia Bogardus, El Reno.

8—Discussion, Miss Ida Ferguson, El Reno.

9—Paper, "The Superintendent of the Small Hospital," Miss Jewel Stafford, Superintendent Muskogee City Hospital.

10—Discussion, Miss H. C. C. Zeigler Superintendent Tulsa City Hospital.

11—Election and Installation of Officers.

12—Adjournment.

Announcements.

Headquarters at Ione Hotel, Oklahoma avenue and Vine street.

Meetings held in assembly room, Carnegie Library, corner of Oklahoma avenue and Ash street.

Registration desk open for thirty minutes before each session. Let everyone register.

Subscriptions will be solicited for American Journal of Nursing and for Trained Nurse and Hospital Record. Copies will be found on Literature table.

Information regarding state registration of nurses may be had upon inquiry at Registration Department.

Inspect the Tuberculosis Stamp System.

Reception Committee will meet all trains.

Nurses taking cases just before the convention should arrange to be relieved during the session.

A GOOD LOCATION FOR SALE.

I will sell for cash my home, consisting of five-room house, one acre of land, concrete storm house 6x8x9, and buggy and team of three horses, with about one hundred dollars worth of drugs, for $800.00.

This includes my practice of about eight miles square in a prairie agricultural country, twelve miles southwest of Duncan and twelve miles northwest of Comanche, Oklahoma. There is no competition, the nearest physician being twelve miles distant. The practice amounts to $2,000 annually, collections good, being 95 per cent. Good schools and lodge, with all churches represented with organization.

Will sell for cash only and will introduce buyer. Am going to take post-graduate work and move to city. If you mean business, write or come, but don't bother if you do not want a good village and country practice. Address Dr. W. G. Brymer, Fair, Route 4, Comanche, Oklahoma.

FOR SALE.

One static machine with all necessary attachments, everything in good order. Price, $75.00; terms if desired. Address Dr. A. E. Davenport, Western National Bank Building. Oklahoma City, Oklahoma.

FOR SALE.

The Journal has tuition to the amount of forty-four dollars in the New York Polyclinic School and Hospital which will be sold at a reduction from the usual rates. Address The Journal.

FOR SALE.

$1,250 cash gets property consisting of three-room dwelling house, barn, stables, pair of horses, good buggy, office furniture and fixtures; $4,000.00 practice gratis; will introduce. Reason for selling going to specialize in Texas. Address Dr. John F. Vick, Fort Towson, Oklahoma.

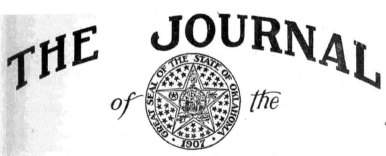

THE JOURNAL of the
Oklahoma State Medical Association.

VOL. 2.   MUSKOGEE, OKLAHOMA, NOVEMBER, 1909.   No. 6.

DR. CLAUDE A. THOMPSON, Editor-in-Chief.

ASSOCIATE EDITORS AND COUNCILLORS.

DR. J. A. WALKER, Shawnee.
DR. CHARLES R. HUME, Anadarko.
DR. F. R. SUTTON, Bartlesville.
DR. G. W. ROBERTSON, Dustin.

DR. JOHN W. DUKE, Guthrie.
DR. A. B. FAIR, Frederick.
DR. W. G. BLAKE, Tahlequah.
DR. H. P. WILSON, Wynnewood.

DR. J. S. FULTON, Atoka.

Entered at the Postoffice at Muskogee, Oklahoma, as second class mail matter, June, 1909.

This is the Official Journal of the Oklahoma State Medical Association. All communications should be addressed to the Journal of the Oklahoma State Medical Association, English Block, Muskogee, Oklahoma.

THE PRESIDENT'S ADDRESS

ANNUAL ADDRESS OF DR. B. J. VANCE, PRESIDENT OKLAHOMA STATE MEDICAL ASSOCIATION, DELIVERED AT OKLAHOMA CITY, MAY 13, 1909.

To the Members of the Oklahoma State Medical Association:

Ladies and Gentlemen: Another year, with its advance and failure, with its joys and sorrows, has passed, and through the kindness of an all-wise Providence, we are permitted to assemble, and receive a cordial reception, in this beautiful city, on this pleasant May day, in the capacity of the Oklahoma State Medical Association, as it is our custom to annually assemble, for the purpose of more firmly establishing our social relations with each other and enhancing our professional usefulness to our fellow man, and while our hearts swell with pride and gratitude, on account of our past success as an organization, we are made sad by the absence of some members of this Association, who have gone from us to that "undiscovered country, from whose bourne no traveler returns." I shall expect the committee on necrology to do full justice to their sacred memory.

Our organization is of a mixed character, social and scientific, both characteristics should enter largely into every physician's make-up. Allow me to suggest that the great object for which this Association was organized was "to federate and bring into one compact organization the entire medical profession of the state of Oklahoma, and to unite with similar societies of other states to form the American Medical Association; to extend medical knowledge and advance medical science; to elevate the standard of medical education, and to secure the enactment and enforcement of just laws; to promote friendly intercourse among physicians; to guard and foster the material interests of its members and to protect them against impositions; and to enlighten and direct public opinion in regard to the great problems of state medicine, so that the profession shall become more capable and honorable within itself, and more useful to the public, in the prevention and cure of disease, and in prolonging and adding comfort to life."

And I propose, in this my annual message, to direct your attention, briefly, to what we, at this time, conceive to be for the best interests of the Association; a brief history of the efforts, difficulties, results and prospects for the future of the Oklahoma State Medical Association, in its campaign for a higher standard of professional efficiency, in the medical profession of Oklahoma, the newest and one of the greatest states in the Union, hoping that we may be the better prepared to understand our duties to ourselves, and our Association, and be able to more intelligently contend for those things, which would be for the best interests of the medical profession and the public good.

The Oklahoma State Medical Association is a component part of the American Medical Association, an institution organized for the upbuilding of the medical profession in America in scientific equipment, whose membership now numbers more than 50,000, and made up of the Associations of the various states of the Union, on the standard plan; hence our constitution and laws should be uniform with every other state association.

The American Medical Association has a committee on Medical Education, and every effort that is to be made, in way of elevating the standard of medical education, is referred to said committee on Medical Education. This committee holds a conference annually to discuss plans whereby they can accomplish the purpose for which they were appointed. Your humble servant had the high honor and pleasure of attending one conference of this committee, as your representative, and was forcibly impressed with the wisdom of the plan and possibilities of the future. There were at that meeting delegates from state associations, state examining boards and medical colleges—all harmoniously advocating the same thing—the elevation of the standard of medical education. So, likewise, does the State Association have a committee on education.

The American Medical Association also has a committee on Medical Legislation, to whom is referred all matters pertaining to medical legislation for their consideration, that they may be able to assist the State Associations, through its representative on the committee, and likewise the State Medical Association of each state has a corresponding committee on medical education to whom is referred everything pertaining to the elevation of the standard of medical education and professional proficiency. And, again, each state association has a committee appointed annually, on Public Policy and Medical Legislation, whose duty it is to "represent the Association in securing and enforcing legislation in the interest of public health and of scientific medicine. It shall keep in touch with professional and public opinion, shall endeavor to shape legislation so as to secure the best results for the whole people, and shall strive to organize professional influence so as to promote the general good of the community in local, state and national affairs and election," and to whom is referred all matters pertaining to Medical Legislation, and this committee, having a representation on the National Committee on Medical Legislation, is brought in direct touch with the work of the National Committee, and as the National Committee on Medical Legislation is a strong factor in shaping the legislative policy of the American Medical Association, so likewise should our own State Committee on Medical Legislation be a strong factor in formulating and promulgating our much-needed reforms which are expected to be wrought out through state legislation in the interest of public health and sanitation. Now, who can doubt the wisdom of such a systematic plan of organization, which is so harmoniously constituted that one part does not conflict with another. The work of one committee, instead of conflicting, works in harmony with and aids the other. All these advantages come of the compact organization, both state and national, which has done so much for the upbuilding of the medical profession and placing it on that high plane of professional excellence, which it so richly deserves.

During the last quarter of a century, by medical research, the medical profession has made greater advances in science and valuable discoveries for the betterment of the human race than any people on earth. We have been brought by medical research from blood-letting to the use of antitoxines, brought to realize that cleanliness is really next to Godliness, and brought to realize the value of electrical theraputics. Research has made possible the building of the Panama Canal, which promises so much to the commercial world, by enabling us to combat disease so prevalent in the canal zone. Medical research has made it possible to limit the ravages of yellow fever, smallpox, dyphtheria, typhoid

fever and rabies. Medical research has enabled us to suppress the bubonic pleague on our Western shores, and by medical research we are encouraged to prosecute a campaign against the Great White Plague. These achievements are not the results of the labors of the quack, nor the mediocre in our profession, who divides his time and attention with other branches of science, religion, politics, or commercial enterprises; but the physician who loves his calling, who devotes his time in season and out, solely to his calling and is loyal to the demands of the public health. When a physician enters any other sphere of scientific, professional or business activity, or engages in politics, necessarily curtailing his hours of medical research, that moment he begins to retrograde in his professional usefulness to his clientele and finally loses his prestige. Then, it is conclusive, that the medical profession is the safest guardian of the public health. If the public could once realize the vast difference between the well trained and cultured physician or surgeon and that of the grossly ignorant boasting quack that often competes with (and sometimes supercedes) him, at the imminent peril of human life, it would be an easy matter to get good wholesome medical laws, with an emergency clause attached.

The policy of the Oklahoma State Medical Association with reference to medical legislation, has always been to favor such laws for the government of the medical profession of the state as would conserve to protect the public health, afford the best protection to the public by elevating the standing of liscensure in the state and improve the sanitary regulations; as the object of all medical legislation is to protect the public health.

And following this line, the Oklahoma State Medical Association offered one medical practice bill to the first legislature, known as the Franklin bill, and it was formulated by the proper authority of our Association on Medical Legislation, the committee on Public Policy and Medical Legislation, aided by the council and others, after due deliberation. This 'bill was a good medical practice act, fashioned after the best medical laws of other states; had no political aspect, gave no chance for graft or greed; required the state's executive to appoint the board of examiners from a list of physicians selected by the State Medical Association, as many other states do, thus eliminating the possibility of any physician being appointed solely on account of political or religious preferment. This was wise, for the state's executives are changed every few years, but our Association will live on and continue the study of these important problems.

Besides, any State Medical Association is far better qualified to select suitable physicians for membership on the Board of Medical Examiners than the executive officers of the state, though he be a physician himself.

We sought to keep politics out of the laws pertaining to the public health, because we know the least politics there is in a medical practice act, the less objection, and the greater endorsement, by the whole people. Had the Franklin bill become a law the standard of medical licensure in Oklahoma would have been on a par with any state in the Union, but instead of elevating the standard, above what it was prior to statehood, it has been said · to have been lowered; yet we are loathe to believe that to be our status. See the report of Dr. N. P. Caldwell, Secretary of the National Council, on medical education, to the annual conference of said Council, April 5th, 1909, at Chicago, and see what others think:

"In only one instance, within the past four years, has a state retrograded in the standard of medical licensure. This occurred during the last year in Oklahoma. A bill for a strong medical practice act was introduced, but so sadly riddled, by the time it came through the Oklahoma legislature, that it provides a lower standard than was formerly enforced in the Territory of Oklahoma."

While Oklahoma can boast of her good Constitution and her many wholesome laws, for the protection of labor and capital, and the splendid guardianship over her natural resources and home industries, for all of which we commend her law-makers, and recognize in these things the blessings of statehood, yet she cannot boast of her safeguards to public health, protection to human life from the ravages of disease. They are not what their importance demands that they should be; they should be greatly improved.

By reference to the report of the legislative committee to this body one year ago, you will find the conditions fully explained. My excuse for dwelling on the questions of medical legislation is the fact that this subject, aside from our scientific investigation, lies nearest the heart of every loyal member of this Association, for if we can get a good practice act, that itself will tend to elevate the standard of medical education. But we should aid the enforcement of the present law. All laws should be enforced. The more rigidly a bad law is enforced the sooner it will be replaced by a better one.

One great problem for legislators to solve, when about to consider a medical practice act, is, who are the safest advisers in matters pertaining to public health? The State Medical Association, aided by the American Medical Association, or the State Board of Health, composed of three members appointed by the state executive? The answer is very apparent to every thinking man, whether he be physician or layman. Just as much propriety in allowing the Supreme Court to dictate the law governing the legal profession, as to allow the State Board of Examiners to dictate a medical practice act. If we succeed as an Association to carry out the purpose for which we were organized, in reference to medical legislation, we must work with the laiety; teach them to know that our cause is their cause. For as a people become educated in matters pertaining to scientific medicine, "quackery" loses its boasted prestige, and the people lose confidence in quack methods, which tends to pave the way for good medical legislation.

To work out these reforms successfully, it is necessary to keep our organization free from political entanglements, in fact, politics once injected into our organic body acts like a deadly poison and disintegration begins at once, and not only limits its influence for the future, but will eventually destroy it. Politics is like the drug and whiskey habit, very insidious and seductive, and when a physician yields to its alluring fascinations, he soon becomes its victim, and it will eventually destroy his professional equilibrium, unless checked.

Let politicians get control of any nonpolitical organized body and begin to make its subservient to the interest of any political party, and that organization will begin to lose its prestige, and finally become disorganized. An examination of the history of all non-political organizations shows that this is true.

In this connection I desire to commend the Oklahoma State Medical Association for the stand it has taken in this matter heretofore and hope it may continue to steer clear of political affiliations. So it will be the duty of every member of this Association who loves his profession better than politics, who desires the welfare of the 'Association, who wants to see medical laws that will reflect credit on the medical profession, who wants to curtail quackery, and who wants the highest standard of excellence established, to see that they are loyal to every undertaking that is put forth for the good of the public health. One of the most valuable characteristic qualifications of our membership is loyalty; loyalty to every effort that is put forth by our Association that is for the upbuilding of our time-honored profession to that standard that it will not be said of us that we are retrograding rather than advancing. Loyalty to every call for the right,

Loyalty to our cause is a priceless gem,
In all our efforts for good through life,
When we walk forth the tide to stem,
To full and complete victory in the strife.

Loyalty stays men on the firing line,
When defeat of purpose seems in sight
Forgetting self, obey orders by word or sign,
Battling boldly for what seems just and right.

If we were loyal to our professional interest as politicians, commercial men, manufacturers, bankers and laborers, and other organized bodies, our profession would soon be the guiding star, that would lead to the enactment of proper medical legislation, for the good of the whole people, and place us on that high plane of medical ethics that our profession so much desires and richly deserves.

The opposition to our purposes should not discourage, but only make us more courageous, stronger like the sturdy oak on the mountain side, that has been made strong by the adverse winds of many seasons during its tender years, causing it to be deeply rooted, so that our Association being fanned by the storms of political opposition will take deeper roots in the hearts of our membership and grow sufficiently strong to surmount all obstacles that are strewn in our pathway that leads to victory.

I recommend that our law be so changed that the committee on Public Policy and Medical Legislation be elected as follows: One for three years, one for two years and one for one year, the president and secretary of the Association being members ex-officio as they are now, for the reasons that they being elected by the Association or house of delegates, they would have more loyal support of the membership because they are elected rather than appointed. Also each would be better qualified after having served a time, and by that means the committee would always have one or more men of experience in their line. I also recommend that you give our Journal your very earnest support. The Journal with proper moral and financial support will become a very strong factor in making our undertakings a success, and it affords us the means of self-protection against the onslaught of enemies of organized medicine.

I suggest to the Council that, in order to make the Journal what it should be, a clean scientific Medical Journal, the articles and advertisements should be closely censored and, furthermore, I believe the salary and allowance of the editor should be increased, as the present amount seems to be inadequate for good service.

I further suggest that the Councillors be more active, that they may be required to visit each county society in their district once a year, or oftener if necessary, for so much depends upon thorough organization in each county, as we cannot admit anyone to membership in the Association, except through the county society. Again, I admonish you, one and all, in selecting officers or delegates, to always select men who are noted for their unselfish zeal and unquestioned devotion to the welfare of the Association, men who regard the interest of the Association above personal matters, that the Association may not suffer for want of official duty performed.

We note with no small degree of gratification that during the last year both of the political parties of the country declared for a National Health Bureau. Hence we feel encouraged to believe that people of this great nation are beginning to feel the importance of a national movement for the protection of the public health, therefore, I suggest that a resolution asking congress to take steps towards the establishment of a Health Department would not be amiss.

I commend to you the work of the Ladies' Auxiliary. That organization promises to be of great service to our Association, as woman's work is always valuable when engaged in any laudable enterprise. Woman has always been man's helpmate, and when we can enlist the Ladies' Auxiliary in our behalf for the public good our success is enhanced manifold. Woman rejoices with man in his ambitions and victories, sympathizes with him in his sorrow. Woman's influence over man is beyond our estimation.

We commend the legislature of Oklahoma for the passage of a bill regulating the registration of trained nurses to care for the sick and injured. Also the defeat of the bill recognizing the chiro-practors as physicians duly registered according to the laws of the state. The action in both of these cases indicates a desire on the part of the legislature to protect the public health.

We commend the action of the present State Board of Health in their efforts towards eliminating incompetent practitioners who were formerly recognized as physicians in the territories prior to Statehood and seek to be recognized under the present law, and pledge our hearty co-operation in all their efforts to elevate the standing of the profession in the state.

I would respectfully urge, that some organized effort be put forth in the state to suppress the Great White Plague, in our borders, thereby not only benefiting the people of our own state, but will lend encouragement to similar efforts in other states.

Another recommendation is, that you so amend our law that the matter of seating delegates will not be a troublesome matter as at this session. Make it specific. A great deal of time could be saved as well as confusion and friction, and possibly it would be a long step toward improving the scientific program.

I regret very much but feel it my duty as presiding officer, to call your attention to one or two things—one, a matter of personal prejudice among some of the members of our Association. Let us get these things out of the Association. Let us harmonize our efforts for the good of the profession. We have one central idea, that is, to elevate our standard of medical

efficiency in the state, and show the other Associations akin to us that we are trying to get on a level with the other states. We have as good medical talent as, I dare say, there is in the Union. Let us utilize it. Let us let these individual matters go; let us strive to keep out all entanglements of a political nature from our Medical Association.

If you will pardon the personality—my father was a physician; my uncle, a physician; my brother, a physician, and my son a physician. So my pride of ancestry and my hope for the future is in the medical profession. Hence I love to see such a noble profession harmonize in the same way as our constitution and by-laws harmonize. If we achieve this "It doth not yet appear what we shall be," but we will be great, especially in the estimation of the medical world.

I thank you, gentlemen, for the trust you placed in my hands a year ago. I promised then that I would make the very best president that could be made out of the material. I have indeed tried to do my best, but I hope that the one that succeeds me will do better. I have found out a few things he ought to know and which I will tell him if he will ask me.

Gentlemen, words fail me to express to you my hearty appreciation of what you have done for me.

I thank you.

THE TREATMENT OF PULMONARY TUBERCULOSIS

BY DR. W. G. LITTLE, OKMULGEE, OKLAHOMA

Read before the Seventeenth Annual Meeting of the Oklahoma State Medical Association, Oklahoma City, May, 1909.

Taking its toll of 150,000 annually from the population of the United States, and

those from the productive period of life, tuberculosis is easily the most stupenduous plague with which we are afflicted. And while these are passing out, there are those who are affected to the extent of being clinical cases, or in an advanced stage of the disease, numbering 500,000 more, who are non-productive because of their illness, and in addition, are a heavy financial tax upon their families and friends. With these facts before us we have easily one of the largest tasks confronting the medical ' fraternity that it has ever been called on to accomplish.

The disease is surely a curable one and also a preventable one. It needs only the proper means to be employed, an awakened interest, and an intelligent application of the knowledge that every physician should have, to accomplish a vast amelioration of the present condition.

The dead house statistics show that from sixty to eighty per cent of people have had tuberculosis, as shown by the healed lesions and where death has resulted from other diseases. We are driven then to the conclusion that the great majority of cases of tuberculosis are never diagnosed. In the clinical annals, the cases coming to the general practitioner have such a tardy diagnosis that the disease is scarcely manageable and usually makes steady progress to an unfavorable end.

LACK OF EARLY DIAGNOSIS.

This lack of early diagnosis is due to two causes: The first is, that the patient does not seek medical aid until he knows he is ill and until he has tried various home and patent remedies with little relief. This covers a period usually of from three to six months after the clinical symptoms have made their appearance.

The next reason for a late diagnosis is that the physician consulted is either too careless, or too ignorant concerning the early recognition of the disease, to arrive at a correct diagnosis until the family and friends have diagnosed the case and have told him, when by investigating he confirms the diagnosis. The average practitioner is probably too careless rather than too ignorant, in regard to this question. The *result*,

however, is the same—a late diagnosis and a long, expensive curative process, or an untoward ending. The economic gain to the body politic being greater, perhaps, in the latter ending.

SYMPTOMS.

The symptoms in the incipient stage are the most important, in that a recognition here may enable the patient to cut short his trouble and secure an early cure. These symptoms are: Emaciation more or less marked, general weakness, pallor of the skin and mucous membranes, a tendency to hypothermia and cold extremities, a rapid pulse with a lowered blood pressure and passive sweating. Add to this the finding of bacilli in the sputum and the diagnosis is made certain. But in the absence of bacilli in the sputum, if there is drooping of the shoulders, lessened expansion, and sinking in of the infraclavicular space, the diagnosis is reasonably sure and should be treated accordingly. Some writer has said: "The case is already past the incipient stage when bacilli can be demonstrated by the microscope." This is probably true for the majority of cases.

TREATMENT.

The treatment of this disease is such that it necessarily taxes to the utmost the ability and ingenuity of the physician, and the patience of the family and friends of the one afflicted. Being an essentially chronic affair in most cases, conditions arise which discourage both patient and physician.

It is not the object in this paper to detail the treatment of this malady, or attempt to cover every point which may arise in the course of the disease, but to outline the treatment and endeavor to stimulate thought and discussion. If we, as a profession, could crystallize our thought into some fixed, rational method, we would accomplish greater results from our efforts. Could this be done, the practitioners in the country towns would be able to treat the patients who come to him in a more effective manner. The majority of these will have to be treated where they are and under the conditions of life that fortune has imposed upon them. So much of our advice in text books is based upon the experience and knowledge of the city physician, who handles his cases in the hospital or sanitarium and so leaves the vast field of operation outside untouched. The country practitioner, thrown on his own resources without a guide for his procedure in adopting ways and means to meet the needs of the hour, is handicapped from the start.

The following is the essential treatment for these cases of pulmonary tuberculosis.

OPEN AIR LIVING.

The outdoor life is of prime importance. The patient should be in the open air twenty-four hours of every day when the weather is favorable. How nearly this can be followed will depend on location and weather conditions. Sunshine in the maximum amount must be secured, and each patient should be instructed to secure all of this available, especially in localities where many cloudy days prevail, for it is not only germicidal in its action, but is also a blood-builder, helps to develop the resistance to infection and improves the metabolic processes of the system. In addition, sunshine puts supreme optimism into the intellectual processes of the patient, producing thus a sort of psycho-therapeutic element.

It is an easy thing to tell the patient to live out of doors or in the open air. He will ask you "How can I do it?" and it will be up to the physician to TELL him how, in detail, as his circumstances will allow. This open air life may be secured by having the sleeping room with the windows wide open all night. The corner of the porch can be utilized for an out door sleeping room by

stretching a canvas on two sides. The out door tent, made especially for the patient, the flat roof of the house, in cities where ground space is at a minimum, may be used, on which to pitch a tent. The physician must see that these measures are carried out, and know that his patient will be in the open air all the time, and where the sunshine can do its beneficient work of purifying and vivifying. The physician must be the mental and mechanical genius to bring into being these agencies for his patient and impress upon him his own great hope and mental outlook.

MEDICAL TREATMENT.

Next the medical treatment; this is not satisfactory or definite. As yet we have no specific for this trouble as there is in diphtheria, malaria and a few other diseases in which a definite remedy has been evolved.

The serum treatment *seems* to be the rational end toward which we look with hope, but as yet it has been a disappointment as a therapeutic agency. Its greatest use at present is for diagnostic purposes. Even in this field there are many of high repute and vast experience throughout the world who are afraid to use it except under extraordinary circumstances and with the consent of the patient. In these latter days, however, many physicians have used the serum abundantly and with many good results, which seemed to have been obtained under other or the old modes of treatment.

Aside from this there are a few other remedies of real value. Of these creosote exerts a healing, stimulating influence. Perhaps, the carbonate is the best form of this drug. Iodine is another useful remedy. The tincture may be painted on the chest for those indefinite, troublesome pains so often annoying to the patient; or it may be used internally with glycerin, especially where there is a tendency to throat complications. Potassium iodid, in increasing doses, beginning at 5 grs., will aid very greatly by stimulating the general metobolic processes, oxidizing the waste products, and increasing the resistance of the individual. For the general care of the case and those symptoms arising from time to time in the course of the disease, the physician must use means which are usually effective for similar manifestations in other maladies, being careful to avoid any measure that would disturb the digestion.

DIETETIC.

The dietetic treatment is simple and easy to follow, viz: Plain, wholesome food, easily digestible. And if the first two principles are followed properly the appetite will usually take care of itself, and need no tempting by dainties and outlandish concoctions found in the domain of the culinary world, but will crave good meat, eggs, milk, bread and vegetables in sufficient quantity to furnish the system with all the necessary material for the upbuilding of the tissues.

HYGIENE.

In the matter of hygiene, a few simple rules suffice. The body should be kept warm, and of an even temperature; warm light garments for cold weather, cool, absorbent ones for warm weather. There should be a warm or tepid bath once or twice a week, or where the patient is robust enough the cold bath might be employed. In this connection, a daily massage with a preparation of salt, alcohol and olive oil, as practiced at Asheville by Von Rucks, will be found especially refreshing and invigorating. Little or no exercise should be taken if pulse or temperature are above normal or the cough is troublesome. The reason for this may be shown by the fact that if a patient had typhoid with a temperature above normal, he would be kept at rest; or if he had a sick hand it would be put in a sling. So with a sick lung, giving the same consti-

tutional symptoms, should be patient also remain at rest.

Where classes for instruction can be formed, this should be done, for the sake of the instruction, for the mental assurance and companionship, and for the general psychic effect, "a la Emmanuel."

CLIMATE.

In regard to climate, there is a mooted question. The mountain men claim everything in sight. The plainsmen claim the same; their statistics show about equal. The fact remains, the great majority have to take treatment at home. More, the home cure is more lasting and beneficial. And if the patient lives the same on the plains in his home that he would under good conditions in the mountains, his recovery would be just as steady and permanent, though possibly not quite so rapid. A locality with especially poor climate is to be excepted, of course.

FOR THE WELL-TO-DO.

For the adaptation of this outline of treatment to the conditions of the patients is a point to consider. For the well-to-do whose means will allow them to have any treatment they want, there are still dangers. Those of this class, as a rule, are not so obedient nor so content with the progress of the treatment in one place, as are the more dependent. They must be "moving on," trying new climes, and new scenes, seeking places where the curative processes are more rapid. As some one has said: "The foot of the rainbow of promise for such as these, rests ever within the boundaries of the spirit land."

THE PATIENTS OF MODERATE MEANS.

For the great majority of sufferers, treatment must be had at home and usually under adverse conditions. Many must work to support themselves or some one dependent on them. They must remain at home, having no chance even for sanitarium treatment for a few weeks only, whereby they may learn to care for themselves properly. They have not the means for any of these luxuries in their illness. In these cases is where the physician is taxed to arrange, if possible, the proper conditions for their treatment. He must contrive ways and means of an inexpensive character whereby the patient may secure the advantages of open air—medicine, rest and relief.

THE INDIGENT.

Another problem is the indigent class. How are they to have proper care? These furnish the greatest menace, perhaps, and the least hope of cure. The reason is: They are not amenable to treatment, are untaught concerning the rules of right living, and are neglected. They spit where they will and spread infection everywhere they go or live. The physician cannot take care of them. The community usually will not. This is a distinct duty of the public or state, it seems to me.

THE RESPONSIBILITY OF THE STATE.

The state has a responsibility in this fight. Its responsibility is measured by the needs of the situation and the duty of the commonwealth to guard the welfare of its citizens. This aid has been very tardy indeed. There is a reason for it, in that the medical men have never brought the matter to the notice of the powers that be (the politicians) in actual facts, measured by dollars. This can be done when the proper laws are enacted and enforced, whereby the number of tuberculosis patients in the state can be ascertained and their whereabouts known at all times. By the last Bulletin of the Health Commissioner, perhaps three hundred cases of tuberculosis are reported in the state. This number would be greatly increased if all the physicians would report all the cases they have under their care.

That would mean that probably five hundred people in the state are afflicted, and that during the productive period of life. This means an actual loss to the state in the present earning capacity of $350,000, reckoning the yearly earning capacity at $700 per annum. Add to this then the average expectancy of life for this number, which would be about twenty years, and the figures reach the enormous total of $7,000,-000. But add to this then the actual expense of caring for these patients through two years' illness and the value of the time required of members of the family to care for them, and this total is greatly increased.

But the state has done not one thing for these unfortunates. We claim to be the greatest state of all, and boast of our attainments and the advanced ideas in public government we stand for, but in this great fight for the lives of our people we are branded as derelicts.

Standing at the fore front in the fight for the suppression of tuberculosis, is the good old state of Illinois, swamped with politics, which yet at its last legislature, laid aside its politics and voted almost to a man for the passage of the Glacken bill, which enables cities or villages to levy a five mill tax to build and support sanitaria for the care of their tuberculous citizens. And be it to their honor, Chicago voted that tax by popular vote of its citizens within a few weeks after the passage of the bill giving the right, and already has its hospital under way.

Why should not our own state lay aside its politics for a few days and pass such a bill for the aid of humanity? Three or four counties might combine and have a union hospital. This would place an institution within easy reach of the afflicted of these counties, thus insuring to them every advantage for cure possible and save to the state the benefit of their earnings during the productive period of life.

I believe the state should provide several hospitals, easily accessible, some for incipient cases, others for advanced cases, of tuberculosis. I believe this Society should have a special committee to work with the legislature for such a provision. I believe this committee should begin with a widespread campaign of publicity and education. I believe every County Society should designate one of its members to make a popular address in each town of his county on this subject and urge the people to work for the suppression of tuberculosis.

PREVENTIVE TREATMENT.

Preventive treatment has a demand in the consideration of this subject, and prophylaxis becomes an element of paramount importance. This goes hand in hand with the active treatment of the individual cases. This makes for the protection of the uninfected as well as for the care of the individual. In this lies the hope for the suppression of the ravages of the white scourge. It will be a slow process; the radiant dreams of those who think this scourge will be conquered in a year and a day are destined to be shattered by a stubborn resistance of the malady through the years to come. But action is in the right direction now and should be given increased impetus by laymen and the profession.

These efforts should be directed along definite lines, such as these:

First—The suppression of quackery: The fake medicine concerns, and heartless vampires calling themselves doctors, having a "sure cure" for consumption, feeding off this credulous class of victims, should be suppressed by a sure and hard hand.

Second—Education: A campaign of education concerning the nature, care and suppression of this malady should be pro-

mulgated for the enlightenment of the public. This could be done by the county and city societies preparing open meetings where this question would be discussed in lay terms, for the education of the masses; or a special popular lecture course might be instituted prepared in an interesting manner, and illustrated by lantern slides or otherwise wherein the disease would be graphically portrayed. This means might even arouse some of the easy going physicians to the extent that they would attend the meetings, and become awake to the importance of care in examining for incipient cases of tuberculosis in their practice, and hence be able to find incipient cases for early and promising treatment.

Third—Sanitation: Certain regulations especially for tenements in cities, should be enforced. And it is possible for private residences, where there is a city building commissioner; at least a certain amount of light should be required in all buildings and no room shut out from the direct sun light. How these measures may be obtained generally, I hardly know, but that they should prevail no one can deny.

Fourth—Legislation: While much beneficent legislation has been enacted in various states, yet the needs have not been adequately provided for. There is need for a law making obligatory the reporting of all cases of tuberculosis to the proper authorities.

Each residence where a tuberculosis patient lives should be reported and cared for properly; and if the afflicted person removes either because of death or change to other dwelling, the premises should be thoroughly disinfected before another occupant is allowed to move in. The Board of Health should also send out adequate printed rules to be given to each consumptive by his physician, as part of the legislative requirements. The dry sweeping of any public building should be prohibited by law, as also the exposing of food products to the action of flies and dust. These things are included in part in the present health laws, but they are not inclusive enough, and the amount of political machinery that has to be set in motion to secure action is too cumbersome—and the proper board to approach in the matter too doubtful.

For *utility* "simplicity is to be sought." The present complexity defeats the purpose of the existing laws in that the physician is unable to find where to report or where to lay complaint.

Members of the Oklahoma State Medical Society, we are standing before the greatest problem of the present age. It is measured only by the opportunity it offers. Let us lay aside all petty wranglings, and narrow bickerings among ourselves, and work together for the mighty achievement the present opportunity holds for the medical profession.

DISCUSSION.

It was moved and seconded that Dr. Turck, of Chicago, be asked to take the floor, which motion upon being put to the house was unanimously carried.

Dr. Turck, Chicago:

The profession is advancing, and we do not see clearly yet, but we are reaching life and light. Nothing would do more good than for others to just peruse that paper and see from the broad predictions in it the spirit of altruism and the nobility of the scientific body who are devoting their lives and interests to the welfare of society, from which they can obtain no personal benefit. The presentation of the more modern methods in the development of anti-bodies in the system has brought to us entirely a new picture. Many may say we are dowdy and that these things were all here before; yes, they were here, and so were all discoveries here, only we now have in our hands every experimental study to more intelligently investigate and to apply all these facts to the protoplasm and therapeutics of tuberculosis. The apparent optimistic tendency that is now so generally prevalent is very different from the pessimistic expressions of a few years ago, and even those who have never done any experimental work haven't even read of the researches that are being made, still see in the very atmosphere the results of these experiments in regard to the anti-bodies and the methods these are reaching. We knew years ago that tuberculosis entered the body; we knew also there were antibodies formed, but we did not know the means by which the anti-bodies were brought out. Now we find sunlight and air. Finert was required by the world and died only too soon, because why? The same sunlight that had been shining for ages was found in a new vision. The affect of open air producing hygiene in the surface of the body and * * * has accomplished its wonderful effect in producing anti-toxics. The effects of dietetics in increasing anti-bodies and the provision of toxin is to decrease these anti-bodies, and this has placed another weapon in the hands of the medical profession. We may say that at the present time we have two important things in our grasp, especially in those conditions in which there are evidences of an impending infection, the * * * from those who are in a healthy state and the treatment and care of all must be in the early stages of tuberculosis.

Now, against the last proposition of sunlight and air. The adjustment of these measures in the hands of whom, the laity? No, they can not do it; no, they had the sunlight for ages. The Christian Scientists? No. The Emanuel Movement, the Osteopaths and the quackeries of this country? No. The highest intelligence of the scientific mind of the practitioner is required. (Applause.) Do not be afraid because now and then you see bobbing up here and there some quacks, some irregulars, some men who do not have an idea of the profession, they must bow, they must go down under the pressure of intellect and science.

Now, the last is the application of dietetics. I wish, ladies and gentlemen, that I could have a few moments on this important thing, as I have been experimenting, but I would simply make this a general proposition and emphasize some of the interesting points brought out.

If I might criticise the paper, it was too extensive, too much, and yet I might say the subject was extensive. It is found that dietetics is one of the most pathological weapons in the hands of we practitioners; air and sunlight are all we have. It is an intrusion. Two things, therefore, are necessary in the question of intrusion. One is the digestive apparatus and the other is the substance to be digested. These two necessary factors must be adjusted to each other with a perfect knowledge, before we attempt treatment in each individual case. The conditions that are found physiologically in the individual must first be established. That can be learned by any general practitioner—not by Christian Scientists, not by quacks, not by those uninformed, but those informed can soon find regular means, and when we find that certain conditions are present in the motor activities of the body, they can bring up and awaken the digestive apparatus to a higher and higher standard.

So, just as a gymnast can be trained, so can the apparatus be taught and educated to increase the power of carrying on the digestion. I might, if I could give a generalization, say, let more attention be paid to secretory conditions than to others and to dietetics. What part of the organism is at fault? The motor activities are at fault. Just as the muscles of the body become weakened, so are the muscles of the tract. Therefore, the deduction is that if the food is finer, it will thus increase the amount of nutrition with less amount of labor. If food is too coarse or too large then food can be reduced to finer properties so that the working apparatus can be carried on. The increase of nutrition is that which furnishes the greatest degree of resistence against toxin of tuberculosis. Can we not see a new era in the scientific treatment of tuberculosis, and this be done to the glory and credit of the open practitioner?

———

Dr. Williams, Wellston:

I hardly feel like following an address like the one just given because of the comparison being too great, but the subject is one of vast importance to us country practitioners. The Doctor's words were surely along lines that we ought to give thought, and not only thought, but I hope it will be brought into effect in Oklahoma. I hope to see the time come when there will be some solution offered for this problem, not only for the benefit of the patient suffering from tuberculosis, but for the protection of the public in general. It is a fact that tuberculosis is an infectious disease, and its patients are allowed to go out and come in contact with the public in general; therefore, I am in hopes that before this medical association adjourns that this solution, offered by the Doctor in his paper, will be endorsed by the Oklahoma State Medical Association. Dr. Turck has told us in his discussion what we should do. I regret very much, gentlemen, that the Doctor didn't have the time to tell us how he would prepare it, but I suppose if we hear his lecture tomorrow he will cover this point. This subject, I will repeat, is one that should interest every practitioner, and one that we should give our assistance to, and see to it that there is some means whereby we can aid the public.

———

Dr. Johnson, Gainesville, Texas:

I am very sorry I didn't hear all of the most excellent paper. I was in the other room and failed to get the first part of it. All the physicians here are well acquainted with the fact that it was at the request of the International Tuberculosis Congress that the local Associations throughout the United States took up this tuberculosis problem to educate and teach the laity as much as possible how to guard against it. I want to say that the Cook County Medical Association, of which I am a member, is one of the very first, I believe, to follow the dictates of the Tuberculosis Congress. We have in the last thirty days had a committee, composed of three or four of us physicians who are most interested in it, and it has been our pleasure and our duty to go out into the smaller towns and lecture upon preventive medicine. We have not confined ourselves simply to the subject of tuberculosis, but we have taken up many infectious diseases; but I wanted to suggest to the Doctors (I presume you are from all over the State of Oklahoma), that when you return to your homes you take this matter up with your Associations, and I want to assure you gentlemen, that when you do this and go out into your little communities you are going to find an intelligent audience awaiting you there. It has been my pleasure to lecture in a few places around my county at home, and they will meet you at the school house, or any sort of a place, because fast the laity are becoming interested, and when you explain to them that one person out of every three dies from tuberculosis, and that one out of every ten succumbs to some form of tubercular trouble, and when you bring home facts of that kind to people, they are going to appreciate it and the time isn't far distant when this matter will become an International proposition and the attempt, as you know, is being made and will be made until it is successful, to have an International officer for this matter. The tuberculosis proposition should not only be International, but it should be a State matter, and it should be looked after by health officers in the city.

———

Discussion closed by Dr. Little, Okmulgee:

I wish to thank these gentlemen for the discussion of the paper which has brought out additional things, and I hope the paper has done some good at least. I thank you.

GYNECOLOGICAL CONDITIONS

BY DR. O. R. JETER, REED, OKLAHOMA

Read Before the Seventeenth Annual Meeting of the Oklahoma State Medical Association, Oklahoma City, May 11-13, 1909.

Mr. Chairman, Gentlemen and Fellow Practitioners:

In the discussion of Gynecological Conditions we have probably the broadest field, and one for the greatest advancement, of any one branch known to the profession today. Gynecological Conditions and who is to blame is the thought I wish to place before you for discussion.

In this paper I wish to mention briefly some conditions found from infancy to the closing day of senility, and in this period I am trying to sub-divide into three periods that come under the observation of the practitioner in his ever-day life. First, we have the child from infancy to menstruation or womanhood. Second, from the age of puberty to the menopouse, or the child-bearing period. Third, through the declining years, or years of atrophy and loss of woman's pride. On an average, extending to about fourteen years, we have but few of the just mentioned conditions that come under our observation, nevertheless those that come are of vast importance to the medical profession, and I will mention some few with their etiology. For instance, we have the imperforate hymen, but as a rule prior to puberty the anomaly does not amount to very much but in exceptional cases. However, there may be an extraordinary mucous discharge secreted which on being unable to escape from the vagina, eventually causes distention, and results in the development of a fluctuating pelvic tumor. As a matter of fact, this tumor, sooner or later, begins to bulge at the vulvo vaginal orifice, and possibly will attain to a considerable size, and will cause more or less interference with defecation and micturation. This will happen in childhood, and as a rule, just before puberty. But who is responsible? Is it the mother, the father, the previous attendant, or either? The poor, backwoods doctor that waited on my wife failed to detect this, for the man in attendance at this time, to unload some of his dastardly work by saying "yes," he, the man, who delivered the child, should have inspected the vagina for any obstruction that might be. I ven-

ture the assertion that there is not one out of every one hundred—no, not one in five hundred—that makes this practice. We have abnormalities too numerous to-mention, but of much less importance, and some etiological factors found after puberty of which we shall briefly speak. We have anatomical causes, hereditary and conginetal causes, civilization, social, educational, unhygienic general and local cleanliness, child-birth, sexual relations, criminal abortion, veneral diseases, accidental infections and traumatism at all periods of life. Women are susceptible or exposed to certain diseases or accidents, beginning at infancy and ending with senility. Some of these conditions we find before puberty, taking them as they come, is it the anatomical conditions with their mal-position or formation that renders the female more susceptible to disease? The hereditary and congenital causes inherited tendency woman is found to be susceptible to certain functional and organic diseases, some we might here mention, dysmenorrhea, uterine, displacement, and even civilization, the natural muscular strength and power to resist disease, is greater in women belonging to savage tribes; who is to blame? There is a marked difference between the working women and the women of higher grades of society as to the frequency of various genitouinary diseases, and many other maladies that might be mentioned under this head. Even our modern system of education has a decidedly injurious influence upon the general and sexual strength of woman, of which our profession should and could be of some aid in relief. Unhygenic conditions, general and local cleanliness, care of bowels and bladder, precaution during menstration, exercise, food, dress, rest, child-birth, injuries resulting from labor also bad management during and after labor, resulting in sepsis. At all ages we are sometimes placed in an awkward position to make a diagnosis. We have gonorrhea in the lady of twenty-five and thirty. She being an innocent party, what must we do, and who is to blame? Ah, can it be, or can't it be the man, her husband, or some other fellow, or did she receive this by accidental infection? Anyway, the doctor is to blame; but we are compelled to make a diagnosis. But in disorders of menstration we have one broad field of gynecology, and of our greatest causes is probably the abnormal condition and position of the uterus, due, no doubt, to the use and abuse of this organ. Amenorrhea to be caused by excessive curettage or cauterization of the mucus lining of the uterus, due to nothing but the incompetent practitioner, and his love for his so-called operation. I shall speak of the one more condition found in menstruation. I hope that your discussion will be full on this point, as I am now wound up in two cases, this being the membranous type of dysmenorrhea. It being characterized by expulsion at the menstrual period of organized membranes, either as a whole or in pieces, its etiology is a matter of dispute. The escape of this membrane can be accounted for by the blood accumulating under it, and dissecting it off. It is forced to pass away. We have for our symptoms severe colicky pains recurring at each period. The flow is often intermittent. The symptoms resemble those of obstructive dysmenorrhoea, and the course is, as a rule, protracted. My severest case begins by fainting, as she terms it, and continues in this state from twelve to eighteen hours; "give me a treatment."

In speaking of all conditions, probably one of the most common in Oklahoma today is laceration of perinaeum, and relaxation of the vaginal outlet, the most common cause being child-birth, either natural or instrumental, but rarely by violence Where we are two hours late, head actively engaged and actually protruding at the vaginal orifice, with face presentation in young women. Please tell me how to prevent perineal laceration. Who is to blame? Three years in the future and at time of next confinement, and Doctor J. is in attendance, and Mr. Smith tells him who attended his wife before. You can guess who was to blame, we find our profession severely censured for the majority of conditions we find—why this? Simply because we have some in the profession that are always ready to butcher our calling.

One more condition, though rarely found in my section, but very necessary to be detected when it exists, and I am through.

Ectopic gestation as a rule is primarily tubal, and we have three varieties: tubal proper, tubouterine in that portion of the tube embraced by the uterine wall. Tuboovarian or pregnancy existing between the tube and the ovary. Abdominal pregnancy was originally tubal, ovarion pregnancy apparently resulting from the impregnation of the ovum, while still in a graafian follicle, can no longer be doubted as a possibility; but the number of cases are still small. It has long been recognized that tubal inflammation, peritoneal adhesions, and pressure upon the tube predisposed to tubal pregnancy. In the case of inflammation, however, not until the tubal mucosas become practically normal is tubal pregnancy likely to occur. Hindrance to the passage of a fertile ova into the uterus will not of itself cause tubal implantation of the ovum. The idea has been advanced that under normal conditions the tube will not undergo the decidual change necessary for pregnancy, but that the tubal mucosa of a few women possesses the property common in many of the lower animals of responding to the stimulus which the fertilized ovum offers by forming a decidual membrane in such individuals, if the passage of the ovum into the uterus is interferred with tubal pregnancy results. And who is to blame? Doderlin states that while there was a history of tubal inflammation in ninety per cent of his cases very few of the number were gonorrhoeal, and that the tubal pregnancy was the first conception but three times in forty-five cases.

' DISCUSSION.

Dr. Gillis, Frederick:

I wasn't expecting to discuss any of the papers and consequently I can not say very much. I enjoyed the paper, though, and it brought out quite a good many more things than we usually handle or more than we generally see in our general practice. I have handled cases on this line and as a rule I don't follow them as closely as the Doctor has. I think all of his suggestions were good and would be well to follow. But as far as treatment for dysmenorrhea, I for one can't give anything much. I think the paper would be well for all Doctors especially the country Doctors, and I think that papers of this kind ought to be extremely interesting on account of making us look after our patients a little more closely and give them all the thought we can, for my experience is the country Doctor is the man that has to do everything and he will get negligent in a great many respects, and papers of this kind, I think. are beneficial because it makes us do a little better. I am very glad I heard the paper.

PLACENTA PRAEVIA

BY DR. M. M. DeARMAN, MANGUM, OKLAHOMA

To discuss before this body more than the treatment of placenta praevia would be a useless waste of time and energy, I will. therefore, pass over the cause, frequency. symptoms and diagnosis without further comment and deal directly with the treatment:

Treatment: There is no single method of treatment in placenta praevia applicable in all cases and at all times, therefore the obstetrician will act most wisely who chooses means corresponding with the special features of the case in hand and the emergencies which arise. Allow me to emphasize the fact that of all conditions which the obstetrician has to deal there is none which comes nearer being a law unto itself than does placenta praevia. The different location of the placenta has to be ascertained, the vitality of the mother, the vibility of the child, the frequence and strength of the uerine contractions all have to be considered and I would say in the life experience of an ordinary obstetrician he would hardly see two cases of placenta praevia that were similar in every respect. Therefore, considering the many different varieties, the infrequency with which it occurs you will readily see that except in large maternity hospitals but few of us would, in the course of an ordinary life's practice hope to become expert in the treatment of this condition if left to experience to gain our knowledge, therefore, there is no condition known in medicine or surgery where the skill and ability of an ordinary practitioner is more surely tried than in placenta praevia. Some of these cases, as I have already intimated, and as I will show you by the record of my first case will, if left to nature, take care of itself nicely with no mortality to mother or child, and I am of the opinion a great majority if left to nature, will terminate fatally, to the child especially, and a heavy majority to the mother. You can only decide which of these cases to interfere with and which to leave to nature by studying well the conditions you have to deal with as they arise and being prepared to meet any emergency, to make this more explicit will give a report of three cases, all that I have ever seen in the accouchement of 1,000 women.

Case One: Mrs. D., age 46 years, mother of twelve healthy children, no history of miscarriage, abortion or peurperal infections; was summoned hurriedly on night of Sept. 9, 1906, by husband, who stated that his wife had had a severe hemorrhage; on reaching the house I found as the husband had stated evidence of profuse hemorrhage on the floor. Apparently from the floor stains and blood in the skirts and on the mattress would say something like one gallon of blood had been lost; on examining my patient I found to my surprise strong pulse, good color, strong and frequent uterine contractions; I found on vaginal examination what I would be pleased to term a central inflammation of the margin of the placenta, that is, the bulk of the placenta attached low down on left side with a portion of the placenta passing over and completely closing the internal os. Having a large spacious vagina and a very nervy patient I was able to introduce my finger well up through the internal os, sweeping it around the os, separated the placenta from its attachment to the uterine walls I was very agreeably surprised to pass beyond the edge of the placenta and have a tense bag of water fill the cervix and protrude into the vagina, which, fortunately for my excited, nervous condition, ruptured with the following contractions, the head descending rapidly into the cervix

completely stopping the flow of blood, the child acting as a wedge, kept the flow in check until the completion of the second stage of labor which was only a very few minutes, the uterus expelling the placenta in ten to fifteen minutes without any aid on my part and without the loss of any more blood. This woman, I feel certain, if left to nature, would have completed her own delivery in a reasonable period of time and without any injury to mother or child. I feel confident that with a very few more contractions nature would have accomplished the same, by dilation of the internal os that I did with my finger after tearing the placenta away and allowing the membranes to act as a tampon to check the hemorrhage.

In this as in a great majority of placenta praevia cases, however, the prognosis as to the termination of labor could only be given after delivery.

Case Two: Age 30, mother of four living children, several early miscarriages. This case I saw in consultation with two of my fellow practitioners, 48 hours after the beginning of a rather profuse but not an alarming hemorrhage, with very poor uterine contractions, while this hemorrhage had been constant for 48 hours, it had at no time been alarming until thirty minutes before I was summoned, when the patient had a rather hard pain and a very free flow of blood, which continued almost uninterrupted regardless of pains. Finding when I arrived at the house patient in an exsanguinated condition. Fortunately the Doctor in attendance had given her stimulants and normal salt and had everything in readiness for interfering with the process of labor. Considering the length of time since the flow began and the very weakened condition of the woman, my efforts were directed to delivering her as rapidly as possible, without thought of the welfare of the child, taking time only to clean my hands and arms, without waiting for the completion of anesthesia, I cleansed the vagina, introduced my hand, dilated the cervix, as rapidly as I could with my finger, tore directly through the centrally implanted placenta, ruptured the membranes, and fortunately found feet instead of the head presenting. Grasping these I brought them down, making a wedge of the thighs of the child which acted as a dilator also for the cervix, which yielded very rapidly, enabling me to complete the delivery in about 25 minutes; contrary to my first case, the uterus did not empty itself of the placenta nor did the hemorrhage cease, but continued to bleed anew very vigorously as soon as the child passed through the cervix, requiring me to introduce my hand a second time and literally dig the placenta away from its attachment, from the excessive manipulation and tendency to continue to hemorrhage I irrigated the uterus with several quarts of hot bi-chloride solution and packed it tight with iodoform gauze, a precaution which I think should always be taken where the hand has been in the uterine cavity for any length of time. The child gasped a few times after delivery, but was unable to resuscitate it; however, I feel confident that had interference been 12 hours earlier the child could have been saved as well as the mother, who made uneventful recovery.

Third case: Aged 24, scond confinement, general septicemia following first labor lasting eight weeks. First evidence of labor at full term was rather hard pain, followed by a continued flow of such an extent that the patient was in an exhausted, unconscious condition when I saw her thirty minutes later; I summoned counsel, gave her a stimulant and getting things ready by the time my counsel had arrived. Upon examination I was able to feel only large clots of blood in the vagina and the cervix which

was dilated to admit of two fingers without difficulty. My method in this was the same as in case 2, dilating the cervix with my finger, until I could introduce my hand, tearing the placenta loose as far as I could reach my finger on either side. Failing to reach a free edge I tore directly through center, ruptured membrane, produced version, brought down the feet and made as rapid a delivery as possible. In this, as in case 2, the placenta had to be removed by my hand on the inside of uterus; no after hemorrhage or infection followed, the baby was slightly cyanosed when it was born, but breathed and cried strong in ten minutes; mother and child both made rapid recovery.

The one and only point I wish to make is this, that any of us are capable of treating placenta previa intelligently if we knew at the beginning the variety we had to deal with, but unfortunately for the mother we cannot be certain of until we have the uterus empty and the placenta where we can examine it, therefore, never sit idly by after you are certain you are dealing with placenta praevia and wait to see what nature will do, but clean up your hands and the woman's vagina, examine and, if possible to introduce your finger in the cervix, dilate, go on through the placenta or to one side, bring down your feet and deliver as rapidly as possible, if done under strict aseptic conditions, you do not jeopardize the life of your patient by leaving her to bleed for hours; you give the child the best chance for its life and run little danger of infection.

As to treatment of placenta praevia early in pregnancy, surely would follow the example of Braxton Hicks of inducing labor as soon as my diagnosis was passed, then you can prepare for your work, have your help and take your time, if left to nature, labor may come when help cannot be gotten, the patient possibly miles from a doctor and the first flow at full term may so deplete your patient that you can never resuscitate her. The high mortality of 60 or 70 per cent as given by large hospitals can be greatly reduced by proper and intel-ligent interference.

DISCUSSION.

Dr. Reck, Hennessey:

I appreciate the paper. It was very good. It has been my misfortune to have two cases in the last twenty-five years and that is the only treatment I know anything about. Of course, it is not always successful with the child. I lost one child, but the mothers both recovered.

Dr. Gillis, Frederick:

I enjoyed this paper. At first I understood the Doctor to say that in a great majority of cases that nature would attend to them all right, but afterwards saw he didn't say that, and I have no issue to make. I wish to say I had one case in consultation with another Doctor. The Doctor asked me to go down in the case with him, and I want to say he was an irregular and I didn't want to go as that was the first and only time I went with an irregular. But when he told me what kind of a case it was I went. He said there was no use to hurry down there for she was doing well and he didn't think it was necessary to try and get down there in such a hurry, but I told him if he was not mistaken in the case I wouldn't be at all surprised to find the woman dead when we got there, and sure enough, when we got there she was almost dead and lived only a few minutes. Another case I had, I saw the case three months before labor and I was pretty uneasy, but I wanted to go the full term if possible, so I had everything ready and I wouldn't leave town without I knew absolutely that she could get attention should

she need it, so in that case I didn't leave and I had everything fixed that she might possibly need, and she went the full term and the child was born all right. I am glad I heard the paper.

Dr. J. J. Dodson, Mangum:

I understood the Doctor to advise the rapid delivery of the woman as soon as diagnosis was made. I suppose he meant at any time during the stage of pregnancy. It is the general rule to give the mother all the advantages possible and if any sacrifice is to be made, it is the child. I think it is a good deal owing to circumstances whether I would advise delivery as soon as diagnosis is made or not, for if they go the whole term there is a chance to save the babies, but when a woman can't have constant care I think it is all right to deliver her, but if she can have constant care and attention. she ought to go the full term for there is a chance to save the child and it is easier to deliver the woman after the whole term than it is before, but sometimes the hemorrhage is so bad, but when she can be placed under care and have attention at any moment I think it best to let her go on as long as possible.

Dr. Donohue, Afton:

I will ask how the Doctor dilates?

Dr. D'Arman, Mangum:

I use my fingers if I can dilate successfully. I think that is all we have to overcome in these cases, is the dilation of the surface, when they have that they can complete the delivery pretty quick, and it is just a matter of complete and proper dilatation of the surface.

Dr. Hulen, Pond Creek:

I have had something over one thousand

cases of that kind, and I have been fortunate enough to steer clear of placenta praevia except in two cases. In one case I never worked so hard or accomplished less in delivery of a seven-pound case. I would get the head down and in a few minutes it would be right back again, and finally I had to resort to the feet. It seems to me that the safer thing to do would be to bore through the center of the placentia if the dilatation is complete or sufficient to allow you to do it. On the other hand if the symptoms are not urgent, let it run until they are. If you have got to encounter a severe hemorrhage and produce dilation at the same time, you are up against a hard proposition.

In regard to the remark the gentleman made in regard to placenta previa in the early stages of pregnancy, unless there are some symptoms urgent enough to cause us to make a local examination, I believe in letting them run. I recall a case that menstruated regularly for six months after conception. There was every symptom of pregnancy yet there was that regularity of the menstral flow. Some one might have taken it for granted that it was a hemorrhage; in any case every night or every second or fourth night there was a little gush of blood like there was pressure there and yet when it was over there was no symptom of hemorrhage. There was no misplacement, no abnormal symptom. And I believe in letting these cases run until there is a demand to do something.

———

Dr. Bardford, Oklahoma City:

It seems to me that it would be safer to wait until nature presses. The child might be lost, but it occurs to me that would save the mother.

———

Dr. Ney Neel, Mangum, Chairman:

Gentlemen, I am glad to see you entering into this discussion. I am only sorry there are no more present for these are subjects that the majority of us will go back home knowing more of.

———

Mr. D'Arman, Mangum:

Mr. Chairman: In cases of placenta previa, I think we are apt to jeopardize the life of the mother unduly trying to save the life of the child. The fact that you have a hemorrhage or the placenta praevia, you have an infection and you will possibly have the mother die from an infection from three to six months before you can deliver the child and for that reason I believe in looking very carefully after the patient. I don't think that Dr. Gillis understood my meaning; I think I wouldn't have much trouble in making a diagnosis during the flowing because during placenta previa they generally have the blood come without pain lasting only a few moments, while in normal flow, it comes with some regularity and certain days apart. I believe Dr. Gillis was a little confused in the beginning, but I intended to convey the impression that a whole lot could be left to nature if they have proper care, on the other hand, are we justified in leaving the patient alone when we might lower the per cent of mortality. And when you start to interfere, you had better complete it at once. I thank you, gentlemen.

THE TREATMENT OF ACUTE ARTICULAR RHEUMATISM

BY LEIGH F. WATSON, M. D., OKLAHOMA CITY

The patient who suffers from acute articular rheumatism should have a quiet room of equable temperature, free from draughts.

Chilling of the body surface is harmful; he should, therefore, be clothed entirely in flannels and put to bed.

Do not allow him to make any muscular exertion whatever, not even to feed himself or move about in bed.

As the object of the rest is to minimize the work of the heart, friends and all forms of excitement must be excluded from the patient's room.

The affected joints should be wrapped in wadding and put at absolute rest, preferably by the use of a splint.

For acute symptoms and to induce quiet the first two days, opiates are to be used, a lead and opium dressing is often useful.

Do not allow too much water, as it increases the work of the heart, and prohibit all forms of stimulants unless absolutely indicated.

The diet should be light and easy of digestion, such as milk, buttermilk, broths, bouillon, egg albumin, chicken jelly, small feedings at frequent intervals are to be preferred.

The treatment is to be commenced by administering a good purgative and securing free catharsis.

Order sodium salicylate 20 to 30 grains every four hours, until pain ceases or symptoms appear? After the acute symptoms have subsided continue the salicylates with diminishing dosage at increasing intervals, being guided by the tolerance of the patient and the severity of the attack.

When the salicylates are ineffectual combine with an equal amount of potassium bicarbonate to alkalinize the secretions. The salicylates prevent the multiplication of the specific organisms in the body.

Give sodium iodide for absorption of fluid around the heart.

When sodium salicylate cannot be borne, or is unsatisfactory, use strontium salicylate 7 1-2 to 15 grains, or aspirin (acetylsalicylic acid), 5 to 10 grains, combined with caffein for depression.

Sometimes salol, salicin, or oil of gaultheria proves beneficial in obstinate cases.

After acute symptoms have subsided use ungeuntum icthyoli, twenty-five to fifty per cent over the affected joints combined with a pressure bandage to hasten absorption.

Two or three small blisters about one inch in diameter used in the left axilla or over the nipple will stimulate the heart reflexly through the intercostal nerves.

Larger blisters above and below the affected joints are useful to relieve the pain.

Hot air at 200 to 250 degrees F. is useful, allowing fifteen to twenty minutes for each application, the joint to be well wrapped in bandages to absorb the sweat and prevent blistering.

The salicylates must be continued two to three weeks, and the rest in bed ten to fourteen days after all symptoms have disappeared, so as to avoid relapse and secure a normal heart.

307 East Fourth Street.

EDITORIAL

MEDICAL DEFENSE FUNDS.

The value of medical organization is no better demonstrated than is shown by the tendency of medical organizations throughout the country to further the interests of the profession not only through the advancement and wide dissemination of new discoveries in dedical treatment and surgical advances, but the equally material interests are being safeguarded by the establishment of medical defense funds in many state organizations whose object is to discourage malpractice suits and defend its members against this class of cases which as a rule have no merit and either have behind them the tentacles of blackmail or are fostered and encouraged by some thoughtless, jealous or ignorant physician.

The proposition usually laid down by these bodies is to assess each member so much annually and from this fund able legal talent is retained for the defense of members who may be unfortunate enough to have such a suit pending against them. The assessment amounts to nothing, $1.50 per annum being the amount raised so far in most states. Its advantages are many.

First: The moral influence created by such a step is very great.

Second: The fact that one set of attorneys are retained to manage these cases speaks well for it, as there is perfection in specialization, such men naturally soon become better equipped to try these causes than even more brilliant men in other phases of the legal profession.

Third: When you consider that you have an attorney to represent you in such a possible contingency and that at a cost of one dollar and fifty cents per annum your conclusion must be obvious.

It should be borne in mind that no man in our profession is too high or low to fall a victim to such suits. One of the ablest surgeons in our state and one of the most universally respected and beloved is now being attacked in a neighboring state, on the grounds that he was guilty of malpractice in the management of a case and recently in England two noted English surgeons were worried with a long and expensive suit of this character.

Immediate steps should be taken by our Association looking toward the establishment of such a branch.

THE STATE BOARD OF HEALTH AND TUBERCULAR PHYSICIANS.

Dr. S. Adolphus Knopf, one of America's leading authorities on tuberculosis, takes sharp issue with the recent ruling of the Board of Medical Examiners of Oklahoma prohibiting, in the future, the licensing of tubercular physicians in this state (see Journal American Medical Association, September 25, 1909), Dr. Knopf is pleased to term the whole matter "A New Type of Phthisiophobia," and at the June meeting of the American Medical Association in the Section on Preventive Medicine, presented a resolution setting forth that "the clean, conscientious, and trained consumptive is not a menace to his fellow man and that the scientific knowledge of tuberculosis has been vastly increased by physicians, past and present, who have been afflicted with the disease."

These premises must be accepted as correct, in the main, but there is always a small element of danger in association with consumptives, even by the healthy and the State Board of Examiners, we presume, assumes that that danger is greatly increased when a consumptive is brought in contact with one who is already run down and open to infection by illness. This conclusion must also be admitted as correct and when one further investigates the matter he must also conclude that all consumptive physicians are not necessarily either "clean, conscientious or trained."

Dr. Knopf points out that Solly, Trudeau, Brehmer and Dettweiler, all concumptives, added greatly to our present success in the management of this disease and added lustre to the medical profession. All this is agreed to, but that does not remove the danger and while it is true that the danger is a minimal one the Board of Examiners are only acting for what they think is best for the protection of the health of the people of Oklahoma.

Considering the humane features of the case Dr. Knopf recalls "indeed, altogether too many (physicians) who become consumptives from overwork and exposure to infection." We conclude from this that there is really some danger from a consumptive physician infecting a patient.

We believe that Dr. Knopf is unnecessarily alarmed at the seriousness of the situation and that the Board will have great difficulty in enforcing its rule in this respect even to a small degree, without taking into consideration the probability of a court holding to the opposite view and preventing them from putting the rule in force.

That there is right and justice in the rule we do not believe any one will deny. As to its final practical utility, this must be determined from the results.

EXCHANGES

ABDOMINAL SURGERY.

F. F. Simpson, Pittsburg (Journal A. M. A., October 9), says that in offering surgical relief we should be prepared to give reasonable and adequate assurance that: (1) The risk is not greater than the danger to life of the condition if not interfered with; (2) if the patient recovers, there is no reason why she should not have the desired relief; (3), the conditions under which the operation is to be done are such that no other combination of circumstances offers less risk or greater security against post-operative complications; (4) in removing the one type of pathology we may be able to avoid substituting another which might cause greater discomfort; (5) no less severe kind of treatment could effect the desired result in a more satisfactory way, and (6) the benefit derived may reasonably be expected to compensate fully for the risk to life, discomfort, loss of time, inconvenience, degree and duration of disability, and the expense and still leave a balance in the patient's credit. According as a surgeon is accurate in his estimates of these factors, will his results be satisfactory. Besides full and accurate knowledge of the general principles of pathology, anatomy, the liability to accident, and estimate of the patient's reserve strength, rigid aseptic technic, wise choice of time, and sufficient manual skill, the surgeon must have full and accurate knowledge of the nature of the disease and its trend, and as far as possible of the actual conditions. A precise and comprehensive diagnosis is especially needed in dealing with inflammatory infections of the genital tract, and a judicious adaptation of time and type of operation to the individual needs of the patient is also essential. Simpson considers the proper oragnization of the surgical service as a large factor in the reduction of mortality, and he gives his idea of the organization as it should be, including the surgical assistant, the skilled anesthetist, the pathologist, and the nursing force. He also lays stress on a minimum amount of anesthetic and considers that the anesthetic and its administration is a most important factor in determining operative mortality. As one thing in the aseptic precautions, is the use of sterile rubber gloves in all cases, and the operation should be so conducted as to be carried out with the greatest speed and precision that are compatible with the other requisites. The post-operative treatment should be made as simple as possible so as to minimize the petty annoyances experienced by the patient.

DIET IN TYPHOID FEVER.

W. Coleman, New York City (Journal A. M. A., October 9), believes that the solution of the essential problems of the typhoid fever diet will be found in the answers to two questions: 1. Shall the typhoid fever patient be given enough food to meet his energy requirements? 2. How much food may be considered necessary for this purpose? The starvation diet, formerly the accepted process for all fevers, has lingered in typhoid, but the practice has gradually advanced from the 300 calories in 24 hours of Graves and Trousseau to the milk diet of Flint furnishing 1,400 calories and the 2,000 calories diet of Bushuyev. There is strong experimental and clinical evidence in favor of giving the typhoid patient sufficient food to meet his energy demands without over-feeding or improperly feeding. Partial starvation lowers the resisting powers and Ewing and Wolf state, in a recent study of the urinary nitrogen in typhoid fever, that the most obvious conclusion of their study is the inadequacy of the diet usually used in typhoid, even in late years. The emaciation which is so characteristic of the disease is, Coleman believes,

largely due to the pyrexia and the toxins, though it is not known definitely how these latter act. Shaffer and Coleman have found in their cases that the losses due to these causes can be prevented by a high caloric carbohydrate diet and the most potent factor of the emaication is therefore partial starvation. A normal man at ordinary rest requires about 33 calories per kilo of body weight each day, and if we add to this the 25 per cent addition to make the febrile increase, which, according to Krehl, is demanded in typhoid, the patient requires 41 calories per kilo of body weight, which for a man weighing 150 pounds would make a minimum diet of 3,000 calories per diem. Coleman has worked out the diet which consists in the main of milk, cream, milk sugar and eggs with the addition of small amounts of stale bread or toast with butter ad lib. The daily quantities were about 1½ quarts of milk, 1 to 2 pints of cream, from ½ to 1½ pounds of milk sugar, and from 3 to 6 eggs. The use of each of these remedies is explained and their use and the reasons for their use. The milk sugar and cream can be given in the form of ice cream, in part at least, or with the eggs in the form of custard. The food has been given at two-hour intervals except that the patient has not been weakened at night. The greater the variety and the more palatable the dishes, the more contented the patient. Meat and meat juices are prescribed by him in the diet and limited during convalescence. The amount of food will, of course, vary with different patients but may be calculated on the basis of 40 calories per kilo of body weight per diem. The article is illustrated.

MASSAGE IN GENERAL MEDICINE.

J. K. Mitchell, Philadelphia (Journal A. M. A., October 9), defines massage as the skillful manipulation of the body for definite therapeutic-ends. In the main, the mechanical results of massage are those of active exercise. We can influence the circulation of the blood and lymph, can improve the tone and in some degree the bulk of muscles, increase the activity of peristalsis and the digestive tract, aid the secretions, and if need be, produce quiet and soothing effects. The superficial nerves can be directly reached and the deeper lying nerves and excretory organs can be, somewhat less immediately, reached. The chief differences between massage and active exercise are that by the former we can not expect to add greatly to the power and volume of the muscles and secondarily it makes no demands on the voluntary nervous system and we can thus avoid drawing on irritable and weak nervous centers. Its greatest value is in diseases that are due to altered metabolism and in which the digestive, absorbing, or assimilating capacity is at fault. Its good effects in hysteria and neurasthenia are due to this fact. The special forms of massage all have their influence, but their combination has more effect than when used separately. Some fancy manipulations used by professional masseurs are deemed by Mitchell more harmful than useful, as they irritate rather than sooth and can not have much effect otherwise on the individual. The vital, useful, alternative movements are the deep ones. After an hour's manipulation, especially after a week or so of treatment when the strangeness has worn off, the patient should be left in a non-disagreeable state of mild lassitude hardly to be called fatigue, usually with moderate drowsiness and feeling of well being. The neurasthenic "tired feeling" should be lessened. Gentle warmth should be felt and a sense of stimulation of the circulation, increase of appetite, improvement of digestion, and sounder and longer sleep. There is a temporary slight increase in temperature in most cases. Too long continued manipulation of superficial rubbing may not have these good effects but may rather irritate the nervous patient. There is an absolute demonstrable increase in the flow of blood in any part, followed by an increase in the amount of urinary excretion and of the digestive secretions, and greater vasomotor control. An increase of red blood cells has been demonstrated. Light rubbing, slapping, and tickling will not produce these desired effects, but slow manipulations for fifty minutes will, and when they are not produced, we may conclude that the right sort of massage was not employed. Among the disorders which are especially benefited by the method, Mitchell mentions chronic constipation, chorea, shaking palsy, sprains, and even peritonitis of which he mentions an example in a patient of Dr. Goodell's in whom laparotomy showed a mass of matted adhesions and good functional activity was produced later by massage. Among other uses of this form of treatment, he mentions its aid to the circulation in early cardiac incompetency, in convalescence from acute and exhausting diseases and in healing of fractures. In conclusion, Mitchell mentions the modern fad of osteopathy which amounts to a sort of ferocious massage. The feelings of the osteopath are, he says, hurt when one calls his manipulations massage, but Mitchell adds "it is rather hard on massage." If massages were properly understood and properly appreciated, however, the osteopaths would never had the success they have had. They have found out and made use of the immense value of massage and, as a result, are teaching the public, without intending to do so perhaps, the important lesson of the value and necessity of bodily exercise, but that they do so in such a manner as to cause frequent damage and almost constant danger is another matter.

MISCELLANEOUS

NOTICE TO MEMBERS OF THE OK-LAHOMA STATE MEDICAL ASSOCIATION.

The United States postal authorities have recently construed the law in reference to second class mail matter, under which the Journal has been admitted in the past, to prohibit the entrance to the mails of publications having for a mailing list members of an Association who receive the publication by virtue of being members rather than being actual subscribers.

This ruling will necessitate one of two things being done. First: As suggested by the Department that the membership and subscription lists be separated so that one could be a member without also being a subscriber to the Journal.

Second: That the Journal be subscribed for separately and independently of the annual dues.

It has been explained to the Department that the dues were raised from $1.50 to the present $2.00 for the purpose of covering the subscription price of each member to the Journal, but the explanation was deemed not sufficient and not entitling us to admission to the second class mail matter.

We are inclined to the suggestion of the Department as being the best solution of the matter, that the lists be separated, but to do this at once would necessitate an overriding of the Constitutional provision of the Association which fixes the dues.

The Secretary has taken the authority to assure the Department that at the next annual meeting an amendment to the Constitution will be offered which has for its object the separation of the subscription and membership lists. The attention of the Department was also called to the fact that the amendment must be offered at one meeting and disposed of at the next regular meeting. If this proposition is accepted the program will be initiated so far as the Secretary is concerned. If, however, it is the wish of the members or a considerable number of them, the two lists will be arbitrarily separated at once; that is, that regular subscriptions be taken for the Journal independent of the annual dues paid then the matter should be inaugurated at once in time for the beginning of the new year. To do this, as previously pointed out, calls for a change of the existing rules of our organization without authority from any one and no one has authority to order such a change to be made.

The Secretary would be glad to have suggestions from the members of the Association and from the County Secretaries as to their wishes in the matter.

CLAUDE A. THOMPSON,
Secretary-Treasurer.

NOTICE TO MEMBERS OF THE STATE MEDICAL ASSOCIATION.

The Committee named by the State Medical Association at its regular annual meeting in May, 1909, at Oklahoma City, to study plans and methods for the eradication of tuberculosis have called a meeting for both physicians and the public to convene at Oklahoma City at ten o'clock A. M. on January 10, 1910, with headquarters at the Threadgill Hotel.

We suggest that before that date each County Medical Society in the State hold an open meeting and discuss this subject with the public and if other arrangements have not been made that this be the subject for your December meeting.

It is the earnest desire that every County Society in the state be represented in this meeting. Every member of the Society should be interested in this subject. We need your assistance. Will you be with us?

COMMITTEE ON TUBERCULOSIS OF THE OKLAHOMA STATE MEDICAL ASSOCIATION.

THE MEDICAL ASSOCIATION OF THE SOUTHWEST, FOURTH ANNUAL MEETING, SAN ANTONIO, TEXAS, NOVEMBER 9-11, 1909.

PRELIMINARY PROGRAM.

Tuesday, November 9, International Club Rooms.

10:30 a. m. General session and addresses of welcome and responses.
Meeting of Executive Committee.
2 to 6 p. m. International Club Rooms, scientific section work.
8 to 10 p. m. International Club Rooms, general session.
The President's Annual Address, Dr. Jabez N. Jackson, Kansas City, Mo.
Oration on Surgery, Dr. M. L. Harris, Chicago, Ill.
Oration on Medicine, Dr. Geo. Dock, New Orleans, La.
10 to 12 p. m. Stag social and smoker.
Wednesday, November 10, International Club Rooms.
8:30 to 9:30 a. m. General session.
9:30 to 12. Scientific section work.
2 to 3 p. m. The Medical Association of the Southwest meeting with the Fifth District Medical Association; an oration of general interest and the election of districts officers.
3 to 6 p. m. Scientific section work.
8:30. Reception and banquet for the doctors and visiting ladies.
Thursday, November 11, International Club Rooms.
8:30 to 9:30 a. m. General session, reports of officers and all committees.
9:30 to 11 a. m. Scientific section work.
11 a. m. to 1 p. m. Election of officers, selection of place for next meeting, etc., and adjournment.

3 to 5 p. m. Automobile ride over city for the doctors and visiting ladies.
Committee meetings will be called as far as possible so as not to conflict with the work of the scientific section.
Special excursion to "City of Mexico" will leave at 1 a. m., November 13.
Sleepers will be ready for occupancy after 9:30 p. m., so that those desiring to do so may retire at the usual time.
Program for Section on Surgery.
Chairman, J. A. Foltz, Fort Smith, Ark.
Vice-Chairman, R. H. Barnes, St. Louis, Mo.
Secretary, E. H. Martin, Hot Springs, Ark.
Some observations of the After Treatment of Abdominal Section, C. A. Thompson, Muskogee, Okla.
Abdominal Operation: Preparation and After Care, Howard Hill, Kansas City, Mo.
Vesico Abdominal Fistula, Le Roy Long, South McAlester, Okla.
Paper, subject to be announced, D. A. Myers, Lawton, Okla.
Consideration of the Operative Patient, H. C. Crowell, Kansas City, Mo.
Some Takes and Mistakes as Demonstrated by the X-Ray, E. S. Lain, Oklahoma City, Okla.
Tubercular Fistula in Ano, with report of cases, E. H. Thrailkill, Kansas City, Mo.
Surgical Considerations of the Pneumococcus, Dr. Blesh, Oklahoma City, Okla.
The Pathological Aspect of the Pneumococci in Surgical Cases, Clarence E. Lee, Oklahoma City, Okla.
Osteophites of the Oscalsis, J. D. Griffith, Kansas City, Mo.
Myomectomy of Large Fibroids, J. J. Frick, Kansas City, Mo.
Retroperitoneal Shortening of the Round Ligaments, W. E. Dicken, Oklahoma City, Okla.
The Value of Surgical Celerity, Chas. Blickensderfer, Tecumseh, Okla.
Tumors of the Breast, F. H. Clark, El Reno, Okla.
Gunshot Wounds of the Abdomen, with report of case, H. L. Snyder, Winfield, Kan.
Non-tuberculous Infections of the Kidney, review of literature and report of cases, C. C. Nesselrode, Kansas City, Kan.
Primary Carcinoma of the Vagina, with report of a case, Jno. T. Moore, Houston, Tex.
Restoration of the Female Pelvic Outlet Based on the Anatomy of the Parts, W. L. Cresthwait, Holland, Tex.
The Classification of Uterine Retro-displacement Cases, with Respect to Treatment, H. S. Crossen, St. Louis, Mo.
Remarks on Floating Kidney with Modified Operation for Its Relief, Adolph Herff, San Antonio, Tex.
The Tendency of Modern Surgery, J. M. Inge, Denton, Tex.
Minor Surgery in Country Practice, D. C. Summers, Elm Spring, Ark.

The Wasserman Reaction, Nettie Kline, Texarkana, Tex.

Fractures of the Femoral Neck, I. C. Chase, Fort Worth, Tex.

A Hitherto Undescribed Operation for Hemorrhoids under General or Local Anesthesia, Wm. Keiller, Galveston, Tex.

Intestinal Obstruction, W. B. Russ, San Antonio, Tex.

My Experience with Formalin according to Murphy, C. M. Rosser, Dallas, Tex.

Acute Dilation of the Stomach Following an Appendectomy, J. E. Gilcreest, Gainesville, Tex.

Uterine Displacements, J. M. Taylor, Fort Smith, Ark.

Congenital Absence of the Gall Bladder, Geo. W. Cale, St. Louis, Mo.

Program for Section on General Medicine.

Chairman, A. K. West, Oklahoma City, Okla.

Vice-Chairman, G. H. Moody, San Antonio, Tex.

Secretary, Louis M. Warfield, Augusta, Ga.

Address from the Chair, A. K. West, Oklahoma City, Okla.

Some of the Newer Phases of the Etiology and Diagnosis of Syphilis, Wm. Frick, Kansas City, Mo.

Sanitary and Moral Prophylaxis, Olive Wilson, Paragould, Ark.

Pellagra, with report of cases, Wilmer L. Allison, Fort Worth, Tex.

Early Diagnosis of Tuberculosis, Theo. Y. Hull, San Antonio, Tex.

The Need for Education on the Question of Sex and Venereal Diseases, Malone Dougan, San Antonio, Tex.

The Diagnostic and Prognostic Possibilities of Blood Pressure Study, D. W. White, Oklahoma City, Okla.

Subject to be selected, K. H. Beall, Fort Worth, Tex.

Program of Section on Eye, Ear, Nose and Throat.

Chairman, F. D. Boyd, Fort Worth, Tex.

Vice-Chairman, J. F. Gsell, Wichita, Kan.

Secretary, A. W. McAlester, Jr., Kansas City, Mo.

Address by the Chairman, F. D. Boyd, Fort Worth, Tex.

Paper, subject to be announced, H. C. Todd, Oklahoma City, Okla.

Recent Advances in Surgery of the Accessory Sinues of the Nose, R. H. Mann, Texarkana, Ark.

Damage Done the Child by Adenoid Growths, J. H. Barnes, Enid, Okla.

When Should Crossed Eyes be Straightened, E. H. Cary, Dallas, Tex.

BOOKS RECEIVED.

International Clinics, Volume Three, Nineteen Series.

J. B. Lippincott Company, Philadelphia and London.

Review.

This volume contains an extremely practical article on the treatment of pulmonary tuberculosis, an article that appeals to the common sense of physicians who deal with this disease and is worthy of careful perusal by all who treat that affection.

An article on post operative complications is well prepared and will be found of use to surgeons.

The work is well written and covers a wide range of subjects.

STEVENS SANITARIUM.

The Stevens Sanitarium at Waurika, Oklahoma, is completed and will be opened in a few days. The institution is modernly built and equipped and will be opened to all reputable physicians.

COUNTY SOCIETIES

COUNTY SOCIETIES.

All County Secretaries who have not been supplied with the card index system for their counties or who have not received them from their predecessors in office should at once write the State Secretary for the system and it will be supplied them immediately and in case they have not been turned over to you with the papers belonging to the Secretary's office you should call on your predecessor for the system.

They are extremely convenient and simple and when put in operation render the keeping of the records of your county society a matter of simplicity.

Many of the newer counties in the Eastern portion of the state have never been furnished the system, while some of the older counties have had them for a long time.

JEFFERSON COUNTY.

Program.

Section on Surgery—Dr. L. B. Sutherland, Chairman, Waurika.

"Acute Intestinal Obstruction"—Dr. J. A. Hatchett, El Reno.

Discussion opened by Dr. G. C. Wilton, Ryan.

"Some Surgical Observations Upon the Pneumococcus"—Dr. A. L. Blesh, Oklahoma City.

Discussion opened by Dr. J. M. Stevens. Hastings.

Section on Eye, Ear, Nose and Throat —Dr. C. M. Maupin, Waurika, Chairman.

"Malarial Keratitis"—Dr. R. E. Runkle, El Reno.

Discussion opened by Dr. Jas. C. Johnston, Waurika.

"Adenoids"—Dr. W. T. Salmon, Oklahoma City.

Discussion by Dr. J. I. Derr and Dr. T. E. Ashinhurst.

Surgical Section, 2:00 p. m.

Eye, Ear, Nose and Throat Section, 7:00 p. m.

Banquet, 10:00 p. m., Steward Hotel. Toastmaster, Dr. L. B. Sutherland.

Response, Drs. Blesh, Hatchett, Runkle, Thompson, Maupin, Cantrell, Stevens, Wilson, Cranfill and Ewing.

President—Dr. W. A. Wilson, Cornish.
Secretary—Dr. F. W. Ewing, Terral.

GRADY COUNTY.

The Grady County Medical Society met in Chickasha, October 1st. Dr. Walter Penquite, who has been absent for several months, presided and the meeting was very successful from all standpoints.

Dr. Paul Vann presented an original communication on Profuse Menstruation and the paper was ably discussed.

Tuberculosis was considered and a committee was appointed to confer with the health authorities with reference to the establishment of a systematic effort for its control and treatment.

Grady County Society will hold regular meetings from now until the summer of 1910.

OKLAHOMA COUNTY.

The first meeting of the above society after the summer vacation was held September 23, 1909.

A paper, entitled "Differential Diagnosis of Fractures of the Hip," was presented and read by Dr. S. R. Cunningham. This paper will appear in some future issue of the Journal.

After the meeting a luncheon was served.

On September 17th the society entertained Dr. H. A. Christian, Dean of the Faculty of Harvard Medical School, with a luncheon after which Dr. Christian delivered an interesting address on the use of Flexner's Antimeningococic serum in the treatment of meningitis. This address is said to have been an extremely able exposition of the use of this treatment.

Oklahoma County will hold regular meetings from this time.

MUSKOGEE COUNTY.

Muskogee County held its first regular meeting after the hot weather, October 11, 1909.

Six new applications were voted and received as members and several new ones were filed for action.

A paper, "Medical Ethics," by Dr. W. M. Nagle, was passed to the next meeting.

A resolution passed to appoint a committee to wait on the City Council and School Board and call their attention to many needed innovations with reference to the reporting of illness in the schools and to devise a general systematic plan for the intelligent inspection of students looking toward the correction and remedying of physical defects.

"Peculiar Manifestations of Typhoid in Oklahoma" was an interesting paper read by Dr. J. T. Nichols, Muskogee. Dr. Nichols invariably uses the agglutination test in continued fevers and states its use shows typhoid present in a large number of cases were otherwise it might not be suspected. He does not favor the use of quinine in cases where the diagnosis is in doubt. This position elicited considerable discussion, many of the profession present using the therapeutic test as a means to diagnosis.

WASHITA AND CUSTER COUNTIES

Joint meeting held at Clinton, Oklahoma, September 29, 1909.

Selective subject—Dr. W. E. Parker, Custer City.

Banquet.

Cystitis—Dr. J. A. Jester, Cordell.

Nephritis—Dr. E. Lamb, Clinton.

A Doctor in Politics—Dr. T. J. Lee, Rocky.

Tuberculosis in Children—Dr. S. C. Davis, Colony.

Report of Case of Hemerrhagic Ascitis Complicating Hypertrophic Cirrhosis of the Liver—Dr. C. Thomas, Weatherford.

Clinical Cases.

President, Dr. W. E. Parkes.

Secretary, Dr. C. H. McBurney.

OKMULGEE COUNTY.

The regular meeting of the above society will be held November 8th, 1909, at 3 P. M., in Okmulgee, and will be followed by a banquet at 7:30. The following is the program:

The Uterine Curette; Its Use and Abuse—Dr. V. Berry.

Puerperal Pyonephrosis—Dr. Weiskotten.

Case Report—Dr. Forbes.

Diseases of Blood Vessels—Dr. A. W. White, Oklahoma City.

President—Dr. Wm. Cott.

Secretary—Dr. W. G. Little.

DISTRICT SOCIETIES.

Program of the Central Oklahoma Medical Association, Guthrie, Oklahoma, Tuesday, October 12, 1909:

Hydrocele—Dr. J. M. Cooper, Enid.

Some Peculiar Conditions Following Malaria; with Report of Four Cases—Dr. C. S. Bobo, Norman.

Adenoids—Dr. J. H. Barnes, Enid.

Auto-Intoxication—Dr. J. M. Postelle, Oklahoma City.

Fractures—Dr. G. H. Thrailkill, Chickasha.

Enterostomy—Dr. A. A. West, Guthrie.

Tumors of the Female Breast—Dr. F. H. Clark, El Reno.

Gangrene, with Report of Case, the

First Ten Days of the Puerpurum—Dr. John S. Hartford, Oklahoma City.

Report of a Case of Ascites from Hypertrophic Cirrhosis of the Liver—Dr. Chas. A. Thompson Weatherford.

Medical Nihilism and Its Effects—Dr. E. G. Sharp, Guthrie.

Prevention of Disease—Dr. T. F. Renfrow, Billings.

PERSONAL MENTION.

OKLAHOMA PHYSICIANS IN EUROPE.

The following physicians are making an extended stay for the purpose of study in Europe:

Dr. D. D. McHenry, Cushing.

Dr. L. J. Moorman, Oklahoma City.

Dr. Horace Reed, Oklahoma City.

Drs. McHenry and Moorman are to return to the United States in December and Dr. Reed will remain until May, 1910.

In this connection it is gratifying to note that of about one hundred American physicians studying in Europe at this time Oklahoma has more than her share by the presence of the above named gentlemen.

Dr. J. C. Mahr, State Health Commissioner, delivered an address at the Alumni banquet of the Medical Department of the University of Kansas, given by the Alumnae Association at the Coates House, Kansas City, Mo., September 15th. Dr. Mahr's subject was on the matter of medical education in Oklahoma.

Dr. J. M. Lemon, who was formerly a member of the Western District (Indian Territory) Board of Medical Examiners,

has located in Oktaha, Oklahoma, for the practice of medicine.

Dr. W. C. Graves, McAlester, has been spending several weeks with the Mayo Brothers, in Rochester, Minn.

Dr. E. B. Mitchell of Anadarko, Oklahoma, has returned from an extended visit to the Pacific coast and the Alaska-Yukon Exposition.

Dr. F. B. Fite has returned from an extended visit to the hospitals of New York, Philadelphia and Baltimore. While absent Dr. Fite made a special study of surgical subjects.

CHANGES OF ADDRESS.

Dr. W. H. Ogden, from McAlester to Toyah, Texas.

Dr. J. T. Manasco, from Non to Tupelo.

Dr. O. T. Robinson, from Hydro to Britton, Okla.

Dr. A. G. Jones, from Byers to Cornish, Okla.

Dr. M. H. Levi, from Oklahoma City to Denver, Colorado.

Dr. J. M. Lemon, from Miami to Oktaha, Okla.

Dr. L. T. Lancaster, from Avard to Cherokee, Okla.

NEW MEMBERS.

Dr. Arthur V. Emerson, Lucien, Noble County.

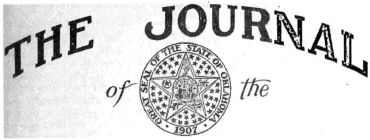

THE JOURNAL of the
Oklahoma State Medical Association.

VOL. II.   MUSKOGEE, OKLAHOMA, DECEMBER, 1909.   NO. 7.

DR. CLAUDE A. THOMPSON, Editor-in-Chief.

ASSOCIATE EDITORS AND COUNCILLORS.

DR. J. A. WALKER, Shawnee.   DR. JOHN W. DUKE, Guthrie.
DR. CHARLES R. HUME, Anadarko.   DR. A. B. FAIR, Frederick.
DR. F. R. SUTTON, Bartlesville.   DR. W. G. BLAKE, Tahlequah.
DR. G. W. ROBERTSON, Dustin.   DR. H. P. WILSON, Wynnewood.
                        DR. J. S. FULTON, Atoka.

Entered at the Postoffice at Muskogee, Oklahoma, as second class mail matter, June, 1909.

This is the Official Journal of the Oklahoma State Medical Association. All communications should be addressed to the Journal of the Oklahoma State Medical Association, English Block, Muskogee, Oklahoma.

GONORRHOEA AS SEEN BY THE GENERAL PRACTITIONER.

BY DR. FLOYD E. WARTERFIELD, HOLDENVILLE, OKLAHOMA

(The admonition given, recently, by the Secretary through the medium of the Journal 'That papers be short and to the point, and as free as possible of text-book material,' is opportune and sensible, and if the hint thus given impresses itself on the mind of each member of this Association as it should it will be productive of much good in that it will tend to give us a more helpful, instructive, as well as a more entertaining class of papers.)

The general practitioner, for the very reason that he is a general practitioner, sees and deals with all manner and kind of disease, and upon his intelligence, tact and skill depends, to a very great extent at least, the future, welfare of the sufferer; whether he is to be conducted safely over the shoals of acute disease, past the maelstrom of complications and on through the eddying pool of convalescence to an harbor of peace and tranquillity in the complete restoration to health and happiness, or whether he is to be passed on from one to another and finally drift into the hands of the designing quack and charlatan to his own material detriment and to the everlasting discredit of the medical profession.

There devolves upon the doctor who first sees the sufferer an even greater responsibility than upon any subsequent attendant, for it is he who lays, in the mind of the sufferer, the foundation for trust, confidence and loyalty, or for distrust, suspicion, indifference and disloyalty.

There are many diseases of so wide spread and frequent occurrence as to be encountered almost daily, or weekly at most, by each practitioner wherever he may live and persue his vocation, and some one of the many complications or sequelae of some of the commoner diseases, which might have been prevented, is most usually responsible for the sufferer seeking aid at the hands of the specialist rather than the primary disease.

To one of these very frequent encountered diseases I am to direct your attention today. I do not expect to tell you anything new, but desire to emphasize in my own way, truths already well known to a great many, and to many unknown or inadequately appreciated.

I feel reasonably sure that there are few diseases more widely disseminated, more far reaching in their ultimate results physically and socially; more productive of domestic and social infelicity; more imperfectly understood and appreciated by the general practitioner, hence more irritationally and illogically managed and treated than is specific urethritis.

Its blighting influences are felt in every community; its baneful effects are abundantly manifest in a great number of the homes of our land; its direful results are ever increasing the responsibilities and financial burdens of the taxpayers of the state.

The general practitioner sees and knows of these conditions as no one else does, and yet he may, and by far too often does, remain passive and absolutely indifferent of his duty.

Let us insinuate ourselves into the good graces of the average doctor, observe him in his work or ascertain in whatsoever way we can, how he meets, manages and dis-

poses of the unfortunate sufferers from this disease who come under his observation and care.

The sufferer may be a young lad who has possibly not had sufficient warning, or who has considered it too lightly, and has been enticed into wrong doing by older and more artful associates; in a short time he notices that all is not right and perchance he goes to the family physician; it may be that it is the old gray haired man, the father of grown-up children who has deviated from the path of moral rectitude and become infected; it may be the young woman who has been insufficiently restrained and imperfectly taught and has loved not wisely but too well and who finds that her partner in libidinous pleasure has imparted to her the fruits of his previous debauches; it may be the housewife and mother who has been pure and chaste through a longer or shorter life of respectability who has been infected by him who styles himself her loyal shield and protector. However, in the great majority of instances, the prospective patient is one who has already consulted his friend, the drug clerk, and possibly the "Boss" also, and has been supplied with a quantity of a favorite prescription that has never been known to fail to effect a cure in a very few days; but it does fail. He then runs the list of favorite prescriptions of friends and associates; then resorts to patent nostrums, without obtaining relief, and with anguish in his heart and a lie on his lips as black as ink, which he hopes will deceive the doctor in making a diagnosis, he presents himself and enlists the doctor's aid in his behalf. He desires to be cured in a few days, yes, and demands that the doctor do so, since it is only a trivial, insignificant matter, only a slight strain perhaps, and he knows of a number who have been cured in a few days and he must be. No matter what the story, whether true or false, the matter is up to the doctor at last, and what does he do?

It is a deplorable fact, observable on every hand, that either from a feeling of self-confidence or complacency, or from a sense of indifference or neglect, a great number of physicians fail to keep step to the march of progress in the scientific investigations and discoveries pertaining to their vocation. When they emerge from their alma mater with their diplomas in hand and the words of council and good cheer still ringing in their ears and go forth to take their place in the great army of medical men to do battle against the foes of mankind, they seem to think that the days of knowledge gathering for them are past. They fail to realize that their real life's work should be, and is, only just beginning. They remember something that their professors said do for this or that disease or condition; they begin and continue for a life time, perhaps, to follow in the footprints of their teachings, although the most cherished ideas they entertained may long since have been disproven and relegated to the junk heap of antiquated notions and more rational and scientific methods taken their place.

The means of acquiring a greater knowledge is within easy reach of every one and may be had for no greater price than the effort of taking, yet many remain ignorant despite age and abundant opportunity.

The doctor hears the story of the sufferer; it may be true or it may be false; he may attach much or little importance to it depending entirely on his state of knowledge. He has no means of either verifying or disproving the statements. He is lacking in pathologic and bacteriologic knowledge. He has not a microscope, and would very likely not know how to use it did he possess one. His imperfect knowledge brought over from his school days, with what he has absorbed from clinical observation is all he has to bring to bear, and he is forced to accept, in a large measure, the statements of his patients in order that he may arrive at a conclusion, not a diagnosis. We should therefore, not be surprised that he speaks lightly of the malady, tells the sufferer that his ailment is not at all serious, in fact, I have heard practicing physicians assert that specific urethritis was not worse than an ordinary cold. Possibly it is not in one case in a thousand. Not every case of specific unrethritis develops complications, but many do. Not every case of rheumatism has as a complication, endocarditis, but many do and when once developed its disastrous results are manifest for the remainder of life should the patient escape death in the primary attack.

The doctor most usually prescribes a balsamic mixture of some kind, a solution of some sort to be used locally, tells the patient to take the one and use the other; thus he continues him in the line of 'dope and gun' victims. The patient is thus doubly confirmed in the belief that his ailment is of very little consequence and exercises himself accordingly. Fortunate, indeed, it would be if this were the last of this case of urethritis; but alas, perchance it is not; its ravages may be manifest many days hence, not only in the individual, but in the person of others: innocent, helpless babes, or helpless, trusting, unsuspecting woman.

In view of this sad, but I am pursuaded true condition in many, many instances, I ask in all sincerity, what should the doctor do?

In the first place: "Every man who enters the profession of medicine assumes an obligation to properly prepare himself for it and in his practice to remember his duty to the public as well as to himself." In the second place his self-pride and ambition to attain the highest possible degree of proficiency in his profession, aside from any altruistic motives, should prompt him to avail himself of every opportunity and means of adding to his store of knowledge. If he is, and is to remain, a general practitioner he should prepare himself to deal intelligently with those more common diseases which are almost constantly confronting him at each turn of the way.

If he feels that he is not prepared, and does not care to prepare himself to deal with any particular disease or class of diseases, he should unhesitatingly announce the fact and not jeopardize the chances to recover health of those who present themselves to him for treatment.

Aesthetically, if he is averse to the treatment of this or any other class of diseases, he should at least possess himself of sufficient information to intelligently instruct the sufferers in a general way, and honest enough to direct them into the hands of someone who is both capable and willing to give them the proper necessary care and treatment.

If he is to take charge of these cases himself there are many things he should know and ever bear in mind, a few of which I wish to mention.

He should know, "That it is illogical to consider the sexual glands as allied to the other glands of the body, and, therefore, their specific activities, except that of their internal secretions, is physiologically intermittent, and prolonged or continued inactivity of their specific functions does not militate against their subsequent ability to perform their normal functions at any time during life." That in the light of this knowledge, if true, and it is reasonable there is no necessity for illicit indulgence; consequently, there is no necessity for acquiring specific urethritis.

He should know that a correct diagnosis cannot be made without a thorough knowledge of the pathological conditions obtaining; that without a knowledge and use of the microscope, endoscope, and other instruments employed, a correct knowledge of the pathological conditions cannot be ascertained, and therefore, a correct diagnosis cannot be made; that until the true pathological condition is known and a correct diagnosis is made no rational or scientific course of treatment can be intelligently instituted.

He should know that he is dealing with a severe inflammatory process, due to, and dependent on the presence of a known micro-organism the biologic characteristics of which are well known, that, notwithstanding, the virulence and tenacity of the micro-organism its manifestations are by no means the same in all individuals.

He should know that many cases of acute urethritis in the female are of short duration and may run their course with little, if any, inconvenience to the patient, and that from these mild cases, quite frequently spring the most virulent type of the disease.

He should know "that there is no physical or microscopical examination that will positively determine that the infecting organisms are not present in the glands and tissues adjacent to the vagina; consequently, even if repeated examinations of the vaginal discharges and secretions discovered no organisms, the inability to infect could still not be guaranteed."

He should know that there is no one way of treating acute urethritis which can be termed the best treatment in all cases; because the success of any method depends in a large measure on the skill and experience of the physician and the willingness of the patient to follow instructions; that in order to secure the best results he must have the greatest amount of co-operation of the patient; that the best way to secure this co-operation, is to be sincere and use every legitimate means of convincing patients that you deal honestly, truthfully, conscientiously, and that you know your business thoroughly.

The doctor should not appear over anxious, but he should use every legitimate means of ingratiating himself into the good graces of the patient, thus making him feel that he is not only his physician but his staunch friend and confidant in time of trouble.

He should know that the consensus of the best opinion is against any kind of local treatment of an active nature during the very acute stage of the disease; that the so-called abortive treatment, even in selected cases, is of doubtful utility; that his main reliance for good results in this stage of the disease should be in those agents calculated to do a minimum amount of harm, and yet capable of doing a maximum amount of good; that rest in bed, local applications of hot water both for hygenic and therapeutic effect, hot baths, light un-irritating diet, and mildly stimulating diuretics and sedatives are of greatest benefit.

He should know that one of the most potent factors for good, in the treatment of any case of specific urethritis, is to deprive the patient, by means of anaphrodisiac medication, of his power of priapism, for he may rest assured that the hoary-haired axium, "that all men are liars" has lost very little of its significance in the class of patients usually affected with this disease.

He should know that in from 60 to 80 per cent of cases of urethritis the posterior urethra with the deeper structures become involved; that it is the tendency of all cases to become chronic; that each case of specific urethritis, like most other diseases is a law unto itself, and should be studied carefully, studied separately and treated

individually in the light of the pathological conditions obtaining.

He should know, that while it is not expected of him that he should be a preacher of moral righteousness to the point of offense, yet he owes it as an obligation to his profession, to himself, his family, his community, his government, and to his God to exert every moral force he possesses to combat the ravages of this physical, moral and social curse and blight.

The doctor should know that of the many pernicious evils confronting him, baring the way to the more rational and successful management and treatment of specific urethritis, the most damaging are, the host of counter prescribers who are exercising the double prerogative of physician and pharmacist; with no knowledge or training at all as a physician, and with an inadequate appreciation of the limitations and responsibility of the pharmacist, and the patent nostrums so widely advertised and so extensively used by sufferers, upon no better authority than of one who knows absolutely nothing of the disease and its complications, or upon another whose sole interest in the patient is to get his money, regardless of what the results of his dope may be.

The doctor should never loose an opportunity to discourage the pharmacist in the sale of private formulae or patent nostrums to these sufferers; he should cultivate friendly relations with the pharmacist and enlist his co-operation in the suppression of these very prevalent evils; he should endeavor to place the pharmacist in such position that he will feel under moral and financial obligations to do so, by according him every courtesy, and using all legitimate means of reciprocation at his disposal.

The doctor should know that many of the time honored, well known and thoroughly tested therapeutic agents always to be found in every well regulated drug store, the different combinations of which can be supplied by every reliable pharmacist, has a wider range of usefulness, more reliable and efficient, much more profitable to the pharmacist to dispense, accordingly of less expense to the patient, than are any of the newer and much extoled preparations on the market.

He should know that it is the opinio of some of our best men that many cases of specific urethritis are incurable, and should not be discouraged if his efforts are not always crowned with success, but press on and remember that it is only the laggard in any vocation who says, enough, awa: with effort.

———

Discussion opened by Dr. H. S. Day of Oklahoma City:

Gentlemen of this section, this paper is one that deserves a great deal of praise. The author has thought, and thought well. In the opening of the paper he stated that this disease was one that was too lightly treated and too lightly considered by the average physician. He could have made no better statement than that. The average physician passes this sort of pathological condition up too lightly. It is usually considered a sort of joke, but to the man who has studied it carefully and thoroughly, he finds that instead of a joke, this is one of the most serious problems that confronts him in his practice. The idea that this disease is not serious and that it can be cured in a very few days time, the idea that some nostrum or some druggist's favorite prescription will relieve it in a few days, is one of the flattest failures that has ever been made.

The use of the microscope in these cases is of exceedingly great value. No case should be treated without the use of the microscope, and yet permit me to say that the absence of the specific organism under the microscope is no evidence that your patient has been cured. It has been thought whenever pus was present that the lymphatic system was involved. I would like to limit that statement just a little at this time: If the lymphatic vessels are as yet uninvolved, we may have pus; if the lymphatic vessels are involved, we have a systemic condition to deal with.

In regard to the question of prognosis, we can not be too guarded. Almost every individual affected by this specific disease is exceedingly anxious to know just when he is permanently cured. It is of vital importance to him. It is not only of vital importance to him. but to others in a social way, consequently he is exceedingly anxious to know when he is absolutely and permanently relieved. You can not be too guarded in your prognosis in these cases, for I firmly believe that this slip-shod carelessness has been the cause of a great many operations that we see in the hospitals. Too many innocent individuals have been the victims of pus and operations because of this slip-shod method of prognosis.

I believe heartily in the outline given by the doctor. He is thorough in the discussion of the subject and imparts to us a message which we never should forget. I thank you.

———

Dr. C. R. Day of Edmond stated that Dr. Frick of Kansas City, Missouri, was present and moved that he be permitted to enter into the discussion. The motion was seconded and unanimously carried.

———

Dr. Frick of Kansas City, Missouri:

I thank the members of this organization.

This subject is a very important one, and I certainly know of no other that is more so. I am glad to see the doctor bring it before the Association, and I think it deserves a full and thorough discussion. I know of no other disease that seems to be so uncertain in a cure as this one. There are some cases we seem to be able to cure easily, while there are others that seem to be extremely difficult. I know that some cases appear to get well, and do get well in the course of a few days' treatment, while there are others that could be treated just as well, just as faithfully, just as conscientiously, and perhaps with the same sort of treatment, and still they will continue for weeks and even months, and then we don't know whether they are well or not. The reason of this seems to be the location that the affected organism assumes. If the affecting organism remains near the surface membranes, then we can combat with it; if, however, they extend into the urethra, down into the prostate, it sometimes takes a long time to cure it. As long as this organism remains in there, some where, we haven't cured our patient. It is a fact that we know to be true that this organism will sometimes hibernate around the inflammation, but the discharge will cease, and apparently our patient is cured; and yet we have hidden the same organism capable of giving some discharge and affecting the organism to do damage later on. This is the reason why it is a particularly interesting subject in a sociological way. This is the reason why we have so many pus tubes, and so many pelvic operations, are because the affection is started by the prior existence of this disease in the partner of the woman. The man has a case of specific urethritis; he believes himself cured; the discharge has ceased, no more pus appears, and he treats the matter lightly. He considers himself cured and the matter is dismissed from the mind of the patient. This patient goes on and gets married. This wife, who is innocent, is soon affected by the former misdemeanors of her husband, and later on this woman comes to the operating table. Numerous instances of these operations are from this cause. I thank you. (Applause.)

Dr. Stinson of Chickasha:

Gentlemen, we have an excellent discussion, and after years of experience, I think we have every advantage in the diagnosis of this disease. Now, the remark made by the gentleman who read the paper in regard to conservative treatment, I want to tell you that everything you can possibly bring to bear against the disease in the first few days of the treatment is worth everything else. Specific urethritis is so common, so prevalent in every neighborhood throughout the entire country, that any one in the medical profession will recognize the disease 99 times out of 100. A good many of us when a patient comes to us with specific urethritis and you let him go with some simple process or another, you fix on that patient a disease that will last him. Gentlemen, what we want to do is to act in the beginning. Just as sure as you go along and treat lightly this disease, 99 times out of 100 you are fixing in that man's system something serious. None of us have ever seen a sufficient number of cases to cover all the ground, but I want to tell you, you want to act in the beginning. You want to put in your time to win.

Dr. Fisk of Kingfisher:

As a matter of fact there is a whole lot about this subject that ought to be known by the people in general. Whenever the women, the wives, mothers and sisters know what we as a profession know about this subject, then the time has come that there will be something done. The medical profession instead of putting a block in the way of this proposition, ought to help. I, myself, have spoken before the Young Men's Christian Association many times, and the Y. W. C. A. have able speakers before them, and in days to come we will find that the women will know something of these things as well as the men; when this time comes, we will have less of these things to look after.

Dr. Burch, Norman:

It will do all very well that there should be such a diversity of opinion about this disease as there is. A bad stricture is worse than a bad case of urethritis. We have simply an inflammatory condition, and we go into that very likely to counteract the inflammatory condition and it is apt to bring about a worse condition. The best authorities that I have consulted say, treat it conservatively at first and then go on with your treatment. It is very natural that the great army of medical men, and men whom I am very proud indeed to be associated with, that there should be a diversity of opinion about a disease as old as this urethritis. But I do believe that the radical treatment in the early stages of urethritis is one of the worst methods that a man ever adopted. I can't help but believe that it is one of the worst things a man ever did.

Dr. Landram, Olustee:

We have a specific for malaria, we have perhaps specifics for other diseases we could count on the fingers of one hand, but we have no specific for specific urethri-

tis. And there is no treatment that will kill the germ without injury to the patient, and the disease is due to a specific germ in the beginning appearing near the surface. If we attack that germ with any germicide, we ruin the soil on which they live, and if we use any form of local treatment, we force these germs further back into the prostate, and I know, and every man knows from experience and from observation and from statistics that it is a dangerous thing to apply vigorous antiseptics. That was a most excellent paper; it was a gem and deserves to be a classic, and the only part that was left out was the part the author had not room for.

Discussion Closed by Dr. Waterfield, Holdenville:

I am very grateful to the Association for the kindly manner in which they received the paper, and the discussion has been worth to me the price of the work I have put on the paper. I hope that the ideas that have been brought out will result in good to you and your patients, because they need every thing they can get from you. I purposely left treatment out of my paper because of the diversity of opinion. Dr. Fisk struck the key note, and I tried to emphasize that fact when I told you that it was entirely under the laws of health and happiness and therefore it was not a necessity to contract the disease in the beginning.

THE NASAL SEPTUM AS A FACTOR IN NASAL CATARRH.

BY DR. S. H. BARNES, ENID, OKLAHOMA

The nasal septum is one of the prime causes of all nasal catarrhs. By its late development and its position being between two well formed hard and non-resisting bones, the nasal and the superior maxillary, it is subject to many malformations and

injuries, which will cause at least 90 per cent of all nasal catarrhs.

So this fact makes the nasal septum the most important part of the whole nasal apparatus as far as disease is concerned.

A short study of the anatomy of the

face and especially the septum and its malformations will convince any one of the above statement.

We find that the text books of only a few years ago on nasal troubles say little or nothing about these conditions of the septum as the cause of nasal catarrh. And many of us have been trying to treat these conditions without removing the cause. In this way we have lead our general practitioner to tell the people that catarrh cannot be cured. So the unfortunate sufferer from nasal troubles have been trying everything that would promise a cure.

I will try to show you that the spurs, deflections and displacements of the septum will cause the three main and most frequent forms of catarrh. These are turgescent, hypertrophic and hyperplastic rhinitis. Then there are others, all kinds of sinus troubles, polyps, tumors and acute colds.

You will notice the two bones and the cartilage that form the septum makes it very susceptible to spurs and deflections.

We will present to you three forms of malformations of the septum; spurs, deflections and displacements. The results of these deformities concern us really more than the condition itself. But we must remember that these pathological conditions are usually the cause of the catarrh and in many cases will have to be removed before the trouble can be cured.

Spurs or ridges is one very common form of nasal obstruction. It is found on either side of the septum, very seldom on both sides at the same time, unless it is due to traumatism. They extend either obliquely upward and backward, horizontally, or perpendicular. They obstruct the breathing and drainage in the lower chamber of the nose and may come in contact with the inferior turbinate completely stopping up the nose on the affected side.

Deflections may be on one side alone just a plain curve in any part of the septum, obstructing one side and leaving the other side very roomy. Then it may be S shaped, deflecting to both sides, obstructing the upper part of the nose on one side and the lower part of the nose on the opposite side. This obstruction is very hard to deal with and causes a great many symptoms on both sides of the nose.

Displacements are usually of the cartilage near the front of the septum. But may be in any part of the septum and very frequently along the floor of the nose. The cartilage is often displaced in the vestibule of the nose causing a complete obstruction on that side.

Then there may be a combination of two or more of these classes of deviations.

The cause of malformations of the septum are two, traumatism and improper development. This last one is the most frequent one and while there are many theories for this cause I want to point you to just one real cause before we take up the nasal troubles that are caused from these malformations.

We have noticed for many years that adenoids in childhood are the fore-runner of catarrh in the adult. It even begins in childhood, we may see the little fellow, with a chronic discharge of muco pus and a habitual mouth-breather with a deformed chest.

Adenoids, by obstructing the nasal breathing will cause a deformity of the hard palate which composes the floor of the nose. The hard palate is pushed up and the arch is contracted, forming a gothic arch in nearly all mouth-breathers of early childhood. The superior maxillary is soft and yielding in infancy and the continual pressure of the air and also the tongue which is placed firmly against the front upper incisors will cause this V-shaped arch. This will then cause the floor of the nose to be higher so that the septum will be deflected in one way or the other and sometimes a double deflection is produced forming a letter S curve. Or it may cause a ridge on some part of the septum. Now, this arched palate will not have to be so pronounced as we have pictured it, or even so we will notice it in the mouth, for it to cause a great deal of deformity in the nose.

The maxillary and the nasal bone are developed before the septum becomes completely ossified, and a very little change in the floor may be the starting of great damage to the septum.

You may see the upper incisors protruding over the lower ones in many of these cases, caused by the pressure of the tongue while the child is trying to breathe through its mouth when it is asleep.

Traumatism may cause any form of deflection, spurs and ridges, more especially displacement of the triangular cartilage in the vestibule at the floor of the nose.

Injury is more often the cause of these deformities of the septum than you at first would think. The little babe gets many falls on its face before it learns to walk, many times its nose is mashed flat and bleeds freely for a time. After a short time there is but little pain and the mother thinks nothing more of baby's nose. So it is with the school boy who first learns to play ball and so on up in life in football and other amusements, as well as the regular duties of life. We don't think of the obstruction many times until there is a constant discharge from the nose, or both sides become occluded so that the child has trouble in breathing while nursing, or in older children, in eating or talking.

There may be some other causes of nasal deflections, but these are the most frequent and you will find on investigating this subject that these two, faulty development and traumatism, take in the greater per cent of them.

The results of these deformities are many and varied and we will be very brief and merely call your attention to a few of these troubles for your consideration.

The most frequent form of catarrh is intumescent rhinitis which you will most often find when the obstruction is near the front of the nose producing a turgescent condition of the inferior turbinates. These organs have erectile tissue in them near the inferior border which are very susceptible to congestion. The increased effort of breathing through an obstructed channel makes a suction through the nose which will cause the erectile tissue to become congested. The constant increased blood supply to the parts will soon cause enlargement of the cells of the mucus membrane, a general thickened condition of the turbinates which is called hyperplastic rhinitis.

Spurs and ridges along the lower part of the septum are often in contact with the turbinates as well as to obstruct the drainage this will cause an increase in the connective tissue which is called hypertrophic rhinitis.

Acute coryza is very common in any and all of these conditions.

When the deflection is high up in the region of the middle turbinates it blocks the openings of the sinuses. It will also cause an enlargement of the middle turbinates which will increase the trouble and cause a constant obstruction and a pressure in the nose often with pain between the eyes simulating eye pain. If you will notice the anatomy you will see that the maxillary sinus, the frontal sinus and the anterior ethmoid cells all empty beneath the middle turbinate and the posterior ethmoid and the sphenoid sinus empty above the middle turbinate. So, anything that causes the middle turbinate to enlarge or obstruct this region will cause one of the most serious and obstinate cases of catarrh we have to contend with. The sinuses are apt to become diseased if the drainage is stopped and there will be a chronic discharge from the nose of pus or muco pus. If the discharge continues for a long time you will often have a crop of polyps.

Catarrh has been until within the last few years a very unsatisfactory trouble to treat. The general practitioner has not got the time to give his attention to these troubles they necessarily require. The laity has been using all kinds of remedies that he can find in our daily papers, or that the quack will guarantee, yet without any results so that it is narrated around that catarrh is an incurable disease. Now, this should be corrected as far as possible for most of these cases can be cured by relieving the obstruction to breathing and drainage caused by the septum.

Just a few years ago the correction of these septal deformities was very difficult and was not always a success, besides, the operation was very painful to the patient, as well as a long continued treatment and a loss of time by him.

Since submucus operations have been worked out by Freer and Killian these cases are all cured and the operation is a very small affair as far as the patient is concerned. He does not lose any time from his work and there is absolutely no pain, and in one week's time we are not able to tell where the wound is in the nose.

The operation itself is not so easy to do as we may expect from the description given by the others, but after the technique is thoroughly understood and with some experience we are able to do this submucus operation with a great satisfaction to our selves and the patient.

Don't understand that all spurs and deflections should be removed in order to cure catarrh, for we are often able to shrink up the turbinates or to remove a portion of the hypertrophied tissue with the very best results.

If the septum obstructs breathing or drainage or comes in contact with the turbinates when the nose is in its best condition then it should be corrected. The septum will cause these various forms of catarrh and not materially obstruct breathing, or drainage itself, and yet not be in contact with the lateral side of the nose except in very severe colds. Very slight deviations or spurs will often cause an enlargement of the turbinates and they will obstruct the nose.

Now to close. the adenoids, by causing a deformity of the mouth, is one of the first causes of septum malformation. Traumatism, especially in babies, is another.

Frequent colds are usually due to septal trouble.

Deflections in front of the nose causes first intumescent rhinitis, which if allowed to continue, will cause hypertrophic rhinitis. Deflections near the floor, further back in the nose, will cause hypertrophic and hyperplastic rhinitis.

If the deflection is higher up on the septum we will have inflammation of one or all of the sinusses.

Polyps are caused by long continued discharge of pus from the sinuss. All deflections or spurs that obstruct drainage or breathing or come in contact with the turbinates should be removed by submucus operation. If we will give our attention to the septum in all cases of catarrh, we will correct the idea among the laity that catarrh is incurable, and the quack will cease to bombard the people with his notorious literature that his medicine used in an inhaler will cure these persistent troubles.

Last, but not least, the treatment of catarrh is surgical.

ENTEROSTOMY

BY A. A. WEST, B. S., M. D., SURGEON TO THE OKLAHOMA METHODIST HOSPITAL,
GUTHRIE, OKLAHOMA

Read before the Central Oklahoma Medical Association, October 12, 1909, Guthrie, Oklahoma.

Enterostomy is the formation of a fecal fistula above the ileo-caecal valve. This operation was done for the first time in 1840 by Nelaton. Notwithstanding the advance made in modern surgical technic, operative interference in acute internal obstruction is still very high. It has varied from 50 to 70 per cent in the hands of different operators. The frequency of intestinal obstruction is estimated by Brinton as one out of 280 deaths from all causes, founded on the results of 12,000 post-mortem examinations. This is probably too high, but they are of sufficient frequency to cause us to be on the alert in making an early diagnosis, for upon this point the mortality rate is computed. It seems, in looking over the report of cases in literature, that women suffer more frequently from intestinal obstruction than men, particularly is this so from certain forms, such as impaction of gall stones or compression of the intestines by tumors, or displaced viscera. I think we may also add those causes from inflammatory adhesions. In 1906, of 100 cases treated by operating in three of the large hospitals of New York, 54 per cent died. Ranzi has collected recently 758 cases from literature with a mortality of 57 per cent.

Now, it is true that most of the patients that present themselves to the surgeon show advanced symptoms of obstruction. We scarcely ever see a patient in a condition when the manipulations necessary to discover the obstruction can be borne. There are two factors that enter into this difficulty; first, oft-times the physician is not called in due time and again he fails to make a diagnosis even when the patient is seen early; second, patients very often refuse the idea of operation until numerous other methods have been tried and valuable time lost. Should we omit even those cases seen in extremis, we would still have a very high mortality rate of 30 or 40 per cent. This mortality rate can only be improved upon by a more early diagnosis and by simpler and more conservative methods of operation.

It is not uncommon to note surgeons of considerable ability open an abdomen and search persistently to discover the obstruction and fail, thus endangering the life of the patient by the long time consumed in the search, and from the great amount of shock sustained by the manipulation of the intestines. There are a small number of patients that are seen in good condition, and in this class of cases, one is justified in picking up the intestine and following it to the point of obstruction, and doing whatever operation seems justifiable. Then there are another class of patients that are always morbid, and with this class there seems to be no contention but that the only relief possible is to open and drain the bowel. Now, there are a middle class of patients which are neither in good condition nor are they in extremis. To this class of patients, and they constitute the large majority, am I making a plea for conservatism.

We all must know the tremendous shock given to a patient by having a loop of intestine twisted upon itself, but this is incomparable to the shock received from the virulent poisons liberated from the retained intestinal contents. Many of the great symptoms are the result of these toxins. I believe them to be a more important factor in the causing of death than the obstruction itself. Hence, it is most desirable that these poisonous substances should be eliminated from the body as quickly as possible. The toxins produced thus have a very depressing action upon the nervous system and the cardias muscles. The great distention of the bowel with the accumulation of gasses, adds its deleterious effects, by embarrassing respiration, by pressing upon the diaphram and by disturbing the circulation of blood in the bowel wall. This in turn is followed by more distention and by the formation of more gasses until I am convinced, the grave symptoms are due to those conditions that follow the obstruction, than by the obstruction itself.

When the significance of these poisons in the intestinal canal began to be recognized, it was thought that, rapid elimination was the best way to rid the body of these substances, by increasing peristalis after the obstruction had been relieved. To this end active catharsis with enemata was practiced. Many patients bear the operation for the obstruction very well, but owing to the rapid absorption of the toxic substances by the healthy gut below the point of obstruction, death has occurred in a few hours. To safeguard this condition some operators emptied the distended loops by aspiration or incision. Others, after relieving the obstruction, drain the bowel above the point of obstruction. The former method is more often practiced today (Elsburg).

In all patients whose strength has been diminished by shock of obstruction and absorption of the toxic materials in the intestine, would it not be better if we were to use the simplest methods at hand? Would we not save more patients if we were to open and drain the bowel, and see less cases followed by collapse by having insufficient strength to withstand the manipulation of the gut necessary to relieve the obstruction?

True, there are some objections. Treves calls it, "A rough and ready operation, extreme, irrational and blindly advised," and declares that such evidence as we possess is in favor of the operation only in "Extreme cases in which the patient can only be submitted to a procedure of the slightest magnitude," however, he recommends the opening of the bowel after the obstruction has been found and relieved, and declares that this addition to the operation has reduced the mortality 50 per cent.

It seems to me that his own argument favoring the drainage of the bowel following an operation for the relief of intestional obstruction, is the strongest evidence possible in favor of the simpler operation on that class of patients where danger of collapse is feared. In many cases it tides the patient over the most imminent danger, relieves all toxic symptoms, and recovery, outside of the embarrassing situation of a fecal fistula, is almost complete and subsequent operation for the relief of obstruction may be done with safety.

No one denies the utility of a simpler enterostomy in desperate cases. It is an operation that can be done in a few minutes and often under local anesthesia, but there are many objections raised in doing this operation on a patient whose circulation is pretty good, and who has not been exhausted by vomiting. They claim; first, that the obstruction is still unrelieved, second, that there may be gangrenous processes remaining in the abdomen and that fecal fistula will necessitate a secondary operation.

These objections have but little force with the class of patients above referred to. It is true that further operative interference is necessary but the rate of mortality is so much lessened with this method of procedure that the division of the operation in two stages, seems justified. Even with the gentlest munipulation I have found that the handling of distended bowel causes enormous shock. Besides the great distention forces the bowel out of the abdomen and difficulty is often experienced and time consumed in preventing it and in closing the abdomen. It means that the operation must be done hurriedly and with the least trauma possible.

As to the objection of leaving the gangrenous material in the abdomen, I believe that this is often taken too seriously and does not happen as often as we are inclined to think. If a gangrenous portion of the bowel is observed during operation, it may be brought out of the abdomen and subsequently treated.

Now as to the technic employed in doing Enterostomy for acute intestinal obstruction there are several methods in vogue. Dr. Stewart of Philadelphia, who is a firm adherent of immediate enterostomy, in acute intestional obstruction, at a recent meeting of the Philadelphia Academy of Surgery, suggested the following method: "After opening the abdomen, the desired loop of bowel is drawn into the wound and emptied of its contents by a gentle milking process. A clamp, the blades of which are covered with rubber tubing, is then placed at either extremity of the loop to prevent fecal reflux, and the whole is surrounded by gauze packing. One-half of a Murphy button is inserted into the empty loop of intestine through a small incision, and the other half is squeezed into the end of a long rubber tube whose caliber is slightly smaller than the flange of the button, over which it projects, like a phymosed foreskin, thus making a tight joint. The two halves of the button are then pressed together, or in other words, a lateral implantation is made between the rubber tube and the bowel. The clamps are

now removed and the feces allowed to drain through the rubber tube into a receptacle on the floor."

Now the above method seems to have been reasonably successful to Dr. Stewart, but it seems to me that it is a trifle more complicated than necessary, and the operation done by Elsburg, of New York, is more simple and as efficatious. His method is to pick up the most distended loop of gut and place two circular sutures in the wall of the bowel about to be opened. A small incision is then made, a catheter inserted; the catheter fixed in the wall of the bowel by a silk stitch, and the two circular sutures then tied. The inner of the sutures is tied first, the catheter being pushed into the bowel. In this manner the canal lined by serous membrane is formed which will close rapidly as soon as the catheter is withdrawn.

The bowel is then attached to the peritoneum along the margins of the abdominal wound by one or two sutures and the abdominal wound closed around the tube. If it is thought necessary a gauze drain may be placed in the small incision. The tube from the intestine is led over the side of the patient's bed into a bottle or receptacle. There is no leakage by the side of the tube and the dressing remains clean. When the tube is withdrawn, the opening in the bowel closes very rapidly.

If the above technic is carefully carried out and if the obstruction has been relieved, a fecal fistula will remain in only a small proportion of patients. If one should result, it can be closed by a lateral enterorrhaphy.

Elsburg from his large practice in Mt. Sinai hospital has drawn the following conclusions:

1. Operative interference for acute intestinal obstruction should very often be divided into two stages.

2. Enterostomy and drainage should be

the operation of choice, not only in the desperate cases, but also in many patients whose condition is still a fair one.

3. Prolonged search for the obstruction and its relief should, in all patients excepting those in very good condition, be delayed until the acute symptoms have been relieved by the opening and drainage of the bowel.

4. The danger of leaving behind gangrenous intestines is a small one, it is smaller than the danger from prolonged manipulations.

5. When gangrenous intestine is present it is preferable to bring it outside of the abdomen and deal with it later; the obstructive symptoms being meanwhile relieved by enterostomy.

6. Enterostomy, thus done, is not an "extreme, irrational and blindly advised"

operation, but one that embodies a distinct therapeutic principle—alleviation of acute symptoms as the first step in the relief of a pathological condition.

7. The operation of enterostomy may permanently relieve acute intestional obstruction.

8. Fecal fistula will remain in only a small proportion of the cases in which enterostomy has been done, if the opening and drainage is made according to the Kader principle.

Bibliography.

1. Elsburg. Annals of Surgery, Vol. 47. No. 5, p. 738.

2. Stewart. Surgery, Gynecology and Obstetrics, Vol. 3. No. 5, p. 677.

3. American Text Took of Surgery.

4. Quain's Medical Dictionary.

ACUTE GASTRIC CATARRH

BY DR. JAMES WHITMAN OUSLEY, KANSAS CITY, MO.

Acute Gastric Catarrh, Gastritis Catarrhales Acuta or Catarrhus Gastricus Acutus.

AETIOLOGY.

We differentiate an idiopathic primary catarrh and a secondary acute gastric catarrh. The latter occurs usually in consequence of other diseases while the idiopathic catarrh is an independent affection but as a whole every catarrhal affection is probably due to the influence of bacteria. Mechanical, thermal or chemical irritations may of course also come into question. Adding to the influence of the bacteria, we will often have patients state that a cold has been the primary cause of the disease. But of course, the most frequent external cause of a catarrh of the gastric mucosa is an insult to the stomach by mistakes in diet either in a qualitative or quantitative sense. During the summer it is probably due more to a qualitative fault in diet.

Raw fruits and beer or other foods that don't agree with each other while during the winter season society life brings

about copious evening meals and thus an overloading of the stomach; a stomach treated in this manner is not able to produce enough gastric juice and even unable to move the food into the gut. On account of this stasis fermentation will arise and all kinds of bacteria will begin to act upon the mucosa.

Foul meat or other foul and bad foods may also produce the acute gastric catarrh. We have to mention also as a cause, the taking of too hot or too cold drinks. On very warm days in the summer the cold refreshment many people take, as cold beer or ice cream brings about the catarrhal affection. The bad habit of many people of eating too hastily is likewise to be accused here. The food comes into the stomach without having been chewed thoroughly which means more work for the stomach. An acute gastric catarrh may furthermore arise if the mucosa of the stomach is irritated by ingestion of foreign bodies or by the invasion of intestinal worms as ascaris, oxyuris, tape worm.

The toxic acute gastritis is chiefly due to an excess of alcohol, sharp spices and certain medicinal poisons, many of course also bring about an acute catarrh. Toxins produced by the body its self, as in uraemia cholaemia or gout or diabetes may cause a so-called auto-intoxication and consequently an acute gastric catarrh. It is also to be mentioned that the nervous system plays a role in the etiology of acute catarrhs. There are patients who are affected by such a catarrh after fright or depression or any other physical influence. People with an idiosyncrasy for special foods or drugs may also get an acute catarrh even if they take these things without knowing it. It is easy to understand that the acute gastric catarrh will occur far more frequently in men than in women, for men will be far more subject to the different noxious influences mentioned before.

For the etiology of secondary acute gastric catarrh feverish infectious diseases have to be mentioned in the first place. In these cases the catarrh is often a prodromal symptom.

ANATOMICAL ALTERATIONS.

That the acute gastric catarrh is a really organic disease has been shown by many pathologic researches. The anatomical alterations are for the greatest part formed at the pyloric portion of the stomach. We find here a mucosa showing all the characteristics of an acute inflammation, the tissue is loosened and swollen, diffusely red and covered with tenacious mucous. Sometimes the redness is not general, but occurs in spots, occasionally blood extravasations are to be found.

SYMPTOMATOLOGY.

The patients consulting us with an acute gastritis complains above all of anorexia and often they even show a perverted appetite for sour and irritating foods. Thirst is mostly increased. In addition to loss of appetite nausea is almost never absent and vomiting is not rare. The stomach contents is mostly vomited in a fermenting and decomposed condition, free H. C. L. is not to be found, but lactic acid and other products of fermentation may be present. Belching of gases with foul or acid odor is another very molesting symptom. The eructation of sharp gases always produce the sensation of pyrosis. The patients commonly also complain of fulness or the sensation of distension and a feeling of pressure or even pain may occur, radiating toward the scapulae and the vertebral column. The objective features of this disease is as can easily be understood, a hyperproduction of mucus on the one hand and a decreased secretion of H. C. L. The function of the stomach is also involved, thus the food remains a long time in the stomach; the tongue is usually coated and salivation is increased, at the same time the patient has a bad odor from the mouth and a pretty frequent occurence is herpes labialis. If urticaria appears we have to suspect a gastric catarrh due to the ingestion of a substance for which the patient has an idiosyncrasy. The bowels are mostly constipated, at least in the beginning, but the usual course of the disease is that the fermenting and noxious substances finally pass into the intestines irritating the mucous membrane here and producing diarrhoea. If a duodenal catarrh ensues the bile duct may be involved and the result may be a jaundice due to a gastro-duodenal catarrh. There is much attention to be paid to the nervous condition of the patients. They complain of a heaviness in the head, headache and throbbing. The patients feel depressed and are mostly incapable of performing mental work. Dizziness also occurs; all these symptoms are very likely due to an auto-intoxication of the brain. The temperature is not always elevated, but in a great number of cases fever rises to 103 F. and higher. The primary acute gastric catarrh continues for a few days as a rule, yet it may even persist for one or two weeks and even tend to relapses. Frequent attacks of this affection may bring about the chronic catarrh.

The symptoms of the secondary catarrh are in the main analagous, but not as pronounced as in primary gastris.

DIAGNOSIS.

It will therefore not be difficult to differentiate between the primary and secondary acute gastritis; other diseases will scarcely come into question for the differential diagnosis.

PROGNOSIS.

The prognosis is always good.

THERAPY.

In the first place we have to treat the primary cause, the superfluous and stagnating stomach contents has to be removed from the stomach; many patients do that instinctively, they feel that the removal of these substances would alleviate them and they excite vomiting by introducing their fingers into the pharynx. If spontaneous vomiting does not occur it is best to insert a stomach sound into the stomach and to wash the latter with warm water. Emetics should be used with the utmost care, not at all in aged people. When using an emetic it is advisable to use it hypodermically or subcutaneously in order not to irritate the stomach, apomorphine hydrochloride will meet the indications. For belching and pyrosis it is best to administer alkaline waters, seltzer water, burned magnesia or

Rx.

Sodii Bicarbonat.	7.7 Grms.
Resorcini.	1.5 Grms.
Sacchari.	7.7 Grms.

M. Ft. Chts. No. X. Sig. One powder every 2 or 3 hours.

Administer laxatives only if we are afraid of involvement of the intestinal mucous membrane, it is however, not advisable to use the drastic means. For severe pains use the hot applications over the epigastrium and in obstinate cases use morphine sulphate hypodermically. It is however best to dispense with all drugs and combat the condition with a rational diet and the diet will be for the first two days nothing but hot peppermint tea, perhaps mild meat soup and gruels. The best is to give the stomach a rest and when the patient begins to eat we will aid his digestion by administering ten drops of dilute hydrochloric acid after meals.

205-6 Argyle Building.

EDITORIAL

THE PREVENTION OF TUBERCU-
LOSIS.

———

Never in medical history has there been such a concerted and unanimous movement toward the control and prevention of tuberculosis.

Aside from the meetings being held and that are to be held in almost every county and city in the United States and by the County Medical Societies during the close of this and the beginning year, many prominent civic bodies are giving the matter their serious consideration.

When one reflects that this is by far the most potent enemy of mankind, doing by far more damage than all armies and navies combined and that all other diseases pale into insignificance when the destructive force of tuberculosis is considered, we then realize it is time something were being done for its prevention. That the final result of clean living and civic cleanliness along broad lines will result in the eradication of tuberculosis no serious thinker doubts for a moment, but to do this calls for almost a revolution of present methods and systems of living. It calls for the overthrow of many prejudices existing in the lay mind and for the highest order of mutual assistance between the lay and professional mind. The people must necessarily be educated and shown the reason for regulations affecting sanitary conditions in order that they may carry them out more effectually and no one is in better position to do this, in fact no one, but the family medical advisor is fitted to point out the proper methods for combating disease.

It should be made the function of every physician to pass no opportunity to advise the families under their care as to the means for the prevention of disease, every thing bearing upon their hygienic condition should be considered and co-operation encouraged for their improvement.

THE MEDICAL ASSOCIATION OF THE SOUTHWEST, MEETING AT SAN ANTONIO, TEXAS, NOVEMBER 9TH AND 11TH, 1909.

At the outset it is not unfair to anyone to say that the attendance at this meeting was not what it should have been by any means; Texas alone should have provided a larger meeting, but with that said all criticism must end for the meeting was most successful from the point of scientific endeavor and offerings and those who were not present are losers by their absence.

The citizenship of San Antonio does not have to exert itself to care for any meeting and hospitality is most natural to them, so on this score alone one was amply repaid for the trip. The hotel accommodations were limited on account of the co-incident meeting of the state fair, but with this all were cared for amply.

The meetings were held in the rooms of the International Club, an institution that is doing much to foster our commercial interests with the Republics south of us and in their rooms everything was at hand necessary for the comfort of the guests.

Two rooms were provided for the use of sections at the same time and St. Anthony's hotel provided space for the various committee meetings.

The social features of the occasion were well attended and consisted of a smoker at the Elk's Club before which the oration on Surgery was delivered by the retiring President, Dr. Jabez N. Jackson, Kansas City, Mo., whose address on "Membranous Pericolitis," together with the pathologic specimens offered of the same affection by Dr. O. L. Castle, pathologist to the Kansas City General Hospital, was received with most marked attention on account of the comparative rarity of the affection up to date or rather its failure of recognition by the profession as a separate entity up to date. Dr. Jackson enumerated twenty-six cases operated by himself and other Kansas City surgeons and one was startled by the fact that in many of these cases operation had previously been done for appendicitis, ovarian trouble or some other abdominal condition without relief to the patient. Attention was called to the fact that the affection was not found in childhood.

An informal dance by the ladies of the city was attended by the physicians and their wives and was pronounced a most

enjoyable affair. The ladies were also tendered a luncheon "a la' Mexicana," this
function produced verdicts according to the
state of the palate describing it, but was
very novel to all attending. The San Antonio fair was visited by many and the
famous old missions of the city called for
a visit from every one of the party, these
old buildings erected early in seventeen
hundred by the far reaching arm of the
Catholic Brotherhoods still stand as a mute
testimonial of the energy of this church
and their ministers, but a more lasting
monument to their enterprise is evidenced
by the fact that practically all of the Span-
ish and Mexican descendants are of this
faith.

Dr. Brumby, State Health Officer of
Texas, exhibited a case of pellagra. Regret was expressed by many at their inability to give this case the proper study
its importance warranted, but the case was
naturally one of interest to all who saw it.

San Antonio, situated as it is at the
meeting point of modern and Latin America, presents everywhere an air of roman-
icism and quaintness; the stylishly dressed
and polished American young lady brushes
elbows with the lowly peon of Mexico, the
virile Texas cowman meets and greets the
suave and educated banker, side by side in
harmony dwell the abode remains of Mexican occupancy of the country with the
modern steel and concrete sky scraper and
under the soft moonlight of the Texan
plain frowns that most historic spot of the
United States, the Alamo. No sign of the
fearful carnage once occuring there is now
evident save the tablets and testimonials
erected by the patriotic and loving Texans
commemorative of the greatest defense
recorded by annals of history. In this
small building the names of Crockett, Fannin, Travis, Bowie and the other defend-
ers will be forever perpetuated by the sons
of Texas and a citizen of the United States
without reference to his birthplace cannot

visit it without a feeling of sadness at
their fate and one of pride in the consciousness that their achievement was the
achievement of his brother American.
Within the walls of this sacred structure a
simple sentence announces that,

"Thermopolae had its messenger of
death, the Alamo had none."

SOME OF SAN ANTONIO'S POINTS OF INTEREST TO MEDICAL MEN.

One of the pleasures of the San Antonio meeting was a visit to Dr. Moody's
sanitarium, an institution now in the sixth
year of its existence and which accomo-
dates on an average fifty patients daily
throughout the season. The buildings are
large and commodious, occupying something like ten acres of ground which ad-
joins the United States army post, Fort
Sam Houston. This ground gives an extensive view of San Antonio and its en-
virons and one is struck with the beauty
of the scene unfolded to the view from any
point of the sanitarium grounds. Nothing
has been left undone to make the institution a complete one. The buildings are
modern and contain all the requirements
called for by an exacting and discriminating clientele; situated on a commanding
eminence the drainage is perfect, and with
the perpetual sunshine of Southwestern
Texas it is a resort to be commended to
any one.

The sanitarium is managed by Drs. G.
H. and T. L. Moody and Dr. J. A. Mc-
Intosh.

SANTA ROSA INFIRMARY.

An institution of 250 beds, which in
the year 1908 cared for more than two
thousand patients, is managed by the Sisters of Charity, with their usual success.
This latter fact is certainly impressed upon
one on entering the buildings, order and
neatness are everywhere apparent. The

building is naturally one of the largest of its kind in the state.

The writer had the pleasure of witnessing operative work by Dr. Adolph Herff on his visit to this hospital. Dr. Herff is the moving surgical spirit of the institution and after seeing his work one is compelled to accede to him this honor.

C. O. THOMPSON.

OKLAHOMA STATE BOARD OF HEALTH.

It will be of interest to the profession throughout the state to know that on the first of January, 1910, the State Commissioner of Health, Dr. J. C. Mahr, will promulgate an order completely revising the rules heretofore published by the Board The revised rules will be practically those called for by the "Model Bill for Vital Statistics" as advocated by the American Medical Association and the blanks for reporting deaths will be similar to those furnished through Dr. Wilbur and the census bureau.

The rule requiring the compulsory reporting of tuberculosis is identical with that in force in New York and these reports are considered as confidential by the Board and are not for the information of the public.

The reporting of typhoid fever and other infectious diseases will remain practically as before.

EXCHANGES

PELLAGRA.

(Reprinted from the Medical Fortnightly, Editorial, St. Louis.)

The recent outbreak of pellagra in various of the Southern states and in Illinois has made an ability to diagnose that unusual disorder a necessity, for there are few of us who have ever seen a case. Quoting Thayer, the editor of the American Journal of Clinical Medicine, describes pellagra as follows:

"The symptoms ascribed to pellagra are: Gastrointestinal—nausea, dyspepsia, vomiting, and especially diarrhoea, marked in the mornings and often obstinate; a severe form of stomatitis with fiery-red mucosa, eating and swallowing being extremely painful; aphthous ulcers extending over large areas, patches of white macerated epithelium exfoliating, leaving a raw, velvety, fiery-red surface, and distressing salivation.

"The cutaneous symptoms are significant. There is erythema on the dorsum of the hands and, in those who go barefoot, on the feet, the palms and soles being rarely affected. These patches resemble sunburn with, however, the margins more sharply defined; they are always symmetrical; they show slight if any swelling, the brilliant-red blush becoming deeper or cyanotic, extending down to the next phalangeal joints and back to the wrist, where it ends abruptly. The affected surfaces soon become dry, scaly and exfoliate in scales, leaving the skin dry, cracked and fissured. Bullae may form on the hands, filled with serum, pus or blood. The epithelium exfoliates in large masses, leaving these skin areas raw and red, thin and atrophied, often glistening, shiny, with slight superficial wrinkles, cracks, deep-red or brownish, and fissures sometimes deep and hemorrhagic. In marked cases the skin over the last two phalanges becomes dry, deep-brown, with bullae and exfoliation. Similar changes take place on the dorsa of the feet in barefoots, and in bad cases they also appear over the cheekbones and the bridge of the nose; occasionally about the neck like a collar.

"While this erythema is influenced by sunlight, it is readily distinguished from the ordinary effects of sunburn. The appearance is not specially prevalent in summer, and children who run naked show the same location of the lesions.

"As nervous manifestations, we have vertigo, and grave symptoms from the cord. In severe recurrent forms we note a general increase in the deep reflexes, especially in the lower limbs; well marked spastic symptoms, sometimes disturbed sensation and sphincter paralysis; reflexes of lower limbs lost, of upper increased; sclerosis, especially in the lateral columns of the cord, lesions of the posterior columns not unusually, and according to and with degeneration of the posterior roots.

"Neusser summarizes the mental symptoms as follows: At first as a rule confusion, weakness of judgment and will, anxiety, disorientation as to time and place, alteration of disposition from slight depression to hypochondria and suicidal tendency; the patient is often silent, dull and serious, looks as if he had forgotten how to smile, with self-depreciation, delusions of persecution, self-accusation; refusal of nourishment; often mania, the depressed patient becoming suddenly emotional and restless, this followed by apathy or catalepsy. Hallucinations of sight and hearing are common. Mutism is frequent. The mental deterioration progresses, and terminal dementia supervenes.

"Clinically, two forms are recognized, namely, the acute typhoidal, and the milder, chronic or recurrent. The first runs to a fatal end in a few weeks, with active delirium, fever and uncontrollable diarrhoea. The second may be prolonged for twenty-five years. With each relapse ane-

mia, debility and emaciation increase, the nervous and mental symptoms advance; the patient becomes cachetic, demented and bed-ridden.

"The onset is usually in the spring. The patient is apt to improve during summer, relapsing in early fall. Apparent recovery may ensue, with recurrence in the spring."

PREVENTION OF MALARIA.

S. Harris, Mobile, Ala. (Journal A. M. A., October 9), finds that statistics show that malaria exists in every state in the union except Wyoming, but the conditions are most favorable to the growth of the anopheles in the states adjacent to the Mississippi, Missouri, and Ohio rivers, where the greatest mortality is shown. The mortality in the year 1900 in the United States from malaria was 14,909, of which 9,320 were whites and 5,589 colored. As the colored population was approximately only one-ninth of the total, it will be seen that they furnished more than one-third of the mortality from malaria to which they were supposed to be more or less immune. This may be accounted for by the unsanitary conditions under which the negroes live and their neglect of treatment of the disease. No race or class is exempt from the disease which destroys more lives every year than have been lost in all the epidemics of yellow fever in the last century; and beyond this the wage earning capacity is affected in millions more. Yet malaria is preventable and quinine is a specific in its treatment. Harris believes that the high death rate from kidney disease in our Southern states can be largely accounted for by chronic malaria. He quotes from history to show what an evil malaria has been in the past and gives Dr. Woldert's estimate of over five million dollars as the annual financial loss to the state of Texas alone from this disease. If it costs Texas that sum, the annual loss to the United States as a whole is at least from fifty to one hundred millions. As regards the possibility of extirpation of malaria he refers to what has been done in Italy, where the mortality rate has been reduced two-thirds in the last five years, and to the work in Havana and the Canal Zone. Malaria should be classed as a reportable disease. Each case should be isolated by netting and the well known measures for the destruction of the anopheles mosquito should be thoroughly employed. There should be a systematic education of the people in malarious districts. Harris advocates the formation of a national association for the study and prevention of malaria, as was done in Italy, with auxiliary state and county societies in the most infected sections. He thinks malaria is of more importance to our country than yellow fever and should receive fully as much attention.

MISCELLANEOUS

THE RESIGNATION OF DR. CHARLES A. L. REED.

The earnest attention of the members of the Oklahoma State Medical Association is directed to the following letter from Dr. Reed. If its advice can be followed even in part great good will result to the profession generally.—Ed.

To the Auxiliary Legislative Committee of the American Medical Association:

Gentlemen:

I beg leave to advise you and, through you, the medical profession of your country, that at a meeting of the committee on medical legislation of the American Medical Association, held at Chicago on October 16, I presented my resignation as a member of that committee to become effective Nov. 15, 1909, or sooner, on the appointment of my successor.

This step has been made necessary on my part, first, because my surgical practice makes it imperative that I decline all engagements that may take me away from my office and operating room, and, second, because the duties of the committee have grown until they can no longer be discharged by any man who cannot devote. if not all of his time, at least more time to them than is consistent with my obligations to my clientele.

I must, however, ask for the privilege of tendering a few final words before I can accept exemption from further sacrifices incident to relations that I have sustained with pleasurable devotion for the last seven years. During that time, by virtue of its splendid organization, the medical profession has been able to assist in the accomplishment of important reforms. Among these reforms may be mentioned the improved status of the medical profession in the governmental organization of the Isthmian canal zone, the reorganization of the army Medical corps, the passage of the pure food and drugs act, the recognition by the government of the heroic services of physicians, the defeat and resulting retirement from office of important personages whose influence was inimical to the welfare of the people along lines represented by the medical profession, the promotion of a sentiment in behalf of state licensure in medicine and the preparation of a model act to that end, the education of the public on questions of medical legislation, the development of a strong public demand for the creation of a broader and stronger national public health service, and, finally.

the development of an organization by which the influence of the entire medical profession can be brought to bear on great questions of legislation and public policy.

It is to be remembered, however, that all great reforms have been and must be effected to the embarrassment if not actual injury of unworthy interests that are thereby prompted to efforts at retaliation. Such efforts are in progress at the present time. Unworthy and discredited manufacturers of impure, adulterated and misbranded foods, fraudulent drugs and spurious liquors are today conspiring with certain equally unworthy and discredited members of the profession to blacken the character of its honored leaders, and thereby disintegrate its organization. The paid representatives in congress of selfish and sinister enterprises, the jealously ambitious members of the public service outside of the medical profession, together with the ignorant and venal pretenders in medicine, are endeavoring to break down the reforms by which they have been adversely affected. In this way the pure food and drug acts is being insidiously annulled by vicious interpretations that are foreign to the purposes of the people and the congress in enacting the measure. An effort is being made to resubordinate the medical service in the Isthmian canal zone to authority that has no technical qualification for the supervision of its functions. Discredited officials are endeavoring to re-establish their power. Ignorance and supernalture,' allied under the guise of cults, are endeavoring to break down the medical practice acts of the states. Mercenary and merciless enterprises, antagonistic to the welfare of the people, are conspiring to defeat the movement for a national department of public health.

To overcome these antagonisms, to maintain the reforms already realized, and to accomplish other reforms, the necessities for which are flagrantly apparent in our national life, is today the first obligation of the medical profession both to the people and itself. Its natural guardianship of the public welfare cannot be ignored or evaded. It can discharge that duty only by an intelligent *esprit du corps* made effective through the instrumentality of far-reaching. well-disciplined and courageous organization. To this end the officers and committeemen of our national body should be unstintedly supported in their altruistic work; the state associations should be strengthened but, above all, the county societies, the units of strength and efficiency, should exemplify in the highest degree the principles of complete organization and disciplined co-operation.

After a consensus has been reached on any question in any county, every member should become the teacher of the public on that question in his respective locality. The public intelligence thus enlightened, public conviction may find expression in public action, if need be at the polls. The medical profession must carry weight, not only by the wisdom of its councils, but by its actual power with the people as the natural conservator of their physical welfare and their normal efficiency. In the exercise of its prerogatives, the county medical societies should hold open meetings to which the public are invited and before which questions of profound general concern should be discussed and appropriate action taken. These questions should pertain to every phase of protection against disease-producing influences in water, food, habitation and personal hygiene. The whole agitation, while not disregarding the defense of existing reforms, should, however, be largely concentrated in the immediate future in behalf of action by the congress to establish an improved national public health service—a measure which, in every form of practical legislation, I am authorized to state has the cordial support of President Taft.

With deepest gratitude that I have been permitted to act as an humble servitor of my profession in carrying out some of these reforms and with assurance that nothing but the inexorable demands of my practice and of my obligations in life could induce me to relinquish the work yet to be done by and through the matchless organization of the American Medical Association, I am

Very sincerely,

CHARLES A. L. REED.

60 The Groton, Cincinnati, Ohio, Oct. 26, 1909.

EXACT, ELEGANT, EFFECTIVE!

These three adjectives have a special application to the alkaloidal and active-principle granules and tablets manufactured and marketed by The Abbott Alkaloidal Company. The remarkable development of this house is undoubtedly due largely to its warm advocacy of the alkaloidal principle —that the doctor should always use remedies which are potent medicinally, concentrated in dosage, accurate in drug-content, easy of administration and in a form convenient of carriage so that they may always be at hand. This is sound common sense. An investigation of the Abbott goods and the Abbott ideas will repay the time and money spent—and not much of either will be required. We suggest that you read carefully the advertisement on back page of cover.

A TUBERCULAR CONVENTION.

The committee, appointed by the State Medical Association, and the State Commissioner of Health of the State of Oklahoma, issue the following call:

On Monday, January the 10th, 1910, at Oklahoma City, and continue for two days, all persons and societies who are interested in this subject, are requested to be represented either in person or by delegates at this time.

Ways and means will be discussed for the prevention and eradication of tuberculosis. Also the care of tubercular patients will be a special feature of this meeting.

Both physicians and the public are invited to participate. Any person, whether a physician or not, who wishes to read a paper or will contribtue to this cause by an exhibit will notify any member of this committee not later than December the 1st, 1909.

We request that all periodicals publish and public meetings announce this call.

H. M. WILLIAMS, Wellston,

J. M. POSTELLE, Oklahoma City,

R. H. HARPER, Afton,

Committee of State Medical Association.

Dr. J. C. MAHR, Shawnee,

State Commissioner of Health.

COUNCIL ON PHARMACY AND CHEMISTRY.

Articles accepted for inclusion as New and Non-Official Remedies.

Perogen Bath (Morgenstern & Co).

Mergal (Riedel & Co.)

Salipyrin (Riedel & Co.)

Suprarenalin Inhalant (Armour & Co.)

Bilein (Abbott Alkaloidal Co.)

Bilein Pills, 1-4 Gr., 1-8 Gr. and 1-2 Gr. (Abbott Alkaloidal Co.)

Iodone Oil (Henry C. Blair Co.)

Iodone Ointment (Henry C. Blair Co.)

Articles accepted for N. N. R. Appendix:

Tablets Atozyl and Iron (Sharp & Dohme.)

Comp. Yellow Oxid and Adrenalin Oint. (M. E. S. Co.) Manhattan Eye Salve Co.

Cocaine and Adrenalin Ointment (M. E. S. Co.) Manattan Eye Salve Co.

Holocaine and Adrenalin Oint. (M. E. S. Co.) Manhattan Eye Salve Co.

Argyrol Ointment 10 per cent. (M. E. S. Co.) Manhattan Eye Salve Co.

Dionin Ointment 5 per cent. (M. E. S. Co.) Manhattan Eye Salve Co.

BOOK REVIEWS

MEDICAL GYNECOLOGY.

The new (2nd) edition, by S. Wyllis Bandler, M. D., Adjunct Professor of Diseases of Women, New York Post-Graduate Medical School and Hospital. Second revised edition. Octavo of 702 pages, with 150 original illustrations. Philadelphia and London, W. B. Saunders Company, 1909. Cloth, $5.00 net; half morocco, $6.50 net.

This work deals in a complete and thorough manner with conditions confronting the gynecologist and general practitioner not usually amenable to operative interference or not in position for such interference.

To the practitioner who exhausts all reasonable means in the way of palliative treatment becofe recommending operative procedures, this work will be found of great value.

Great stress is laid on the treatment of inflammatory conditions, such as gonorrhoea, cervical catarrh and endometritis and especial attention is given to displacements subinvolution and their prevention. Much attention is given to troubles of neurotic origin and the chapters devoted to the exercise and massage treatment or constipation are worthy of close consideration.

BOOKS RECEIVED.

Note: Notice of the receipt of publications will be made under this heading upon their receipt. Their review will follow from time to time at some later date whenever time is found for the work.—Editor.

MEDICAL GYNECOLOGY.

By S. Wyllis Bandler, M. D., Adjuct Professor of Diseases of Women, New York Post-Graduate Medical School and Hospital. Second revised edition, W. B Saunders Company.

A TEXT BOOK OF OBSTETRICS.

(Including Related Gynecologic Operations). The new (6th) edition, by Barton Cooke Hirst, M. D., Professor of Obstetrics in the University of Pennsylvania. Sixth revised edition. W. B. Saunders Company

AMERICAN ILLUSTRATED DICTIONARY.

The new (5th) edition, by W. A. Newman Dorland, M. D., with 2,000 new terms. W. B. Saunders Comapny.

W. B. Saunders Company, Philadelphia and London.

PERSONAL MENTION.

MARRIED.

Dr. Harold Blake Justice of Sapulpa and Miss Shirley Louise Monck were married in Morrison, Illinois, November 7th, 1909, and will make their home in the future at Sapulpa. The many friends of Dr.

Justice congratulate him and wish he and Mrs. Justice great happiness for the future.

———

Dr. and Mrs. A. K. West, Oklahoma City; Dr. and Mrs. Carl Puckett, Pryor Creek; Dr. Claude Thompson, Muskogee, visited the City of Mexico after the meeting of the Medical Association of the Southwest in San Antonio, Texas.

———

Drs. F. Messenbaugh and M. Smith of Oklahoma City have been spending considerable time at the clinic of the Mayo's, Rochester, Minn., and with Ochsner and Murphy in Chicago.

———

Dr. L. Dresren Bruton, formerly of —————————, Missouri, has located in Muskogee. He is associated with Dr. A. W. Everly.

———

NEW MEMBERS.

Dr. J. Z. Barnett, Quinton.
Dr. Lambertus Kuntz, Perry.
Dr. Fred J. McComb, Pocasset.
Dr. Fred R. Disney, Pocasset.

———

A GOOD LOCATION FOR SALE.

I will sell for cash my home, consisting of five-room house, one acre of land, concrete storm house 6x8x9, and buggy and team of three horses, with about one hundred dollars worth of drugs, for $800.00.

This includes my practice of about eight miles square in a prairie agricultural country, twelve miles southwest of Duncan and twelve miles northwest of Comanche, Oklahoma. There is no competition, the nearest physician being twelve miles distant. The practice amounts to $2,000 annually collections good, being 95 per cent. Good

schools and lodge, with all churches represented with organization.

Will sell for cash only and will introduce buyer. Am going to take post-graduate work and move to ctiy. If you mean business, write or come, but don't bother if you do not want a good village and country practice. Address Dr. W. G. Brymer, Fair, Route 4, Comanche, Oklahoma.

———

FOR SALE.

A 1909 Model "Gleason" K. C. Car, four passenger, 16 H. P., good clearance. In first class condition. Reason for selling want to buy a larger car. Guaranteed to be all right and will sell at a bargain, if sold within the next thirty days. Don't write unless you mean business. Address
DOCTOR,
Box 44, Holdenville, Okla.

———

FOR SALE.

$1,250 cash gets property consisting of three-room dwelling house, barn, stables, pair of horses, good buggy, office furniture and fixtures; $4,000.00 practice gratis; will introduce. Reason for selling going to specialize in Texas. Address Dr. John T. Vick, Fort Towson, Oklahoma.

———

FOR SALE.

———

One static machine with all necessary attachments, everything in good order. Price. $75.00; terms if desired. Address Dr. A. E. Davenport, Western National Bank Building, Oklahoma City, Oklahoma.

———

FOR SALE.

———

The Journal has tuition to the amount of forty-four dollars in the New York Polyclinic School and Hospital which will be sold at a reduction from the usual rates, Address The Journal.

COUNTY SOCIETIES

TO ALL COUNTY SECRETARIES.

Gentlemen:

You are advised that beginning with January 1, 1910, the membership and mailing lists of the Oklahoma State Medical Association and the Journal will be separate and distinct, that is membership will not carry with it subscription to the Journal and vice versa.

In collecting membership for the year 1910 you will notify each member that he is to pay one dollar and fifty cents for membership and if he wishes to become a subscriber to the Journal fifty cents more is to be collected for the purpose of covering the price of the Journal to members.

You are urged to call the attention of each new member to the importance of his being a supporter of his state Journal and to the fact that the publication is easily worth the amount paid for it.

The above procedure is necessary on account of the ruling of the postal authorities, who decided that membership in an organization could not permit the creation of a mailing list by reason of such membership and that the mailing and subscription lists should be separated in order to permit the entry of the Journal as second class mail matter.

In conformity with the above you will be sent a supply of blank forms for taking subscriptions and as fast as these forms are sent the Secretary with the remittance, publication will be made of such name under the head of new subscribers.

Your attention is directed also to the fact that the above is an arbitrary ruling of the Council which was made necessary by the ruling of the postal authorities.

CLAUDE A. THOMPSON,
Secretary.

OPEN MEETINGS FOR COUNTY SOCIETIES.

The attention of all county secretaries is called to the following resolutions unanimously adopted at the Atlantic City session of the American Medical Association, June 10, 1909:

Whereas, The American Medical Association, not only as one of its declared purposes, but by numerous lines of activity, many of them connected with the section on hygiene and sanitary science, stands committed to the education of the public with respect to the nature and prevention of disease, and

Whereas, The demand for such popular education with respect to tuberculosis, cancer, typhoid fever and other decimating diseases has become urgent; therefore, be it

Resolved, That all county, district and other local medical societies be and they are hereby requested to hold annually one or more open meetings to which the public shall be invited and which shall be devoted to a discussion of the nature and prevention of disease and to the general hygienic welfare of the people.

OPEN MEETINGS OF COUNTY, DISTRICT AND OTHER LOCAL MEDICAL SOCIETIES.

(Extract from the minutes of the House of Delegates of the American Medical Association, Atlantic City, N. J., June 10, 1909.)

Whereas, The American Medical Association, not only as one of its declared purposes, but by numerous lines of activity, many of them connected with the section on Hygiene and Sanitary Science, stands committed to the education of the public with respect to the nature and prevention of disease; and,

Whereas, The demand for such popular education with respect to tuberculosis, cancer, typhoid fever and other decimating diseases has become urgent; therefore, be it

Resolved, That all county, district and other medical societies be, and they are hereby, requested to hold annually one or more open meetings to which the public shall be invited to attend and participate and which shall be devoted to a discussion of the nature and prevention of disease and to the general hygienic welfare of the people.

It was moved that the resolution be adopted.

Seconded and carried unanimously.

GEORGE W. SIMMONS,
General Secretary American Medical Association.

POTTAWATOMIE COUNTY.

PROGRAM
Three Months Lecture and Quiz Course of the Pottawatomie County Medical Society
Beginning Saturday Evening,
October 2, 1909.
Saturday Evening, October 2.
Meeting at Earlboro, Okla.
Drs. Cullum and McAlister Entertaining.
Lecture—Malaria...Dr. J. B. Ellis, Shawnee
Quiz—Hernia...Dr. H. A. Wagner, Shawnee
Saturday Evening, October 9.
Meeting at Dr. Trigg's Office, Shawnee.
Dr. Trigg Entertaining.
Lecture—General Surgical Considerations
.....................Dr. J. M. Trigg
Quiz—Malaria.............Dr. J. B. Ellis
Saturday Evening, October 16.
Meeting at Dr. Ellis' Office, Shawnee.
Dr. J. B. Ellis Entertaining.
Lecture—Influenza.........Dr. J. B. Ellis

Quiz—General Surgical Considerations...
.....................Dr. J. M. Trigg
Saturday Evening, October 23.
Meeting at McLoud, Okla.
Drs. Kaylor and Reynolds Entertaining.
Special Program.
Saturday Evening, October 30.
Meeting at Dr. Trigg's Office, Shawnee.
Dr. J. M. Trigg Entertaining.
Lecture—Appendicitis......Dr. J. M. Trigg
Quiz—Influenza.............Dr. J. B. Ellis
Saturday Evening, November 6.
Meeting at Dr. Cannon's Office, Shawnee.
Dr. J. S. Cannon Entertaining.
Lecture—Dysentery........Dr. J. S. Cannon
Quiz—Appendicitis..,.......Dr. J. M. Trigg
Saturday Evening, November 13
Meeting at Dr. Sanders' Office, Shawnee.
Dr. T. C. Sanders Entertaining.
Lecture—Gall Bladder Surgery..........
.....................Dr. T. C. Sanders
Quiz—Dysentery..........Dr. J. S. Cannon
Saturday Evening, November 20.
Meeting at Dr. Cannon's Office, Shawnee.
Dr. J. S. Cannon Entertaining.
Lecture—Small-pox.......Dr. J. S. Cannon
Quiz—Gall Bladder Surgery...........
.....................Dr. T. C. Sanders
Saturday Evening, November 27.
Meeting at Dr. Sanders' Office, Shawnee.
Dr. T. C. Sanders Entertaining.
Surgery of Stomach.......Dr. T. C. Sanders
Quiz—Small-pox....,.....Dr. J. S. Cannon
Saturday Evening, December 4.
Meeting at Dr. Scott's Office, Shawnee.
Dr. J. H. Scott Entertaining.
Lecture—Scarlatina and Rubeola.......
.....................Dr. J. H. Scott
Quiz—Surgery of Stomach..Dr. T. C. Sanders
Saturday Evening, December 11.
Meeting at Dr. Sanborn's Office, Shawnee.
Dr G. H. Sanborn Entertaining.
Lecture—Surgery of Intestines.........
.....................Dr. G. H. Sanborn
Quiz—Scarlatina and Rubeola..........
.....................Dr. J. H. Scott
Saturday Evening, December 18.
Meeting at Dr. Scott's Office, Shawnee.
Dr. J. H. Scott Entertaining.
Lecture—Cerebro Spinal Meningitis.....
.....................Dr. J. H. Scott
Quiz—Surgery of Intestines.... ......
.....................Dr. G. H. Sanborn
Saturday Evening, December 25.
Meeting at Dr. Mahr's Office, Shawnee.
Social Meeting.
Saturday Evening, January 1, 1910.
Meeting at Dr. Sanborn's Office, Shawnee.
Dr. G. H. Sanborn Entertaining.
Lecture—Surgery of Kidneys..........
.....................Dr. G. H. Sanborn
Quiz—Cerebro Spinal Meningitis........
.....................Dr. J. H. Scott
Wanette Meeting, Extra.
Program Committee.
J. M. Byrum, Chairman; T. D. Rowland,
J. A. Walker, H. H. Wilson, W. C. Bradford,
Secretary.

HUGHES COUNTY.

"What to Do in Appendicitis," Dr. G. W. Patterson. Open Discussion, Dr. Leo J. O'Shaughnessy. General discussion.

'Some Observations in Treatment of Pneumonia," Dr. Vanderpool. Open Discussion, Dr. A. J. Pope. General discussian.

"Anesthesia," Dr. H. A. Howell. Open Discussion, Dr. J. D. Scott. General discussion.

"Clinic," Dr. A. L. Davenport.

Thirty Minutes Quiz: "Femoral Artery," its relation, its branches, and their distribution, Dr. A. M. Butts.

"Patent Medicines," Dr. T. J. Cagle.

"How to Prevent Tuberculosis," Dr. Troy of McAlester.

Dr. Troy will gladly answer any question relative to the subject asked by any member present.

MAJOR COUNTY.

Program for the meeting to be held December 14, 1909:

Address by Dr. B. F. Johnson, President, Fairview,

Treatment of Typhoid Fever, Dr. W. L. Gleason, Fairview.

Pneumonia, Dr. W. J. Taylor, Chester.

Gunshot Wounds, Dr. P. F. Herod, Alva.

Fractures, by Dr. N. S. Mayberry, M. D.

At this meeting the organization of Major, Blaine and Alfalfa counties into a Tri-County Medical Society will be considered.

KAY COUNTY.

Program for meeting to be held December 8, 1909, at Newkirk:

"The Aseptic Management of Normal Labor," Dr. Gearhart, Blackwell. Discussion opened by Dr. Johnson, Peckham.

"State Board Examinations and Reciprocity," Dr. Mathews, Braman.

"Retroversion of the Uterus," Dr. Risser, Blackwell. Discussion opened by Dr. Robertson, Ponca City.

A. S. Risser, Secretary, Blackwell, Oklahoma.

PUBLIC MEETING LINCOLN COUNTY MEDICAL SOCIETY, WELLSTON, OKLAHOMA, DEC. 8, 1909.

10 A. M.

Early Diagnosis Pulmonary Tuberculosis, Dr. J. Z. Maraz, Prague.

Open Air and Diet Treatment of Tuberculosis, Dr. C. M. Morgan, Chandler.

Tubercular Sinuses, Dr. W. D. Baird, Davenport.

Surgical Aspect of Tubercular Glands, Dr. J. O. Glenn, Stroud.

Tuberculosis in Public Schools, Supt. O. F. Hayes, Chandler.

Tuberculin—Its Use, Dr. A. M. Marshall, Chandler.

Tubercular Glands, Dr. J. J. Evans, Stroud.

How Can We Care for Tubercular Children of Oklahoma, Dr. Lelia F. Andrews, Oklahoma City.

Review of County Work, County Health Commissioner, Dr. F. H. Norwood, Prague.

Paper, Ladies' Club of Wellston, Mrs. A. H. Taylor, Mrs. J. S. Ross.

Tuberculosis from Editor's View, Messrs. D. L. Bathurst. Wellston; H. B. Gilstrap, Chandler; Geo. Smith, Chandler; Geo. Barger, Tryon; Geo. Walbright, Stroud.

Tuberculosis in Charitable Institutions and Prisons, Miss Kate Barnard, Guthrie.

Specific Tuberculosis, Dr. F. W. Noble, Guthrie.

Recent Scientific Tubercular Researches, Dr. J. M. Postelle, Oklahoma City.

Legal Aspect of Organization Against Tuberculosis, Hon. Ira E. Billingslea, Wellston; Dr. R. H. Galyen, Chandler.

Address, Dr. W. C. Bradford, Shawnee.

Tubercular Meningitis, Dr. F. B. Erwin, Wellston.

The Church and the Great White Plague, Rev. G. H. Hilmer, Wellston; Rev. J. L. Granthem, Wellston.

Hygiene and Physical Culture as a Preventative, Miss Havergal Wickham, Wellston.

Organization from Medical Standpoint, Dr. H. M. Williams, Wellston.

Business Session, (Election of Officers).

7:30 P. M.

Illustrated Lecture (Auspices Ladies' Club), Com. of State, Dr. F. K. Camp and others.

Work of the Women's Federated Club, Mrs. Nina Hill Johns, Chickasha.

All who are interested in this subject are invited to attend this meeting.

F. B. ERWIN, Pres.

H. M. WILLIAMS, Sec'y.

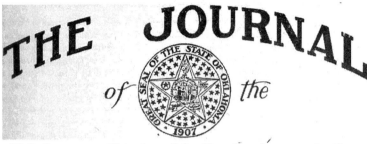

THE JOURNAL of the

Oklahoma State Medical Association.

VOL. II.	MUSKOGEE, OKLAHOMA, JANUARY, 1910.	NO 8.

DR. CLAUDE A. THOMPSON, Editor-in-Chief.

ASSOCIATE EDITORS AND COUNCILLORS.

DR. J. A. WALKER, Shawnee.	DR. JOHN W. DUKE, Guthrie.
DR. CHARLES R. HUME, Anadarko.	DR. A. B. FAIR, Frederick.
DR. F. R. SUTTON, Bartlesville.	DR. W. G. BLAKE, Tahlequah.
DR. G. W. ROBERTSON, Dustin.	DR. H. P. WILSON, Wynnewood.

DR. J. S. FULTON, Atoka.

Entered at the Postoffice at Muskogee, Oklahoma, as second class mail matter, June, 1909.

This is the Official Journal of the Oklahoma State Medical Association. All communications should be addressed to the Journal of the Oklahoma State Medical Association, English Block, Muskogee, Oklahoma.

DIFFERENTIATION OF FRACTURES OF THE NECK OF THE FEMUR

BY S. R. CUNNINGHAM, A. M., M D., OKLAHOMA CITY, OKLAHOMA.

Lecturer on Fractures and Dislocations Epworth Medical College, Member of the Surgical Staff St. Anthony's Hospital and Oklahoma City Dispensary.

Read Before the Seventeenth Annual Meeting of the Oklahoma State · Medical Association, May, 1909.

To anticipate and to some extent disarm criticism, let me state now that there is little, if anything, original in this brief paper. I am addressing men younger and older than myself; men poorer and richer in clinical experience.

To the first class let me make this statement of facts: I left college with my ideas, as probably yours were, in hopeless con-fusion as to the pathology of fractures of the femoral neck. My confusion came, as probably yours does, from a conflict of opinion, and hopeless disagreement between teacher and teacher, and between teacher and text book. So that, except that some fractures were within the capsule, and some were without, and that in the latter cases, bony union resulted, and in the former not, there did not stand out clearly in my mind *one single fact* or *symptom* upon which I could base even an *approximately* accurate differentiation between these two kinds of injury. Under these circumstances, I was forced, as you have been, or will be, to analyze the symptoms, and to ascertain as well as I could their relative value. I have proposed to myself to present these matters to you tonight, trusting that the symptoms on which I have relied for the last several years may prove as valuable to you. To men of greater age and wider knowledge, I offer my clinical experience, that they may compare it with their own, expecting criticism, correction or corroboration, as may be deserved at their hands.

Concerning this differentiation several questions arise, as first, is it worth while to make it at all? Many good men say not, alleging that the treatment is much the same in every fracture of the neck, and that it is unusual to see a case in which a positive prognosis, favorable or otherwise, can safely be made. With all due deference to these distinguished men and their supporters, I must beg leave to differ as to both propositions. First, because there is scarcely a single practitioner today who would not make a distinction between the treatment of a fracture clearly intracapsular—unimpacted, and one as clearly extracapsular—impacted. The habit of treating all cases alike has for its corner-stone a doubtful diagnosis. It matters not so much whether the fracture is intra- or extra-capsular, but rather *is it impacted?*

Certainly we do *usually* get bony union in extra-capsular, and *as certainly* we *often* get bony union in intra-capsular fracture.

As to the second proposition, I believe that a positive differentiation, and consequently a positive prognosis, can be made in nineteen cases out of twenty. But aside from treatment, we have a strong inducement to leave untried no chance of accurately locating the seat of injury.

When a patient employs a surgeon, he has a right to expect not only the utmost exercise of that surgeon's skill in diagnosis and treatment, but as well to receive such consolation, and relief from mental suffering, as may come from the confident hope of a favorable termination to his case; and, on the other hand, such warning as to the future disposition of his affairs as may come from a less favorable prognosis. Fractures of the neck of the femur, in the lay mind, as well as in the professional, are divided into two great classes, the *one* leaving as a net result, even though it be after weeks of suffering, a limb shortened, deformed, with lessened motion, but still serviceable, even strong enough to help earn a living for its owner and his family; *the other* leaving a state of affairs little short of practical helplessness.

Here is now a sufferer, probably already stricken in years, suffering from a painful injury, his hold on life none too certain, particularly prone, as most of these cases are, to melancholy and gloomy forebodings, possibly with his ambition not yet satisfied, his family not yet provided for; he may be oppressed with a dread of coming upon ungrateful children or the public for support. These people, and their friends, from the minute we look at the case, *anxiously* and *rightfully* await a word of *comfort*. I hold that the surgeon *who*, confronted by these conditions, a favorable prognosis being *possible*, fails to ally his patient's mental anxiety by giving it, but allows a tardy convalescence to decide the patient's future, is fully as blameworthy as he who unskillfully or negligently treats the physical ailment.

Can this differentiation be made in all, or nearly all cases? It all depends, in my judgment, on whether the so-called extracapsular fracture is impacted. If we except the impacted fracture at the base, it is impossible during life, by any *justifiable* examination, to decide what part of the neck is broken, or whether the fracture has occurred within or without the capsule. I have been in the habit of dividing injuries of the neck of the femur into the impacted fracture of the base of the neck, and the impacted fracture of the rest of the neck.

without regard to the capsule—a practical classification, embracing a majority of the cases, and to which the other lesions may be regarded as exceptional.

I assert that, probably *all* fractures in which the cervix femoris is detached at its base are impacted, and that the impaction is entirely wanting only in those exceptional cases in which the great trochanter forms part of the upper fragment.

Admitting then, for the sake of argument, that at the moment of occurrence all extra-capsular and mixed fractures are impacted, and most intra-capsular not, we come to the third and last question: How can this differentiation be made?

By settling the question of impaction first of all, for upon the maintenance of this condition depends our security of best future results. All violent manipulation, extreme flexion, hyper-extension, rotation, or standing the patient on his feet, are to be avoided. Surgeons have long since called attention to the fact that the certainly and rapidly fatal cases were those which had been roughly handled.

One watching the *common* diagnostic methods in these cases, advocated by high authority, too,—ceases to wonder that surgeons are skeptical about impaction, as it is often broken up under manipulation before they think of looking for it. As a matter of fact, preternatural mobility and crepitation, *invaluable symptoms* under ordinary circumstances, should be kept in the background, since a search for them is prejudicial and often fatal to impaction.

To make this diagnosis it is not necessary even to lift the limb from the bed, to make any great amount of extension, or more than slightly and gently to rotate the limb.

The behavior and appearance of the great trochanter is the key-note to the situation. This may be examined first, or what is perhaps better, the surgeon's mind may be prepared by the preliminary consideration of several minor circumstances. As first, the patient's age. Although it can scarcely be said that authors agree "as touching any one thing" in this connection, there can be no doubt that the extra-capsular fracture affects younger victims than its great rival, generally under say 65. Intra-capsular fracture rather appears over 60. The period between 60 and 70 is, however, debatable ground, in which neither can be said to have obtained the ascendancy. The direction and character of violence or force is worth considering. As a rule a fall on the trochanter will produce an impacted fracture of the base of the neck, and the force is usually great. On the other hand, a force less in amount and acting at right angles to the neck will produce an unimpacted or intra-capsular fracture. The patient is often unable to tell, however, how the fall occurred. Besides, the fall may be the consequence rather than the cause of the bone giving away, as when a patient slipping from a curbstone receives an intra-capsular fracture, and then confuses the diagnosis by falling upon his trochanter. Eversion of the foot is of little practical differential value. It may be present, either slightly or markedly, in either variety. If there is any difference it may generally be shown that in impacted fracture the eversion is of a positive character, impressed on the limb by the interlocking of the fragments, and does not yield to any moderate force. In non-impacted fracture, on the other hand, the eversion is due to the weight of the limb, or contraction of the external rotator muscles, and is, therefore, not so persistent.

In the amount and character of the shortening we have the first symptom of positive value. With regard to this feature of the case, you will find among authorities the greatest difference of opinion. Some assert that it is greater in one variety, some in the other. It all depends on the presence or absence of impaction.

If a fracture at the base of the neck be un-impacted the shortening would very probably increase from day to day, and, being entirely free from capsular restraint, might reach an amount scarcely attainable in a fracture within the capsule, unless this capsule were extensively lacerated. Impaction, however, is only compatible with shortening certainly not exceeding an inch in amount. Practically, in such cases, the shortening is almost invariably about three-quarters of an inch, due partly to the telescoping of the fragments, and partly to the lessening of the angle between shaft and neck.

Moreover, the shortening in impacted fracture is constant from day to day, and is not to be increased or diminished by a moderate and safe force. The pull required to bring the limb to its proper length is said to exceed, on the average, forty pounds. In the unimpacted fracture the shortening, at the first examination, may be nothing, or an inch or more, can be readily increased or diminished, and generally increases from day to day.

It is, however, to the larger trochanter we must look for convincing evidence as to the nature of the injury. The foregoing symptoms are valuable as proving the existence of a fracture of the neck, but with the possible exception of shortening, are of little worth in determining the kind of fracture. Some author has said that the diagnosis for fracture of the femoral neck could often be made from an inspection of the foot alone. I am certain that the result has often justified a differential diagnosis based upon an examination of the trochanter alone.

What now are these important trochanteric symptoms? In a fracture wholly within the capsular ligament the trochanter can be changed only as to its position and relation to other parts. In the impacted fracture at the base of the neck, on the con-trary, the trochanter is always split, often comminuted, and, we must add, therefore, in such cases, changes in its appearance and behavior. For this part of the examination the patient should be on the back, close to the edge of the bed, with hips and both lower extremities naked (if a man) ; covered only with a tightly and smoothly drawn sheet, if a woman. The surgeon, kneeling or sitting by the bed, should put one hand on each trochanter and examine like points at the same time. For example, as one must begin somewhere, let the question of the distance of each trochanter from the crest of its corresponding ilium be settled once for all; while at the same time, the limb, being *gently* pushed and pulled by an assistant, we may determine the presence or absence of impaction. The amount of reliable information to be gained by this system of simultaneous bimanual examination of like points, the importance of which is not sufficiently understood as a rule, is truly remarkable. In both fractures the trochanter is or may be above its proper level. *Here the likeness ceases. In the intra-capsular variety, the trochanter, no longer propped out by the neck, is drawn by the muscles attached to it, whose entire pull is inward, toward the medium line,* and in well marked cases is tucked under the flange of the ilium, becoming, of course, less prominent and allowing the hip and buttock of that side to flatten. On the other hand, in the impacted fracture, the trochanter is higher by an amount which is constant, unless due force is used. It is also markedly prominent. One of the effects of the fracturing force is to lessen the angle between neck and shaft, causing it to approximate a right angle. As the trochanter rises, therefore, it is at the same time pushed out, a result only partly neutralized by the telescoping of the fragments. As now the surgeon's hands are passed down the patient's sides, the hand over the affected side, instead of gliding smoothly along the tense fascia between the iliac crest and the trochanter, and over the latter, almost unconscious of its presence, suddenly falls into a depression below the crest of the ilium, the fascia lata being relaxed by the elevation of the trochanter, and is as suddenly checked at the lower part of the depression by the prominent lip referred to, behind which in thin individuals the fingers may even be slightly inserted. By this raising and widening process, not only is the hip made fuller and rounder than the opposite presumably healthy side, but obtains a shape noticeable to the hand, and in some cases to the eye also, which I call, for want of a better name, "square shouldered." This condition can scarcely escape observation, and its meaning seems to me unmistakable. The prominence does not yield to lateral pressure; while in the unimpacted fracture the flatness of the hip can sometimes be increased by pressing the unpropped trochanter still further inward.

In these impacted fractures, as before mentioned, the trochanter is nearly always split or comminuted. Its antero-posterior diameter is therefore increased, first by the mechanical wedging apart of the fragments, which increase is afterward made still greater, and this in all diameters, by inflammatory deposits.

The splitting or other injury to the trochanter naturally increases the sensitiveness of its outer surface, so that complaint of pain is made when pressure is exerted upon it. A good plan is to compress the trochanter antero-posteriorly with thumb and finger. In this way it may be clearly made out whether the tenderness is in the trochanter itself or is more deeply seated. Care must also be taken not to press upon the overlying soft structures, in all cases when these are contused. Some tenderness over the injured trochanter may be found by pressing upon it within an hour after injury. It increases as inflammation is set up in the periosteum and other fibrous tissue surrounding the trochanter, reaching its maximum only after several days. It will be noticed therefore, that the trochanteric symptoms grow more and more marked for several days, at least, so that a diagnosis somewhat doubtful at first may soon be confirmed by a little careful observation.

Bryant's and Nelaton's lines—good but not reliable in my hands.

Should there be no impaction present in fracture at base of the neck I should consider a positive diagnosis almost impossible, but should try to base it on age, direction of force, rotation of femur on its own axis, and signs of injury to great trochanter.

A word about the peculiar medico-legal aspect of these cases. Suits against surgeons for failing to secure bony union in intra-capsular fractures, or on account of the deformed, shortened and partially crippled limbs resulting from the impacted variety, are not uncommon. I am convinced that by a little foresight on our part these suits can be avoided. The first recommendation I would make is the careful differentiation of the varieties, with a view to accurate prognosis. On the basis of this clear diagnosis, let a prognosis equally clear be made in plain language, and in the presence of reliable witnesses. Not one patient in a thousand is dissatisfied with a result which was foretold from the day or perhaps hour of injury.

I would even go farther than this, however, and carefully and patiently explain, as I have done for years, both to patient and friends, aided by rough sketches or pictures in text-books, the exact location of the fracture and the absolute necessity of the results, whatever they may be. Honesty between surgeon and patient never pays better than in this instance. I should advise also that we claim no special credit for good results in such cases. If we do, now how are we to escape the logical conclusion on the part of patients that we are responsible for bad results? Taking this view of the matter, therefore, I tell my patient: You have suffered from a fracture of the neck of the thigh bone; the break is in such a place; the fragments are in such a relation to each other; the result, if you live, will probably be so and so. I am utterly powerless to affect this result for better or worse. All I can do is to relieve your pain, look after your general health, and carry you as comfortably as possible through the period of confinement and suffering which necessarily follows your injury.

305-307 Majestic Bldg.

CHANGES OF METABOLISM IN DIABETES MELLITUS

BY DR. ROBERT H. HARPER, AFTON, OKLAHOMA

Read Before the Seventeenth Annual Meeting of the Oklahoma State Medical Association, May, 1909.

In this paper, no originality will be claimed nor assumed, as the data are from the writings of various workers, and from the literature; nor will any detailed account of the disease be given, as this may be found in any good text-book; but any description of the etiology and pathology of the disease that is more than four or five years old is out of date, the truth of which a perusal of the literature of the past ten years will convince any one.

Definition. A persistent variation from the normal metabolism of carbohydrates and fats, in which an excess of glucose is present in the blood, and is excreted in the urine; usually characterized by loss of weight, thirst, polyuria, and a tendency to a fatal termination.

The carbohydrates of the food undergo a series of changes during digestion, as a result of the action of the diastatic ferments in the saliva, pancreatic juice, and succus entericus. Starchy food is acted upon to a limited extent by the ptyalin of the saliva; the molecules of starch are hydrolyzed by the addition of a molecule of water, and the end result of successive stages is that the starch is converted into maltose and dextrin; this process is limited on account of the short time that the ptyalin has to act, except that some of the food of an ordinary meal may remain in the fundic end of the stomach an hour or more, untouched by the acid of the gastric juice, which promptly stops the action of ptyalin. It is not known that the action of ptyalin is changed in diabetes.

In the stomach, the dextrin, formed by the action of ptyalin, is probably absorbed; but most of the starch and sugar foods are passed on, unchanged, into the small intestine, where the important processes of digestion and assimilation occur. As the carbohydrates are acted upon by the pancreatic juice, the source of this secretion will be considered. It is now established that the effect of the contact of the acid secretion of the stomach upon the duodenal mucous membrane and its secretion is to convert what is known as pro-secretin into an active form, secretin, which is absorbed into the blood, reaches the pancreas through its artery, and stimulates the pancreatic cells to secrete the ordinary pancreatic juice. This, it is interesting to note here, does not contain trypsin, the proteid digesting ferment, but a potential form of it, known as trypsinogen; the duodenal or jejunal mucous membrane in its turn, secretes a substance, enterokinase, which, combining with the trypsinogen, forms trypsin as needed; trypsin is such a powerful digestant of proteids that were it not for this method, an excess of it might digest the mucous membrane itself. Lipase and amylopsin are probably formed in the pancreatic juice ready for immediate action. Amylopsin is similar or identical to ptyalin; it hydrolyses starches into dextrin and maltose, which is further converted into dextrose and levulose, the former being by far the larger in amount.

Cane and milk sugars are di-saccharids, $C_{12} H_{22} O_{11}$, and cannot be used as such by the body tissues. By the action of an intestinal secretion, invertase, they are hydrolysed, by the addition of one molecule of water, into dextrose and levulose. Any excess of the di-saccharids above the converting power of the amylopsin, is absorbed unchanged and excreted in the urine. The dextrose and levulose formed from the sugars and starches are absorbed by the small intestine, enter the portal vein, and are carried to the liver, where, by a process of dehydration, they are changed into glycogen $C_6 H_{12} O_6 + H_2 O - C_6 H_{10} O_6$ This, when needed by the tissues, is re-converted into glucose, probably by the action of a special enzyme secreted by the liver cells. But if dextrose reaches the liver faster than it can be changed into glycogen, it causes an increase of the amount in the blood, and when this exceeds 1 to 2 per cent, it escapes in the urine. The renal mechanism seems to be adjusted to this physiological limit; this accounts for transient glycosuria, after the ingestion of a large amount of sugar in the food, and is a normal method of getting rid of the excess of sugar.

Glucose and glycogen are formed from proteid food, to a small extent, in health. and in diabetes, this becomes abnormal, even the body proteids being converted into dextrose.

The liver is capable of storing up glycogen to 14 per cent of its own weight. Taking the average at 55 ounces, for the adult liver, this would mean 7.7 ounces, nearly 1-2 pound, of reserve glycogen.

An important point to note here is the fact that glycogen is liberated from the liver "probably by the action of a special enzyme produced by the liver cells." As in the case of trypsin and secretin, this enzyme may depend upon some other secretion for its formation, and if, this potential enzyme were lacking, or in excess, the action of the liver in normal metabolism would be interfered with.

We will now trace the normal course and role of glucose in the tissues. By the blood, it is carried to the muscles, where probably a small part is used at once, but by far the larger part is changed into glycogen, and stored in the muscle cells. This, the evidence shows, is effected by a special ferment, or part of one, secreted by the muscle cells, but depending upon another ferment that probably comes from the pancreas. As needed for energy production, this muscle glycogen is re-converted into dextrose, passing from the form of dynamic to kinetic energy, being oxidized in the muscle tissue into carbonic acid and water. Glycogen cannot be used as such by the muscle cells, nor can dextrose be stored either in the liver or muscle tissue. The amount of glycogen the muscles are capable of storing may equal the liver in weight, or .5 to .9 per cent of the weight of the essential muscle tissue.

Here, in the muscle cells, is another place where the normal metabolism may be disturbed. Some secretin, in excess or deficiency, may prevent glucose from being converted into glycogen, and so increase the amount in the blood above the normal limit of .2 per cent; or after being so stored, may cause it to be liberated faster than it can be used, or prevent it being used at all by the muscle cells to produce kinetic energy. The last is the most probable derangement of metabolism.

In 1903 and 1904, and again in 1906,

Otto Cohnheim made some very enlightening experiments on carbohydrate metabolism. He obtained juices from the pancreas and muscles by pressure. Each juice, when added to a solution of glucose, was inactive. When muscle juice and glucose solution were mixed, and pancreatic juice added, there was rapid and eventually complete conversion of the glucose into carbonic acid and alcohol. He believes that both the pancreas and muscle cells produce substances that are necessary for carbohydrate metabolism. Notice the conversion into carbonic acid and alcohol. The experiments of Lepine, of Paris, show that alcohol is probably a product between dextrose and final oxidation into carbonic acid and water, in the muscle tissue. Also note that this has a special bearing on the treatment of special cases of diabetes. This theory is advanced by Carl Ramus, in a paper in the Journal of the American Medical Association, February 6, 1904. Cohnheim's experiments prove that there is a special ferment in the pancreas that enables the muscle cells to use glucose in the production of energy; what is this special ferment? In 1889 von Mering and Minkowski removed the pancreas from animals, and found that in all cases, the operation was followed by glycosuria, even if carbohydrate food is withheld from the diet. There is also an increase in the amount of urine, and of urea, thirst, hunger, emaciation, muscular weakness, and death results in from 2 to 4 weeks. But if a portion of the pancreas is left, one-fourth or one-fifth, of its bulk, no glycosuria follows, even if the remnant has no connection with the duct, or it may even be transplanted to the abdominal wall. This proves that it is not the ordinary pancreatic juice that controls the amount of glucose in the blood; considerable evidence has accumulated to show that it is not the pancreatic cells of the secreting tubules that is concerned in carbohydrate metabolism, but a special product of the islands of Langerhans; in man, these islands are scattered through the pancreas, forming spherical or oval bodies, that may reach one millimeter in diameter. The cells in these bodies are polygonal, their cytoplasm pale, finely granular, and small in amount; the nuclei possess a thick chromatin network, which stains deeply; each island has a rich capillary network which resembles a glomerulus of the kidney. Ligation of the pancreatic duct is followed by atrophy of the pancreatic cells proper, while those of the islands of Langerhans are not affected, and glycosuria does not follow, which is the condition when the whole organ is removed. Obviously, these islands secrete a substance which controls the formation, or the liberation, or the consumption of dextrose, either in the liver, or in the muscles. This was worked out by Opie, in Welch's laboratory, and published in 1900 and 1901, and independently by Sobelow, in 1901. "Hyaline degeneration of the islands appears to be the characteristic lesion in pancreatic diabetes in which they are not destroyed secondarily to an interstitial pancreatitis."

The essential and principal variation of metabolism in diabetes is an excess of glucose in the blood; the normal amount varies between .1 and .2 per cent, but in diabetes it is always more than this, and may reach 0.6 or 0.7 per cent. There is a failure of the liver to store up glycogen, as the amount in the liver is always reduced, and may be absent entirely. There is a demand for an extra amount of food to make up for the loss occasioned by the glycosuria, and consequently, there is excreted an excess of nitrogen in the form of urea; this becomes pathological only when the nitrogen excreted exceeds that taken in the food, showing that in addition, the nitrogen of the tissues is being used. There is also a decrease in the ability of the tissues to oxidize fats, and beta-oxybutyric acid, and its derivatives, diacetic acid and aceto-zone, arise as a result of the incomplete oxidation of the fats.

The presence in the blood of an excess of glucose means one of two things: Overproduction, or under-consumption; there is no evidence that there is more glucose formed from a certain amount of food in the diabetic than in the normal individual, but there are some data that lead to the belief that there is a lowered power of the tissues to oxidize glucose, and, to some extent, fats.

A very suggestive theory may be based on the fact that when the pancreas is removed, there follows a glycosuria; now, if the adrenal secretion is inhibited, there is no glycosuria; and again, if adrenal secretion be injected in a normal individual, glycosuria results; this seems to indicate that some principle in the adrenal secretion, if present in the blood, in excess of some other secretion of the pancreas, most likely the secretion of the islands of Langerhans, than there is an under-consumption of glucose by the muscle tissue; this, in its turn, seems to depend upon the proper proportion of the pancreatic and adrenal secretion, on the one part, to combine with a muscle-cell secretion on the other, and that when the balance is disturbed, normal oxidation of glucose does not take place, the muscle cells are unable to decompose the glucose molecule, the amount in the blood reaches the limit to which the renal mechanism is adjusted, and it is drained out in the urine. Sweet and Pemberton conclude from their experiments that there is a principle in the adrenals and the nervous part of the pituitary gland that, in excess, suppresses the secretion of the pancreatic juice, and probably also, the secretion of the islands of Langerhaws; this has been found in no other tissue, is independent of the principle that causes a rise of the blood pressure. This is very suggestive that the adrenals, or the hypo-physis, or both, hold the key to the pathologic changes in diabetes.

CONCLUSIONS.

The internal secretion of the islands of Langerhans seem to be essential to normal carbohydrate metabolism; this seems to be controlled by the adrenal, and probably also, the pituitary secretions; a special product of the liver and muscle cells is also essential to the process.

The glucose in the blood may be prevented from being converted into glycogen by the liver by the deficiency or excess of a special enzyme or secretion, probably the product of the pancreas, the adrenals, or the hypophysis.

From the same reason, the liver may give up its glycogen faster than demanded by the muscle cells; or, the liver mechanism may not be deranged at all, the demand of the insufficiently supplied muscle cells causing it to give up an excess of glucose.

Deficiency or excess of some special secretion seems to prevent the consumption of glucose by the muscle cells, or prevent its conversion into glycogen; again, the same cause may allow muscle glycogen to be converted into glucose faster than it can be oxidized, or this final oxidation process may be prevented, which last seems the most probable.

Deficiency or excess of some special secretion seems to prevent the consumption of glucose by the muscle cells, or prevent its conversion into glycogen; again, the same cause may allow muscle glycogen to be converted into glucose faster than it can be oxidized, or this final oxidation process may be prevented, which last seems the most probable.

There is some evidence that alcohol is an intermediate product between the dextrose resulting from the conversion of muscle glycogen and the end products of carbonic acid and water.

A CASE OF SUPERNUMERARY OVARY

BY F. W. NOBLE, M. D., GUTHRIE, OKLAHOMA, SURGEON TO OKLAHOMA METHODIST HOSPITAL; SURGEON TO
FT. SMITH & WESTERN RY. AND EL RENO & WESTERN RY

SUPERNUMERARY OVARY.

My excuse for reading you a paper on Supernumerary Ovary is that this condition is so rarely reported that all authentic cases should be placed on record. Engstrom defines a supernumerary ovary as an additional gland, which is independent but equally important to the normal ovary. He defines an accessory ovary as a mass of ovarian tissue, which has been cut off from the normal ovary as a result of certain conditions obtaining in fetal or post-fetal life. He further states that the supernumerary ovary has its origin in early embryonic existence, during the time the sexual glands are being differentiated from the uro-genital ridge. The accessory ovary he believes is a portion of the usual ovary which has become separated from the ovary as the result of some disturbance, frequently peritonitis or an inflammatory state which has arisen during fetal or post-fetal life; so that may be merely fission, probably on the same principle that bands within the amniotic sac cause spontaneous amputation and other deformities.

An accessory ovary may be intra-peritoneal or retro-peritoneal, the former being apparently of more frequent occurence. The reported instances of retro-peritoneal accessory ovary or isolated portions of ovarian tissue show that they are often best placed between the layers of the broad ligament, but occasionally, as exemplified by a tumor containing ovarian structure, they are met with under the peritoneum of the posterior pelvic wall or behind that of the abdominal parietes.

Up to the present time no instance of normal accessory ovary or ovarian tissue in these latter locations, is reported in every instance degenerative processes having taken place when the adventitious organ was discovered. Perhaps the explanation of this lies in the fact that so small a body as the ovary, in such positions as those cited would be very difficult to recognize until attention had been called to its presence through symptoms arising from pathological changes.

Manton reports a case of multiple operation with appendectomy, total ablation of the left appendages and resection of the right ovary, who was operated upon the second time for pain in the right iliac region and more severe backache than ever, in whom he found cystic degeneration of the remains of the right ovary, and behind the uterus, buried in the tissues of cervicovaginal junction and distinctly below the peritoneum, a small mass the size of a filbert could be outlined and pressure on it caused severe pain at the "spot" as the patient said. It consisted of a mass of friable tissue more than one inch long and three quarters of an inch thick and when this was removed the symptoms subsided.

Gibbs of Detroit said it was composed of an ovarian stroma with a few Graffian follicles.

It is not of so rare occurence to find one ovary absent and when this occurs the corresponding half of the uterus and also tube of that side and very often the kidney will be found lacking. Rarely however do we find mention of either actual accessory or supernumerary ovaries; although not rarely a constricted portion of an ovary has been mistaken for the real thing. Accessory ovaries immediately adjoining a normal ovary and contained usually within the same epithelial covering have been found at post-mortems and at operations; but actual accessory or supernumerary ovaries situated at a considerable interval from the other ovaries seem positively rare. *It is probable that incomplete removal of all the ovarian tissue is the cause of recurring flow after total ablation of the uterine appendages and not the presence of a third ovary because Bland Sutton deems these extra glands so rare that he says there is no established case of an accessory gland quite distinct and separate from the main gland; but Grohe reported a case of supernumerary ovary and mentioned a second case described by Klebs, where a constriction band cut the ovary in two halves, each rudimentary. An autopsy on a new born babe which showed six appendages to one normal ovary and while one of these showed normal ovarian tissue, the remainder was cystic, Kochs and also Lumniczer described supernumerary ovarian finds. Winckel reports a case between the uterus and bladder.

The case I wish to put on record is the following: A spinister 30 years old, residence Guthrie, Okla., occupation, teacher. Family history negative except one aunt died with tuberculosis. Personal history contains nothing of note except that at sixteen years of age she suffered from a "breaking out" on the neck and at this time she also had—an attack of continuous nausea accompanied by severe pain in the neck and face lasting three weeks, which was followed by facial paralysis lasting for six months. She complains that menstruation comes on every three weeks, lasts two or three days, is profuse and clotted and that she suffers greatly with pain especially before and after the flow. She also complains of pain down the inner side of the thighs on the outer side of the hips in groins and sacral region which are increased at the menstrual period. She suffers from insomnia, vertical headache, slight

*Since writing this paper I have seen an article on "hemorrhagic uterus" that may have some bearing on this point.

cough, deafness, lassitude, anorexia, belches gas after meals, bloating of the stomach after meals.

She tires easily, especially in the back, wakes up unfreshed in the morning, there is a bandlike sensation around her head, memory is poor, she finds difficulty in planning, worries all the time, cries easily, all the reflexes are exaggerated and wrist jerks are present.

An examination of the pelvis demonstrates a retroflexion of the uterus and two tender ovaries. The diagnosis was Neuresthenia, Retroflexion of the Uterus with probable Cystic Degeneration of both Ovaries. An examination of the stomach contents showing chronic gastritis.

I advised operation and later opened the abdomen by low median incision and found the diagnosis of cystic ovaries confirmed as well as retroflexed uterus and an enlongated appendix containing fecal concretions was removed. The ovarian cysts were incised and the lining membrane of the cysts wiped out according to Watkins technique and the wounds of the ovaries sutured with fine catgut.

I was surprised to find a well developed ovary about the size of a wren's egg situated about an inch posterior and inward from the left ovary which microscopically consisted of normal ovarian tissue. It lay in the broad ligament an inch posterior and inward from the left ovary. The retroverted uterus was corrected by Ventral Suspension.

References: Gray, Flint, Piersol, Kelly, Bland Sutton, Penrose, Manton, American Textbook of Gynecology, Dudley, Spencer Wells, Leidy.

It is more than likely that a rule abolishing the common drinking cup upon railroad trains, interurban cars, depots, public buildings and public schools will be announced to take effect the first day of April.

THREE ECTOPICS AND THREE OPERATIONS IN THE SAME PATIENT IN FOUR YEARS

BY DR. J. HUTCHINGS WHITE, MUSKOGEE, OKLAHOMA

In a series of ectopic cases reported in the January, 1909, number of the Kansas City Index-Lancet, I gave a history of the second ectopic in the following case. Since that time the third tubal pregnancy has taken place:

Mrs. H., age 33 years, married 16 years, a fleshy woman, suffered from one attack pneumonia since childhod. During childhood suffered from whooping cough and measles. Periods began about fourteen years of age, suffered no pain, flow normal, periods lasting five days. Has given birth to three children; one now living, five years old; one miscarriage. No complications arose at time of births or after miscarriage.

Two weeks prior to her first operation, on November 27, 1905, she was seized with pain in lower abdomen and bloody discharge from vagina. She did not skip a period, however. On the above date the cul-de sac was opened and a quantity of blood evacuated. Recovery uneventful.

Two and one-half years later she failed to menstruate in April, and on May 25th was suddenly taken with severe cramps in lower abdomen, temperature 101° F. Pain and tenderness in pelvis on examination. The following day patient suffered from considerable shock and abdomen became rigid. She rallied from this and improved up to the 29th, four days after onset, when she again suffered much pain. I saw her first in consultation with Doctors Joblin and Adams, May 1st, and operated same day removing left tube and ovary. The abdomen was filled with a large quantity of blood. Recovery uneventful. On examination of the tube we found a scar the seat of rupture of first ectopic.

May of this year patient again skipped her period, and in June was seized with a sudden sharp pain in lower abdomen. Nauseated and suffered shock. Abdomen became swollen and very tender. Her condition was too grave to move to hospital at once. She rallied from the shock and gained enough strength to be carried to a hospital two days later, where abdominal section was performed, and the right tube and an ovary removed. Recovery uneventful.

I would like to call attention to the fact that the second and third operations were performed five days and four days respectively after primary rupture.

THE VALUE OF BISMUTH VASELINE TREATMENT IN TUBERCULAR SINUSES AND ABSCESS CAVITIES

BY A. A. WEST, M. D., GUTHRIE, OKLAHOMA

Read before the Lincoln County Medical Society.

The failures in the treatment of tubercular infections, both of the bone and soft tissues has been so appalling, and the multitude of patients going from one surgeon to another seeking relief, only to be disappointed, and finally giving up, with perhaps a half dozen discharging sinuses had almost caused a panic amongst surgeons both in this country and Europe.

The numerous methods in vogue at one time or another have all become obsolete after time and practical demonstrations proved them worthless.

You are all acquainted with the later. methods of treatment, no doubt, such as was originated by Professor Senn, of using decalcified bone chips in abscess cavities of the bone in which the removal of large portions of bone was necessitated.

The Moseliz-Moorhof plug was a very favorite treatment for a time and the still later method of the iodoform emulsion in glycerine, has still many advocates today. Undoubtedly many cases have yielded to these treatments, but there is a large class of cases that have not improved under any of the above treatments.

Dr. Emil Beck (1) of Chicago has recently given us a new method of diagnosis and treatment of tubercular sinuses and abscess cavities, which seems to be gaining great headway among the surgeons in treating this class of cases. Besides answering every purpose in the treatment of long neglected tubercular sinuses, it furnishes us with an excellent method of diagnosis as well. In the last six months I have treated a number of tubercular sinuses by this method and all have given me the most flattering results with one exception, and in this case the destruction of bone was so great, I was compelled to amputate the leg.

I will briefly give you the formula and the method of injection as used by Dr. Beck, and I have only varied the formula in a few instances as in my judgment it seemed necessary.

Formula of paste for diagnosis and early treatment:

Rx.   Bismuth Subnitrate ....30!
      Vaseline ....60!
   Mix while boiling.
   Formula for late treatment:
Rx.   Bismuth Subnitrate ....30!
      White Wax .... 5!
      Paraffine .... 5!
      Vaseline ....60!
   Mix while boiling.

As to the method of injection, I will give it verbatim as Dr. Beck describes it.

"The fistula should be dried out, if possible, by packing into its depth a strip of plain gauze, one-half to one inch wide. This gauze is removed just before the injection of the paste. The emulsion is sterilized before using, and the syringe is charged while the emulsion is hot and liquid. (It is sufficiently cooled by allowing cold water to run over the springe until the contents are of the right consistency.) A glass syringe with a nozzle similar to that of the Valentine irrigating tip should then be loaded with the bismuth paste and tightly pressed against the fistulous opening; the emulsion is forced in very slowly, until the patient complains of pressure. The syringe is then removed and a small gauze sponge is quickly pressed against the opening to prevent the escape of the paste until it has hardened sufficiently. An icebag may be applied to hasten the hardening of the material. I inject the bismuth-vaseline paste until the discharge ceases, and then use the harder preparation containing wax and paraffine, after which it usually remains closed. The injections are painless and produce no dangerous symptoms, such as hemorrhage, sepsis, embolism, etc."

Dr. Beck in his first paper laid stress on the drying out thoroughly of the cavity when possible, and checking the hemorrhage before injecting with the bismuth paste, but in one case that we had in which there was considerable oozing of blood after an extensive curettage of the diseased bone, we injected the paste and had excellent results. Since then, Dr. Beck has found this to be unnecessary, but where possible, I think better results are obtained if care is taken to have a clean cavity before injection.

The composition of the two formulas given may be modified to suit the case you are treating. For diagnosis and early treatment, I make use of formula No. 1, and for later treatment and large open cavities, I use formula No. 2, and if deemed advisable, more paraffine and wax may be added giving it still more solidity when cooled.

I do not attempt to clean the cavity with any antiseptic solutions of any kind. It is of no particular value and it is often harmful. In mixing and sterilizing the paste great care should be taken to keep out any water from getting in the paste, and the syringe to be used should be sterilized by some dry process. The plunger should then be removed and dipped into a little sterilized olive oil.

Of the value of bismuth-vaselin paste in tubercular sinuses there can be no doubt. Dr. Beck in his first contribution on this subject gives a series of thirteen cases in which he injected bismuth-vaselin paste and a sufficient length of time has now elapsed to have proved its efficacy.

These cases cover a large variety of tubercular lesions. The first case he describes as a sinus following a psoas abscess in a child four years old. The injection was made more for diagnostic purposes than that any actual benefit should accrue, but in a few days after the injection, the child returned and the sinus was found to be closed and has remained closed ever since.

I would be glad to have you all secure the Journal of the A. M. A., Vol. L, No. II, and read the reports of Dr. Beck's cases, in which he has used the bismuth-vaseline injections. In this short article I have neither time nor space allotted me to give in detail a report of these cases, but I believe if this treatment is properly carried out and given in conjunction with the electro-therapy, fresh air, fixation and bacterial vaccines, all of which are necessary adjuncts to the treatment of any tubercular process, that all tuberuclar sinuses can be healed out and patients given the relief they are seeking.

I wish to report a case in which a period of six months has elapsed and in which no evidence of the recurrence can be seen.

Case 1. F. D., male, single, 23 years old. Family history: Brother died of pulmonary tuberculosis. Previous history: When a child 3 years old he had tuberculosis of the hip joint which lasted over a period of four years, during which time there was a number of sinuses discharging from different parts of the hip. There was the usual destruction of the bone seen in these cases, ankylosis, and deformity. These sinuses all closed and he was in apparent good health until in November, 1907, when he again complained of pain in the knee joint with some tenderness when pressure was made over the great trochanter. An abscess formed which dissected its way and opened at a point on the outer thigh about four inches below the hip joint. It had followed in the tract of one of the previous sinuses. As the hip joint was already ankylosed there did not seem to be any necessity for further fixation. I operated on May 5, 1908, opening the abscess and curetting the sinus, but it continued to discharge until the following August 1st, when I injected 100 grms. of bismuth. On August 10th, he came to the office with the sinus entirely closed. He is now able to get about without the aid of crutches; all the pain and tenderness gone, and his general health has greatly improved. I have several other cases to report at a future date but I wish a suitable length of time to pass that I may be more certain of the results.

The use of the bismuth-vaseline paste injection in the treatment of suppuration of the ear, nose and throat, have been well tested out by Dr. Joseph Beck (2) in which he has treated over three hundred cases with excellent results. In this class of work he uses two other formulas adding considerable more of the paraffine and white wax.

The good results ascribed to the use of bismuth paste in this special field are very likely due to several causes. Dr. Emil Beck in his recent article read before the International Congress on Tuberculosis says:

"Many factors undoubtedly contribute to the healing process, but I am convinced that the bactericidal effect of the bismuth subnitrate is the most prominent one. In nearly every case treated we have noted that the injections are followed by the gradual diminution and final disappearance of the micro-organisms. Tubercle bacilli are no exception. This fact was discovered in a case of tuberculous empyema, and corroborated by another typical case. Whether the bismuth subnitrate destroys the bacilli by its chemical action or whether it exerts a chemotactic power has not yet been definitely determined. I am inclined to believe the latter to be the case. The fact that the number of tubercle bacilli at first increase in number, and are found mostly in the interior of the leucocytes, while the injections were started they were scanty and mostly extraleucocytic, supports the chemotactic theory."

Its value in the treating of abscess cavities of the lungs is fully demonstrated in a case that Dr. Beck treated by this method. The case was a boy 19 years old that in January, 1907, had a severe attack of bronchitis. This resulted in an empyema which on March 19, 1907, necessitated an operation in which two ribs were resected, the put cavity evacuated and drainage established. The young man was referred to Dr. Beck the following December with a fistula discharging two to three ounces of pus each day. The cavity was injected with bismuth-vaseline daily and though it kept on discharging, the quantity diminished, and after ten injections the wound

ceased to discharge and remained dry for three days. Fearing there might be some retained pus, a tube was passed and the patient ordered to close his mouth and nostrils and distend his lungs as much as possible. This brought out the material in a semi-liquid state which hardened immediately in the basin. This indicated that the body temperature had kept the bismuth-vaseline in a liquid state, and the wax and paraffine were added to the next injection. This was done Jan. 10, and the fistula closed up entirely the next day. There were no unpleasant symptoms following except the patient coughed up some of the paste through the mouth. This proved that there was an abscess of the lung as was suspected by the character of the discharge.

As yet I have had no occasion to use bismuth-vaseline in abscess cavities of the lung, but the report of this case alone is sufficient evidence for me to give it a trial in the first case that presents itself. The benefit to the patient by this method seems to me to far exceed the more radical operations and the relief is almost spontaneous.

The use of this method of treatment does not lessen your obligation in using any other means to effect a cure. In fact I may be too sanguine as to its value in the treatment of tubercular sinuses but from the reports of Dr. Beck's numerous cases, and the widespread popularity with which it has been received by surgeons everywhere, and the results obtained in my own cases, give me some ground for my belief.

The amount of bismuth that we are enabled to inject without danger of poisoning our patients seems to be a matter of some discussion among the various authorities, that it exerts some toxic effects seems possible when given in large doses into the pleural cavities or given intraperitoneal.

Schuler (3) and von Bardeleben (4) claim it is non-toxic and Professor Muhlig (5) has administered as much as 300 grs.

daily without producing any poisonous effects.

As early as 1793, we have reports of poisoning by bismuth, but these are thought to be due to the impurities of the drug. Kocher (6) in 1882, observed that in using bismuth where there was a large surface for absorption that it seemed to produce poisonous effects, the symptoms of which were similar to those of lead poisoning. Similar cases have been reported by Professor Petersen (7). Professor Muhlig (8) reported the following case: A man 26 years of age, received a burn on both arms, hand and neck. The same were dressed with oil for three days and the pure bismuth subnitrate applied. Two weeks later a black border around the teeth appeared and within five days more, the whole mouth and uvula were grayish-blue and slightly ulcerated. The urine remained normal, digestion normal. Recovery took place after wounds were curetted and freed from bismuth.

Dressman (9) reports a similar case and Worden, Sailer, Pancoast, and Davis (10) reported two cases in which two to four ounces were administered in one dose. In both cases symptoms of bismuth poisoning developed.

The first fatal case was reported by Bennecke and Hoffman (11). A child three weeks old was given forty-five grs. of bismuth subnitrate in buttermilk to diagnose a pyloric stenosis. The child died three hours later. Postmortem revealed small quantities of bismuth in the liver and in the blood.

Professor Hefter suggested that the death might have been caused by nitrate poisoning as nitrites were found in the blood and pericardial fluids. Bismuth could not be found in the liver or blood. These findings prompted Dr. Bohme (12) to determine the true cause of bismuth subnitrate poisoning. His results were as follows: A number of pure cultuers of the

bacterium coli were found to liberate nitrites in every case when applied to bouillon to which some bismuth subnitrate was added. The controls of bouillon treated the same way but without the addition of bismuth remained free from nitrites.

Collishon (13) reports two cases of accidental nitrite poisoning in which sodium nitrite instead of sodium nitrate was given. The symptoms were cyanosis, extreme weakness, and a grayish-blue discoloration of the mucous membrane and the tongue. The symptoms were so severe as to produce collapse but cleared up after the drug was discontinued. Binz (14) injected a dog with a small dose of nitrite causing death in a few hours with symptoms of gastroenteritis.

Harnack (15) killed a cat in five minutes by administering five grammes of sodium nitrite.

The blood in all these cases presented a condition of methaemaglobinaemia which appears to be a factor in producing the cyanosis, dyspnoea, diarrhoea and cramps. As the sudden change in the blood impairs the internal or tissue respiration and the patient dies with symptoms of suffocation.

The injecting of large cavities with bismuth-vaseline paste in which a large part of the bismuth subnitrate is retained, the question naturally arises: what becomes of the bismuth? In many instances as the cavity itself closes, the bismuth is forced out, but in many other instances it becomes encapsulated and absorbed. This has been demonstrated by taking radiographs at frequent intervals. Harnack (16) states that bismuth subnitrate is slowly absorbed and slowly eliminated. Bergeret (17) and Wood (18) detected bismuth in the urine after its administration also proving that it is absorbed and eliminated very slowly.

The reports of these cases by men of advanced professional standing, signals a note of warning in the indiscriminate use of bismuth especially in extreme doses. I have given from 30 to 50 grms. of bismuth subnitrate for a prolonged period of time without noticing any toxic symptoms.

In the Beck clinic in Chicago over 2,000 bismuth paste injections have been given, some as much as 300 grms, without encountering a true case of poisoning. He suggests, however, that not more than 100 grms. be given at the first injection which can then be subsequently increased, when the resistance of the patient has been observed.

When occasion demands the administration of large doses of bismuth subnitrate, either by mouth or injection of sinuses or abscess cavities, I would advise that the urine be examined frequently for casts, and the blood tested for haemaglobin, and if any toxic symptoms appear, discontinue its administration. When symptoms of poisoning do occur, it is best to remove the bismuth paste and for this purpose Dr. Beck has contrived a special suction apparatus. This is accomplished much easier by injecting into the cavity some sterile olive oil.

Since writing this paper, two cases of bismuth poisoning with one fatality following injection of bismuth-vaseline paste have been reported by David and Kauffman (19). The symptoms were those produced solely by the bismuth constituent of the subnitrate, no nitrite symptoms such as syanosis, dyspnoea, etc., being observed.

Case 1. Patient, W. E., an American, aged 24, single, bookkeeper, entered Cook County Hospital Aug. 31, 1908, on Dr. Ryerson's service. He gave a history of discharging sinuses about the left hip, which had existed since an injury twenty-one years previously. Examination showed an ankylosed hip with healed and discharging sinuses anteriorly and posteriorly. A clinical diagnosis of tuberculous hip was made.

Bismuth Treatment.—On September 8. three ounces of 33 1-3 per cent bismuth

vaseline paste was injected into the sinus on the posterior aspect of the hip. On September 28, a second injection of about six ounces of bismuth paste caused considerable immediate pain to the patient.

Effects of Bismuth.—Pain continued through the night so severe that the patient got scarcely any sleep. On the next day the temperature, which had been normal, rose to 101° F., but returned to 98° in the course of forty-eight hours. The sinus remained open and discharged some pus and small amounts of bismuth paste. Eleven days after the second injection the patient complained, on awakening, of pain in the mouth. From this time on an intense stomatitis rapidly developed. Pain and burning were very severe, and increased so much on attempted mastication and deglutition that the patient took very little of even liquid diet. The gums were swollen and extremely sore. The teeth became loose. A gradually widening, heavy greenish-blue line showed on the gums and on the tip and margins of the tongue. On the left side of the tongue small superficial ulcers apperaed, which increased and coalesced until larger than the thumb-nail; the ulcer was covered with a dirty blue black membrane. The fauces and throat showed the same swollen and pigmented condition. Salivation was constant, intense, and very distressing. Accompanying the stomatitis was some headache and a very marked constipation. The general condition remained fairly good with normal temperature, running to 99° F., only occasionally.

After reaching its height the stomatitis gradually subsided so that at the end of six weeks the ulcerations and salivation had entirely disappeared and the patient was again on regular diet.

The patient complained of continued pain in the hip. An X-ray examination showed deposits of bismuth about the joint and a small necrotic focus in the great trochanter, which was removed by operation on December 7. An abscess which formed in the thigh six days after the operation but which had no demonstrable connection with the operative wound, was aspirated twice under 2 per cent cocain and and finally freely incised. Large amounts of bloody pus and later masses of reddish discolored paste was discharged.

On Dec. 21, several days after cocain had been used, the patient, who previously had been quiet, and well-mannered, became suddenly rather noisy, restless, and unable to sleep. During the day he was irritable, ugly, abusive to the nurse, and at times irrational. He also became negligent about his person, showing a complete change in his temperament.

At present, five months after the first injection of bismuth paste, the patient's general condition is much improved: the sinus is closed; the abscess nearly healed, and mental condition almost normal. The bluish deposit still remains on the gums in a deep blue line a little more than an eighth of an inch in width, extending to the very margin of the gums. Both the labial and lingual surfaces of the lower jaw are involved; more than those of the upper. Points of teeth contact on lips show blue canines. The tongue-lip and lateral margins extending to the under surface show areas of bluish discoloration solid to first glance, but made up of punctate spots of bluish deposit slightly larger than a pin-point.

At no time was there any palpitation, dyspnoea, cyanosis or dizziness.

Case 2. Patient, H. F., well-nourished white man, 21 years old, freight handler, entered Cook County Hospital on the service of Drs. Kahlke and Keyes, Dec. 31, 1908, complaining of lameness and presenting a sinus above inner third of right Poupart's ligament. The clinical diagnosis of a tuberculous hip was made with some difficulty; but a skiagraph revealed an irregular area on the head of the femur. The patient's temperature varied from 98.6° to 103° for a few days after admission, depending somewhat on amount of pus discharged. Pulse was 80 to 90; respiration, 20.

Bismuth Treatment.—Six ounces of a 33 1-3 per cent bismuth-vaseline paste were injected into the sinus on Jan. 19, 1909; a skiagraph taken on the same day showed the bismuth shadow leading to the diseased head of the femur.

Effects of Bismuth.—Ten days after the injection the patient complained of soreness of his gums and an increased flow of saliva. An examination of the mouth revealed a light greenish-blue discoloration of the gums, linear in character, about one-sixteenth of an inch from the incisor teeth on the lower jaw. The line was composed of pin-point puncta at first, but later became solid. There was increased flow of saliva at this time and subjectively, some nausea and anorexia. The next two days saw a further progress of the stomatitis. The blue line extended over the gums of the lower jaw, involving both the lingual and labial surfaces and remaining a little way from the margin of the teeth and gums. There was also on the lower lip opposite the incisors and especially on the lateral edges of the tongue a distinct blue discoloration of the mucosa, which seemed to follow the configuration of the teeth contiguous to them. At this period the salivation was extreme, the patient lying with his head over the edge of the bed drooling and groaning. His breath was becoming foul and he was taking no diet but liquids and this only when forced on him. His temperature was 98.6° to 99.6°; pulse 80 to 96; respiration, 20. He had some headache and nausea, but no dyspnoea, tinnitus aurium, palpitation, or syanosis of mucous membranes, ears, nose or finger-tips. On Feb. 2, the patient was nauseated and vomited several times. There was then some superficial ulceration on the lateral surfaces of the tongue and labial mucosa. The blue line had become darker, a grayish-blue. There were a few erythemic blotches on neck and face. The patient was restless and did not sleep; took diet with difficulty.

In the following week the stomatitis increased greatly in severity and the general condition of the patient for the first time was bad. The tongue was swollen, about

peared on the fauces and right tonsil. The lower lip and face were edematous and salivation was marked. There was some tenderness over the parotid glands but no swelling; moderate cervical adenitis. The patient complained of pain in the mouth and great weakness. Speech was difficult. He groaned constantly; was becoming very emaciated, had no appetite, and was constantly nauseated. He had slight epistaxis once. His breath was putrid. The pulse

Fig. 1.—Metal syringe for use in injecting bismuth paste into the ear, nose and throat.

Tip A.—A silver canula that can be bent to suit each individual case and is used in the injections of the various sinuses after their openings have been made accessible.

Tip B.—A finer silver canula, which is used for injection into the regions of the nasofrontal duct, sphenoidal sinus region, and the upper, narrowest portions of the nasal cavity; that is, before any operation is done; also into the tonsillar crypts, supratonsillar fossae, and into the incised peritonsillar abscess cavity.

Tip C.—Olive-shaped tip for injecting ear paste into the perforations and beyond, even through the tube into nasopharynx.

Tip D.—Fits into a Eustachian catheter; used for injecting tube and middle ear by the nasopharyngeal route. Also used to fill the cavity of the mastoid process after the simple operation.

Tip E.—Eustachian catheter with large bull-ons end.

Tip F.—Very fine canula for injecting tear ducts and fine fistulas.

Collapsible Tube G.—For the patient's own use for home treatment. While the result from its use will be insignificant, because not all the parts can be reached, it is convenient and necessary in some cases. The conical tip is introduced either into the nasal vestibule or external auditory meatus, and the paste expressed.

Glass Syringe H.—The same that is used for general surgical work; is practically for the use of the paste in injecting the general nasal cavity, and also the ear after the sinuses, as well as the middle ear have been filled by the metal syringe. After the various operations on the turbinates and septum, this syringe is used with good effect; in other words, for general application, as the dressing for the nose and ear.

twice the normal size, and showed marked areas of necrosis on the lateral surfaces, corresponding to the teeth imprint, with central gray sloughing area and blue margins. The labial mucosa on lower lip became much pigmented, with irregular areas of superficial necrosis. The gums showed necrosis at the junction of the teeth, and the blue line was darker. Blue pigmentation and irregular superficial ulceration appeared

was weak, 100 to 120; heart, lungs, abdomen negative; 99° to 100°; respiration, 20 to 24.

From this time on the general condition of the patient became progressively worse. Nervous symptoms, as marked restlessness, choreiform movements and insomnia developed. Involuntary defacation and urination supervened. The patient's mentality gradually became less acute and for two days before his death he was constantly ir-rational and in continuous motion. Decubitus sore developed on the sacrum and over the hip in spite of every precaution. At the time of his death, twenty-seven days after the injection of the paste and seventeen days from the date of the first toxic symptoms, his tongue was almost twice the normal size and its lateral surfaces was the seat of ragged dirty blue areas of necrosis which were also present on the lower lip and on almost the entire inner surface of the cheek which came in contact with the teeth. The fauces and tonsils were partially covered with blue pigmentation. The gums of the lower jaw were soggy and ulcerated but still showed the almost black line. The upper jaw, except on the lingual surface, was not affected at any time to the same extent as the lower jaw. Salivation had ceased. The breath was very foul. The face and lips were swollen. The patient's body was markedly emaciated. Temperature was 104° F., just prior to death, but until a few hours before death had been almost constantly 99° to 100°; respirations, 24 to 26, and pulse 120.

CONCLUSIONS.

1—The administration of bismuth subnitrate either by mouth or injection into abscess cavities in small doses is harmless.

2.—After the injection of large quantities of the bismuth paste into abscess cavities, symptoms of nitrite poisoning may appear.

3.—The symptoms produced by nitrite poisoning are cyanosis, collapse, methaemoglobinaemia and may terminate fatally.

4.—Bismuth subnitrate given internally

or used as injections is absorbed very slowly and as slowly eliminated.

5.—The injection of bismuth-vaseline paste into tubercular sinuses and abscess cavities, with the proper technique, has proven the best treatment for these conditions.

6.—Children are more susceptible to nitrate poisoning than adults.

7.—The prolonged use of bismuth subnitrate is very apt to cause nephritis, gingivitis, ulcerations of mucous membranes and diarrhoea.

8.—That we need to employ some other preparation of bismuth than the nitrate.

1. Beck—Journal A. M. A., Vol. L, No. 2, p. 868.
2. Beck, Joseph C.—Journal A. M. A., Vol. LII, p. 117.
3. Schuler—Zeitschrift fur Chirugie, 1885.
4. Von Vardeleben—Deutsche medizinische Wochenschrift, 1901, No. 23, p. 544.
5. Muhlig—Munchener medizinische Wochenschrift, 1901, No. 15, p. 592.
6. Theodore Kocher—Volkmann's Klinische Vortrage, 1882, p. 224.
7. Petersen—Deutsche medizinische Woghenschrift, June 20, 1883.
8. Muhlig—Munchener medizinische Wochenschrift, 1901, No. 15, p. 592.
9. Dressman—Munchener medizinische Wochenschrift, 1901, No. 6, p. 238.
10. Davis—University of Pennsylvania, Medical Bulletin, 1906.
11. Hoffman—Munchener medizinische Wochenschrift, 1906, No. 19.
12. Bohme—Archiv fur experimentelle Pathologie und Pharmakologie, p. 441, 1907.
13. Collishon—Deutsche medizinische Wochenschrift, No. 41, 1889.
14. Binz—Archiv fur experimentelle Pathologie und Pharmakologie, XIII.
15. Harnack—Ibid, 1908, p. 246.
16. Harnack—Arzneilchre, 1883, p. 883.
17. Bergret—Journal de l'anatomie, L873, p. 242.
18. Wood—Transactions of the American Neurological Association, 1883, p 23.
19. David and Kauffman—Journal A. M. A., Vol. No. 13, p. 1035.

THE ETIOLOGY, PATHOLOGY AND THEORIES OF GLAUCOMA

BY DR. EDWARD F. DAVIS, OKLAHOMA CITY, OKLAHOMA

(*Read before Seventeenth Annual Meeting Oklahoma State Medical Association, May, 1909.*)

In primary glaucoma, the immediate local cause is a compression or other occlusion of the angle of filtration, brought on by a combination of predisposing and exciting causes.

Among the predisposing causes, come first, perhaps, age as glaucoma is distinctly a disease of advanced life. This may be explained, in part, by the fact that while the eye reaches its full development in size and capacity early, the lens continue to grow slowly and as it increases in size, the fibres of the zonule of zinn become relaxed. The lens is thus held less securely in position and it may easily be forced against the iris and encroach on the space of the anterior chamber in the case of any disturbance which might cause a rise of pressure from behind.

The majority of glaucomatous eyes are hyperopic and on account of the excessive effort required to see, there is an unusual development of the ciliary body. Hyperopic eyes are small as a rule but as this does not involve a reduction in the size of the lens, the circumlental space through which lymph must flow in passing from the vitreous to the aqueous chamber, is narrowed. In case of an increased secretion in the vitreous chamber, there is a damming back on account of the restricted circumlental space and the tension in this chamber rises, forcing the lens forward with the iris and producing a shallowness of the anterior chamber.

Owing to a compensatory out-flow through the canal of Schlemm, and the crypts of the iris, there is no general increase of tension at this time but a strong predisposing cause is present and a sudden obstruction to the excretion through swelling of the iris on account of venous stasis or infiltration, will bring on an acute attack.

Race has little influence on the liability to glaucoma although the idea that Jews are particularly prone to it, has long been almost a classic.

Probably there may be some hereditary predisposition.

Glaucoma occurs more commonly in women than in men on account of the circulatory disturbances connected with the generative system.

The exciting causse are those conditions which produce a congestion of the vascular system; sudden emotional excitement, fatigue, loss of sleep, exposure to wet and cold, hunger, heart weakness, fits of coughing or sneezing, chronic constipation, etc.

The cause of secondary glaucoma are less obscure than are those of the primary form, although the production of the increase of tension is the same in either case in that there is a lack of equilibrium between the secretion and the excretion within the eye.

Annular posterior, synechia, resulting from iritis, with exclusion of the pupil, by checking the flow from the posterior to the anterior chamber, causes the iris to be forced backward against the cornea and abolishes the filtration angle.

A total synechia between the iris and lens may have the same result but in this case, the lens also is forced forward.

In serous cyclitis, there is an alteration in the composition of the fluid secreted by the ciliary processes in that the albuminous elements are increased. This comparatively thick fluid can not escape freely through the iris crypts or through the pectinate ligament into Schlemm's canal and it collects in the anterior chamber, gradually forcing the lens and adherent iris backward, deepening the anterior chamber. With the exception of the increase in depth of the anterior chamber, the conditions are the same as those in glaucoma from other causes.

Annular synechia between the iris and cornea from perforation of the latter, show no special results in this connection so long as the wound remains open but on closure, the escape of the aqueous is shut off through adhesions.

An increase of tension may result from any form of cataract operation, either with or without preliminary iridectomy. In this case there may be some incarceration of the iris or the capsule of the lens in the wound closing the angle, the pupil may be closed through inflammatory exudates or the hyaloid membrane may be adherent to the scar. To acertain extent, this condition is present in all cases but fortunately it is in only a small percentage that the involvement of the angle is of sufficient extent to materially alter the excretory process.

Simple wounds and confusions of the lens and the needling operation may increase the tension through swelling of the lens and consequent pressure of the iris against the cornea or incarceration of some of the lens fragments in the channels of excretion.

The lens may be dislocated and wedged in between the ciliary body and the vitreous.

Intra-ocula tumors will eventually set up a glaucomatous state. In sarcoma of the choroid, pressure on the choroidal vessels, causes an exudation of serum which detaches the retina forcing it forward into the vitreous. The tension is not increased at first, for as the vitreous chamber is encroached upon, there is a transudation of its fluid through the hyaloid membrane into the posterior and anterior chambers and out of the eye until the retina is completely detached and is forced against the hyaloid membrane and further filtration is impossible. Then it is that the lens and iris are pressed forward into the angle of the anterior chamber.

Glioma of the retina brings about much the same condition.

Tumors of the iris should be mentioned also.

PATHOLOGY.

The most important pathological changes are those of the uveal tract. In recent cases, there is an infiltration and swelling of the iris, the veins are congested and there may be many extravasations of blood. The ciliary processes are particularly swollen and press the iris against the posterior surface of the cornea where it soon becomes agglutinated.

There is a great infiltration of the pectinate ligament by pigment from the pigment cells of the iris and ciliary body. In case there is an anterior peripheral synechia it is pigmented also. This region later loses the pigment on account of its being carried by the leucocytes into the general circulation and into the anterior surface of the iris. According to Levinsohn, this alteration in the pigment epithelium is due to the hypertrophy of Mueller's muscle and the ciliary processes by pressure and possibly by a certain trophic influence. This hypertrophy may produce a dislocation of the saggital edge of the ciliary body and the root of the iris and in this way produce a shallowness of the anterior chamber.

After the high pressure has continued for a time, there is an atrophy of the smooth fibres of Mueller's muscle and the sphincter, but Brucke's muscle and the dilator of the pupil seem particularly resistant and may even undergo a permanent hypertrophy which accounts for the obstinate dilation of the pupil. The ciliary processes share in this atrophy, their secretion ceases, the tension becomes reduced and the eye shrinks. The retinal pigment layer is especially resistant but with the exception of this and the hypertrophy of the dilator and Brucke's muscle, there is a general atrophy of the whole uveal tract. The iris becomes thinner and narrower and its vessels almost entirely disappear as have the fibres of the sphincter and there is little of its former structure left but the retinal pigment layer. The pectinate ligament becomes fibrous and Schlemm's canal disappears.

In the choroid, the vessels have disappeared, particularly in the regions of the points where the vasa vortocosa pass into the sclera and in the papilla. The choroid becomes firmly attached to the sclera which is thinned and bulges outward. There may be a total obliteration of the lumen of the vasa vorticosa. At the papilla, the layers of the lamina cribrosa are compressed and it is displaced backward until it may lie beyond the outer surface of the sclera and have overhanging edges.

Aside from the pressure atrophy of the optic nerve, there may be an atrophy of the trunk also in which the nerve fibres have given way to the increase of the connective tissue of the trabeculae.

THEORIES.

Many theories regarding glaucoma have been advanced only to be found faulty and discarded.

Intra-ocular pressure is dependent on the rigidity of the envelope of the eye and the volume of its contents. The volume of the contents is determined by the relation between secretion and excretion. As the cornea and sclera are very resistant to pressure, an increase of secretion is physiologically disposed of by an increase of excretion on account of the impossibility of any increase in the volume within the eye. The increase of tension is, therefore, due to an interference with excretion only. The chief channel of excretion is through the pectinate ligament and it is here that the obstruction must be-expected.

The onset of an acute attack of glaucoma is due primarily to a stasis of blood in the general circulation. This manifests itself in the eye, principally in a swelling of the ciliary processes, which is the case of a naturally predisposed eye, compress the angle of filtration. In addition to this, the circumlental space in encroached upon and the lens is pushed forward aggravating the condition.

A sudden dilation of the pupil, in an eye with a shallow anterior chamber, by producing a thickening of the iris, may block the angle. If the swelling of the ciliary processes and increased thickness of the iris is transient, it is possible that on their restoration to their normal condition, the angle may be opened again and the pressure fall, but-when the iris has been in contact with the cornea for any considerable time, an agglutination takes place and the tension will remain permanently elevated.

EMBOLI, WITH REPORT OF A CASE

BY DR. THOMAS H. FLESHER, EDMOND, OKLAHOMA.

Read Before the Seventeenth Annual Meeting Oklahoma State Medical Association, May, 1909.

Mr. President and Gentlemen of the Oklahoma State Medical Association:

It is not my purpose to attempt bringing out anything new regarding the pathology, symptoms, diagnosis and treatment of this subject, but more particularly to report that came under my observation a few months ago.

An embolus may be defined as any body transported by the circulating blood and capable by its physical characteristics of obstructing the flow of blood in any part of the vascular system. Oil and air, though not solid bodies, may be impacted within the capillaries and hence may constitute emboli. The transportation and lodgment of these bodies with the resulting changes constitute embolism.

The composition of emboli varies; they may be composed (1) detached thrombi, (2) fragments of cardiac valves or endocardial vegetations, (3) calcareous plates, (4) fragments of morbid growths torn from tumor masses and penetrating the blood-vessel walls,)5) purely extraneous bodies, such as bubbles of air and pieces of bone from fracture, (6) certain parasites, as echinococcus, filiaria, etc. They may be spoken of as arterial, venous and capillary, however, the most important classification is (a) simple, (b) infective. The former being aseptic, the latter containing bacteriae.

The functional importance of the tissue involved scarcely merits more than mere mention, thus it will be evident that a small embolus involving cutaneous, subcutaneous or allied structures may induce so little change as to escape detection, while an embolus of the same size involving the coronary or pulmonary artery or a cerebral area might produce instantaneous death. The possibility of at once establishing collateral circulation to supply nutrition to the area determines to a large extent the subsequent changes. With the sudden stoppage of the circulation the distal portion of the artery empties itself of blood and an area of ischemia is thereby induced; the sudden and persistent diminution in the intra capillary pressure favors the influx of blood from adjacent capillaries whose blood is directed in the line of least resistance, coincident with the changes just mentioned, dialation of the anastomasing or collateral arteries occurs, increasing the amount of blood traveling through those vessels. When the anastomosis between the artery involved and the artery whose circulation still remains intact is sufficiently free, there is quickly formed a circulation adequate to maintain nutrition in the previous ischemic area. In the absence of sufficient collateral circulation, degeneration or necrotic processes occur; especially liable to this condition being certain brain areas a portion of kidney, and spleen, the nutrition being derived from terminal arteries. The area beyond the plugging of a blood-vessel is called an infarct and is usually wedge-shaped but may be modified by a collateral circulation.

If the area is very large the center may undergo fatty degeneration, as found in cerebral softening, or it may be converted into a cyst. Repair not uncommonly takes place if the area is small. An infarct is very liable to infection while undergoing necrosis owing to the lessened resistance offered by the tissues and not infrequently a simple may be converted into an infected embolus and such diseases as pyaemia and general tuberculosis may be disseminated in this way. Amebic abscesses in the liver are most probably brought from intestinal legions through the portal circulation. Thus it may be seen that from parasitic, neoplastic and infected. emboli, secondary thrombi may form and again emboli may become detached and continue the process of dissemination.

The symptoms, diagnosis, prognosis, etiology, pathology and treatment may be determined by the area involved and the character of the embolus.

Report of the Case: I was called in consultation with Dr. M., December 6, 1908, to see Mrs. A., aged 21. Previous health good, mother of one child, aged 18 months, and healthy. Patient was about three months pregnant and as her previous labor was severe with instrumental delivery, she decided at the solicitation of her friends to try a friend's "cure-all" for such troubles and had her husband procure a soft rubber catheter, which was introduced into the uterus by herself in the erect posture. Her husband attempted to blow some quinine through the catheter into the womb. No sooner had he given the first blow she fell to the floor and lapsed into unconsciousness and died about fifteen hours later.

On physical examination no hemmorrhage was present either internally or intraperitoneal. Lungs showed passive congestion, heart action rapid, 160 to 180 per minute with a general cyanotic condition. Diagnosis was an air embolus as the priamry cause of death, gaining entrance by way of the uterine sinus and carried to the right side of heart, producing a thrombus or going still farther by way of the pulmonary artery to the lungs and producing oedema of the lungs.

The treatment was strychina, atropine, heat, foot of bed elevated and general supportive treatment.

I would be glad to hear if any other physicians present have had a similar case and if they agree on the diagnosis.

THE TREATMENT OF FRACTURE OF THE CLAVICLE

BY LEIGH F. WATSON, M. D., OKLAHOMA CITY

The large number of dressings that have been suggested for the treatment of fracture of the clavicle proves conclusively that no one method is applicable to all cases.

Gurlt says there have been about seventy dressings devised for drawing the shoulder upward, outward and backward.

Pilcher has remarked, the fact remains that those methods that are efficient are intolerable and those that are tolerable are inefficient.

Sayre's (15) is the most popular dressing; others frequently used are Moore's (14), Velpeau's, Desault's and the Hippocrates position where it is especially desired to minimize deformity in women.

A plaster paris splint is used by O'Connor (1) and Stimson.

Curtis (2) used a wooden crutch fastened to a belt extension bar with a set screw, the belt is supported by a strap over the shoulder.

Harris (3) and Pick used a four tailed bandage.

Henson (4) used a shoulder cap over shoulder, elbow and forearm of affected side, over this Sayre's modification of Velpeau dressing.

Birdsall (5) used a Moore's dressing, over this is put an elastic bandage around elbow and over affected shoulder.

Botkin (6) used a leather or binders' board splint to fractured side and over this a bandage.

Colomb (7) used a bandage 2½ in. wide and 3 yards long; start at hand then under affected forearm around elbow and up over forearm and sound shoulder, then around neck and down in front on opposite side and fasten to starting point.

Russ (8) used a plaster paris dressing over front of chest extending just above and below clavicles, a pair of suspenders are secured in the plaster and buckled behind.

The arm of injured side is supported by a figure of eight cravat.

King (9) used two strips of adhesive plaster, the first strip beginning at inferior and of scapula up behind and over affected shoulder, then down in front under axilla and transversely across back around body to midsternal line.

The second strip begins at free border of ribs anteriorly and runs up over tilted end of inner fragment then down back to several inches below the scapula, a Velpeau bandage is worn for two weeks.

Manning (10) used a shoulder and elbow cap with Sayre dressing.

Underwood (11) used a padded collar around each shoulder fastened and tightened by adhesive straps behind.

Kinnaman (12) used a bone peg.

Johnson (13) used catgut sutures, Langenbeck wire sutures and Roberts nails the broken ends.

The barrel-hoop splint as suggested by Dr. Spohn of Corpus Christi, Texas, I believe to be the best dressing that has been devised for the treatment of these fractures in children and in selected cases it is applicable to adults.

.Its advantages over other methods are: Simplicity, ease of application, no discomfort to patient, no detention from light work nor from school in the case of children, no possibility of shoulder or elbow joint adhesion as an after result.

Case 1.—Fred W., aged 10, was struck by a street car on June 4, 1908, and sustained a complete oblique fracture of the middle third of the left clavicle.

He was admited to the New York Polyclinic hospital and treated in the service of Dr. John A. Bodine.

A splint was made from a wooden barrel-hoop long enough for the ends to fit snugly into the infraclavicular fossa while the shoulders are drawn upward, backward and outward.

A short piece of the hoop was fastened to the inner surface of each extremity of the splint. (Fig. 1.)

The nails were left projecting to prevent the bandage slipping.

This extra piece made immobilization firmer and allowed free movement of the chest in breathing.

The ends of the splint were then padded with cotton and a cotton pad placed in each axilla to prevent chafing.

While the assistant held the shoulders upward, backward and outward the fractured ends were approximated and the splint applied and firmly secured by a figure-of-eight bandage. (Fig. 2-3.)

Long strips of adhesive plaster were applied over the bandage to prevent loosening from slipping and stretching.

The patient had no pain at seat of fracture while wearing the splint, and used the arm of the affected side as freely as the other.

Union was prompt and without deformity.

Case 2.—Verde B., aged 20, teamster,

while driving over a railroad crossing he was struck by a locomotive.

Besides an extensive scalp wound he sustained a complete fracture of the middle third of the right clavicle.

He was treated in the service of Dr. J. B. Rolater and the barrel-hoop splint was made of double thickness and applied in a similar manner to case 1. (Fig. 4.)

Recovery was without pain or deformity.

Bodine (16) has recently reported several cases successfully treated with the barrel-hoop splint.

BIBLIOGRAPHY:

1.   O'Connor—British Medical Journal, 1883, I, 406.
2.   Curtis—Medical Record, N. Y., 1890, XXXVIII, 491.
3.   Harris—Chicago Medical Recorder, 1896, XI, 147.
4.   Henson—Maryland Medical Journal, 1897-8, XXXVIII, 453.
5.   Birdsall—Internat. Journal Surgery, N. Y., 1898, XI, 169.
6.   Botkin—Medical Sentinel, Portland, Ore., 1904, XII, 223.
7.   Colomb—N. O. Medical and Surgical Journal, 1905, LXIII, 509.
8.   Russ—J. A. M. A., 1905, XLV, 1084.
9.   King—St. Paul Medical Journal, 1906, VIII, 82.
10.   Manning—Practitioner, London, 1906, LXXVIII, 301.
11.   Underwood—International Journal Surgery, N. Y., 1906, XIX, 268.
12.   Kinnaman—Medical Record, N. Y., 1892, XLII, 214.
13.   Johnson—Annals of Surgery, Phila., 1903, XXXVIII, 99.
14.   Moore—Buffalo Medical and Surgical Journal, 1888-9, XXVIII, 363.
15.   Sayre—Archives of Pediatrics, N. Y., 1898, X, 215.
16.   Bodine—N. Y. Polyclinic Journal, Nov. 1908.

ABSTRACT OF PROCEEDINGS OF THE MEDICAL ASSOCIATION OF THE SOUTHWEST, MEETING AT SAN ANTONIO, TEXAS, NOVEMBER 9, 10 and 11, 1909.

Meeting of Executive Committee with Drs. Jabez N. Jackson, E. H. Martin, C. W. Fassett, J. D. Griffith and F. H. Clark present. Dr. Jabez N. Jackson, President, was invited to read a paper on Membranous Pericolitis in place of the address on surgery by Dr. M. L. Harris of Chicago who was absent. A committee composed of Dr. J. D. Griffith and E. H. Martin was appointed to audit the books of the Secretary-Treasurer.

2:30 P. M.

Call to order by Dr. G. H. Moody, Chairman, Committee on Arrangements.

Adderss by Honorable Bryan Callahan, Mayor of San Antonio.

Address of Welcome Dr. W. B. Russ, San Antonio.

Address for the District Association, Dr. W. A. King.

Address for the Bexar County Society, Dr. T. Y. Hall.

Dr. J. N. Jackson in the Chair called upon Dr. C. Lester Hall, Kansas City, to respond to the addresses of welcome.

Paper—The Need of Medical Inspection in the Public Schools, by Dr. F. D. Boyd—Chairman of the Section on Diseases of the eye, ear, nose and throat.

Dr. E. H. Martin in the Chair, Section on Surgery.

Paper—Some Observations on the After Treatment of Abdominal Section, Dr. Claude Thompson, Muskogee, Oklahoma.

Paper—Abdominal Operations and after Care, Dr. C. Howard Hill, Kansas City.

Paper—The Value of Surgical Celerity, Dr. Chas. Blickensderfer, Shawnee, Okla.

The three papers were discussed by Drs. Griffith, Kansas City, Paschal, San Antonio, Keiller, Galveston, Pettue, Eldorado, (Ark.,) Still, Brownwood, Tex., J. N. Jackson, Kansas City, C. Lester Hall, Kansas City and Wolf, San Antonio, Discussion closed By Drs. Thompson, Hill and Blickensderfer.

Paper—Damage done the Child by Adenoid Growths, Dr. J. H. Barnes, Enid, Okla.

Discussed by Drs. J. F. Gsell, Wichita, G. W. Maser, Parsons, J. N. Jackson, Kansas City, Boardman, Parsons, E. H. Martin, Hot Springs, Keiller, Galveston, and F. D. Boyd, Ft. Worth, Discussion closed by Dr. Barnes.

State Delegations selected the following nominating committees:

Oklahoma—D. A. Myers, E. S. Lain, A. W. White, H. C. Todd, C. A. Thompson.

Missouri—C. W. Fassett, R. H. Barnes, Wm. Frick, Robt. L. Neff, C. L. Hall.

Arkansas—J. T. Henry, E. H. Martin, J. A. Foltz, C. S. Pettus, A. J. Vance.

Kansas—C. E. Bowers, G. W. Maser, E. W. Boardman, C. C. Nesselrode, S. S. Glasscock.

Texas—F. D. Boyd, E. H. Carey, M. L. Graves, J. S. Turner.

8:30 P. M. Elks Hall:

Dr. Joe Becton, Greenville, introduced the President Dr. J. N. Jackson who delivered an address on Membranous Pericolitis, illustrating the same with pathologic specimen. The address received marked attention.

International Club Rooms, 8:30 A. M.

Report of the Secretary received. The Secretary called attention to the objects of the Association which he stated were purely those in keeping with the advancement of medical and surgical science in the southwest. One invitation and sometimes two are sent annually to each member of the State Associations comprising the parent body to unite with the Association of the Southwest.

A membership of 491 in good standing was reported.

November 11, 8:30 A. M.

The nominating Committee through the Chairman Dr. S. S. Glasscock reported the following nominations for officers for the ensuing which report was adopted and the officers declared duly elected:

President—Dr. G. H. Moody, San Antonio.

Vice-Presidents—Missouri, Howard Hill.—Kansas, G. W. Maser, Parsons.—Oklahoma, D. A. Myers, Lawton.—Arkansas, A. J. Vance, Harrison.

Secretary-Treasurer—F. H. Clark, El Reno, Oklahoma.

Wichita, Kansas, was chosen as a meeting place for 1910.

Resolution of thanks to the citizens of San Antonio and to the Press of the city was introduced by Dr. A. L. Blesh, Oklahoma City, carried. Drs. E. H. Martin, Hot Springs, Ark., J. D. Griffith and S. S. Glasscock, Kansas City, were appointed to visit the next annual meetings of the State Medical Associations of Louisiana and Colorado and invite those states to affiliate with the Medical Association of the Southwest.

Dr. J. A. Foltz, Ft. Smith, Ark., introduced the following resolution:

"Resolved that it is the sense of the Executive Committee of the Medical Association of the Southwest to frown down upon and to do all in its power to prevent the publication of the scientific papers of the Association in Journals which advertise flagrant nostrums which make claims so as to be a disgrace to our profession if in any way we should associate with them or countenance them." The resolution was discussed and adopted.

Meeting adjourned.

The following Oklahoma Physicians were in attendance: Drs. A. L. Blesh, Oklahoma City, W. E. Dicken, Oklahoma City, E. H. Troy, McAlester, B. J. Vance, Checotah, E. S. Lain, Oklahoma City, H. C. Todd, Oklahoma City, A. W. White, Oklahoma City, D. A. Myers, Lawton, F. H. Clark, El Reno, C. F. Woodring, Bartlesville, Chas. Blickensderfer, Shawnee, J. H. Barnes, Enid, A. K. West, Oklahoma City, C. A. Thompson, Muskogee.

EDITORIAL

ANIMAL EXPERIMENTATION.

The activity of the Council on Defense of Medical Research of the American Medical Association is strongly attested by the recent issuance of several publications—rather briefs or arguments on the questions involved, which cover in a complete manner all points at issue between the regular medical profession and the rampant cranks comprising the Anti-Vivisectionist Associations.

The following comprises a list of the agruments presented by the various authorities who have undertaken the work and each member of the profession in Oklahoma should procure copies of the work, by request from the American Medical Association, in order to thoroughly familiarize himself with the matter for future use if ever needed in this state.

The articles are thorough, exact, scientific and worthy of a place in the files of your office.

Animal Experimentation and Cancer, Dr. James Ewing, New York.

The Ethics of Animal Experimentation, Dr. James R. Angell, Chicago.

The Role of Animal Experimentation in the Diagnosis of Disease, Dr. M. J. Rosenau, Washington.

Animal Experimentation and Tuberculosis, Dr. E. L. Trudeau, Saranac Lake, N. Y.

Vaccination and its Relation to Animal Experimentation, Dr. Jay Frank Schamberg, Philadelphia.

PREPARING FOR THE ANNUAL MEETING AT TULSA IN MAY.

The Tulsa County Medical Society has already begun preparations for the entertainment of the Annual Meeting which is to occur in their city May 10th, 11th and 12th, 1910.

An Executive Committee, to have exclusive control of all matters pertaining to the meeting, consisting of Drs. C. L. Reeder, F. S. Clinton, W. E. Wright and Ross Grosshart, was appointed and Dr. Wright was named as permanent Secretary of the Committee.

Any one desiring any information about this meeting will do well to communicate with Dr. Wright who will cheerfully assist them in whatever way he can.

A KNOWLEDGE OF REFRACTION.

The letter published below is given for the purpose of calling the attention of the profession of the State to a matter that has long needed remedying at its hands and the hands of the State Board of Examiners. The custom of itinerant peddlers, traveling quacks and other persons of poor ability or none at all, who go about the state making one day stands and promiscuously fitting glasses or pretending to fit them should come to an end.

These conditions especially prevail in the smaller towns and localities far from the reach of the specialist and naturally the class of people affected are of the poorer and ignorant class as a rule and it is for this class that medical legislation and rules are peculiarly beneficial, in that they protect him from his own gullibility.

A person having anything to do with the live human being should be required to show evidence to the State Board of Medical Examiners of his fitness and the suggestion embodied in the letter that the Board of Examiners incorporate a rule requiring knowledge of refraction as one of the tests of registration is a good one and it is to be hoped will be adopted at some future date.

Nov. 13, 1909.

Dear Doctor:

At the late meeting of the Ophthalmic Section, A. M. A. (eleven hundred members,) the undersigned were appointed a Committee to promote *a working knowledge of simple refraction* among family physicians.

It has secured abundant evidence that such knowledge has been acquired and is now used by many physicians, so proving that all medical men can do likewise, if they so desire.

But that the practice may become uniform, it is necessary that the State Board of Registration require it for license and medical colleges teach it in course.

Recognizing its importance, the Michigan State Board of Registration, on Feb. 12, 1909, notified medical colleges, that thereafter, it would grant license to practice only to such applicants, as demonstrated, on a living subject, with simple spherical lenses and test types, their working knowledge of simple refraction.

Your committee is confident, that every State Board of Registration, would make a like requirement, if it grasped the situation: and then all medical colleges would qualify their students therefor.

Recalling the fact, that our system of medical education, makes no adequate provision for training the family physician in simple refraction, and that it be impossible for experts to meet the needs of all the people in this respect; it is plain that this class of cases had no source of relief other than the optician. But if the State Boards

require a working knowledge of simple refraction for license, the needs of all the
people will be fully met by qualified physicians, and the optician resume his normal
vocation as a spectacle merchant.

Recognizing your great influence in
medical affairs, and assuming your vital interest in enlarging the field of family practice, your Committee confidently ask your
active endeavor to persuade your "State
Board of Registration" to require "a working knowledge of Simple Refraction" from
each applicant for license.

Each member of your Committee stands

ready to assist you to a fuller understanding of the situation, or to co-operate with
you in seeking its relief.

With thanks for your aid, and a report
of your success, we remain, Dear Doctor,
Sincerely Yours,
LEARTUS CONNER,
Detroit, Mich., Chairman.
A. R. BAKER,
Cleveland, Ohio.
J. THORRINGTON,
Philadelphia, Pa.
91 Lafayette Boulevard,
Detroit, Michigan.

EXCHANGES

IODID OF POTASSIUM.

G. Dock, New Orleans (Journal A. M.
A., November 13), reports his opinion as
to this drug which he says is a striking example of the uncertainty, unrest, and dis-
satisfaction characterizing the therapeutics
of the day. He says we have here a good
example of the value of empiricism as a
guide to wider knowledge as well as a
refuge and comfort in time of need. First
he speaks of the necessity of knowing how
much of the remedy to give and says some
of the ideas entertained by some members
of the profession at present are an example
of imperfect education as regards dosage.
Any one who thinks that more than five
or ten grains at a dose is dangerous in
syphilis is hardly fit to judge of the qualities of the medicine. As regards the prescribing of the remedy, imperfect ideas are
also entertained, some thinking that it can
be given in one way, and some in another.
There are other vehicles that can be con-
veniently used than the compound syrup
of sarsaparilla. Dock has found giving the
drug in a solution of a grain to a drop of

water and using milk as a vehicle most
satisfactory to him when used to produce a
marked effect. A bad taste does not necessarily discourage patients from taking a
remedy, and he speaks of the freedom of
the method from gastric irritation as one
of its advantages. Iodism is most frequently seen in patients who have been taking
small doses such as one or two grains at a
time, and in the form of inflammatory
lesions of the skin and mucous membrane.
Lack of cleanliness is responsible largely
for the skin infections and local infections
may be supposed to play an important part
in the mucosa lesions. The iodin "drunk"
and iodin mumps he has never observed.
Edema of the glottis should be borne in
mind but it is probable that in the reported cases there were other more important
factors than the iodid. In rare cases iodid
causes symptoms due to idiosyncrasy and
it is possible that some of the cases of iodin
coryza and iodin headache belong to this
class. The more general symptoms credited to iodism, with nervousness, emaciation,
tachycardia, etc., are not really due to
iodids but to thyroid intoxication. He has

used the potassium salt almost exclusively as he finds it better for the constitutional effect, but he would like to see sodium iodid tried further. He has been convinced that it has no decided advantage as regards taste and effects on the stomach are concerned. Of the special preparations on the market he does not speak with any confidence, nor does he recommend the various combinations as being of advantage. He concludes by saying: "Potassium iodid can be taken easily and safely and in adequate quantities by most patients who need it. Other preparations of iodid may prove to be better, but need to be tested, and recommendations based on the inferiority of potassium iodid should be looked on with suspicion."

CYSTOCELE.

G. R. White, Savannah, Ga., (Journal A. M. A., November 20), says that the reasons for failure of operations for the permanent cure of cystocele seems to be that the normal support of the bladder has not been sought for and restored, but that instead, an irrational removal of part of the anterior vaginal wall has been depended on for this purpose. The bladder rests on the anterior vaginal wall to which it is slightly adherent. The support of this wall is due to its attachment to the symphysis pubis for pubic bones in front, laterally to the white line of the pelvic fascia and ischiatic spine, and above and behind to the uterus. The uterus itself, being freely movable, is of little importance as a support and the real support of the vagina comes from its attachment to the white line of the pelvic fascia and especially a thick bundle of fibers attached to the spine of the ischium and radiating out on the anterior and posterior surfaces of the vaginal tube. If the fibers along the white line, and especially those from the spine, are divid-

ed, the vagina falls down and a cystocele results. It is easy to see how this can happen in difficult deliveries and he has had it occur under his eyes in a case of instrumental delivery. In the operation he describes: "The vagina is held open by two retractors, the ischiatic spine is located by palpation, and an incision from one to two inches long is made throught the mucous membrane, parallel to the white line, and extending well up the vagina. The bladder is separated from the vagina by blunt dissection until the spine of the ischium and white line are reached and can be felt uncovered beneath the finger. Hemorrhage is seldom troublesome and can be controlled by a fey minutes' pressure. The sutures, which are of chromicized catgut, are passed under guidance of the finger by a Decchamps handle-needle. The first suture goes back of the white line just as it joins the spine of the ischium. The handle-needle is taken off, and each end of the suture threaded on a separate needle; one needle is passed from within out through the median edge of the incision, taking a firm hold on the vagina; the other needle is passed in a similar manner through the lateral edge of the incision. The two ends are then clamped and are ready to be tied. A similar suture is placed half an inch lower down on the white line, and when this is in place both sutures are tied, bringing the lateral sulcus of the vagina in contact with the white line of the pelvic fascia. Should there by any prolapse at the outlet of the vagina, the incision may be extended down alongside of the urethra and the vagina sutured to the dense fascia covering the pelvic bone. The opposite side is treated in a similar manner and when both sides are tied the anterior vaginal wall is drawn up in a normal position, and has no tendency to sag, even when the patient coughs or strains. The vagina reaches across from one ischiatic spine to the other, without any tension; it collapses when the retractors are removed and normal relations of the parts are restored." The advantages claimed for this operation are the restoration of the normal supports, no sacrifice of tissue; rarity of recurrences, and the fact that it can be done without interfering with any other plastic work about the vagina. In fact such work has been performed in connection with the operation in all the nineteen patients so far operated on. The article is illustrated.

SALT-FREE DIET IN NEPHRITIS.

V. C. Vaughan, Ann Arbor, Mich., (Journal A. M. A., November 27), says that the following points seem fairly well established: "1. Urea and uric acid are not important constituents of the urine so far as their toxicity is concerned. I mean to say that neither of these can be regarded as the active agent in the causation of those symptoms that result from failure to function on the part of the kidney. 2. About 85 per cent. of the toxicity of the urine is due to its inorganic constituents, the most toxic of which is potassium chloride. 3. There are present in normal urine certain organic poisons, the nature of which has not yet been ascertained. 4. Although the inorganic constituents, notably potassium chloride, are markedly poisonous, they cannot be regarded as standing in a direct causal relation to that complex of symptoms which we designate as uremia. A small fraction of a grain of potassium chloride, as I have frequently demonstrated, injected into a ventricle of the brain of an animal, may cause prompt death, but neither the symptoms nor the post-mortem findings are those of uremia." He is confident that withholding salts does not touch the real cause of uremia. It seems possible that the inorganic salts of normal urine and its organic constituents may neutralize each

other party. At least it has been repeatedly found that the ash of urine is decidedly more toxic than the whole urine and he thinks that there is room for more research on this point. There is evidence also that an absolutely ash-free diet may disturb the health and this also needs further study. In dogs, long-continued feeding of a salt-free diet materially reduces the acidity of the gastric juice and it has been repeatedly shown that there is a minimum of salt content in the living tissues below which it is impossible to go. Single organic salts may be more poisonous than a combination, and therefore there is reason for suspecting that the inorganic constituents of the urine may neutralize each other. Vaughan shows that salt retention is not proved to be the cause of nephritis or of its edema, and it seems to him that the greatest good is to be secured by restricting salt in the diet of patients who may be called prenephritics, and there are many of this kind; he is in the habit of advising such individuals to have their food prepared without the addition of salt. He is positive that we eat too much highly salted food. With unsalted food we drink less and the kidneys are relieved of excessive work; otherwise, he has never been satisfied that he has seen any benefit in any form of nephritis in denying the patient the satisfaction of his thirst. It seems good sense to limit the consumption of food in nephritis, so far as possible without distress to the patient.

THE PALLIATIVE TREATMENT OF UTERINE CANCER.

W. B. Chase, Brooklyn, (Journal A. M. A., December 4), holds that the early radical measures have about reached their limit in the treatment of uterine cancer and that the palliative treatment is not receiving the attention it deserves. His statements have more reference to cancer of the cervix than cancer of the body but the same principle applies to both. When the disease has reached the adjacent structures it may be advisable to limit the treatment to the superficial area of ulceration. After long personal observation and experience he is convinced that no palliative treatment is so effective as the thermocautery, which has the advantage of thoroughly closing the lymphatic vessels. Whether its superiority over caustics is due to the influence of heat on the diseased cells beyond the area of cell destruction is a matter of opinion, but he is inclined to think it probable. He specially emphasizes the fact that it is rare for the patient to suffer pain after the use of the thermocautery if the mucocutaneous surfaces are not injured. This requires tact and experience. He has usually found it easiest to protect the surfaces from injury by the use of strips of asbestos paper of proper size and shape. He alludes to Dr. John Byrne's method of the use of the galvanocautery, which he calls the correct one, and which consists in the gradual eating out of the diseased tissue of the uterus nearly to its peritoneal covering by the use of a platinum wire loop for the cautery and curetting away the burned tissue. Skill with this method consists in not going far beyond the area of involvement and having the cautery just hot enough to burn the structures but not to disintegrate them too rapidly. If proper heat is not maintained troublesome hemorrhage may follow. He has seen patients with cancer, far advanced, of the cervix and body, showing signs of grave systemic infection, who lost their cachectic appearance after themocautery operation. The greatest gentleness should be employed in all manipulation of the parts after operation and a bivalve speculum should not be used as a rule, as it is likely to infringe on the burnt area. Daily vaginal douches with permamganate of potassium or compound solution of cresol are the best intiseptics. In hopeless cases this local treatment of galvanocautery is essential for the patient's comfort and the skilled hand of the attending physician is the most satisfactory in applying the dressing. The local use of cocain, frequently repeated, is sometimes useful in relieving pain, or rectal suppositories of cocain and hyoscyamus are advisable. Later, increasing doses of morphine may be used. He has not been so fortunate as Dr. Bryne in thus preventing the local recurrence of the disease, which may be due, he says, to his less skillful technic. There is no reason why in recurrent cases the thermocautery can not be repeatedly used with benefit. He gives the history of four patients, two of whom after periods of from four to eight years, according to accepted standards, were cured, and the other two were greatly benefited and their lives prolonged for years with very litle suffering— a result unobtainable, so far as he knows, by any other treatment. He regrets that he can not give in this paper more than passing mention of the utility of x-ray and radium treatment in uterine cancer. His experience with either of these has not been sufficiently extensive to enable him to speak authoritively as to their value, but, as far as his experience goes, he regards radium as far the most useful, since after its use granulating surfaces take on a more healthful activity than after the use of the x-ray and this he believes is in accordance with recent observations.

NEW MEMBERS.

Dr. J. Paul Gay, McAlester.
Dr. A. W. Harris, Muskogee.
Dr. H. T. Balentine, Muskogee.
Dr. J. G. Noble, Muskogee.

MISCELLANEOUS·

COUNCIL ON PHARMACY AND CHEMISTRY, NEW ARTICLES ACCEPTED FOR INCLUSION.

Articles accepted for N. N. R:
Orphol (Schering & Glatz.)
Orphol Tablets, do.
Arsen-Triferrin, (Knoll & Co.)
Arsen-Triferrin Tablets, do.
Arsen-Triferrol, do.
Lactophenin, (Merck & Co.)

AMERICAN MEDICAL ASSOCIATION, SPECIAL CONFERENCE ON MEDICAL EDUCATION AND MEDICAL LEGISLATION.

To the Officers and Members of State Medical Licensing Boards,
To the Officers of State Medical Associations,
To Members of the National Legislative Council,
To University Presidents, College Professors and others interested in Medical Legislation,

GREETING:

A special conference on Medical Education and Legislation will be held at the Congress Hotel (formerly the Auditorium Annex,) Chicago, Monday, Tuesday, and Wednesday, February 28, March 1 and 2, 1910, the session to begin at 10 o'clock Monday morning.

Monday, February 28th.

On Monday the Council on Medical Education will hold its Sixth Annual Conference. A report will be presented showing the present status of the medical colleges in the United States and another report giving practical tests in state license examinations. Other important topices bearing on medical education will be discussed.

Tuesday, March 1st.

On Tuesday there will be a joint Conference on Medical Education and Medical Legislation, at which the essentials of a model medical practice act will be considered.

Wednesday, March 2nd.

On Wednesday the Committee on Medical Legislation will hold its Annual Conference, discussing a National Bureau of Health, vital statistics, pure food and drugs, expert testimony, and other live topics.

You are cordially invited to attend this conference and to participate in the discussions.

Council on Medical Education
N. P. COLWELL, Secretary.
Committee on Medical Legislation
FREDRICK R. GREEN, Secretary.
Chicago, Ill., Dec. 1, 1909.

ADRENALIN IN A NEW PACKAGE.

In addition to the ounce vials in which it has hitherto been supplied, Adrenalin Chloride Solution is now being marketed in hermetically sealed glass containers of 1 cubic centimeter capacity. "Adrenalin Ampoule" is the name used to designate the new package, and the solution is of the strength of 1 to 10,000 (one part Adrenalin chloride to 10,000 parts physiologic salt solution.) In their announcement of the ampoule Parke, Davis & Co. have this to say:

"Adrenalin Chloride Solution has become a necessity in medical and surgical practice. The most powerful of actringents and hemostatics, it lends itself to many practical uses and at little risk of injury in reasonably careful hands. Since the time of its introduction it has been marketed in ounce vials, and of the strength of 1:1000. Experience has shown, however, that a weaker solution is much more frequently required than the "full strength;" and while it is generally an easy matter to dilute with water or normal saline solution, in certain emergencies an already fully diluted preparation is to be preferred. While the danger of deterioration from occasionally opening a vial containing a solution of Adrenalin Chloride is not great, still, in consideration of the fact that a dose is needed now and then for hypodermatic injection, it is believed that the small hermetically sealed package will be welcomed because of its greater convenience and security."

As will be apparent from the foregoing the Adrenalin Ampoule is intended for hypodermatic use. It should be of great value in such emergencies as shock, collapse, hemorrhage, asthma, etc., or where prompt heart-stimulation is desired.

THERAPEUTIC SERMONETTE.

By Dr. Geo. F. Butler.

At the onset of acute tonsilitis the bowels should be cleansed by calomel, podophyllin and bilein followed by saline laxative. Defervescent compound (No. 1 or 2 according to age,) every half hour until the temperature reaches 100 degrees F. or less. If much hoarseness and soreness of throat, potassium bichromate gr. 1-67 in in a teaspoonful of water should be given every two hours. As the acute symptoms subside these remedies should be replaced by calx iodata (Calcidin) gr. 1-3 given in a teaspoonful of hot water every hour or two as indicated. The throat should be sprayed three or four times a day with an antiseptic solution (Menthol Compound, Abbott, 1 tablet, glycerine 1-2 ounce, water 12 ounces.) The urine should be frequently examined, and if there is evidence of acidemia sodoxylin and salithia should be given in plenty of water until the condition is overcome. A light diet should be given and the child kept in a room moistened with steam or the air medicated with a vapor of cresoline or with antiseptic oils. By all means keep up free elimination through bowels, skin and kidneys.

BOOK REVIEWS

American Illustrated Medical Dictionary. The New (5th) Edition. Dorlands American Illustrated Medical Dictionary. A new and complete dictionary of terms used in Medicine, Surgery, Dentistry, Pharmacy, Chemstry, Nursing and kindred branches; with new and elaborate tables and many handsome illustrations. Fifth Revised Edition. By W. A. Newman Dorland, M. D., Large Octavo of 876 pages, with 2,000 new terms. Philadelphia and London. W. B. Saunders Company, 1909. Flexible leather, $4.50 net; indexed, $5.00 net.

This work will be found most useful to the Medical Student and as a work of easy access and one that covers the field well; it will be found to be of great value to the general practitioner as well.

Many of the new illustrations are in colors and the charts on bacteriology and those showing the appearance in the exanthmatous conditions, arterial and venous systems, pathologic conditions and anatomic structures are very beautiful and most attractively gotten up.

The work is well worth the price and will be very popular with profession.

A Text Book on Obstetrics, Including Related Gynecologic Operations. The New (6th.) Edition, Barton Cooke Hirst, M. D., Professor of Obstetrics in the University of Pennsylvania. 992 pages, with 847 illustrations, 43 being in colors, 1909. Cloth, $5.00 net; Half Morocco, $6.50 net.

W. B. Saunders Company, Philadelphia and London.

This work is too well known to the profession to require an extended description or discussion. It takes rank as one of the leading text-books on this subject and deserves the careful consideration of the general practicioner as well as the student of medicine. It will appeal to the general practicioner on account of being most thorough in the consideration of complications arising from the puerperal state and much space being devoted to the operative work following such complications. Vaginal, uterine, abdominal and all classes of work confronting the Gynecologist and Obstetrician are given attention.

Much space is devoted to the preparation and after care of the operative case. The technic and details are carefully entered into and the advice as to operations of selection is good.

The work will be found of use to every general practitioner who will take even a short time to give it the perusal and reflection it richly deserves.

BOOKS RECEIVED.

The Physician's Pocket Account Book. By J. J. Taylor, M. D., bound in full leather, 24 pages of practical instructions for physicians, 216 pages of accounts. Price $1.00 per copy; published by The Medical Council 4105 Walnut Street, Philadelphia, Pa.

PUBLIC HEALTH

Rules relating to tuberculosis will be changed, and the law will require compulsory reporting of this disease. The forbidding of the occupancy of a house having been infected either by removal or death of a tubercular patient until the same has been fumigated or disinfected; and the free examination of sputum of a tubercular patient by the State Board of Health will be adopted as rule governing the Oklahoma State Board of Health. The rules relating to vital statistics will be amended so as to conform and meet the requirements recommended in the Model Bill of vital statistics prepared by the Committee of the American Medical Association and the Census Bureau at Washington.

On the first day of January, 1909, the State Commissioner of Health will promulgate some new rules as follows: pellagra, hook worm, anterior poliomyelitis of infantile paralysis will be included in the list of diseases that it is necessary to report to the State Commissioner of Health.

NEW AND NON-OFFICIAL REMEDIES.

Published by the Council on Pharmacy and Chemistry of the American Medical Association for free distribution to members of the American Medical Association, complete to January, 1909.

Second supplement to New and Non-Official Remedies issued by above named Council and complete to and including September 11, 1909.

Published by Press of the American Medical Association, Chicago, 1909.

COUNTY SOCIETIES

TO COUNTY SECRETARIES.

As your annual elections are well under way and in many instances have already been held I think it proper to call your attention to some of the conditions, a remedy of which may be found in your co-operating with this office by promptly sending in your reports for the coming year. This letter is prompted by the fact that in many instances no communication whatever has been received from the county secretaries since my incumbency in office in May, 1909, and to all intents and purposes the county society to which they are accredited as secretary does not exist except on paper and in the imigination.

The function of a county secretary has previously been outlined in these columns and it is only necessary to say that promptness in sending in reports of your county society transactions, movements of your local profession and other matters of interest generally are a part of your duties which should be attended to. This caution is not necessary in the case of many of the secretaries as some of them have been more than prompt and efficient and very kind in giving the state secretary all the aid in their power in the work, which at best is very hard and difficult of execution.

It occurs to the secretary's office that if a county secretary cannot fulfill the obligations of his office he should resign and make room for some other person who has more time or taste for the work. NOW if you propose to retain your office without having war with the state secretary please send me a list of your officers elected for 1910, Presidents, Vice-Presidents, Secretaries and Delegates, and send all the transactions of your society as rapidly as completed.

Respectfully,

C. A. THOMPSON,

Secretary.

BRYAN COUNTY.

Bryan county held its annual election for officers for 1910 with the following results:

President, Dr. J. L. Shuler, Durant.

Vice-Presidnt, Dr. J. F. Park, Durant.

Secretary-Treasurer, Dr. D. Armstrong, Mead.

Censors, Dr. H. E. Pappolee, Caddo, one year; Dr. W. L. Kendall, Durant, two years; Dr. W. F. Clifton, Durant, three years.

MUSKOGEE COUNTY.

The Annual election of officers of this county occured December 13, and resulted as follows:

President—Dr. H. C. Rogers.

Vice-President—Dr. S. W. Aiken.

Secretary-Treasurer—Dr. H. T. Ballantine.

Delegates, Drs. P. P. Nesbit and I. B. Oldham.

Delegates to Oklahoma City Tubercular Convention, Drs. J. O. Callahan and G. A. McBride.

A spirited discussion arose on the question of the county society employing additional legal help to aid in the case of Muskogee County's prosecution of Chiropractors. Some of the members present taking the position that the county should assume all expense and initiative in the prosecution as it does in other criminal cases, while others held to the view that the county society should not only aid in a moral way but should also appropriate money for the prosecution as is done in many important cases where it is necessary to have legal assistance to aid the regularly constituted authorities. The matter was not disposed of and will come up at a special meeting later.

An elaborate banquet was indulged in after the meeting at the Turner Hotel, about sixty people being present.

HUGHES COUNTY.

Program for the meeting to be held December. 30, 1909, at Holdenville.

What to do in Appendicitis, Dr. G. W. Patterson.

Some Observations in Treatment of Pneumonia, Dr. Vanderpool.

Anesthesia, Dr. H. A. Howell.

Clinic, Dr. A. L. Davenport.

Quiz, "Femoral Artery" Its Relations, its Branches, and their Distribution.

Patent Medicine, Dr. T. J. Cagle.

How to prevent Tuberculosis, Dr. Troy, McAlester.

The last paper will be illustrated by stereopticon pictures by Dr. J. C. Mahr, State Commissioner of Health who will also show some pictures of Pellagra.

The question of ridding the county of illegal practitioners will also come up for consideration and the annual election of officers for 1910 will be held.

PITTSBURG COUNTY.

The Annual election of officers for 1910 resulted in the following officers being chosen:

President—R. I. Bond, Hartshorne.

Vice-President—R. K. Pemberton, Krebs.

Secretary-Treasurer—H. E. Williams, McAlester.

Delegates to Annual Meeting, LeRoy Long, McAlester, R. L. Mitchell, Dow.

PERSONAL MENTION.

MARRIED.

At Chickasha, Oklahoma, December 3rd, 1909, Miss Zenobia Cuthbertson to Dr. Fred R. Disney of Pocasset, Oklahoma, at the residence of Dr. Glenn.

Miss Cuthbertson was formerly from Liberty, Mo., and Dr. Disney is comparatively a new man in Oklahoma, having come here from the Augustana Hospital, Chicago.

The best wishes of the medical profession of Oklahoma are extended to them.

Dr. C. B. Bradford of Oklahoma City was recently elected Chairman of the Board of Freeholders of that city. They are to draft a new charter for Oklahoma City and it is to be hoped that its Public Health Department, which is now inferior to none in the state, will be well looked after.

Dr. J. M. Byrum, President of the Pottawatomie County Medical Association, has just completed a post-graduate course at Chicago, and a visit to the Mayos.

Dr. G. W. Colvert, of Shawnee, will take post-graduate work in St. Louis this month.

Dr. O. E. Templin has changd his location, having movd from Darrough to Alva, Oklahoma.

Dr. W. S. Works of Matoy, Bryan County, Oklahoma, has reported four cases of infantile paralysis to the State Board of Health.

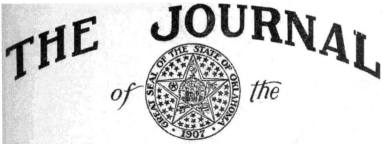

THE JOURNAL of the

Oklahoma State Medical Association.

VOL. II.	MUSKOGEE. OKLAHOMA. FEBRUARY. 1910.	NO. 9.

DR. CLAUDE A. THOMPSON, Editor-in-Chief.

ASSOCIATE EDITORS AND COUNCILLORS.

DR. J. A. WALKER, Shawnee.
DR. CHARLES R. HUME, Anadarko.
DR. F. R. SUTTON, Bartlesville.
DR. G. W. ROBERTSON, Dustin.

DR. JOHN W. DUKE, Guthrie.
DR. A. B. FAIR, Frederick.
DR. W. G. BLAKE, Tahlequah.
DR. H. P. WILSON, Wynnewood.

DR. J. S. FULTON, Atoka.

Entered at the Postoffice at Muskogee, Oklahoma, as second class mail matter, June, 1909.

This is the Official Journal of the Oklahoma State Medical Association. All communications should be addressed to the Journal of the Oklahoma State Medical Association, English Block, Muskogee, Oklahoma.

TUBERCULOSIS

AN ADDRESS BY DR. H. M. WILLIAMS, WELLSTON, OKLAHOMA, CHAIRMAN OF THE COMMITTEE ON TUBERCULOSIS OF THE OKKAHOMA STATE MEDICAL ASSOCIATION

It has been but a few years since, that the instigators of a gathering of this kind, would have been called heretics. It is only during the last one-half century that people have become to realize, that things that were once said to be impossible are now recognized as a reality. It is within the memory of the present generation that many of our most valuable articles of commerce, when predicted that such a thing would exist was said by those who classed themselves as the conservatives to be an

(*Read before First Anti-Tubercular Convention, Oklahoma City, Jan.* 10 *and* 11, 1910.

impossibility. That the mind of man could not conceive and think out a machine that would carry man to and fro at his will, yet today we witness the obedience of the automobile and electric car to the will of man. Coming close behind the automobile is wireless telegraphy flashing messages from one continent to another, by this method the world is constantly informed as to the events that are taking place. It will be but a few more days until we witness man go flying through space on every side, all due to the workings of the mind of man.

These facts are familiar to all as through our daily papers we are constantly informed as to the commercial advancement of the world.

Those of us who are fortunate enough who take the advantage of the opportunity to listen to the precepts and doctrines taught by the clergy. We are readily convinced that their knowledge of the Bible and its teachings are more clearly defined than that of our fathers. Daily we witness the spiritual growth of man.

The educator can readily demonstrate to us, by his methods of objective illustrations, and mechanical appliances that, he too has kept pace with the times and that through a systematic process the world is rapidly advancing in educational lines.

The deliberate and careful manner in which justice is dealt out to our fellow man is evidence of the advancement of the legal profession.

The time of this meeting could not have been better eselected, coming as it does following so close our Xmas festivities, held in remembrance of the birth of Christ, the imitation of whose life makes all men more charitable. The beginning of the new year the time when all good men and women, if not openly secretly vow to be a better man or woman during the coming year and thus are greater benefactors to mankind.

The place of this meeting could not have been better chosen than, this, the largest city of our state. Which is absolutely cosmopolitan in its citizenship, modern in construction, whose citizens are noted for their charitable acts. Whose physicians are honored for their scientific researches have invited us to congregate here as physicians and laymen to study the "Great White Plague," a disease which is costing 200,000 lives annually, 400 daily and our own state about three per day or at about the rate of 1,000 annually.

The cause of this meeting is due to a resolution that was introduced in the State Medical Society, at this place in May of last year, calling for a committee to be named, who should study plans and ways for both physician and layman to pursue to eradicate tuberculosis from our state.

Meetings not unlike this in many respects have been the occasion for the coming together of the most learned men, of the communities, states and nation since the beginning of events. In order that they might be better prepared to combat the diseases to which man is subject. From the history of medicine it is concluded that the ancients knew very little of pathology, anatomy, and their surgery was of the most crude nature, and antisepsis was not practiced. The first authentic history of any real medical knowledge is found in the Biblical history of Joseph's request that he be embalmed. An art in which his people excelled. Although four thousand years have elapsed we are unable to restore this apparently lost art. The ancient Hebrew race have given the world some excellent rules of hygiene in the writings attributed to Moses which is hard to improve upon of today but these people have left no works on this subject outside of those of the scriptural records. While in the library at Alexandrea a number of treaties of medicine were found by Egyptians, with arrangements and completeness that rivaled the Hippocrates collection which they antedate by one thousand years, the latter being recognized authority of ancient medicine.

Of all ancient races of people the Grecians furnish us with the most complete remains of the history of medicine and supplies the names of the ancients whom the science of medicine reverence. To Aesculapes, the Greek god of medicine, we find temples dedicated in numerous places. The priest, as a rule, presided over these temples and the most learned men of the age came here for knowledge and treatment; people made regular pilgrimages to these resorts from all parts. They were here placed upon a restricted and well regulated diet, pure air, sunshine, temperate habits, and sea-baths. "History speaks of cures that were affected in this manner that would be considered marvelous even in our day." Though no authentic account is given, it is possible that tuberculosis was successfully treated in this manner, as we find that phthsis was known to the Greeks as a wasting disease. A custom practiced by these people of no little importance, was their method of physical culture which was made compulsory. They, by this means, built up a nation of athletes, a people of rugged constitution among whom disease was almost unknown. An example after which our own legislature would do well to pattern.

Having in a manner briefly reviewed the history of ancient medicine, we will now turn to modern with which we have to deal.

There are those whose names to our profession are prominent, because of scientific researches, have made themselves great benefactors to humanity. And yet these same men are unknown to the outside world. It was in the sixteenth century that the medicinal world was aroused by the announcement of Dr. Wm. Harvey, that he had made the discovery that the blood did actually circulate through the body, which completely revolutionized the field of medicine. Following Harvey was a completion of the process of inoculation or vaccination by Dr. Edward Jenner, who has made it possible for us to go among those affected with the once dreaded disease, smallpox, with but very little danger of contracting it. The next area of importance is that of the pathological investigation in which the pathological changes that takes place in the cells and tissue in the process of disease are noted and tabulated. Drs. Klebs, Loeffler and Koch names are prominent in this connection.

In this field the microscope is brought into active use.

The next discovery in this line, that was of benefit to mankind, was that of general anesthesia, and is pronounced by the surgeon as a "God send," has been in use for only about fifty years.

Following close to general anesthesia and perhaps second in importance, is the recognized use of asepsis and antisepsis. The names of the men who first made its use practicable are that of Drs. Pasteur and Lister by means of antisepsis surgical operations are successfully performed today that a few years ago would of been criminal to of attempted.

Is it any wonder that we who have come here today should take an optimistic view of the eradication of tuberculosis, when we consider the great advancement, that recent years have made for bettering the physical condition of man? What he now needs most of all is to be educated.

It will only be necessary to recall what is being done in the way of advancement in the commercial and scientific world to realize what is doing in the medicinal. Compare if you will our crude methods of transportation of one hundred years ago with that of today and by this method you will get a fair idea of the medicinal advancement of the last hundred years.

It has been but a few years since when that once dreaded disease diphtheria made its appearance in the home, it was considered almost certain death to some member of that family, but of recent years we all agree that we have a remedy, if properly administered, removes that dread to both the physician and family, and has in this one disease greatly reduced the death rate.

By careful application and the microscope we have been able to isolate the germ that is the cause of consumption and find that which destroys its growth. Is it any wonder in view of the above that we believe that affective improvement can be had in a majority of cases of tubercular; and almost all incipient cases cured.

We have come together for the purpose of not only educating ourselves, but that we might adopt some plan that all the working forces may act in unison to combat tuberculosis. Other states are engaged in a similar warfare, and some have been for years. We believe that much good has been accomplished and that many states through their legislatures are making liberal appropriations for the combating of the white plague. During the last year fifteen different state legislatures made appropriations in some form to aid in this cause.

In our own state we are glad to note much interest has been aroused during the past months by the efforts of our State Health Commissioner, the Women's Federated Clubs, the State Medical Association and many other working organizations toward a campaign of education. However, we find that much remains yet to be done. It is not an uncommon circumstance for a physician in his daily rounds to find some member of a large family who has contracted this disease. And of his or her own resources are unable to change their surroundings, thus exposing the entire family by sleeping together in overcrowded and poorly ventilated rooms. Circumstances of this kind are a very common sight to the family physician. To help this class of people would be a blessing, not only to the victim of this disease, but to those who have to daily come in contact with this unfortunate, thus exposing them to this dreaded disease, which is both contagious and infectious.

The medical profession are willing to do their part in this campaign toward eliminating this condition, but we of ourselves can do but little without the aid of the public, for the people who must come to our assistance in this struggle for better conditions. Our knowledge so far as scientific investigation is as to cause, prevention and cure of this disease, we freely give to you without price. We would that we possessed the power to say to these, "Go wash in the pool of Siloam," and be healed, but it seems as though the Creator of the universe, in his supreme wisdom, did not find it advisable to bestow that power upon the peculiar, if you wish to call them such, school of medicine represented here today. To us we must deal with cause and effect. The cause of tuberculosis is due to a micro-organism of veritable origin, though its existence has long been known. It is only of recent years that the infection and contagious theory has been fully accepted, however, in the early part of the last century physicians refused to hold autopsies on subjects who died of this disease, because they believe it contagious. It was not until 1883 that Dr. Robert Koch, a Berlin physician, was able to isolate this germ completely and announce to the world the direct cause of tuberculosis. To him much honor should be given as a benefactor of mankind. Since the complete isolation of this germ there has been a never ceasing war waged upon it by able men of the medical profession, and we feel to a large extent their efforts have been rewarded. This will be fully explained by those who will follow on this program.

As before stated we are not alone in this campaign. At a recent meeting of the State Medical Association of the state of Minnesota the following was suggested as an outline of the working forces that should enter into the "anti-tubercular campaign:" "The Governor, the State Medical Examiners, the Board of Health, the State Medical Association, the public schools, the Dairy and Food Inspectors, the Woman's Federated Clubs, the Commercial Clubs, the Labor Organizations, the Charity Organizations, the Municipal Leagues," (we would suggest the adding of the clergy, the press and the legal profession to the above list) "the uniting of these forces upon public health matters would constitute a working force if properly organized that would in a short time reduce the death rate to the minimum in our state and it would be but a few years until there would be a single case where today there are scores. The Association further suggested that the State Medical Association could reach the people through lecturers and through the County Medical Societies. Pubilc health lecturers should be in the field constantly, the tubercular exhibit should be a traveling exhibit and a liberal appropriation should be made by the legislature of the state to carry on this campaign of education to the people. We believe that much could be accomplished by the ministry and the press by informing themselves upon this subject and through their respective channels assist in this campaign of education. Permit me to quote from the address of Mr. Jones, editor of the Minneapolis Journal, before the State Medical Association of his state the latter part of October, 1909: "The press represents a great responsibility to the country as does the medical profession. I think that the medical fraternity have been governed too long by their laws; that the people know too little what they are doing. We have only to listen to papers on occasions like this. Physicians would be surprised to know what little the people know of what is going on regarding the care of the health of the people. I think that if we could come together a little more we would reach an understanding." He called the attention to the willingness of the papers to take up the work from an educational standpoint rather than from a general news. In conclusion he urges the society to take up the campaign and pledges the support of all good newspapers which is our most popular means of education.

The State Medical Association of Kentucky, which convened the same month, though a distance of more than a thousand miles from the above state, having this same subject under consideration, Dr. Jacob Glahn, of Owensboro, Ky., made the following statement relative to the existing conditions of his state: "There are recorded between six and seven thousand deaths annually alone in the state of Kentucky during one year. If we multiply this by five we have over 30,000 ill with tuberculosis at this time, and there is no telling how many obscure cases are existing that are not reported." In his conclusion the doctor makes a strong plea for legislature appropriations for county and state Sanatoria.

The Department of Health in a recent bulletin gives the approximate cost of tuberculosis to the people of Chicago during 1908, "as $23,635,190, distributed as follows: The money value of lives lost amount to $19,571,950. Wages lost by decendants, $1,336,200. The cost of illness to those who died, $707,040. Loss of wages to patients, still living, $1,120,000, and the cost of illness of 10,000 living patients $900,000. During the first nine months of 1909, 3,024 new cases were reported to the Health Department of the Board." After showing the class of people who are affected it is found that by far the greater per cent is among the poor people, making the class who are least, able, having the burden of expense for this sickness to bear.

The Metropolitan Life Insurance Company of New York recently filed papers in courts of that state asking the courts to order the State Insurance Commissioner to explain reasons for refusing to grant the company a permit to buy land upon which to establish a tubercular sanitarium, holding it is a proper purpose for a company to conserve its assets by cutting down its death rate.

Life insurance companies have carefully studied this subject and have estimated that about 75 per cent of all cases of tuberculosis can be prevented; that all cases are curable, if taken in the incipient stage. With this thought in view they are building numerous sanitariums, where they will cure their policy holders free of cost.

We have endeavored to show that tuberculosis is one of the most destructive diseases known to man; it kills more people than the most fierce battle known in the same length of time. It is found in all civilized countries. Until recent years the death rate has been on the increase; that climatic conditions have but little to do as to its development, will be seen. The percentage of deaths are larger in the cities than in rural districts. Life insurance companies whose responsibility ends by the paying of the policy, are preparing sanitariums for the cure and pay the patients cheaper than it can permit them to die.

Our state, according to meager statistics, has a death rate of three each day, or about one thousand annually. A large per cent of those who are affected are unable to change their present condition without financial assistance. Our condition at present, or present death rate per 100,000 is not as great as many states, yet it is costing our state over one-half million dollars annually. If conditions are allowed to continue it will be but a short time until this will greatly increase. It has been accurately estimated that 75 per cent of all cases are preventable; that all uncomplicated, incipient cases are curable. Life insurance companies can cure policy holders to permit them to continue to pay assessments, who have no responsibility to the family other than paying of the policy. Would it not be an economical problem for the state to care for her sick and provide a way for a cure? The most affected is between the age of 25 and 45, making the affected class the bread winners, who at death will leave a family of orphans a charge to the state, when within such a short time, if beginning properly and with proper methods, so many cases can be cured, thus prolonging the life of the bread winner, who will be able to care for his family until they reach their majority and can care for themselves. That the matter relative to a state organization might be carefully considered I would suggest that a committee be chosen from those present at our first session to devise a plan to persue and report back to this body for definite action before the adjournment of this meeting.

SURGICAL ASPECT OF TUBERCULAR UTERUS AND APPENDAGES

BY DR. CHARLES NELSON BALLARD, OKLAHOMA CITY, OKLA.
Formerly of Chicago, Ill., Associate Professor of Gynecology at College of Physicians and Surgeons Medical Department of the University of Illinois;) Surgeon to Marion Sim's Sanitarium, Chicago; Attending Surgeon to West Side Hospital, Chicago; Attendant in Gynecology, West Side Dispensary.

We are not here today to vie with each other in a political contest; we are not here to listen to attorneys discuss some

(*Read before First Annual Meeting of the Oklahoma State Anti-Tubercular Association, Oklahoma City, Oklahoma, January 10-11, 1910.*)

hypothetical question; we are not here to see some surgeon exhibit his skill; neither are we here to hear the whys and wherefores of the suffragettes but we are here to discuss the ways and means of defense against our most dreaded enemy, the White Plague.

The most destructive disease of the

human race today is consumption or tuberculosis, being the cause of one death in every seven occurring among our people.

It is said that in Germany alone, there die yearly, from this disease 100,000 people.

Our efforts in the great crusade now being made by all civilized nations, is to devise some means of preventing the spread of the disease. People must be instructed as to what is the most potent factor in its production; through what medium it is most frequently transported; and how we are to prevent its gaining vantage ground. We find it in both sexes, at all ages, in all climates, in all vocations, among the rich as well as the poor, and not confined to any special organ, but disposed to migrate from one to the other, affecting all in proportion to their ability to resist disease.

The pathologist teaches us that the bacillus tuberculosis takes the stain slowly but surely. This is characteristic of its actions where ever it is found. Its invasion is slow, but only too surely does it master the situation while its enemy sleeps.

They also teach us that this germ strongly resists the decolorizing action of mineral acids, demonstrating again its ability, when properly emplanted within the entrenchment of tissue inactivity, to gradually advance without interference, with any, so far known, remedial agent.

It behooves us to be active in our effort to prevent its becoming so securely entrenched beyond our control. We are not to allow it to gain the vantage ground Much good must be accomplished by our teaching those who are not aware of the manner of its spreading, or the gravity of being exposed.

We must begin teaching the fathers and mothers. In fact the instruction must begin before this, as we are aware that tuberculous parents produce offsprings, if not tuberculous at birth, are fit subjects to

very readily contract it. They are weaklings—unfit to cope with any disease. They become subjects of charity, and finally must be cared for by public institutions . Then is it not our duty to prevent the birth of such children? If so, we must prohibit, if possible, the marriage of-tubercular people.

In some foreign lands, where the laws in many respects are less severe than ours, they require a certificate of health before the marriage ceremony is performed.

A tubercular mother is unfit to nourish her babe. She should be prevented from placing it to her breast.

Medical men have learned and learned it well, by actual observation, that not only parturition but lactation is hazardous to the tubercular mother. If she nurses her babe she allows it to sap her life away more rapidly, and only too surely lays the foundation, in the babe, for the ready ingress of this most dreaded disease.

This leads us to a delicate point for the legal profession to handle. Is it possible to pass laws that will prevent the marriage of tubercular subjects, if not we will be compelled to cope with the disease in infants. This is a starting point of vital importance in preventing the spread of the disease. The organs within the field limited to my subject, when once overcome by this disease, must usually succumb to the surgeon's knife. By this means the tissue or organs so effected may be removed, cutting short the destruction of adjacent organs, crippling the onward progress of the disease. This gives time to strengthen the tissue, about to be invaded, by more palliative means.

The surgeon can only hope to be a means to an end. He can only open the way, in advanced cases, for what must follow to successfully combat the disease. He can stifle the enemy but more must be done.

When he has exhausted his skill the patient is not now, as formerly to be placed in a hospital, surrounded on all sides by higher buildings, shutting out the rays of the sun so all important to his final success, but will make use of that greatest enemy of the tuberculosis bacilli, the rays of sunlight.

I think it is becoming recognized, more and more, that all forms of tuberculosis must be treated along the same general hygienic, dietetic lines, and that tuberculin is coming more and more in favor, especially in surgical cases.

The old plan of performing an operation on a tuberculous patient and placing him in a stuffy room in a stuffy hospital, I am sure will soon be among the things that were.

The post-operative treatment of this class of cases should be substantially the same as with pulmonary type. This leads me to suggest that the hospitals of the future will be constructed with a view to giving patients more light, more air and better food.

In order to accomplish this it will become necessary to take the hospitals to the country, or at least to the suburbs of large cities.

The time will come when only emergency hospitals will be maintained in congested districts.

One thing is certain, and that is that the profession are recognizing the valuable aid of fresh air, and sunshine in the treatment, not only of tuberculosis, but of all forms of disease.

But few outside of the medical profession are aware that tuberculosis can exist in any other organ except the lungs. This is a reason for many forms of the disease being neglected until far advanced. It may be making its inroads felt in some vital internal organ, without being visibly manifest.

The female genital organs are exposed to infection secondarily, from some other organ or primarily from without. The first form may be transmitted through the blood, lymphatics or by contiguity of tissue, while the latter is usually introduced by the use of unclean instruments or hands. The patient may infect herself on the train, in hotels, or baths by the careless and promiscuous use of towels and bed clothing. The public bath is a fruitful source for infection when every sanitary precaution is not carefully carried out. These are only a few of the means of introduction of infection from without that are of special interest to the surgeon.

How many times the little school girl pale and emaciated, poor appetite, no energy for study or play, is compelled to attend school and neglected because she does not cough, and make plain that one definite symptom of lung tuberculosis, yet her life is being destroyed by unsuspected tuberculosis of her reproductive organs. In inflammation of these organs in the young girl, tuberculosis should always be suspected until proven to be of some other source. Oftimes only a slight inflammation of the tubes may be beginning tuberculosis. About 15 per cent of all infections of the tubes are tubercular.

It is stated that fully 75 per cent of the cases of tuberculosis operated on at John Hopkins' hospital are of this unsuspected type.

They are diagnosed only by the use of the microscope previous to or following the operative procedure. It is not just as important that proper means be used to diagnose the disease of the genital organs in the young school girl, as that of the lungs or any other organ from which infection can take place. This is a point, I am sure, wholly neglected by many who are to carefully examine the school children. If these cases are diagnosed early and proper hygienic and dietetic treatment instituted, together with the use of tuberculin, we can give them much encouragement as to a final, complete recovery without surgical intervention. If neglected, surgical interference is the only hope.

We must not forget that tuberculosis of the lungs may cause tuberculosis of the uterus and tubes or that of the tubes and uterus cause tuberculosis of the lungs.

The symptoms of tuberculosis of the uterus and adnexa are never positive but are not unlike those of ordinary inflammation of these parts, but if occurring in a weakly, especially unmarried woman, with a tuberculous family history; a continuous slight afternoon temperature, are suspicuously indicative of the tuberculous character of the affection. If neglected, it tends to a fatal termination by localization or extention to more vital organs.

The age at which the disease is most active if existing in the female genital organs is between 20 and 30 years.

This is the period of greatest activity of these organs as well as the time of their most frequent exposure to disease. Their vitality may be lessened by accidents incident to their reproductive activity or their exposure to other forms of infection.

If the infection begins in the pelvic organs and palliative means do not suffice then we must resort to radical surgical means to cut it short and prevent its spreading to more vital organs. By this means we will remove the source of supply of the infective germs and prevent their being carried to the more remote parts of the body and being implanted where medical and surgical skill is of no avail. A carelessly cared for consumptve not only endangers those about him but continuously reinfects himeslf; new tissue is infected by the newly introduced germs; new fires are being lighted by neglect, as the old ones are extinguished by medical or surgical skill.

Surgical tuberculosis is pre-eminently a disease of the very young. If diagnosed early the firse decennium will furnish the majority of the cases; the second, one-fourth of the total number, and the balance will come after twenty years. Of all the diseases to which the negro and North American Indian have fallen heir, tuberculosis in all its forms has proven the most fatal. Years ago these two races were not as subject to the disease as the whites, but since their change of living from out-door life to the stuffy, unsanitary huts in the cities the disease is found three times more frequently than among the whites. The surgeon notes this change in these people in particular, as their generative organs are especially subject to the disease. Observing the effect of the change in the manner of living of these two races, teaches us again the importance of fresh air and sunshine.

Statistics show that the change of the Indian girl from the tent to the school room produces a noticeable increase in the disease.

The change of the peasant girl, when she comes to this country and lives the life of a domestic or a factory worker is made note of by the specialist in diseases of women in particular as her generative organs are the ones seemingly first to suffer. The tubercular bacilli is always ready and waiting to take advantage of this diseased condition and tuberculosis of the reproductive organs is the result.

Patients too frequently expect surgery or medicine to restore them to perfect health. When once disease has practically destroyed the tissue we can not hope by any human power to replace such tissue as perfectly as it was before it was diseased. Could we teach them that after this disease has become far advanced in the uterus or adnexa that they can only hope for assistance, and that it will be due to their untiring effort in following instructions given them to finally accomplish the desired results.

The surgeon may cut the disease short by the use of the knife; the medical expert may diminish its progress by the use of tuberculin; but the patient, himself, must be the principal factor in conquering the disease.

In operating on tubercular patients I am very careful to inform her of her actual condition, explaining the gravity of the disease and the importance of her observing carefully the instructions given, not only for her protection but to protect those who are compelled to be about her. Without her knowledge of the existing disease, her co-operation can not be obtained.

More depends upon our ability to instruct and the patient's willingness to make proper use of the instruction given, than to all medical nostrums at our command. It is true that medicine is very necessary when actually needed, but it is not the important factor in a cure.

Surgery must be resorted to when the condition demands it, but both medicine and surgery are too promiscously used in tubercular affections.

Well do I remember a case, a young married woman of 30 years, who had passed through six weeks of what was supposed to be typhoid fever. She was attended by one of the best internal medical diagnostitions in this country. She did not recover satisfactorily and drifted to my clinic in the East, where from the scrapings of the endometrium, examined with the microscope, a diagnosis was made of tuberculosis of the uterus. A tubal complication existed. It was decided to do a complete removal of all the internal genital organs which I did. She made an uneventful recovery, and was free from disease five years subsequent to the operation. The disease was evidently primary—not having extended to adjacent organs.

Tuberculin was used and proper hygienic and dietetic precautions taken after the operation.

I cite this case only to show how easily the disease may be overlooked in these organs, how seldom thought of by the general practitioner, and yet how important when a diagnosis is made early enough.

The disease being primary the principal distributing point was removed and a better opportunity given to check its progress.

We conclude then,

That it is our duty to protect the public from contamination with the now existing disease.

That it is our duty to prevent the marriage of tubercular people.

That our hospitals for the care of consumptives should be placed in the country.

That our babes be protected from the tubercular nurse.

That the disease of the genital organs of the young school girl be as closely watched as that of any other part of the organism.

TUBERCULIN

BY DR. CHARLES BLICKENSDERFER, SHAWNEE, OKLAHOMA.

The chief principle involved in the

Read Before the First Annual Meeting of the Oklahoma State Anti-Tubercular Association, Oklahoma City, Okla., January 10-11th, 1910.

treatment of tuberculosis is now and always will be preventive.

This is manifest from the fact that tuberculosis is caused from infection by a low grade parasite, the tubercle bacillus, such infection being made possible by conditions of lowered tissue resistance, results of various personal vices of the organism receiving the infection.

Among these may be mentioned, hereditary predisposition, which does not infer an actual communication of disease from mother to child, but the disease in the parent so affects the growth and development of tissues in the child that they are rendered fertile fields of low resistance to the specific agent, the bacillus.

Those who are thus disposed often show peculiarities of body structure, notably those in which the conformation of the chest or thorax give us the phthisical chest. In this we have a thin, long, and sometimes, stooping chest. The transverse diameter of such a chest may be of good dimensions, but the antero-posterior diameter is usually short. These individuals usually have a lowered vital resistance to the tubercule bacillus, although at times showing a high resistance to the invasions of some of the other agents of infection.

Other types of inherited predisposition are scrofula, the status lymphaticus and others who show no peculiarities of either type, yet having a condition of inherent lowered tissue resistance that is not manifest upon inspection or the ordinary means of physical examination.

There are two types of scrofula recognized; the one, phlegmatic, is the most common, with a stolid expression, thick neck and lips, coarse hair and features, muddy complexion, slow in movement and awkward in gait. The other, is sanguine, not so common, is seen most often in children, some of them beautiful, with fair, clear skin, light complexion, light silky hair, blue eyes, long silken lashes and long, slender bones. These children are precocious, graceful and subject to nervous influences.

Lymphatism, a term devised by Potain, is a condition frequent among children in which there is a strong tendency to disease of the lymphatic structures. This condition usually, but not always, exists in scrofula. These children most often have enlargement of the glands of the neck, enlarged tonsils and adenoids. They are frequently and easily invaded by the bacillus. These types may be acquired as well as inherited.

Other causes predisposing to this disease, and which are more or less related to the personality are race, age, sex, position in life and occupation. Extraneous causes are occupation, environment, habits and diseases inducing a state of lowered vitality. The most important of these are intemperance in eating and drinking, lack of sufficient food, fresh air, sunlight and cleanliness. In other words, poverty is a great factor in the production of tuberculosis.

From these facts it is easily seen that tuberculosis is a disease that can and should be treated most successfully by preventing the conditions that lead up to it. After the bacillus has effected a lodgement, it naturally follows that something should be done to cure the individual attacked, or at least, ameliorate his condition to such a state as will make his existence as comfortable as possible.

The popular idea concerning tuberculosis is, that it is essentially a disease of the lungs, (consumption) and when once contracted, cure is impossible. Nothing is farther from the truth, and lung tuberculosis is but one of many manifestations of this disease. The popular term, consumption, is no doubt due to the wasting away of tissues and vital resources of the victim, literally consuming him and rapidly reducing his body to a wasted frame of skin and bones.

The treatment of tuberculosis is rapidly approaching a degree that is wholly rational. To the medical profession there are two different reasons for treatment of diseases. One of these is based upon a knowledge of physiology, and changes effected by disease in the organism, and the physyiological and curative action of drugs. This is rational treatment.

In the other, which is known as empiricism, a drug may be used in the treatment of diseases without a clear knowledge of *how* it acts in effecting a cure, the only thing known concerning its use being, that in some way its action is curative. In tuberculosis, treated as it should be, this treatment is rational, for we know the reasons for the things we do.

One of the newer old remedies now being extensively used is tuberculin; but to better understand our reasons for employing this remedy you must know that the body in health, has several auto-protective faculties inherent in the organism, that serve, in one way or another, to destroy or throw off the many varieties of disease germs with which we are constantly assailed.

The blood of the body has three ways of resisting the invasion of bacteria or disease germs:

1st. Bacteriocidal, the power the blood has of destroying bacteria.

2nd. Antitoxic.

3rd. Phagocytic.

The last two concern us principally. What is said of the antitoxic action of the blood may as well be said of the body as a whole, and refers to a cellular action of certain and perhaps nearly all of the active cells of the body, by which is manufactured an antitoxin that in its chemical and physiological action is directly opposed to those of the toxins or poisons that are the products of bacterial activity. This phase is exemplified in diphtheria and its antitoxin.

The phagocytic action of the blood is one in which the white blood cells or phagocytes attack, devour and thus destroy the germs of disease that find lodgement in the body. There is a class of diseases that must be cured by *antitoxins,* whether introduced by design or manufactured by the body cells of the person diseased.

Another class, of which tuberculosis is a very prominent member, depends for its cures upon the proper stimulation of the phagocytes or white blood cells to the destruction of the particular bacteria in question. These phagocytes, in some instances refuse to do the work required of them, the reason for which is now quite well known. In the blood of a normal individual there is floating around little chemical bodies, which Wright has termed opsonins. The word 'opsonin is a derivation of the word opsono, which means "I cater to" or "I prepare food for."

The diseases in the phagocytic class all have opsonins peculiar to each, the function of which appears to be in some way, chemical or otherwise to satisfy the germ with which it comes in contact, after which the white blood cell attacks and destroys the germ. When there are, for any reason, an absence of opsonins in the blood, the white blood cells or phagocytes are unable to thus destroy the germs, and the function of the physician is to stimulate the production of opsonins in the patient's blood until the disease germs are destroyed or rendered powerless to continue their destructive processes.

It is well known that under ordinary conditions, an infection by a germ of this class stimulates the blood and body cells to the production of opsonins. The amount of opsonins in a patient's blood is known as his opsonic index. In reference to tuberculosis this would be his tuberculo-opsonic index. We can therefore, readily see that if an individual of average good health be infected with the tubercle bacilli, the toxins manufactured by the bacillus would stimulate the cells of the body to manufacture the tuberculo-opsonin, and the white cells would thus be enabled to destroy the bacillus, the result then being a higher resisting power to subsequent invasions of this particular germ. This condition is known as immunity, and may be natural, or acquired, partial or complete.

There are a number of tuberculins on the market differing somewhat in their methods of preparation. Their physiological action, however, is practically the same, differing only in degree.

As my personal experience has been almost altogether with that known as "Old Tuberculin," what follows will naturally refer to this preparation. 'Old tuberculin contains all of the soluble secretion products of the tubercle bacillus in a 50 per cent solution of glycerin."

The bacilli are cultivated artificially, killed by steam, their soluble secretions dissolved out and kept in the glycerin solution above mentioned.

From the foregoing it will be seen that the tubercle bacillus by the presence of its toxins or poisons in the body, stimulate the cells of the body to the secretions of opsonins, without the very objectionable presence of the germ itself. This is a very apparent advantage to the individual treated.

It has been definitely determined after many years of experimentation and research, that all animals infected with tuberculosis are acutely susceptible to exceedingly small doses of tuberculin, and respond to the same by a definite line of symptoms known as the reaction. This fact would at once suggest the usefulness of tuberculin as a diagnostic agent.

Tuberculosis is usually a focal disease, and with the exception of miliary tuberculosis, in which you have a general systemic infection, the reaction of thereapeutic doses of tuberculin would represent the physiological action—moderate reaction.

In focal tuberculosis, whether it be of the lungs, joints, glands, ovaries, testes, skin, bones or otherwise, a dose of tuberculin induces a change marked by increased leucocytosis. The cells immediately around the center of infection are intensely stimulated to the production of opsonins, antituberculin and agglutinins, accompanied by a great influx of phagocytes. Macroscopically there is congestion of this area, and more or less liquefaction of the diseased tissue with absorption of the residue. This absorption causes fever and increase of pulse and respiratory rate.

The opsonic index due to the introduction of the tuberculin at once becomes lower to be followed by a decided rise, due to the products of increased cell stimulation.

The clinical or observed symptoms of tuberculin reaction are marked by fever, increased pulse and respiratory rate, increase of cought and expectorated matter, a feeling of lassitude, pains in the muscles, loss of appetite and a sense of weariness.

These symptoms should not be induced to a marked degree by the use of tuberculin, since they are an indication of over-dosage. The same changes occur to less extent and to the increased manufacture of opsonins and other anti-bodies when the dose is kept low and within the physiologic tolerance of the patient. When overdoses are given the presence of the tuberculin, added to that of the bacilli, overpower the cells whose function is the production of opsonins, so that none is produced, and you have then the symptoms of an aggravated tuberculosis infection without any beneficial results accruing.

Physiologically the reaction is caused by the presence at the same time and in the same serum of anti-bodies—opsonins or anti-tuberculins and tuberculin. It is believed, and is no doubt true that in individuals not infected with tuberculosis there are no anti-bodies and as a result an injection of tuberculin would provoke no reaction, whereas an injection practiced upon a tubercular subject would be followed by a reaction more or less pronounced. In subjects far advanced in the disease, the body cells have been exhausted by over stimulation and are unable to produce anti-bodies. There is therefore, no reaction resulting from an injection of tuberculin. In my opinion this is the only class of tubercular subjects in which a diagnosis cannot be made by the use of tuberculin.

The physiological actions of tuberculin may then be briefly stated as follows:

1st. A stimulation of all the cells of the body capable of producing opsonins and other anti-bodies, and particularly of those cells immediately surrounding the zone of infection.

2nd. An enormous migration of phagocytes towards the zone of infection, and the subsequent destruction of great numbers of the bacilli.

3rd. The liquefaction, absorption and expectoration of tuberculosous foci, with a great increase in the number of bacilli expectorated, i. e., in pulmonary foci.

4th. There is increased cough and expectoration, the sputum being softer and more easily expelled.

5th. The temperature and with it the pulse rate is increased, the latter being increased in frequency and but little in force.

6th. There is headache, malaise, loss of appetite, wandering pains in the muscles and limbs, lassitude and increased hoarseness.

The dose of tuberculin must of necessity be small at the beginning and cautiously increased. The mistake has so often been made of giving too large and frequent dosage, coupled with too rapid increase in the size of the dose, that it seems unnecessary to again refer to it. However, upon the careful and judicious administration of this agent depends its usefulness.

The maximum dosage of Old Tuberculin should never at the beginning exceed .001 Mg. or it may with propriety be made even smaller than this, the object being to get the maximum opsonic effect with the least possible physiological disturbance.

The dose may be repeated again after an interval of three to ten days after the reaction (should there be any) has subsided. Should the patient show a proper tolerance the dose may be increased .001 Mg. and so on until complete tolerance has been established. Manufacturers are placing tuberculins on the market in serial dilutions. Mulford's Old Tuberculin is put up in 1 gm. vials of five or six serials. Two minims of No. 1 is equivalent to .001 Mg. and represents the average dose at the beginning of the treatment. I refer to this manufacturer because I have used their tuberculin products exclusively and in justice to them can say that the potency and action have always been uniform and satisfactory.

THERAPEUTICS.

One-seventh of all deaths in the world are caused directly by tuberculosis, or in other words, during a year five million people in the whole world die of this disease.

The most important feature in the treatment is an early diagnosis. Treatment instituted early in the disease will almost always result in cure. Hence, the exceeding great value of tuberculin as a means of diagnosis.

There are a number of methods employed for this purpose, the most prominent of which are:

1st. By injection of tuberculin, obtaining the reaction.

2nd. Ophthalmic reaction from local application.

3rd. Von Pirquiet's.

4th. Moro's test—O. T. & Lanolin equal pts.

They are all in the nature of a vaccination resembling in many ways that against smallpox.

Personally I prefer Von Pirquiet's method, as the reaction is seen only at the point of introduction, and is not accompanied by constitutional symptoms. Besides, this is a very delicate test. The local changes taking place in the skin tests, serve to show that opsonin producing cells are probably distributed throughout the whole of the body. Objections have been raised to Von Pirquet's test, because such a large per cent of individuals are found who are responsive to it, but when due consideration is given to the prevalence of this disease, and that in almost every building of whatsoever kind tubercle bacilli in great numbers and varying virulence are constantly found, it should excite no wonder that a large per cent of the people should suffer from a variety of tubercular infections. Tuberculosis is primarily a local disease, and large numbers are thus infected annually. Of this number a certain per cent are enabled by their natural protective powers to successfully dispose of the infection. Another class will harbor the infecting agents for a length of time, their natural resources being insufficient to completely eradicate or destroy them, though being sufficiently potent, for a time, to hold them in abeyance. Of this class a certain per cent will by their own means eventually get well, while the remainder will finally succumb to the ravages of tuberculosis in some form. There is no doubt but that this class furnishes by far the greatest number of patients afflicted with pulmonary and other forms of this disease.

Still another class furnishes us with examples of rapid advances of the disease process from quite recent infections, but this class is small. It will thus be seen, that by far, the greatest number of individuals who present themselves to us, victims of tuberculosis, are derived from a class in whom the disease has been latent for a long time, and can only be demonstrated by using tuberculin in time to prevent an actual destruction of a life.

In the treatment of tuberculosis, tuberculin, like all remedial agents, has its special fields of application. It also has its limits. It is specially adapted to all latent forms, whether it be pulmonary or otherwise.

Glandular tuberculosis, for which a great deal in the past has been done surgically, will in almost every instance, yield to the influence of the tuberculin treatment, and when we refer to this treatment, we do not wish to be understood that we countenance the neglect of other essential modes of treatment now in vogue, for without them it would be next to useless to depend upon tuberculin. Good results from this treatment can only be reasonably expected when it is combined with the open air, dietetic, hygienic and tonic treatments, the reasons for which are apparent.

Tubercular peritonitis or tuberculosis of bones, joints, beginning infections of the lung tissue, or anywhere else are almost without exception suitable subjects for this method of treatment.

All forms of tuberculosis become less and less amenable to this or any treatment as the disease progresses. In pulmonary types after cavities are formed, and especially when the infection is mixed with other forms of bacteria, exceeding great care must be used in exhibiting this remedy, for experience has shown that while some individuals may respond favorably, a large number will rapidly grow worse. It is in this class of cases that least can be expected from this remedy. However, in many instances tuberculin, when used judiciously, will prove beneficial, even curative in some of these cases.

It has been shown that in advanced pulmonary tuberculosis the tuberculo-opsonic index is usually low. This fact accounts for the violent reactions following the injection at times, of even minute doses of tuberculin. The determiantion of the opsonic index therefore, in these cases, is more imperative than in latent forms. This, however, is a complicated process, and for practical purposes among the poor, is, as a rule, not available. The absence of the opsonic index need not interfere with the treatment, since we know that a marked reaction following a dose of tuberculin is an indication that such dose was too large; that is, out of all physiologic proportion to the patient's tuberculo-opsonic index. With a knowledge of the index the dose can be more accurately determined as well as the time for its administration. A lack of this foreknowledge has compelled us to be exceedingly careful, in both size of dose and frequency of administration. It is customary with us to begin with a very small dosage at intervals of six or seven days, increasing the size of the dose, or not, according to the symptoms. We rarely give five days, more often every six days, our experience having shown that smaller doses less frequently given are better and safer than to increase either or both simply for the sake of expedition. We divide the tuberculin more frequently than once in symptoms of reaction into two classes; physiologic and pathologic. The first may not be clinically discoverable; they are an increase of cough, temperature slight, increase of expectorated material and perhaps of bacilli, lassitude and headache, etc. The second class is an exaggeration of the first, and is pathologic, because no therapeutic results ensue, the action being that of increased toxemia.

To obtain the physiologic reaction is not entirely unobjectionable, because we know that the patient's extreme tolerance so far as physiological results are concerned, has been reached, and it is good practice to keep the dose within these limits.

By knowing the tuberculo-opsonic index one can so gauge the dose that increased phagocytosis and elaboration of anti-bodies can be obtained without the manifestation of the clinical symptoms of reaction. Without a knowledge of the index a mild reaction is a sufficient and safe guide to indicate the size of the dose.

We usually begin the treatment by the injection of two minims of the first serial dilution. This is doubled in six days, and so on until twenty minims have been given at a dose. If, during this time the symptoms of reaction are prominent, the dosage is reduced to one-half the size of the dose causing the reaction. The remaining series are gone through in the same manner, the same precautions being used. After an injection of tuberculin, it is well for the patient to lie down for an hour or two.

Patients with high temperature, symptoms of hemorrhage, and with large cavities, are, if treated at all with tuberculin, kept quiet in bed and given exceedingly small doses, the results being carefully watched.

In mixed infections good results have been obtained by using conjointly, the antícocus serum indicated by the findings. Our experience has been that the good results from tuberculin treatment come slowly, the greatest obstacle being lack of intelligent co-operation of the patient, who expects and demands immediate results. With one or two exceptions our best results have not been plainly evidenced sooner than from three to six months.

There seems to be quite a diversity of opinion regarding the frequency of the administration of tuberculin. In our practice we rarely give it oftener than once in six days, often once in seven and in some cases the patient seems to gain faster while receiving the dose twice or three times per month. Children appear to require more frequent dosage than adults.

Violent reactions are to be avoided, since the vital resources of the organism are called upon to overcome them. The excretions are stimualted to the extent of an increased waste of anti-bodies, the result of tuberculin stimulation, besides other losses incident to increased heat production and waste.

Reactions are more pronounced and oftener provoked by too frequent dosage than where five or six days are allowed to elapse between them. It appears to me that the chief object to be attained is to gradually produce immunity by increasing.

phagocytosis, although there may be a class of cases whose immunity is to be gained by acquiring immunity to large and frequent doses of tuberculin. Both of these phases ultimately produce the same result, immunity to tuberculosis; and the question naturally arises, whether or not the best results cannot be obtained, in some instances, at least, by the gradual increase of the size and relative frequency of the dose

---

THE SURGICAL TREATMENT OF TUBERCULAR GLANDS

BY DR. WILLIAM T. TILLY, PRESIDENT, OKLAHOMA STATE BOARD OF MEDICAL EXAMINERS, MUSKOGEE, OKLA.

Never before in the history of medicine has a more vigorous fight been made than is being waged against the tubercle bacillus. Our vital statistics for the last few years show the number of deaths and the individuals infected through this country in such appalling numbers as to be almost inconceivable; but with a co-ordination of work from all sources, better sanitary surroundings and environment, and with a clearer knowledge of proper hygienic and mode of living, we will place the White Plague far down the list of diseases that go to make up our heavy mortality.

There is practically no organ or tissue of the human mechanism exempt from invasion by the tubercle bacillus, and next to the lung the lymph nodes are the ones most frequently invaded.

Tubercular glands or the commonly so-called scrofula among the laity, is the invasion of a lymph gland and its subsequent degeneration. No region of the lymphatic tract is exempt and all are equally susceptible, but some are more frequently invaded than others from their greater exposure to infection.

(Read before the First Annual Meeting of the Oklahoma State Anti-Tubercular Association, Oklahoma City, Oklahoma, January 10-11, 1910.)

Nearly one-third of the autopsies show that tubercular lymph nodes exist somewhere in the body. The majority of instances include the bronchial, the mesenteric and the retro-peritoneal nodes. These are not usually recognized during life. Of the surgical forms the cervical nodes come first, the axillary next followed by the inguinal. This is due to the extent of area which they drain.

The majority of cases occur during the first three decades of life but more frequently during the first. The bacillus enters through an abrasion of the skin or mucus membrane into the tissues, is taken up by the lymphatics and carried along until arrested by the first lymph gland that it encounters. In other words the membrane absorbs, the lymph vessels carry and the lymphoid material harbor the bacillus.

Dowd, of the Jenners Children's hospital in Berne, found that the throat was the most common portal of invasion, or almost 86 per cent of the cases were traced to this source. The recognition of tubercular glands in early life can not be over estimated as statistics show that in 20 per cent of tuberculosis pulmonalis, the cervical lymph nodes were the first in which the infection manifested itself. Carious teeth, fissures of the lips, ulcers of the tongue and buccal surfaces, chronic affections of the scalp, catarrhal conditions of the nares and pharnyx all allow and contribute to an infection.

An unsettled question and one of importance is whether the presence of the bacillus tuberculosis produces the inflammatory changes or whether it was engrafted upon some other micro-organism which produced the inflammation. I think the disease or inflammation may begin in both these ways. While in the majority of glands the bacteriological findings show a mixed or multiple infection, yet some cases show a purely tubercular condition and it is highly possible that in the mixed infection the later one followed the original tubercular invasion.

The glands of surgical interest are those of the neck, the axilla, and the inguinal region; owing to their relation to the deeper and more important structures. The first symptoms noticed is a simple enlargement or hypersplasia of the gland or glands; these vary in size from a pea to a marble. The node shows signs of a slight inflammation without any marked constitutional symptoms. The chronic nature of the process is probably due to the low virulence of the bacillus.

This hypersplasia may last for some time with any apparent change due to the bacillus being situated in the peripheral end of the node and in the lymph cord. The course of a tubercular gland tends to destruction by liquifaction, the degenerative process extending over a long period of time. The surgeon rarely ever sees them until they have existed for some months, or liquefaction has taken place; an abscess formed and a discharging sinus being present.

A tubercular gland may be mistaken for the glandular enlargement of Hodgkins disease in its earlier stages, syphilitic infection or sarcoma; all these conditions

showing the chronic manifestations. But the lack of the constitutional symptoms shown by the latter troubles usually lead to a correct diagnosis even before excision with its pathological findings are resorted to.

I am a firm believer in the early and complete removal of these infected glands as soon as they show signs of breaking down; I do not mean by this that all cases should be operated upon; far from it; for in children, general constitutional treatment, good hygienic surroundings, nutritious food, with fixation and complete rest to the glands involved with local applications as an adjunct will some times clean them up. For in no stage of the disease is a spontaneous cure impossible, especially in children. Yet on the other hand the chief danger in allowing a tubercular gland to remain is that the bacillus may push its way through and into the adjacent tissues and cause a great amount of damage elsewhere. When the enlargement is progressing rapidly and the inflammatory changes show the formation or presence of pus, or even in the chronic condition when an exacerbation occurs with a slight temperature; then surgical interference is indicated. In this condition with a free incision it is an easy matter to shell the glands out of the surrounding tissues but after the gland itself has broken down into a fluxuating mass the only practical thing to do is to drain freely and treat as an ordinary abscess cavity.

Yet no matter how careful the surgeon may endeavor to eradicate the foci of pus by destroying the capsule, careful curettment, and asepsis the wound some times leaks, the cavity refills, and the sinus develops which requires months to heal.

The technique of an operation for tubercular glands is based upon the location of the infection, the extent of the degenerative process, and the involvement of the surrounding tissues. Cosmetic reasons demand careful work and results in the glands of the neck, for an old leaking sac with its fistulous opening leaves a very irregular and unsightly scar. It will be frequently found that the pus comes from a suppurating gland beneath the deep fascia and that the discharge has burrowed through this and appears under the skin. So it is imperative that every nook and crevice of the cavity should be thoroughly explored for existing sinus that might lead to a deeper involvement. When found they should be opened and treated the same as the superficial focus.

In all cases where pus is found the incision should be large enough to thoroughly expose the glands involved and at the same time show the least deformity. Carefully dissect out the glands if they are intact and suture wound with drainage.

If a cavity has formed clean out very carefully, doing your work thoroughly and treat as an ordinary abscess. Where one gland only is infected, you may aspirate and inject into the cavity thus created a 5 or 10 per cent emulsion of iodoform. This with fixation to the parts will some times suffice. But careful excision of the gland or glands is much surer and more satisfactory. The cases where peritonitis exist the operation requires a more careful and delicate dissection to free the glands from the more important structures.

But taking, all in all the successful treatment of tubercular glands and the cardinal factors to bear in mind to an early termination and gratifying results, is the early excision, the building up of the patient's general condition, proper hygenic surroundings, an out-door life with plenty of sunshine, and cleanliness and regularity as to his mode of living.

MEDICAL EDUCATION OF THE PUBLIC ON TUBERCULOSIS

BY DR. J. M. POSTELLE, PRESIDENT OKLAHOMA ANTI-TUBERCULAR ASSOCIATION

War in the East, war in the West, war in the North and South, and victory will crown it all. Such is the slogan against tuberculosis. Every three minutes in the day of these good United States of America some one pays the death penalty assessed by tuberculosis. Ten times this number of death penalties are assessed each day by this same disease, but are remitted by the kind hand of medical sciences which embraces sanitation. Scientific research has made wonderful progress for the past few years in the prevention and cure of tuberculosis. The laity is becoming educated along medical lines, medicine is not looked

(*Read before the First Annual Meeting of the Oklahoma State Anti-Tubercular Association, Oklahoma City, Oklahoma, January 10-11, 1910.*)

upon by the masses as hoodism and myths as it has been in the past. The public is indebted to the medical sciences through the physicians for all our laws governing sanitation and the prevention of disease and the good done for humanity along these lines is immeasurable; however the public in the past has not accepted the doctor's efforts and judgment willingly and we have had to convince first our lawmakers who in turn by legislation has, by enacting material laws, municipal, state and national, has brought about this compulsory education of the public mind, until we are now on the threshold of a great advancement in preventative medicine. The public is waiting, their education has been brought up to the point where they are anxious to receive more and to put into action that which they have learned. The next step in the education of the public should be the compulsory study in the public schools of the county, in church and literary societies, through the public press and in every way possible to reach the public the important relationship existing between the penalties paid in the violation of material and physical laws, penalties paid for violating material laws might be termed direct, or paying when assessed by the courts, penalties paid for the violation of physical laws might be termed indirect, and paid to the doctors and undertakers with pain and death thrown in for good measure. As soon as the public mind has grasped this idea and begins to figure on an economical basis it is then that our average longevity will have been extended many years. Many of the present and prevalent ills of humanity will have been forgotten; sorrow and grief can be given wider berth; homes be made more happy; higher education better obtained, all because of the commercial value obtained by obeying physical laws. What a revelation! and it is not far distant. The relation existing between disease and the physical laws governing health are well understood and it will be only a litle time when necessary legislation will be enacted; governing and regulating the health of the individual as it is done in the protection of the health of the domestic animals. A great deal has already been done in the prevention of tubercular and other diseases in animals, the protection of which effects in a direct way our industrial economy and adds more to the commercial wealth of the nation, how much more would the nation be worth in dollars and cents if the same legislation could be made to protect the human family. The health of each individual has a commercial value, why not protect it? What is a man worth to his family and country when he is sick? Our physical infirmaties are an asset to poverty by reason of which

we are lowered in the scale of society and the commercial world. Valuable lives are blotted out, loves most sacred ideals are blasted, bereavement, sorrow and grief change places with happiness, wealth and contentment, this word picture is the realities of life, in the young, middle and old It is a natural consequence in the aged because we are born to die, in the young and middle aged such consequence to a large degree should be avoided by the proper protection of our health. It is not the office of this paper to go into detail with reference to the necessary legislation, but will say that this can be worked out step by step along economic lines, with a saving to the country of millions of dollars per year. We need detention hospitals, quarantine farms and villages where those effected with tubercular and other communicable diseases can be kept isolated and treated, we need laws governing architecture so that our homes may be safe guarded with ventilation and sunshine. Modern research in the study of tuberculosis has proven beyond any doubt that it is a preventable and curable disease, but without the necessary weapons to fight with and without the co-operation of our legislative assemblies the victory will never be won, but if the public will insist this co-operation will come at once.

Fully one-half the deaths are caused by communicable diseases and in which can be demonstrated living germs, these germs are transferred from one individual to another in various ways, some are inhaled through the air, others gain admittance to the body through the drinking water and the foods we eat and others from direct contact. All depend upon a suitable soil for their development and growth. When these germs are implanted in living tissue they at once begin to multiply. From a few hundred germs planted on a culture media in a test tube and kept at the body temperature from twenty-four to thirty-six hours millions will have developed where we only have started with hundreds. Just in this same way they grow and multiply in the human body and are passed out through the excretions of the body to reinfect some one else.

As long as our present quarantine regulations exist, the infected people not protected and their living regulated, just so long as these conditions prevail we will be surrounded with these germs and will be prone to infection.

The most tender tie to the average family is the afflicted one no matter what the affliction. If these families could be taught the importance of isolation and disinfection it would go far toward the controlling of the spread of disease germs.

Tuberculosis is the most common of all infectious diseases and almost every one are exposed to these germs, but all people do not take it for the reason that their health and mode of life produces in their blood a resistance to infective agents.

We have in our veins blood, this blood is composed of several different bodies or elements. The two distinct bodies are called cells. The office of the red cells is mainly to carry oxygen to the different parts of the body, the white cells carry nutrition throughout the body and protect the body from disease. Behind the white cells in the blood stream we have another element called opsonons. These opsonons govern the action of the white cells and lend to them nerve energy or power and our resistance to disease is measured by the power of our opsonons or the power of the white blood cells had to attack and destroy disease germs. When the germ enters the body it is absorbed into the blood and at once there is a battle set up between the white cells and the germ, if the cells have sufficient power the germs are destroyed, eaten and digested by the blood

cells, but if the opsonons are deficient the resistance of the cells are lowered, they have not the power to fight and the germs are victorious, then it is we have unmolested in our blood stream disease germs. All of these germs do not remain in the blood stream, but in their circulation through the veins they select for their lodgment tissue most suitable for their growth, and in case of a tubercular germ they have a preference for the lung. Soon after their abode is established, if it is in the lung, it is called consumption, if it is in the skin lupus, if in other tissue or bone it is called tuberculosis. Wherever the germ finds lodgment they grow and multiply in proportion to the vitality or resistance of the individual, if from good care and treatment the individual's resistance or index can be raised high enough so that the blood cells have sufficient power to keep up their warfare and overpower the germs he gets well, otherwise the disease progresses. The amount of damage done to the living body and the number of deaths is not always caused by the amount of tissue lost, but by the poisoning of the blood from toxine which is manufactured by the tubercular germ and circulates in the blood throughout the body poisoning all the nerves and tissues of the body, this excites the brain and all the forces of the body, the heat centers in the brain and all the defensive organs of the body are thrown into a state of excitement in trying to eliminate the poison, fever results and the tissue wastes under its burning influence, if from remedial agents the vital forces can be sustained; that is if the power of the opsonons can be raised, which is called raising the opsonic index of the blood a new element is manufactured in the blood stream called antitoxine. This anti-toxine neutralizes the toxines in the blood, the blood cells have the power of digesting the germs that are present and the individual gets well. This is the mode of operation in most all infectious and contagious diseases, such as smallpox, mumps, measles, etc. The opsonons or resistance of the white blood cells is raised so high that the body is forever thereafter protected from these germs and individual has the the disease but once.

Scientific research has worked out these truths so well by experimentation upon animals infected with the different disease germs that we can at a certain stage withdraw their blood, separate the serum from the cells and use it together with its increased opsonons as an anti-toxine. This antitoxine injected into the blood of the individual as in case of diphtheria hastens the action of the blood cells by its increased opsonons and neutralizing properties arrests the disease almost at once.

With the knowledge we have gained through scientific investigation we are prepared to go still farther into the sciences and deal with diseased conditions in a new light, we now know the true cause of every contagious and infectious disease, we are familiar with the habital and physical properties of most all infective agents, in fact the scientific investigator or up to now doctor knows by sight and name, nearly all pathogenic or poisonous germs and the preventative of disease or preventative medicine that the physician will become the true humanitarium, his service will be sought in time of health; his reputation for good will become famous in proportion to his skill in preventing disease; he has become a teacher of the law, physical law, and his pupils the masses of humanity; then the value of man to man will be measured not alone by his mental capabilities and personal accomplishment, but by good health in the bone and sinew as well, while his increased power will still be measured by his increased intellectualities.

HOW BOVINE TUBERCULOSIS IS TRANSMITTED TO MAN AND ITS PREVENTION

BY DR. LOUIS A TURLEY, NORMAN, OKLA., PROFSSOR OF PATHOLOGY IN THE OKLAHOMA STATE UNIVERSITY AND STATE BACTERIOLOGIST.

The transmission of bovine tuberculosis to man, so far as investigation has gone, is confined to two of the ordinary paths of infection. These are through wounds in the skin, and through the gastro-intestinal tract.

Transmission through wounds in the skin occurs almost entirely in adults and among those who handle cattle or raw meat. Such persons as butchers, both those who slaughter animals and those who serve customers in meat markets, and cooks, veterinary surgeons and men employed on cattle cars, in cleaning cattle cars, or in stock yards. When infection by bovine tubercle bacteria takes place in wounds, the result-

(Read before the Anti-Tuberculosis Association of Oklahoma.)

ing lesions are usually confined to the site of infection, or the infection extends to neighboring tissues by contiguity, and in the majority of cases induce verrucose tuberculosis or tubercular tumors. This form of tuberculosis is rarely very serious although Ravenel has reported fatal cases from accidental skin inoculation.

Bovine tuberculosis is transmitted to man through the alimentary canal by meat, milk and milk products. Ordinary meat, i, e., muscle tissue, rarely if ever contains tubercle bacilli, but it may be contaminated by being smeared with the contents of glands, or other tissues containing tubercular lesions, during the process of slaughtering or cutting up the carcas. Glands, such as kidney, liver, sweet-breads and lymphatic glands in other cuts of meats may contain tubercular lesions and if the meat is not thoroughly cooked, living tubercule bacilli will be set free in the alimentary canal.

But by far the most frequent and most dangerous means of transmission is by milk and milk products. And this is true because the diet of children, who are far more susceptible than adults to bovine tuberculosis, is largely made up of milk, especially in early childhood and because in milk the bacteria are usually surrounded by fat droplets and in this way are not acted upon by the acids in the digestive juices but are taken unharmed into the lymphatic and blood streams.

Milk may become contaminated in two ways. First, from tubercular lesions in the cows producing the milk. It was formerly believed that it was necessary for the cows to have tuberculosis of the udder in order to contaminate the milk, but Rabinowich, Kempner and others have found by experiments that 71.4 per cent of cows reacting to tuberculin, without tuberculosis of the udder, give virulent milk. The cream of tubercular cows almost always contains tubercule bacilli. And Mohler, Washburn and Rogers found that tubercle bacilli in butter and other milk products retain their virulence as long as one hundred and fifty-three days.

The second source of contamination of milk is from the skin of the cows while being milked. Cows suffering from tuberculosis eject the bacilli by coughing, sneezing and in their excreta. The tubercule bacilli ejected in this way get on the hair and udder by the cows lying down in the stalls or barn yard, or by their rubbing against the timbers about the barn or corral, or are deposited by flies which have picked them up where ejected by the cow, and are scraped into the milk by the milker. Schroeder and Cotton believe that the most fruitful source of contamination by and transmis-

sion of bovine tuberculosis through milk is from the fells of cows suffering from the disease.

To summarize: Bovine tuberculosis may be transmitted to man, first, through wounds in the skin by handling tubercular cattle and contaminated raw meat, and in cleaning cars or places where cattle have been confined. It may be transmitted through the alimentary tract by ingesting the tubercule bacilli in food stuffs such as meat, milk and milk products.

I will say in concluding this part of my paper that infection by the first means, i. e., through the skin, is confined, so far as reported, to adults, as children rarely come in contact with cattle or raw meat. But on the other hand, infection by the second means, i. e., through the alimentary tract by the ingestion of the tubercule bacilli in food, is confined largely to children. Klebs and Rievel report the case of a young man who assisted them in their experiments. He was in the habit of drinking the milk of tubercular cows used in the experiments. He contracted tuberculosis with a fatal outcome. But few other authentic cases of bovine tuberculosis in adults contracted by eating contaminated food have been reported. Dr. W. H. Park, of New York, states that 23 per cent of the fatal numbers and 17 per cent of the fatal cases of tuberculosis in children that have come under his observation have been of bovine origin and Von Bering maintains that most of the ordinary forms of tuberculosis in adults are from latent foci formed in childhood from bovine sources. This statement, while its truth is quite probable, is nevertheless speculative and unproven. But the figures of Dr. Park cannot be controverted. And whether we take the figures of the British Royal Commission that 23 per cent of the cases of tuberculosis are bovine or whether we take the conservative estimate of Dr. Theobald Smith that 1.5 per cent to

2 per cent of the cases of tuberculosis are bovine, no one would say that a cause resulting in from 2,000 to 5,600 deaths annually in the United States was to be neglected as Koch maintained.

This brings us to the second part of this paper: how may the transmission of bovine tuberculosis to the human subject be prevented? And I shall consider it from the standpoint of the paths of infection.

The prevention of skin infection naturally falls under two heads; personal precaution and public precautions. First, every one who has to handle cattle or raw meat, or who has to clean places where cattle are kept and confined should take precautions by sterilization and protection of wounds, against contamination. And any wounds received in the discharge of their functions, whether slaughtering cattle or cutting up meat or cleaning after cattle, should be thoroughly cleansed and sterilized as soon as possible.

And secondly, the authorities by laws and rigid inspection should prevent the slaughter for meat of tubercular cattle and the keeping and sale of meat from tubercular cattle. This would also remove the danger of infection through the alimentary tract from infection carrying meat.

The prevention of infection through the gastro-intestinal tract would consist of obtaining a sterile food supply especially a non-infection carrying milk. To obtain this strict laws should be made regarding dairies and these laws should be rigidly enforced. All dairy herds, and in fact all cattle, should be thoroughly inspected and all tubercular cattle, especially the dairy cows, should be slaughtered and the carcasses burned. And this process of eradication should be repeated often enough to be sure that these herds were kept free from tuberculosis. Pasteurization of milk as commercially carried out does not kill the tubercle bacilli.

Whenever a herd is found to contain a tubercular animal, the entire premises should be cleansed and disinfected.

Dairy barns and corrals should be kept immaculately clean and should be disenfected several times each year.

The sides and udders of cows should be washed at least with warm water and soap; better still with 1-10,000 Hgcl 2 solution just before milking.

The persons employed in milking should sterilize their hands just before milking and should have uniforms to wear at this time and these should be used for nothing else. These garments should be frequently laundried.

Flies from the barn or cow yard should not be allowed to come in contact with the milk, for it has been proven that flies can and do digest tubercle bacilli and excrete virulent tubercle bacilli for several days.

And lastly, no person suffering from tuberculosis should be allowed to work about a dairy nor come in contact with milk from the cow to the consumer.

These precautions may sound speculative and impossible to accomplish but they are thoroughly practical and as thoroughly effective, for in the first place, these precautions would remove the source of infection, viz., the tubercular animal, and in the second place, prevent contamination from outside sources. The measures here mentioned may be summarized in two brief statements. (1) A little extra care and very little expense on the part of the dairyman. (2) Watchfulness on the part of the authorities to see that the care is taken, and the removal by them of the cattle.

MARRIED.

On the evening of December 22nd, at the residence of the bride's parents, Captain and J. W. Everage, Grant, Oklahoma, Dr. Edwin Ayres Kelleam to Miss Ophelia Everage, both of Grant.

TUBERCULOSIS OF THE TONSIL

BY DR. J. H. BARNES, ENID, OKLA.

The tonsil is a small gland just behind and at base of the tongue between two folds of mucus membrane, called pillars of the tonsil. It is made up of several small bodies placed together something like a strawberry. Each one of these bodies are covered with a peculiar membrane, leaving a small space between each one of the small bodies which goes clear through the whole tonsil to its posterior capsule, which is a thick membrane that covers the back part of the tonsil and is attached to the anterior and the posterior pillars in front. There are eight to a dozen of these crypts as they are called and they are the part of the tonsil that becomes diseased in acute or chronic tonsillitis.

The tonsil is very abundantly supplied with blood and is the beginning of lymph channels that empty into the cervical glands as shown in the drawing, and from there into the general system.

The function of the tonsil is not known. It is supposed to be protective in childhood but how this is done we do not know. This we do know, that when the tonsil is diseased that those crypts retain a foul cheesey pus that is a menace to good health, and that the infectious material is carried directly into the lymphatic circulation.

The tonsil is subject to all kinds of infection being located as it is in the mouth where it comes in contact with everything that we eat and drink, and in those children who are mouth breathers it comes in contact with the air that they breathe, which may contain dust and dirt that is heavily laiden with the most devitalizing

(*Read before the First Annual Meeting of the Oklahoma State Anti-Tubercular Association, Oklahoma City, Oklahoma, January 10-11, 1910.*)

and destructive germs. I mention this fact because many of our children and some adults are constant mouth breathers because of some obstruction in the nasal passage, the true and proper respiratory channel.

Now while the tonsil is the seat and origin of many infectious diseases, we want to speak of only one, that is tuberculosis, more especially the result of the drainage into the glands of the neck.

Tuberculosis of the tonsil may be primary or secondary. That is the tonsil may be the first and only place of the disease in the body, or it may become involved after some other organ of the body, as the lungs or the larynx, then it is called secondary. The symptoms and the patology and the treatment are the same whether it is primary or secondary, but the prognosis is more favorable in the primary form.

The tonsil may be either large or small and the infection produces a foul, irregular ulcer that shows no tendency to heal with the most persistent treatment. There is considerable pain.

Then again the tonsil may be diseased so that it has no protective power and the tubercular bacillus be lodged in the crypts and from there be carried into the lymph glands in the neck, producing what was once called scrofula. The ulcerative form is not so bad as the effects of the absorption into the other organs.

It is a certain fact that coloring material injected into the tonsil will soon be found in the lymph channels and the lymphatic glands of the neck, and from these to the deeper glands, the bronchial, and from these to the lungs. But this is not a very frequent route of tuberculosis to the lungs, as the infection usually takes a more direct route.

The lymphatic glands are a frequent source of tubercular infection from the tonsil. In fact the diseased tonsil is always the cause of larged diseased anterior cervical glands. These glands often break down one after another till all the glands of the neck are envolved.

I want you to notice on this drawing how the infection is carried from the adenoids, the third tonsil, and the pharyngeal tonsil to these glands, and in severe infections to the posterior cervical glands.

The lymphatic glands all over the body stand guard to any infection entering the system, but like the watchman of our national armies, they often have to give up their own lives in trying to protect the body. This is always the case when such an enemy as the Koch's bacillus invades the field, for it never crosses the Rubican but once, all bridges are burned behind, and victory is theirs.

There is a way to prevent this dreaded and terrible enemy from coming down on our posterity and destroying our robust boys and girls, yes for the strong as well as the weak are attacked by this disease.

There are two things to consider in the prevention of tuberculosis in the tonsil. One is the field of infection which is the diseased tonsil, and the other is the germ that causes the disease.

The tonsil is a normal gland of the pharynx, should atrophy by the time the child has reached maturity and leave only a vestage of the old tonsil. The normal tonsil is not large and should not become diseased. They become large and diseased in those children who have adenoids, and if the adenoids are large enough to obstruct nasal breathing, the child is going to breathe through its mouth and then with the diseased tonsil constantly being in contact with contaminated air we are sure, sooner or later, to have some kind of infection of the tonsil.

Second: If the Koch bacillus is in the air you can plainly see the result. This bacillus is very light and is carried through the air on small particles of dust. Now you may ask the question how does the germ get in the air? Only one way, and that is by those who have the disease, constantly spitting on our floors and carpets, and in street cars, and on the sidewalks and other public places.

Drinking cups have been known to spread the disease. We don't know these days who have consumption. In fact autopsies demonstrate to us that many have tuberculosis who die of other disease and have never been suspected of having lung trouble. These two questions answer themselves. What to do with the field? and how can we keep the germ out of the air? To solve either one will prevent tuberculosis of the tonsil.

If the child is a mouth breather, remove the obstruction and allow it to breathe through the nose. Did you know that we would have no consumption of the lungs if we had proper breathing space and would breathe right? The respiratory apparatus begins with the nose and not the mouth. So air to be moistened, warmed and filtered must go through the nose.

If the tonsil is diseased remove it in its entirety. Don't cut them off, eneculate it and leave no part of the diseased tonsil. Then we are sure of having no infection in to the tonsil or the glands of the neck if the work is done soon enough. Then we must stop the spitting in public places and on our private floors. In many of our cities we have ordinances to prevent expectoration in public places but it is seldom enforced. There is no law to prohibit us spitting in our homes. Here is where we need to educate the people as well as the importance of proper breathing and the care of diseased tonsils.

HOW CAN WE CARE FOR THE TUBERCULAR CHILDREN OF OKLAHOMA?

BY DR. LEILA E. ANDREWS, OKLAHOMA CITY, OKLA.

There is every reason to believe that if Oklahoma really decides to wage war against tuberculosis, she will win the fight.

With her own peculiar degree of earnestness and enthusiasm, emanating as it does from the press, the doctors, the woman's clubs and the clergy, the education of the public can surely be accomplished and this question disposed of in the same manner as Oklahoma is in the habit of disposing of other matters of great importance.

It would be gratifying, indeed, to believe that from purely a humanitarian motive we expect to blot out this disease. But such will not be the case.

In our campaign for education, we must present for consideration, every side of this question; for I am sorry to say, that, knowing as we do the disregard that even our government shows in dealing with the health and lives of its constituents, we shall be obliged to appeal through that most vulnerable point, the pocket-book, before we shall expect due governmental aid.

It is a fact in economics that it pays in dollars and cents to spend money to keep people good. Good people not only cost the state nothing, but prove valuable assets to the communities in which they live. One murder costs the state enough money to build a church or library. Reasoning along this same line, it will pay this state in dollars and cents to spend money to prevent tuberculosis; for one case, prevented, will save enough money to the state to keep several thousands from becoming infected.

I wish to speak today of a class of pa-

(*Read before the First Annual Meeting of the Anti-Tuberculosis Association of Oklahoma, Oklahoma City, January* 10-11, 1910.)

tients not often considered, yet they are appealing to us just as strongly for help— tubercular children.

As we become better acquainted with the tubercle bacillus, we find it to be the cause of death in a much larger percentage of children than was formerly supposed.

The predisposition to tuberculosis is either hereditary or acquired. It is hereditary in the sense that the child inherits tissues that are more or less receptive to, and which provide a favorable material for, the development of the tubercle bacillus.

The predisposition is acquired by attacks of the various diseases resulting in a great reduction of the vitality, and in certain of the acute infectious diseases as measles, whooping cough and lagrippe. Repeated attacks of the catarrhal inflammations of the mucous membranes of the nose, throat and bronchial tubes, or of the intestinal tract, render these tissues more vulnerable.

The lesions of tuberculosis are very numerous, and in the child do not differ materially from those found in the adult. However, the ordinary chronic lesions met with in the adult are rarely seen in children. The younger the child, the more likely is tuberculosis to be located in the lung. As the child grows older, the meninges, or the covering over the brain and spinal cord, are commonly affected, and later the intestinal tract, and finally in late childhood, the bones and joints are most commonly the seat of infection.

The good we can do these little patients with the acute attacks involving lung, or the digestive tract, is very little, comparatively speaking, for the cases are very fatal; but in the losses we are now having from this class, we must, by the unnecessary sacrifice of these innocent children, use the stories of their short lives to arouse ourselves to a study of the means of prevention of the disease in the children in the future, for the only solution of the problem of treating this type, is in the prevention of it.

Let us think for a few moments of the prophylactic means we have at hand, were we to make good use of them. First, our climate, our altitude, our great number of hours of sunshine in this state give us a natural advantage decidedly conducive to health. This is our best weapon in our war of prevention.

If we understand, ourselves, and are glad of the opportunity to teach others; that milk from tubercular cows can, and does, cause intestinal tuberculosis in children and is thus responsible for a countless number of deaths of these children, if we systematically take up the education of the mothers and fathers of the state to show them that by the regular systematic inspection of cattle we can discover the infected ones, kill them, and thus control·the source of infection, therefore preventing this sacrifice of innocent children, the people of this state would surely demand that not one tubercular cow be found living in Oklahoma.

If we can present the knowledge we possess—that children who creep on the floor or who put anything available into the mouth (and where is the child who does not), are in direct danger of infection either to the lung or the digestive tract, where is the mother who would persist in wearing long dresses or dresses with trains, if she knew that the dust she carried about from hall or floor, from walk or street, was likely to be saturated with the dried sputum of a careless consumptive.

I believe that we could find that fashion could be changed, if mothers knew how their own children were in danger of being made sacrifices to its foolish demands.

How anxious parents usually are to hurry the little youngster back to school as soon as the law permits, after an attack of measles, pneumonia or lagrippe—the diseases so easy to leave fertile soil on which the tubercle bacillus thrives and grows. They should be taught the value of an abundance of fresh air, good wholesome food, sunshine, pure water, and when necessary, a short change of climate in the restoration of that little body from convalescence to its normal condition.

The state can care for these types, the most quickly fatal in children, by the prevention of the disease among them. First, by providing. a pure milk supply, clean streets, walks and alleys, with working laws against spitting in these places, a clean means of transportation and a good medical inspection of schools. Then, and by all means the most important, the education ot the residents of the state upon the necessity of these preventive measures and their value as weapons in the fight.

We have with us, in our cities, in the country, among the rich and poor, a class of tubercular children that are amenable to treatment. I speak of children suffering with tuberculosis of the bones and joints. Of all the types of the disease affecting childhood, these reward us with the best results. The most common sites are the hip joints, knees and those of the spine. How much joy and usefulness in life is denied these little patiènts by the early recognition of the handicap that is theirs throughout life!

There are several reasons why these cases should not be cared for at home. The treatment requires not only the mechanical apparatus necessary to put the joint at rest, be it hip-splint, brace or plaster jacket— but it also demands plenty of fresh air and sunshine, good food and water, regular habits, kind but firm discipline, skillful medical and surgical attention.

Real dutiful love is so often overcome·

by sympathy and pity, for it is hard indeed to have a child in a plaster cast or in bed with weights to the leg, or with an unsightly splint or brace on the body. These are therefore just the reasons why the cases should be institution cases. Children do not feel a disability or a deformity nearly so keenly if there are other children associated with similar conditions. It is easy to keep a child cheerful and happy, during the long period of treatment, for nature is slow in bone and joint work, if the child has the advantage of attention to its mental growth with the treatment to its body.

The Home for Crippled Children in Chicago was opened several years ago, and for its beginning, a very modest dwelling was used. What a blessing this has proved both to the rich and poor, for there is no difference made, and many are pay cases.

For several years the children cared for at that place were much the same as it a hospital. Some were in beds, some on crutches, some were in braces and jackets and some in little wheeled chairs.

A large play-room and play-ground with toys were provided. Later a kindergarten was established and again later there grew out of it a school as a branch of the city city schools of Chicago.

The Home for Crippled Children of Chicago has changed the feeling toward tubercular bones and joints of a countless number, from one of pessimism to one of optimism.

The doctors who have been graduated by the hundreds from the various medical schools of that city, have been enthusiasts by watching the transformation of some of these cases. A straight spine, with only so slight a deformity as to be scarcely noticeable, certainly rewards the use of a cruel-looking jacket made of plaster, even if it must be worn over a period of two years.

There is much we can do for these patients. We must provide a home for them. If we decide to build tubercular sanitaria or pavillions or even cottages it is just as urgent to care for these unnecessarily deformed and crippled children.

It is almost with shame that, a few days ago, I read in a newspaper of the appropriation of several thousands of dollars for the study of the habits of a parasite affecting the cotton plant, with a view to its extermination. The writer pointed with pride to the fact that some of the European countries were much interested in the splendid work that is being accomplished here in America in our Department of Agriculture, and that in many instances our methods of dealing with the diseases of fruit and forest trees, of field and garden plants, were being adopted abroad with glowing results.

The writer surely does not know the Germans well enough, to know that Germany regards the health and the life of her population of far greater importance than she does the health of her vegetation or of her animals.

Germany, for instance, would be a good pattern in many ways for our government, for since the cause of tuberculosis has been known, Germany has regarded it as a preventable disease and has spent thousands of dollars in preventing it, with a result that in only fifty years at the rate they are progressing now, tuberculosis will have been stamped out in Germany.

There are many forces at work in this war in our state. We have begun this fight to win. We should be proud of our State Commissioner of Charities and Corrections, she is the person for the work and is making good.

The Medical Societies, National, state and county have not only done much of the real work, but propose to take the role of teachers.

That powerful body of women, the

Women's Clubs, have been identified in the movement. These with the public and professional press, are all united as a unit in this great fight, and I have confidence enough in the efforts that shall be used, to believe that it will not be many years until Oklahoma will not only be known as the best state of the Union, but as the *first* state in which tuberculosis would not be allowed to live.

TUBERCULOSIS IN THE PUBLIC SCHOOLS FROM A MEDICAL STANDPOINT

BY DR. W. G. LITTLE, OKMULGEE, OKLAHOMA.

There occurs about one thousand deaths a year in our state, due to tuberculosis. About 75 per cent of these persons dying are under twenty-five years of age. Putting aside all consideration of the cost of caring for these, the actual expense during illness, and the deprivation of the state of their earning capacity for a life expectancy of twenty years, we still have a factor seldom counted in these graphic figures with which we pile up arguments for making a financial showing. In addition to the preceeding, we are educating a large number of persons who die just when their education is accomplished and before they have really entered on their years of usefulness.

This phase of the subject is not a popular one, neither is it a usual one. Inasmuch, however, as it is estimated there are in the United States 257,000 children, between the ages of eight and fifteen, who are actually afflicted with tuberculosis, the question should be one of vast import. With all these tubercular school children there are in the United States only eleven Open Air Tuberculosis Schools for them. These are located as follows: Three in New York City, two in Washington, and one each in Providence, Boston, Rochester, Hartford, Pittsburg and Chicago.

In Stockholm investigation showed 1.61 per cent of children actually afflicted with tuberculosis. On this basis, in our own country, about every city of the first class should have a provision for tubercular and backward children. By this means a large number would be guaranteed a recovery and a life of usefulness, and all would be rendered more comfortable. The results in the few schools so conducted amply prove this statement.

The work in this line is handicapped because of the ignorance and indifference of the laity, the lack of appreciation on the part of school men and school boards, the inefficiency of funds to institute the work, and the dearth of volunteers, where no money is forthcoming to pay trained help. The burden of all this falls on the medical fraternity, whose gift of time and trained thought and self-imposed duties requiring untiring energy in a mighty achievement, is one of the glorious heritages belonging alone to the wide awake medical men of the country. Of such as these, Kipling is writing, when he says:

"Only the Master shall praise us and only
    the Master shall blame,
And no one shall work for money, and
    no one shall work for fame,
But each for the joy of working."

But *others* should have a part in this great work, by being receptive to the teachings of the medical profession of the country in their efforts to enlighten and save; by applying for school purposes to further the interests of the child, handicapped by physical deficiences, and in helping to enact proper legislation by the election of

(*Read before First Annual Meeting of the Oklahoma State Anti-Tubercular Association, Oklahoma City, Oklahoma, January 10-11, 1910.*)

men to frame laws, who can lay aside political entanglements and 'work for the joy of the working" in their efforts to serve the people.

Many Elements: There are many elements to consider in this regard and I would call attention to some of them and trust that the matter will be of sufficient merit to find consideration at the hands of the "Committee of Plans" and also meet the approval of this body of men and women which has at heart an earnest desire to heed "the cry of the children," and enlist the energy of all in one of the most beneficent movements in our present history.

The Child: The child is one of the first considerations. I have stood in amazed wonder when parents have deliberately chosen to let their children suffer permanent and irreparable ill under the heartless, but to them very wise assertion of "Well, we will let the matter go, maybe he will outgrow the trouble." If the father's horse, worth a hundred dollars, were as sick, he would hire a horse doctor to care for him. But it is only a boy or a girl, so "we will see if he will not outgrow the trouble."

Our great United States government appropriates millions of dollars to doctor hogs and cattle, but not one dollar goes to help "mere humans." Our state, as political measures, has appropriated hundreds of thousands for its hogs and cattle, but its citizens are of so little value, being "mere humans" that nothing is done for their health. It seems inconceivable that parents will let the future happiness, well being and mental equipment of the child entrusted to their care, to be put in jeopardy, thinking they are saving a few dollars, when on other matters they are wide awake and even humane.

In all our homes and schools are children with adenoids, enlarged tonsils, throat trouble, catarrh, the effects of rickets, and with mental hebetudes. Perhaps 90 per cent of these could be relieved by the outlay of a few dollars to a wise physician, and the exercise of some care and common sense on the part of parents.

It is largely from this class that the ranks of the tuberculous are recruited. And all these years we have been trying to check the stream where it empties into the sea, instead of going to the fountain-head, and have been doing so by the silly nonsense talk of heredity and Povidence and other like imbecility. Pasteur says, "It is in the power of man to cause all germ diseases to disappear from the world." Only in these late years have we been seeking the fountain to make it sweet, and have we had physicians in a body willing to spend and be spent "for the joy of the working."

School Age: The children are all sent to school too early. To put little tots into the kindergarten, unless it is conducted in God's out of doors, is wrong. It is only a snare and delusion and a sin against the child; and often, only for the sake of relieving the home of their care for a few hours each day.

To send the child to the public schools before he is eight years old is also essentially wrong, except in instances or localities, such as the crowded slums of cities. Every child should be allowed to claim his God-given heritage of childhoods happy years in which to grow, and smile, and laugh, and frolic; with the grass, the leaves and the flowers, the sunshine and the blue sky to put blood in his veins and a mighty impulse in his heart.

The old Greek who took his pupils out across the meadows and taught them the great lessons from God's open book is yet the ideal, and in eight cities only of our great and progressive nation do they have such schools, and these are so inadequate in number that only a pitiful few of the teeming thousands needing them, can be accommodated. And those schools have to depend mostly on gifts of charity for their maintenance. Oh! shame on our servility and inhumanity!

The School: In regard to the school building; call is made on several professional departments wherein scientific knowledge is required. Dr. Evans, Health Commissioner of Chicago, says: "The sanitary engineer has earned his right to a post of honor along side of the civil engineer, the mechanical engineer and the numerous other engineering professions. But the ventilating engineer has thus far utterly failed to make good. As a proof of this let us recall the numerous shops, factories, office and public buildings of which we know, and consider the small number of ventilating systems which really ventilate."

Very few schools rooms are properly ventilated. The child, or the teacher, or both, are so thinly clad that to admit fresh air from the outside that is cool, is too cold. To open the windows is to invite the rage of the "powers that be" because it "deranges the ventilating system." The children and the school room exist for the purpose of demonstrating "ventilating systems," which must not be deranged.

Dry Sweeping: The school rooms in most places are dry swept—that is, the dust, accumulating during the day, is thoroughly dislodged and with the windows open, a part is blown out, while some of the grosser parts are removed on a dustpan. The remainder is allowed to settle in an even coating over ledges, seats and furnishings. The result is, an amount of thoroughly mixed infective material over everything, the worst kind of infection that can be introduced.

Drinking Cups: Again there is the common drinking cup to which the children of a hundred homes resort, and which furnishes water to the "clean and the unclean" alike. Using a trite present day economic term it is a "common carrier" and should be so declared by the legislature in its august deliberations.

Seating: Seats are provided. Perhaps most children would be better off were they not so favored. A certain room has seats of a certain size and the pupil must fit the seat. The desk is a certain height. A short child has his book up under his chin. The tall child drops into the droop shouldered, sprawling attitude with consequent deformity and restricted breathing capacity, and all because some alert agent of the school supply trust has bribed a few legislators or hoodwinked a school board, which board usually is devoid of members who have ever studied child needs from a mental, moral and physical standpoint.

The Remedy: There is a remedy for these conditions, and since this is a "how and why" convention, and looking for a "way to do things" a few suggestions along the proper lines will be given, with the hope they may be of value to those who are to shape the course for action in the coming months.

I. *Medical Inspection*: Medical inspection of schools should be a part of the procedure in every school, especially in cities and towns of the first class, and where it can be done by resident physicians. Until the legislature can so amend the school laws that a physician may be employed by the board at a nominal salary, I would advise that the county societies throughout the state be asked to appoint an inspector, who will give his services gratis, and that an alert man be chosen for this position, one who would do his work well.

II. *Lectures*: That lectures on Hygiene and Preventive Medicine be given regularly in the schools by a competent physician, especially lectures regarding tuberculosis. This might be a service in which teachers, pupils, and the physician might all receive an untold benefit. Such an office would require a physician who keeps himself in touch with "up to date work" in this line; and graduated from the antiquated hygiene and nonsensical writings that occur in most of the school hygienes. To this end, I would further advise that a committee of physicians be appointed whose duty it shall be to compile or write a suitable, authentic text-book on hygiene in general, and concerning tuberculosis especially, and that this committee be made a "Legislative Committee" also, to have the law enacted whereby the schools of the state would be furnished this text for general use, and where it may, if possible, be taught at times by a competent physician who would elucidate much of the general phenomena of disease that would be unsuitable for text-book work in the common schools.

III. *Exclusions* An exclusion act should be passed, not a "Chinese exclusion act," but a tuberculosis exclusion act, whereby all pupils and teachers having advanced tuberculosis, shall be excluded from the public schols, or admitted only after having had an extended and thorough course of training in caring for themselves and others properly.

IV. *Out Door Room*: An out door room should be provided in each school for pupils of this class, and for all classes of backward pupils, this room to be in charge of a competent nurse-teacher. The details of such a room and such work to be along the lines obtainable from any of the cities where the out door work is in operation.

V. *Society Work*: The organization of an Anti-Tuberculosis Society in each city school, the members to be made up of teachers and pupils. This society to meet at stated intervals, to consider the question of tuberculosis and each member to wear a litle button of artistic appearance and emblematic of the work; these buttons to be inexpensive and an obligation on each member. I believe this would be a measure of vast educational value.

VI. *Seating*: The adjustable seat and desk for all pupils in school, so that proper comfortable attitudes at study may be maintained.

VII. *Ventilation*: Open windows, out door ventilation, with proper clothing should be used as against the inefficient "patent ventilation" which does not ventilate.

VIII. *Individual Drinking Cups*: This measure I understand is to be ordered into the schools by the State Commissioner of Health as a Board of Health rule, and is a very commendable measure indeed and in keeping with the Commissioner's advanced work.

IX. *Sanitary Sweeping*: Dry sweeping of all school rooms should be prohibited absolutely. Some moist substance should be put on floors—antiseptic in nature and which would keep any dust from rising. This may be inexpensive, as sawdust and carbolic acid water, or formaldehyde water would answer.

Members of this Convention: I believe there is enough splendid and reliable material in this state to put in motion a great work for the schools, and let us all expect great things in the coming months from the interest derived here.

Dr. R. N. Donnell of Malvern, Arkansas, has located in Muskogee after a postgraduate course in Chicago.

Dr. K. D. Gossom of Custer City, County Superintendent of Public Health for Custer County, has reported a case of hook worm at Clinton, Oklahoma, to the State Board of Health.

TUBERCULAR MENINGITIS

BY DR. F. B. ERWIN, WELLSTON, OKLAHOMA.

This is a disease of the nervous system which the general practitioner sees seldom and one which is more often diagnosed improperly than almost any other disease which he meets. Yet it is not necessarily the physician's fault entirely because the symptoms, or many of them, are in common with the leading symptoms of many other diseases. Therefore it requires a very close differentiation to be able to absolutely make the diagnosis sure. And the general practitioner has a very broad field to cover to keep the leading symptoms of all diseases in mind at all times.

This disease is a form of acute tuberculosis in which the membranes of the brain and sometimes of the spinal cord, are attacked. At a certain stage of the disease an excess of cerebro-spinal fluid is secreted, on account of the inflammation, which fluid produces pressure symptoms as a secondary effect. It is sometimes called acute hydrocephalus or commonly, "water on the brain." It is a disease which is usually basilar, never purely purulent. It affects chiefly young children; has prodromata and an irregular course.

Robert Whytt, of Edinburgh, in 1768 first gave a complete description of the symptoms and called it "dropsy of the brain." The pathology became known about 1830. Papavoine showed that the morbid process consisted of deposition of tubercles in the membranes but considered the excess of fluid in the ventricles as of minor importance. Bricheteau first suggested that the condition be called tubercular meningitis.

(*Read before the First Annual Meeting of the Oklahoma State Anti-Tubercular Association, Oklahoma City, Oklahoma, January* 10-11, 1910.)

The relation between the clinical symptoms and changes found in the brain, post-mortem, are not wholly clear. It seems that early in the disease the inflammatory condition has the power to irritate the nerve elements to over activity, for in this stage considerable paralysis may be found, while only insufficient changes in the brain are demonstrated. The paralysis later on can be accounted for as due to pressure of cerebro-spinal fluid or damage to nerve centers by the inflammatory process.

However, on examination of the brain, post-mortem, two distinct conditions are shown. One is the deposition of miliary tubercules in minute gray dots, sometimes difficult to see, or if caseating, then opaque and yellowish in color. The other, is an inflammatory exudation. Sometimes miliary tubercules are plentiful, and lymph scarce and vise versa.

The surface of the brain is injected or engorged. The most pronounced cases are basilar. When the base is affected the effusion is found chiefly in the triangular space bounded by the cruri cerebri and optic tracts. It may also be found on the ventral surface of the pons and medulla as well as along the fissure of sylvius and may also extend down the spinal meninges.

The miliary tubercles are usually most pronounced along the course of blood vessels. Small hemorrhages may occur in the pia and brain.

The rigidity of the muscles is due to irritation of the cortex, crus, pons, medulla or maybe spinal cord. Affection of the cranial nerves is due either to irritation or destruction by inflammatory processes at the base of the brain. The face and tongue symptoms may be due to a cortical lesion and such lesion be accountable for irregularity of pupils of the eyes and strabismus.

Tubercular meningitis occurs chiefly between the ages of two and ten years. Males are more susceptible than females.

As this disease is nearly always found in some other part of the body, pre-existing, it is carried to the meninges by the the blood and lymph vessels, when so found.

The indirect cause which possibly stands pre-eminent is tuberculosis in other portions of the body, as—lungs, liver, pleura, intestines, kidneys, bronchial, or mesenteric glands, bones and joints. The most direct cause probably is traumatism; then comes hereditary tendencies, impure air, unwholesome or insufficient food, lack of exercise, and acute diseases as—diarrhoea, enteric fever, whooping cough, bronche-pneumonia and measles. It is practically unknown before six months and in advanced years.

There are four stages of this disease, namely: premonitory, exciting, depressant and comatose. The premonitory symptoms may last for two or three weeks or longer or more. About the first thing which is noticed is, that the child is easily irritated in play, becomes fretful, wakeful at nights, somewhat emaciated, slight headaches, some vomiting, disorder of the digestive system, slowness and irregularity of pulse, giddiness, squinting or drowsiness.

Then comes the first stage which is probably ushered in by convulsions or severe vomiting. Then comes general irritability, temperature begins low in the morning gradually rising in the evening until it reaches 103° F., severe pain in the head which is paroxysmal and most constant in children but some times absent in adults, bowels are constipated, hyperesthesia of all senses, squinting or double vision. The mental faculties are clear at first but gradually become dull, pupils usually contracted, pulse quick which gradual-ly becomes slow, later irregular, respirations are rarely alterated.

Child gradually passes from this irritated stage to restful or depressant stage. This condition is due as a rule to the pressure of the effusion on the brain. The fever abates, irritability is replaced by apathy, vomiting ceases, sleeps continuously but can be aroused for medicine or nourishment, breathing becomes irregular and often assumes the Cheyne-Stokes variety, the sharp cry or hydrocephalic cry, head slightly retracted, *tache cerebrale*, boat shaped abdomen, immobility of the pupil or eye-ball. The ophthalmascope may reveal optic neuritis, pupils equally or unequally dilated, bowels incontinent. Gradually the child passes from the depressant stage to that of a comatose condition. Convulsions are frequent, temperature is higher but irregular, coma is profound, unable to arouse the patient, pupils dilated unequally and react little if any to light, paralysis becomes pronounced if present.

Some times a day or two before death there is a seeming general improvement, but the pulse does not share in this improvement.

The symptoms which I have given are of a typical case of tubercular meningitis in children. Seldom, if ever, do we find all these symptoms well marked in any one case, but there are a few cardinal symptoms which are always found in a true case of tubercular meningitis. There are severe headaches, which do not cease as delirium comes on, projectile vomiting, hydrocephalic cry (this is a sharp piercing cry which the child gives at irregular intervals without any apparent cause) and constipation.

The symptoms in adults are similar to those in children with few exceptions. The delirium is more pronounced and comes on earlier, generally convulsions are uncommon, sometimes marked paralysis is the first symptoms, emaciation, to any marked extent in adults does not occur except in some pre-existing disease.

This disease is frequently confounded with acute bronchitis, acute non-tubercular meningitis. In tubercular meningitis headache presists when delirium comes on, while in general diseases it ceases. On account of the cerebral and digestive symptoms it is frequently diagnosed as typhoid fever. Widal's test will differentiate in this case; otitis in children sometimes is hard to distinguish. In tumors paralysis develop gradually while in tubercular meningitis, suddenly. However, the presence of optic neuritis, limited convulsions or paralysis point to cerebral lesions.

The prognosis is always grave, there should always be taken into consideration the liability of mistaken diagnosis. Early coma is very grave; if three weeks pass without loss of consciousness the chances of ultimate recovery are improved. A few cases of recovery have been reported, yet there might be a doubt expressed as to the true diagnosis.

The diagnosis depends upon hereditary history, age, existence of tuberculosis in any portion of the body, and prodromata. It requires a very close differentiation to make the diagnosis absolute. If drowsiness, headache, vomiting and constipation are found following a week or more of malaise or petulance, then the diagnosis can be almost certain. Also if the tuber-

cle is found ni the retina or tubercular bacillus is found in the spinal fluid then it is certain.

As to the treatment not much can be said as to the curative side. The best is the preventive. In all tubercular conditions the best is the hygienic side as is demonstrated by all the societies and organizations who have been or are engaged in the work. In the first place as this is a disease of childhood, all mothers should notice any of the above named prodromal symptoms and at the first appearance of any of them they should take their children at once to a competent physician as to the best course to pursue. Better to err a half dozen times in taking them too early as to err on the other side and wait till too late. The treatment in general is symptomatic. Hygienic, good nourishment, hot water treatment, keep bowels well cleansed, kidneys free and quiet. Tuberculin may be tried as well as many other remedies. While there are many other suggested remedies yet none have proven a success so that the treatment for cure are theoretical, not demonstrated. We, as physicians, hope that in the near future, when we meet a case of tubercular meningitis to say to the patient or relatives as we do in many other diseases that we have a cure for them instead of standing patiently by and calmly await the fatal results which are most sure to follow.

GOVERNMENT SUPERVISION OF TUBERCULOSIS

BY DR. G. S. BARGER, WAYNE, OKLA.

It is not my object in this paper to go into the scientific part of tuberculosis; that I leave to others. Neither do I claim these

(Read before First Annual Meeting of the Oklahoma State Anti-Tubercular Association, Oklahoma City, Oklahoma, January 10-11, 1910.)

suggestions as perfection even along this line, only submit it for thought and comparison, and, if possible, create some interest in government supervision of tubercular patients.

We all know and must admit beyond a doubt, that tuberculosis is contagious, that being associated with it we subject ourselves to its dangers. We also know that the more crowded and unsanitary the conditions and the greater the poverty the worse the ravages, and more widely spread the disease.

Now, this being the case, why not begin at the fountain head of this great malady and there try and check the spread, instead of trying to cure the great ocean waves of suffering after the overflow of contagion?

Take the crowded districts of the East and the cities, see there families where one by one they succumb to the disease until almost the entire family have died, then you will see occasionally one who will suffer for years perhaps, sowing broadcast the germs to be picked up by the innocent and in turn scattered again. So goes the endless chain of contagion with death, poverty and woe following in its wake.

Why can we not with the great interest that is now being taken in the eradication of this great plague, create an interest on the part of our government? Let us make a united effort along this line and see the great good that can be accomplished. Let us hand down to posterity that which will ennoble our human race, good health.

The strength of our government depends upon the people that constitute it and if we are weaklings from any constitutional cause, our government will retrograde. So let our first aim be for the betterment of our human race.

My plan for the eradication of tuberculosis is isolation. Now how may this be accomplished? My plan I believe is simple and would be to a great degree if not entirely effective, and that is to have the government build sanitariums in the West and Southwest where there is plenty of sunshine and pure air, build irrigation dams, set apart some of the vast deserts of the West and Southwest and there colonize the tubercular suffering.

Now this may seem expensive to our government, and no doubt does as it is for human beings, but if it was for hog cholera or ticks on the longhorns, it would be but a small item. This only goes to show the knowledge of the average legislator of this terrible disease.

But let us compare for awhile and see if it is costly. Let us compare it to the vast and worthless expenditure "so far as the public is concerned," of the cost of the Philippine islands and the Panama canal. The Philippians have cost up to date $800,-000,000. The Panama canal will when completed cost about $350,000,000. The two you see is $1,150,000,000. The Roosevelt dam in Arizona will when complete cost $8,000,000, and will irrigate 160,000 acres of land. Spend one-fifth of this large sum for irrigation and you will have 230 of these large irrigation projects the size of the Roosevelt and provide homes for 9,000,000 people, to say nothing of the towns and cities that would spring up, of men of different occupations and trades.

Then spend another $1,000,000 building sanitariums and you have left for maintaining them $921,000,000.

This is of course much more than would be necessary, but I only make this comparison to show how grossly the government is neglecting the people for the dollar, and how needlessly and willingly the government has and is spending large sums and yet our people needlessly dying by the thousands each year.

Let us make a bloodless war, let us average disease as well as insult, let us direct the attention of our government to the great and everlasting good that could be done.

There is not a physician who has practiced his profession long who has not been called to administer to the suffering of this class of patients, and your hearts have been filled with sorrow when you think of the good possible to accomplish and yet it is not available.

With the great variation of climate from Colorado to California you can have any climate you desire if you have the money, and with the government supporting you know this difficulty has been overcome and instead of people being sent far away from home with but little means, as often occurs, or left to suffer and die at home under unfavorable conditions, spreading the disease, they could go away feeling that they were sure of the necessaries of life, and for they that have the money let them have luxuries according to their wish.

To exile may seem cruel, but to bury our friends at the prime of life is sad; so let us give to the suffering the greatest care possible, and to the non-suffering the greatest protection possible. It is easier to prevent than cure.

God has done all things well, he gave us the snow covered mountains, the fertile valleys, the days of sunshine and pure air, of the great Southwest and it is for a purpose. Let us utilize it as He has intended, let us convert it into a vast garden, and instead of death, penury and woe, let there be life, beauty, and joy.

EDITORIAL

THE OKLAHOMA STATE ANTI-TUBERCULAR ASSOCIATION.

The above association, which is destined to be the greatest factor in the prevention, treatment and control of tuberculosis and of incalculable benefit to the dissemination of knowledge to all classes on the subject; perfected an organization at its first annual meeting held in Oklahoma City January 10th and 11th, 1910; pursuant to a call issued by Drs. H. M. Williams, Wellston, J. M. Postelle, Oklahoma City, and R. H. Harper, Afton, a committee appointed at the May meeting of the Oklahoma State Medical Association to co-operate with the state health authorities and civic bodies looking toward the intelligent control of tuberculosis, and Dr. J. C. Mahr, State Commissioner of Health, Oklahoma City.

The Federated Association of Women's Clubs was represented by Mrs. Nina Hill Johns, of Chickasha; the state officially, by Miss Kate Barnard, Commissioner of Charities for Oklahoma; the State University by Professor L. A. Turley, Norman, and

the medical profession by physicians from the state generally.

The attendance was not as large as it should have been considering the importance of the meeting and its object.

Many papers were read which will appear in the Journal of this date and the various phases of tuberculosis were given extended attention by various medical and lay writers.

A permanent organization was perfected with the following officers elected:

President, J. M. Postelle, Oklahoma City.

Secretary-Treasurer, Mrs. Ed F. Johns, Chickasha.

A Vice President from each Congressional District: First, E. O. Barker, Guthrie; Second, Rev. M. D. Reed, Weatherford; Third, Mrs. Geo. M. Ransom, Muskogee; Fourth, Mrs. G. W. Phillips, Pauls Valley; Fifth, W. C. Bradford, Shawnee.

An Executive Board was selected as follows: J. H. Barnes, Enid; O. K. Benedict, Oklahoma City; Mrs. W. G. Little, Okmulgee; Sydney Suggs, Ardmore; Rev. Thomas H. Harper, Chas. L. Doer, Miss

Kate Barnard. Governor Chas. N. Haskell and Honorable Bill Cross were elected honorary members of the association.

It is contemplated that there will be organized at once in each county in the state an auxiliary body which will work in conjunction with the parent organization.

The National Tuberculosis Association was present with their striking display on tuberculosis. The display called for the closest inspection from all attendants. Practically every sanitarium in the United States is given space in this display and many of the special features used in various institutions for the treatment and prevention of tuberculosis were shown.

The association starts out with a great purpose before them and the earnestness displayed at the organization augurs well for it.

That the Oklahoma State Medical Association as an organization and its members individually will support it in every way is not doubted.

THE LITTLE EDITOR.

An irate physician, one known personally to the editor as an able and conscientious one, sent a clipping recently to the Journal from the editorial columns of the Vinita (Oklahoma) Leader, in which the director of the department of health and charities in Philadelphia claimed that many physicians in that city purposely prolonged cases of diphtheria in order to charge for more visits and suggests that an alleged custom from that most highly enlightened land, China, be adopted, where it is said fees are paid only so long as the patient is well.

Ordinarily such a mean little squib would be unnoticed, but bearing in mind the nature of this issue of the Journal one cannot help but call attention to the falsity of the article and prove it by a comparison of its spirit and the movements of the last sixty days of the medical profession in Oklahoma.

The pen, paper, press; in fact everything in connection with the little editorial was made, marketed and used subject to patent regulations. Is the public charged any great sum for the vaccination that protects it from smallpox? For the antitoxin that saves an infant's life? For any of the thousand and one improvements in medical and surgical treatment? No; it is freely given over to the saving of life, often without hope of reward.

It is fitting that some notice be taken in this particular issue of such a matter, even if it is small and otherwise not worthy of notice, but when you remember that every advancement of medicine is surely limiting the field of work and income of the physician, and that such advancement comes only through the labor of the physician himself and his unselfishly handing it over to the world, then one concludes that the spirit criticising such a profession is small; too small entirely to notice.

THE LAITY AND THE PROFESSION A UNIT ON TUBERCULAR QUESTIONS.

The Oklahoma City meeting of the State Anti-Tubercular Association developed one gratifying fact and that is that the laity who think of such matters are a unit with the profession of medicine in their efforts to devise ways and means for the suppression of tuberculosis.

The papers and opinions delivered at this meeting appear elsewhere in this Journal and the thought given the subject by the contributors evidences their deep interest in it.

Medical thought today is rapidly being focussed on the idea of prevention. It is a reasonable proposition to say that it is better to prevent disease than to have it and rely on treatment afterward for its control. A large percentage of our present day affections are preventable ones and tuberculosis is one of them. The treatment of this disease is necessarily prolonged, the outcome doubtful and in any event it is costly from the standpoint of money and time; requiring practically sole attention to that and no other affair of life for its control. Many people are not in position to undergo treatment of the disease and to such prevention should appeal especially.

The train of evils following tuberculosis, social, financial and economical should cause every thinking man to devote some of his brains and energy to prevention.

Naturally it is among the uneducated and unthinking that its ravages are greatest, it is however, surprising to become aware of the apathy and ignorance among the more intelligent regarding the trouble.

This organization starts out right. It proposes to put before the public its condensed and accumulated information and to demand of the people who must necessarily assist in their co-operation.

ONE WAY TO GET CONSIDERATION.

Having requested the prosecution of Woody Grissom on the ground that he was practicing medicine without a license and deeming that the case was so handled by the county attorney that conviction was not had the Hughes County Medical Society adopted and published in the local paper a resolution condemning County Attorney W. P. Langston for "perpetuating and permitting such a fraud on the people, society and the laws of the state."

We venture the opinion that the next time Hughes County Society wants something done that it will not have as much cause to complain.

Physicians are great at getting together, resoluting, condemning and then letting the matter drop. When they begin to go right to the people with their troubles their cause will be sustained. From many counties in the state comes the complaint that county attorneys will not prosecute violations of many of the medical laws on the ground, usually, that no funds are provided for such prosecutions. We believe that these cases are of more importance to the body politic than the prosecution and conviction of an occasional ilicit vendor of liquors or some other petty criminal.

The county societies of the state should uniformly demand the enforcement of the law. The medical profession is one of this state's strongest assets. It supports the laws in the payment of taxes and from a moral standpoint and its demands for enforcement should be heeded.

BOOK REVIEWS

An acknowledgment of books received will be made on their receipt; their review will follow when time is found for the work.—Editor.

A TEXT-BOOK OF THE PRACTICE OF MEDICINE.
Ninth Revised Edition.

A Text-Book of the Practice of Medicine, by James M. Anders, M. D., Ph. D., L. L. D., Professor of the Theory and Practice of Medicine and of Clinical Medicine, Medico-Chirurgical College, Philadelphia.

Ninth revised edition, octavo of 1,326 pages, fully illustrated. W. B. Saunders Company, 1909. Cloth, $5.50 net; half Morocco, $7.00 net.

THE PRACTICE OF GYNECOLOGY.
New (4th) Edition, Thoroughly Revised.

A Text-Book on the Practice of Gynecology. For Practitioners and Students, by W. Easterly Ashton, M. D., L. L. D., Professor of Gynecology in the Medico-Chirurgical College of Philadelphia. Fourth edition, thoroughly revised. Octavo of 1,099 pages, 1,058 original line drawings. W. B. Saunders Company, 1909. Cloth, $6.50 net; half Morocco, $8.00 net.

PRACTICAL STUDY OF MALARIA.

A Practical Study of Malaria, by William H. Deaderick, M. D., member American Society of Tropical Medicine; Fellow London Society of Tropical Medicine and Hygiene. Octavo of 402 pages, illustrated. W. B. Saunders Company, 1909. Cloth, $4.50 net half morocco, $6.00 net.

EXAMINATION OF THE URINE.
The New (2nd) Edition.

Examination of the Urine: a Manual for Students and Practitioners, by G. A. De-Santos Saxe, M. D., Intructor in Genito-Urinary Surgery, New York Post-Graduate Medical School and Hospital. Second edition enlarged and reset. 12 mo. of 448 pages, illustrated. W. B. Saunders Company, 1909. Cloth, $1.75 net.

W. B. Saunders Company, Philadelphia and London.

The Committee on Tuberculosis of the State Medical Association wishes to thank all who contributed to the recent meeting in Oklahoma City, at which time a State Anti-Tubercular organization was formed.

H. M. WILLIAMS,
Chairman Committee.

| PERSONAL MENTION. |

Dr. G. Griffin, Resident Physician for the Norman Insane Hospital, and Dr. Walter Hardy of Ardmore, Oklahoma, have both reported cases of pellagra to the State Board of Health.

Dr. D. C. Gamble will change his location from Alva to the County Seat of Cimarron County, Oklahoma, the first of the year.

Dr. M. M. DeArman, Mangum, President of the Greer County Medical Society, was operated on for appendicitis January 6th by Dr. McFerrin, of Childress, Tex.

Dr. Francis B. Fite, Muskogee, is attending the clinics in Baltimore.

FOR SALE.

A 1909 Model "Gleason" K. C. Car, four passenger, 16 H. P., good clearance. In first class condition. Reason for selling, want to buy a larger car. Guaranteed to be all right and will sell at a bargain, if sold within the next thirty days. Don't write unless you mean business. Address

DOCTOR,
Box 44, Holdenville, Okla.

FOR SALE.

$1,250 cash gets property consisting of three-room dwelling house, barn, stables, pair of horses, good buggy, office furniture and fixtures; $4,000.00 practice gratis; will introduce. Reason for selling going to specialize in Texas. Address Dr. John T. Vick, Fort Towson, Oklahoma.

FOR SALE.

The Journal has tuition to the amount of forty-four dollars in the New York Polyclinic School and Hospital which will be sold at a reduction from the usual rates. Address The Journal.

ENTERONOL.

The Journal A. M. A., November 20, states that it has received a circular from The Enteronol company offering to take a fourth or half page advertisement in The Journal for the year at the regular rate if payment will be accepted in stock at par, or in the product itself, and saying that a number of medical journals had accepted the proposition. It mentions the journals of which it has record that they print the enteronol advertisement, saying that it might be inferred that they are being paid with enteronol stock or the nostrum itself, as proposed in the circular sent. It adds "as we have previously shown, however, the veracity of the enteronol advertising matter is by no means unimpeachable." Enteronol was exposed by The Journal, March 12, 1908, and its extravagant claims refuted. The formula given is understandable, with the exception of one ingredient "Latalia rad.," which is unfindable and unknown to experts. The first analysis made also failed to disclose a trace of bismuth subnitrate or caffein which are also included in the formula published in the literature, but did find that the tablets contained an amount of iluminum oxid corresponding to over twenty-five per cent of crystalized alum which is not even hinted at in the formula given. Attention is called to the curious discrepancy between the formula as printed on the label and that given in the literature. The Food and Drug Act, it will be remembered, makes lying on the label illegal and therefore dangerous but it does not control statements made in the advertising matter that does not accompany the product. On the label the formula does not contain "Latalia rad.," the marvelous Himalayan plant ingredient on which so much stress has been laid, and the label further shows that opium is an ingredient, about which the literature is curiously silent. The Journal asks why this discrepancy and implies that the answer might be interesting. For the purpose of determining how nearly the product as it is now sold compares with statements on the labels, another analysis of enteronol was made in the Association's laboratory. The absence of caffein and bismuth—in appreciable quantities—was again demonstrated. We are told that at present the Enteronol company manufactures two products: a castor oil preparation known as fig-ol and enteronol; very shortly, however, the company expects to "add seven equally efficient products." Other quotations are, "The average cost to manufacture, ready to ship, a dollar's worth of these goods is less than ten cents." "In enteronol alone, the company has fortunes and the only thing needed to bring tremendous results and dividends of 100 per cent. is the proper amount of judicious advertising." We are told elsewhere that about four-fifths of the outstanding stock is held by the medical profession alone. The Journal adds that we are sometimes in danger of being too optimistic in regard to the results of the propaganda for reform in proprietory medicines.

STANDING COMMITTEES OKLAHOMA STATE MEDICAL ASSOCIATION.

Public Policy and Legislation—Dr. David A. Myers, Chairman, Lawton; J. H. Scott, Shawnee; J. A. Hatchett, El Reno; F. S. Clinton, Tulsa; Claude A. Thompson, Muskogee.

On Medical Education—Drs. B. J. Vance, Checotah; A. K. West, Oklahoma City; E. O. Barker, Guthrie.

On Scientific Work—Drs. Floyd E. Waterfield, Holdenville; P. A. Smithe, Enid; Claude A. Thompson, Muskogee.

On Necrology—Drs. C. S. Bobo, Norman; H. M. Williams, Wellston; M. A. Warhurst, Remus.

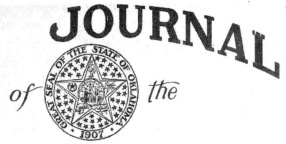

THE JOURNAL of the

Oklahoma State Medical Association.

VOL. II.	MUSKOGEE, OKLAHOMA, MARCH, 1910.	NO. 10.

DR. CLAUDE A. THOMPSON, Editor-in-Chief.

ASSOCIATE EDITORS AND COUNCILLORS.

DR. J. A. WALKER, Shawnee.
DR. CHARLES R. HUME, Anadarko.
DR. F. R. SUTTON, Bartlesville.
DR. G. W. ROBERTSON, Dustin.

DR. JOHN W. DUKE, Guthrie.
DR. A. B. FAIR, Frederick.
DR. W. G. BLAKE, Tahlequah.
DR. H. P. WILSON, Wynnewood.

DR. J. S. FULTON, Atoka.

Entered at the Postoffice at Muskogee, Oklahoma, as second class mail matter, June, 1909.

This is the Official Journal of the Oklahoma State Medical Association All communications should be addressed to the Journal of the Oklahoma State Medical Association, English Block, Muskogee, Oklahoma.

THE SURGICAL ROLE OF THE PNEUMOCOCCUS

BY A. L. BLESH, M. D., HORACE REED, M. D., AND C. E. LEE, M. D., OKLAHOMA CITY, OKLA.

In the evolution of the germ theory of disease causation, the idea that a specific germ is the sole cause or etiologic factor in a given disease, obtained a fixed hold of the professional mind. That a given germ manifests a predilection for certain organs is true but this is not the extent of the truth. The simplicity of this belief was fascinating and even yet some of us are loath to let go of it. It is true that as our

(Read in part before the Jefferson County, Okla., and the Marshall County Medical Societies, and in full before the Medical Association of the Southwest, at San Antonio, Tex.. Nov. 9-11, 1909.)

understanding of natural phenomena enlarges we are often amazed at the simplicity of nature's methods, which at first seem so very complex and mysterious. But we often misinterpret this simplicity and always in the direction away from the real largeness of it. The simplicity of nature is always a comprehensive one. In approaching it we are obliged to reason from effect to cause and so, frequently in following a single ray of light leading from the illuminated center, we mistakenly believe that this one ray which leads us to the blazing central truth, is the only ray eminating from it. After our eyes become accustomed to the light we marvel at the fact that other rays innumerable are issuing from the same illuminating source. Then the largeness of nature's simple directness dawns upon us.

The pneumococcus (1) has been so long associated with the pathological process known as pneumonia that the mention of the one instantly calls up a mental picture of the other. To many of us the fact that it has any pathological affinity for any other organs, comes to our minds as a surprise.

Outside of the relation it bears to the lungs in pneumonia, the literature of it is not plethoric.

That it is a surgical factor of no little importance, will be the endeavor of this short paper to demonstrate. We are convinced that many operations have been performed in the past in which this germ has been the determining surgical factor but in which it was not so recognized by the surgeon.

For convenience of description we will consider the organs seriatim which may be and frequently are infected with it and in which it gives rise to its peculiar pathology for, be it constantly borne in mind that the pathologic processes it occasions are the same wherever it may be situated, modified only by the peculiar histologic formation and physiology of the tissue itself.   •

That the pneumococcus is closely related by family ties to the genera of cocci, or pus producing organisms, is well known to the bacteriologist in special and to the profession in general. So here at once its surgical aspect becomes manifest.

THE PLEURA.

Empyema as a secondary complication of pneumonia, is a surgical phase of pneumococcic infection familiar to all. The surgical treatment of it is likewise familiar

so by the mere mentioning of it we will pass it.

THE PERITONEUM.

That the peritoneum is susceptible to a pneumococcus infection is not so generally known. In a paper read before the May, 1909, meeting of the Oklahoma State Medical Association we read a paper in which we briefly and incidentaly reported a case of pneumococcic peritonitis. This case we will again later in this paper, use for the purpose of illustration.

The pneumococcus is found, according to Sternberg, in a large percentage of the mouths of normal persons. Their number and virulence is increased during an attack of pulmonary pneumonia. In children it is usual that the expectorate is swallowed after being raised from the lungs to the mouth. Digestive processes are disturbed by the large quantities of mucus alive with bacteria, thus thrown into the digestive tract, as well as by the high temperature and toxemia incident to the disease. Thus the natural antiseptic action of the digestive ferments is put out of commission and the bacteria laden mucus is passed along the tube from mouth to anus. Jensen (1) has frequently found the pneumococcus in the feces of patients suffering from pneumonia.

Pneumococcic peritonitis is more frequent in children than in adults.

A rational interpretation of these facts would lead us to believe that the most frequent source of infection should be considered to be the intestinal tract. Again we know that there are natural points of weakness along this tract, where, in the evolutionary process taking place, nature has, in a fashion, let the bars down so to speak. These weak points are the appendix (an organ undergoing evolution-elimination), the gall bladder and pyloric re-

---

1. In this paper we refer simply to the pneumococcus of Frankel.

1. Archives f. Klin. Chirurgie (Langenbeck) Berlin, Vol. 70, No. 1, page 526.

gions. Later we shall cite two cases briefly, illustrating the appendix as the source of infection, the one showing the infection well advanced to a diffuse peritonitis which was localized by treatment, the other showing the infection as yet limited to the appendix.

Knowing that a pneumococcic bacteremia (1) is common, we must also consider the blood as a possible source of infection but probably an uncommon one. If the infection is hematic its localization would probably be determined as is most hematic infections, by trauma.

Pneumococcic peritonitis may be localized or diffuse. Owing to the tendency to fibrinous exudation characteristic of this germ, the localized form is the most common. The mortality rate from the diffuse type is very high, Von Roos (2) giving it in a series of his own cases as 77 per cent.

The weight of opinion consequently is for late operation, preceded by efforts directed toward localization. This is accomplished by the same treatment as in the ordinary diffuse form of the disease.

Case. G. G. Hosp. No. 1108, Aet. 11, family history negative.

Personal History: Negative except that she had always been a delicate child and had had the ordinary exanthems of childhood with a good recovery.

About one month before the present attack she had had a light attack of pneumonia with characteristic sputum. From this attack she was sick about ten days but made an apparently good recovery.

Present Trouble: Began one week ago. Pain at first general over the abdomen and the lower part of the chest, localizing after a few days over the appendix. Nausea and vomiting were present. Temperature touching 101. Great tenderness and rigidity of

1. Rosenow, J. A. M. A., Vol. 49, pp. 1799.
2. Archiv. f. Kinderheilkunde, Stuttgart, Vol. 46.

musculature, especially over the appendiceal region.

Physical Examination: Blonde girl, weight 60 pounds, pulse 130, temperature 102. Examination negative except for the abdomen which is tympanitic, sensitive to pressure, rigidity general with an especial hardness over the appendiceal region.

Diagnosis: Diffuse peritonitis.

Treatment: Usual localizing treatment. This was continued for two days with the result of a well defined localization about the region of the appendix. Operation at this time resulted in the evacuation of a large quantity of flocculent pus resembling the pus of an empyema.

Microscopic Findings: Pneumococci in almost pure culture. Patient died two days after operation from an acute endo- and peri-carditis.

This case demonstrates two things quite clearly, viz: 1st. The route of infection by the appendix, and 2nd, the tendency to metastatic infection. In this case the heart being involved and was responsible for the fatal termination. At the time of the death the abdomen was soft and comparatively flat.

Case II. Aet. 7, Hosp. No. 643.

Family History: Tuberculosis but no nearer than maternal grandmother. Paternal grandmother died of carcinoma of the uterus.

Personal History: As a little child had chronic bowel trouble from which a good recovery was finally made. Exanthems of childhood were all well recovered from.

Present Illness: Began ten days ago with vomiting and loose bowels for which he was treated by a physician. One week later another physician was called and found pain and soreness and rigidity over McBurney's point, nausea and vomiting, temperature 100-102, pulse 100-120.

A few days later the writer was called in consultation and verified the above findings and confirmed the diagnosis of acute appendicitis and agreed with the recommendation for immediate operation.

Operation: Usual incision for appendix which was found acutely inflamed but contained no pure pus but a muco-purulent substance. Wound closed without drainage. Within twenty-four hours of the operation a frank pneumonia of the right lung appeared, followed very soon by free pus expectoration.

Microscopic examination of the appendix showed an almost pure pneumococci culture in the contents, a few communis coli were present. The pneumococci were also found in the pus from the lung. The patient made a prompt operative recovery but a tedious one from the lung disease.

A study of this case shows two things very clearly: 1st. The appendix in an active stage of infection, the free peritoneal cavity not yet involved and the appendix as in the previous case as the atrium of infection. 2nd. That there was a pre-existing, or at least a co-existing pneumonia of the lung, undiagnosed at the time of operation, the clinical picture being overshadowed by the intensity of the appendix syndrome.

These two cases have been selected because they demonstrate clearly the most common atrium of infection and the clinical course of the disease. Also they forcibly call our attention to that type of pneumonia so often spoken of as abdominal, or with referred abdominal symptoms. Our work is more and more convincing us that the field of reflex manifestations must be more carefully circumscribed. Had the diagnosis of pneumonia in the second case been made first and the patient had recovered without operation, it would doubtless be classed among the so-called cases of pneumonia with abdominal symptoms. It is probably that this has often been done in the past. Is it not quite probable that all these so-called abdominal types of pneumonia are really cases of pneumococcus infection of the peritoneum?

THE KIDNEY.

In the literature of the subject we have found but few references to pneumonic infection of the kidney. Our experience is limited to two cases the pathology of which is very interesting and will be fully considered by Dr. Lee.

When the right kidney is involved in any pathologic process it is often, without the exercise of the greatest diagnostic acumen, mistaken for appendiceal trouble. Especially is this true when dealing with the pathologic retrocecal and undescended appendix. It must also be borne in mind that both may be simultaneously involved in the same process and from the same infecton. This is the source of the infection in the case which follows.

Case I: F. F. Aet, 39, German, farmer, Hosp. No. 613.

Family History: Negative except for present trouble which began when the patient was 16 years of age, with attacks of severe pain vaguely described as in the right side, no nausea, but little soreness or fever. The first attack lasted for a few days, recurring every two or three years.

Present Illness: Began six weeks ago with pain just above McBurney's point, fever, soreness, but little nausea and *no rigidity*. After three weeks the pain moved upward and toward the back at which time urination became more frequent and occasionally slightly bloody. The pain over the kidneys grew progressively worse and was attended by a progressive emaciation and the fever remained high.

Physical Examination: Small man, normal weight 155 pounds, but has lost a great deal during this last sickness. Pronounced soreness over right kidney and upper right quadrant of abdomen with tumefaction which lay just above McBurney's point. No muscular rigidity.

Diagnosis: Primarily chronic kidney disease of long standing. Present attack beginning as an appendicitis in a retro-peritoneal undescended appendix and ending as an infection, by continuity, of the chronically diseased kidney with probable nephritic abscess.

Operation: Appendectomy, appendix retro-cecal, the tip pointing upward and adherent to the tissues in front of the kidney. The pre-kidney structures were infiltrated and the entire appendix was buried in adhesions. Nephrotomy, usual loin incision exposing a mere shell of a kidney filled with pus. Drained.

The urinalysis in this case showed a few hyaline and granular casts, leucocytes, cylindroids, a few pus cells and squamous epithelia. It is to be regretted that a cystoscopic examination was not made, for the operation demonstrated that the ureter was occluded. This explains the apparently negative urinary findings. The cystoscope would have determined these facts and thus have materially aided in the diagnosis.

Blood Examination: Leucocytes 11520, polymorphonuclears 71.4 per cent.

Microscopic Findings: From both the kidney and appendix, pneumococci in abundance.

It is quite clear in this case, from the history of it, that there was a long standing pathology of the kidney, the exact nature of which was not determinable at the time of the operation, the newer infection covering it over. Following this he had had several attacks of appendicitis leaving in their wake the adhesions found at the operation and which attacks the patient interpreted as his old kidney trouble, the appendix being located retro-peritoneal and in close proximity to the kidney, on the other hand the intensity of the appendix

symptom obscured the kidney lesion in the mind of the attending physician who referred the case to us for operation.

It is also quite clear that his last attack began as his old trouble with the kidney, but after three weeks, an acute attack of pneumococci appendicitis came on with extension to the kidney by continuity. (1).

Case II: A. L. D., housewife, Aet, 27, Hosp. No. 801.

Family History: Negative.

Personal History: During childhood negative. Menstruation normal up to two and one-half years ago when a pelvic pathology developed which has no bearings on the subject of this paper so will not be considered at this time. Backache for the last two years has been continuous and has been especially severe on the left side, radiating over sacrum and down the thigh. Urination has been frequent and painful and sometimes contained a little blood. This symptom worse at night and when lying down, often nauseated. has lost twenty pounds in weight but has had no night sweats.

Physical Examination: Tall, spare, blonde woman, weight 124 pounds, fairly well nourished, extremely nervous type and given to attacks of hysteria. Temperature 99, pulse 80. Chest and heart negative, abdomen the same except for the left upper side and loin. The kidney area on the left side in front and behind and the ureter along its course, extremely sensitive to pressure. The lower pole of the kidney palpable because of probable enlargement.

Cystoscopic Examination: Urethra small, bladder irritable, trigone injected; this injection being much more pronounced

---

1. In passing permit us to again call atention to the fact that a retro-cecal appendix when inflamed does not give the symptom of overlying muscular rigidity. The lesion that invokes this must involve the parietal peritoneum. These contain the sensory ednorgans of the abdominal cavity so to speak.

on the left side forming an intensely red zone around the left ureteral meatus. Left ureter catheterized the urine from which contained pus. Cells from the pelvis of kidney abundant and contained pneumococci. Right kidney working normally.

Diagnosis: Pneumococcus infection of left kidney.

Operation: Kidney removed by the usual loin incision. Enlarged, measurements, long transverse diameter 5.75 cm, polar length 10 cm. Split section (3) showed pelvis dotted with hepatized areas resembling hepatized lung tissue, platinum loop slides from which contained the pneumococcus. The entire kidney showed the same mottled dark appearance. Time of operation, twelve minutes.

But little comment is needed further on these two cases. Suffice it to say that in both these cases the infection was thoroughly worked out and in case one the route of it as well.

THE MENINGES.

This infection may become surgical in view of the modern treatment of tapping the canal to relieve pressure. The usual source of infection is the mouth, nose and accessory sinuses (1) and usually follows pneumonia.

THE BRAIN.

Here it usually manifests itself in the form of abscesses and is generally fatal and undiagnosed during life. Green (2) reports ten cases, one of which was his own. Route of infection, otitis media 2, secondary to pneumonia 3, chronic pulmonary condition, character not stated 1, nasal infection 1, trauma, character not stated 1, cause unknown 2.

1. Darling, J. A. M. A., Vol. 47, pp. 1561.
2. J. A. M. A., Vol. 50, pp. 1799
3. See cut.

THE JOINTS.

The pneumococcus manifests a predilection for the serous membranes. Luse (1) cites a case of abscess of the right knee occuring during the course of a pneumonia. Large numbers of pneumococci were found in the pus evacuated from it.

The infection of the joints is probably hematogenous and the localization is probably determined by trauma. These as in the case of all infected joints, are very painful (2).

THE BONES.

In children, Meyer (3) shows that the germ manifests a specially pyogenic tendency, hence osteitis, osteo-myelitis and periostitis following pneumonia is not to be counted a rarity.

REMARKS.

It will be seen from what has been said that scarcely any tissue or organ of the body can be said to be exempt from the attack of the pneumococcus. Eyre (4) gives the following list in which it has been the recognized causative factor; meningitis, ulcerative endo-carditis, suppurative peri-carditis, pleurisy, otitis media, arthritis, peritonitis, diffuse and local, conjunctivitis, epiphysitis, osteo-myelitis, periostitis, and necrosis, thyreoiditis, parotiditis, tonsillitis, gastritis, nephritis and perInephritis, and endo-cervicitis.

With us its most interesting phases from the surgical standpoint, have been its manifestations in the kidney and peritoneum.

Robbers (5) has shown that the peritoneal type manifests but little tendency to spontaneous recovery, but does endeavor to localize itself.

1. British Med. Journ., Vol. 2, pp. 1182.
2. Roswell Park, J. A. M. A., Vol. 48, pp. 720.
3. M.tteilungen a. d. Genzgebeiten, Jena, Vol. 2.
4. Lancet, London, Feb. 22 ,1908.
5. Deuasche Med. Wochenschrift, Berlin and Leiusic, Vol. 32, No. 23.

Ferraud, (1) in a child of six years, found multiple localizations. These were most severe in the kidneys and were trivial in the lungs and pleura where they were supposed to be secondary. Papillon (2) reports a similar case in which the kidneys were the dominating feature. But these cases were of so acute a nature that the patients both died, while on the other hand ours seem to have been of a more chronic nature and surgery was the means of restoring both to health .

Munter (3) reports a case of fatal pneumonic phlegmonous gastritis, in a man of 33. Dieulafoy an Fuller three similar cases (4).

McGregor (5) reports a case of gangrene of the fingers necessitating amputation, during an attack of pneumonia. He accounts for it in the following way: 1. Pneumococci bacteremia with increased agglutinating power of the blood which occurs progressively up to the crises but does not then cease. 2. Weakness due to acute fever and cardiac asthenia. 3. Pneumococcic pericarditis and endo-carditis giving rise to clots and vegetations which may act as emboli. 4. Pneumococcic phlebitis. 6. Pneumococcic endarteritis.

The pneumococcus, so-called, is biologically really a compromise between the cocci and the bacilli. It resembles and is named because of its resemblance, the cocci, but at times having a capsule, it is not unlike the bacilli. .

One of the most important properties of the pneumococci is the production of an acid reacting toxin. This can be demonstrated by growing them on litmus-nutrose or inulose agar.

1 Bulletin de la Societie de Pedriatriae, April, 1908.

2. Ibid.

3. Deutsche Med. Wochenschrift, Berlin, Vol. 81, pp. 1337.

4. Ibid.

5. Glasgow Med. Journ., Aug., 1908.

There seems to be no doubt now that pneumococci, a priori, are distinctly non-capsulated organism. When cultivated it produces no capsule excepting on a gelatin containing media. ·

Leucocytosis: The presence of a leucocytosis tends toward a favorable prognosis when the affection is confined to the thorax. In pneumonic infections elsewhere the only clinical significance of leucocytosis is to ascertain the severity of the process, as regards suppuration or inflammation.

Phagocytosis: Pneumococci isolated from the blood of patients, during or after crisis, are not taken up (in vitro) by the patient's blood; or by any other blood.

In view of the fact that pneumococci isolated from the blood, are not taken up by normal or pneumococcic serum and leucocytes, the phenomenon of crisis and healing in primary pneumonic affections, cannot be attributed to phagocytosis. It is our contention that the successful resistance to and recovery from, pneumococcic invasion is: first attenuation of virulence brought on by too rapid proliferation of the pneumococci; second, by the increased alkalinity of the blood in the affected part.

Reaction: The reactions of the blood in the presence of pneumococci are: oxidation and reduction, hydration and dehydration and simple addition (methylation). When the blood is more alkaline its bactericidal powers as regards pneumonic infection, is increased. The variety of reactions and the variety of defensive substances are both markedly small in number.

Protective Substances: First and most important of all, the alkalies of the blood, proteids, hydrogen sulfide, di-sodium phosphate, sodium hydrate, sodium carbonate, etc. In a lowered state of resistance there is found a lessened amount of these (alkaline) properties, and an increase of urea, bile acids, glycuronic acid, sulfuric acid, glycocoll, etc. This can have but little .

bearing on any except such cases as have been styled "pneumonia with abdominal symptoms." In other words, these changes of and in metabolism, cannot take place rapidly enough to prevent infection when a virulent type of pneumococci invade.

Infections: We have positive evidence

The kidneys at the very best have but a poor circulation; they have constantly present a large amount of blood that is more or less impure. Given then, a colony of virulent pneumococci allowed to remain practically stationary for a time in the smaller capillaries of this organ and you

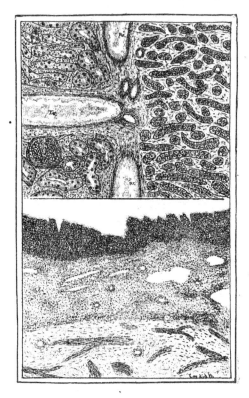

Upper Figure; Iv. Inter-lobular Vessel. Ar., Ar. Terminal Arteries.
Lower Figure; "Hepatized" Mucosae, Pelvis of Kidney.

that infection takes place along the course of blood vessels, lymphatics, nerve sheaths, or by localization of pyogenic micro-organisms floating in the blood stream, in *locus minora resistentiae.* This brings us again to the most important points in the paper.

have the common phenomenon of inflammation with succeeding micro-biotic changes. (Fig. 1.)

Owing to the remarkable lack of drainage, the histologic arrangement of its blood vessels and the richness of its lymphatics, the same argument applies to the appendix.

In the majority of instances where we have a pneumococcic (metastatic) affection, the microbic invasion is hemal. It may also be carried by the lymphatics as in some cases of so-called idiopathic peritonitis.

In pneumococcic meningitis the invasion is, no doubt, through the nerve sheaths.

Infarction: This is the most important of renal lesions that occur during or following infection. It is not to be presumed that there is only one etiologic factor in this condition.

The infarctions, as they occur in the kidney are, as a rule, small and involve chiefly the cortical portion on account of the causative embolus lodging in one of the terminal or interlobular arterioles.

The renal vessels have no arterial anastomoses; therefore when a renal arteriole is blocked by an embolus, infarction is sure to result. Infarction with subsequent pathologic changes, given later, does not exist in the kidney without the presence of both micro-organisms and their toxins.

The histologic demonstrations of an infarct (infected) is not possible without early diagnosis and surgical interference. Instead of multiple, small, infarcts, the entire cortical portion of the organ may assume the appearance of a diffuse process. This happens only in pneumococci invasion, when there is an extreme amount of virulent toxins and bacteria present at one time, and when the circulatory functions of the kidneys are at the same time impaired. In such a case the following changes occur in their regular order, tabulated with corresponding clinical symptoms:

PATHOLOGIC CHANGES.	CLINICAL SYMPTOMS.
1. Bacterial invasions; producing.	1.
2. Virulent toxins; followed by,	2. Pain in lumbar region.
3. Diffuse hyperemia; with,	3.
4. Diffuse nephritis.	4. Albumin and mucin.
5. Hemorrhagic infiltration;	5. Blood in urine.
6. Suppurative phlebitis, and local arteriosclerosis.	6. Puss cells in the urine.
7. Necro-biosis; causing,	
8. rrest of anabolic metabolism;	
9. Complete necrosis; and final.	
10. Suppuration.	

ANIMAL HEAT

BY DR G. H. THRAILKILL, CHICKASHA, OKLA.

Animal heat may be defined as the thermic energy stored up in animal body under both normal and pathologic conditions as measured by the thermometer. These units may be similar but not identical, for the same animal species; since each individual of the same species may, technically speaking, have its own standard so that in studying this complex physiologic mechanism, we must needs compromise science on some general average for

(Read Before Grady County Medical Society, September, 1909.)

the warm-blooded animals; also for the so-called cold-blooded animals; while we are compelled to reverse the position in this classification under certain external surroundings of the so-called cold-blooded animals, since their range of temperature may be very much lower or very much higher than the warm-blooded animal.

Cold-blooded animals have been frozen by the surrounding media, and have been resuscitated after this suspended animation, and their temperature raised. Surrounded by a liquid media, to a temperature beyond the possibilities of the warm-blooded animal; thus, it may be readily seen, that no general average can be fixed even for the same species of the cold-blooded animal; while for any species of the warm-blooded animal a general average temperature can be approximately determined.- The youth of warm-blooded animals sustains a higher general average than the aged of the same species; while the general average of the different species would each have its own general standard; this general average of the different species would have its own general standard; this general average also differs in the sex of the same species, females being higher than males. Studying all species of warm-blooded animals, the general average of each species gives us a wide difference of general averages; so, also, the temperature in any warm-blooded animal for any given time differs for the different parts of the animal anatomy from which the temperature is taken, the liver being hottest, the cutaneous surface the coldest. The lowest average general temperature among warm-blooded animals is that of the Duckbill Plohbus, which is seventy-six degrees F., while the highest is that of the Sparow, which is 110 degrees F., while we note averages ranging between these for the different species, we also note that there is a daily remission and exacerbation, varying from a half a degree to a degree and a half, in the same animal, in a comparatively quiet state. Physical exertion, increased respiration, accelerated heart action, the ingestion of a hearty meal, excitement, mental exertion, physical trauma, toxic reaction, metabolism and so on, increase body temperature. In the human species man has an average normal temperature varying from 98 to 99 1-2 degrees F., with a daily incursion of 1 1-2 degrees, F., this general average normal temperature is subject to minimum variations constantly.

Hyperthermacy is any temperature of the body above normal; hypothermacy is any temperature of the body below normal. These points, as we readily see, must be determined in a general way to be practical; yet they must necessarily differ by 1 1-2 degrees F. between the low temperature and high temperature. They must necessarily, at times, occupy common positions.

Thermogenesis is today a speculative field for the physiologist. Yet many facts have been proven, demonstrating that in the base of the brain, we have thermogenic centers which control the heat mechanism of the body, through the reflex or sympathetic system; that we have afferent and efferent nerve centers and nerve fiber which to their possessor unknowingly control heat production and heat dissipation. Thermogenesis, or heat production, being excited by all pathologic toxines, physical violence, as an electric current producing a spasm of the skeletal musculature of the body, or a chemical violence, as the increased muscular tone resulting from physiological action of drugs, as strychnine, digitalis, curara, or any drug, increasing or decreasing physiologic function of an organ; the venom of any serpent, insect, cold or heat, increase oxidation and stores heat energy in the animal body; nature's method resisting extrensix intrusion, thus, waging a battle for the survival of the fittest.

The factors of heat and cold first manifest themselves on the sensory nervous system; the following being a good example: About twelve years since, while passing over the mountains at an altitude of about 11,000 feet above sea level, one cold winter night, your humble essayest was caught in a mountain blizzard; found it impossible to urge the team against the cold wind, or get his breath while facing it, stopped and turned around to breathe, and in a short time experienced the pains of severe cold, which were replaced in a short time by a comforting glow of warmth and a self-satisfied physical condition, which forced itself upon him; and, except for the mental agony of the knowledge that he was freezing, could have lain down and gone to sleep; however, my destination was finally reached, due to calming of what had been a severe but short blizzard; for four or five weeks after this the nerves of sensation were so injured that tactile sensation was lost in the fingers of both hands. The thermogenic centers had saved my life.

The thermogenic centers may be classified as acceleratory and inhibitory centers. Thermolysis employs the inhibitory centers and efferent nerves and diminishes body heat, as follows: By radiation, perspiration and respiration; while the extrinsic factors of absorption by surrounding media aids nature's battle; shock and syncope assist at times in diminishing temperature by temporarily suspending animation. . Thermotaxis is that nervous control that regulates hyperthermacy and hypothermacy, and does so by either increasing, excretion, or diminishing excretion, by exciting inactivity of the skin, kidney, or alimentary canal; thus storing up heat in the animal economy. The appearance of so-called goose flesh is a guard against loss of heat, and stores up, temporarily, heat energy in the animal body; while flushing hastens elimination temporarily; both is a kind of momentary reflex and produces a hysterical action of very short duration.

Heatstroke (insolation) is followed by high temperature; due to internal congestion, and may involve vital organs, as the stomach, heart, liver, spleen, kidney, or may be followed by evidence of central nerve exhaustion, as evidenced by mania, melancholy, neurasthenia, neuritis, and even insanity; due to high temperature affecting nerve centers, nerve tracks, and improverishment of blood corpuscles; when the person so affected survives the stroke; while persons dying of insolation die in collapse, and a low temperature maintained throughout; a moderately high temperature in heatstroke, prognosticates recovery, while a low temperature is eminent of collapse.

Fever is a result of a pathological change going on in the animal economy and is pathognomonic of a diseased condition.

When called to the bedside of a patient with a thermometric record above or below normal, we should decide at once that there is a diseased condition, and search for the same; the disease may be toxochemic or toxobicrobic or physical in origin, thus requiring diagnostic acuteness, which may require several visits to determine and locate. We may never locate the pathologic conditions; however, we may be always assurred there is one. A subnormal temperature is just as positively a pathognomonic index as a super-normal temperature, and should demand as careful examination; it may mean impending brain or circulatory lesions; it may be the result of pathogenic toxines recently thrown into the circulation by a very recent fission of pathogenic germs, as in the early rigor of a pernicious malaria or a very malignant diphtheria or erysipelas. The experience of all bacteriologist confirms the lowering of body temperature when a pathogenic toxine or vaccine is first injected into the circulation, followed soon, however, by a rise of temperature. The rigor being nature's method of resisting the invasion, and the beginning of nature's battle for the survival of the fittest.

In conclusion on this point when we have a patient with temperature above or below normal, we must at once look for a pathological condition, for such surely exists. Thermometers do not lie. The temperature may be ephemeral or may be hysterical, but a pathologic condition has called it forth; and it is our duty to so acquit ourselves as to be able to intelligently search out the etiology. Let us hope that the day of systematic treatment is nearing an end. Whatever good it may have served us in the past, it is but an acknowledgment of a condition not yet thoroughly investigated. An open admission of ignorance, a frank acknowledgment of indolence and mental turpitude, a poor apology for a frank I don't know.

I hope the day shall soon come when we shall cease to hear such misnomers as lung fever, bilious fever, brain fever, hay fever, puerperal fever, remittant fever, as ordinarily used, scarlet fever, splenic and yellow fever, et al. They mean nothing within themselves, and have no pathological significance. The sooner we drop them, the sooner shall we begin to know something of the pathology of fevers and the morbid anatomy of disease. Let us consider all fevers of having a pathologic origin, and soon these meaningless terms will be obsolete, and we will be correcting pyrexias by other means than cold tar derivatives; that are fraught with dangers and must only reduce temperature at the expense of an already weakened physiological body; as a result of a pathogenesis.

Cleinically, fevers may be classified as remittant, intermittent and continuous, as they relate to the normal average temperature and with this meaning only; remembering that their excursions on the fever chart will show variations between the youthful and the aged.

Last but not least let us endeavor to assist the termogenic mechanism in the control of body heat in accord with physiological processes; namely by keeping in mind the metabolisms of the normal physiological animal body.

Chickasha Oklahoma April 7th 1909.

THE SOCIAL EVIL

BY DR. M. A. WARHURST, MAUD, OKLA.

The public does not appreciate the fact that the immense majority of the victims of venereal diseases are the young and inexperienced and the irresponsible through ignorance. While it may be said that society is under no obligation to protect those who voluntarily expose themselves to contagion. Can the young who have been brought up in entire ignorance of such matters be said to voluntarily expose themselves to dangers which they may not know exist? Society is to blame for this faulty training or rather absolute lack of training which exposes them to these dangers. The attitude of society is not merely one of apathy or indifference, but it seriously endeavors to cover and conceal existence even of these diseases. Society frowns on all efforts for its enlightenment, it resolutely closes its eyes to the dangers that threaten the social body from the venereal plague. The attitude of the medical profession which around these diseases the sacred circle of the medical secret, tends to keep the public ignorant of their prevalence and dangers. We hear that this secret is more binding than any human law. It relaxes none of its vigor, even when confronted with the alternative of a crime about to be committed. When for example a syphlitic man is about to marry with the practical certainty that he will infect an innocent woman and her offspring. This same reticence and concealment are not only observed in private practice, but dominate the attitudes of governing boards of our general hospitals. If the venereal patient is admitted to a hospital his disease is baptized under a different name. The methods adopted by our hospitals is calculated to conceal the extent of venereal morbidity. Venereal diseases masquerade under various names. This policy of concealment follows the patient with venereal diseases to his grave. The cause of death is concealed under some compromising title. In view of the dangers which menace the public health and interests of the family and society from venereal diseases, it is time to break down the barriers of concealment and silence behind which these diseases propagate and flourish, to dissipate the dense ignorance of the public, by turning on the light of knowledge to do away with the mystery and secrecy which have always surrounded them and put aside the ridiculous prudery which regards all knowledge of sexual matters as profane. Young men should be educated in a knowledge of sexual hygiene, they should be instructed as to the dangers incident to the irregular exercise of the reproductive function; they should be warned of the pitfalls and dangers which beset the pathway of dissipation; they should be instructed in the knowledge that venereal diseases are the almost invariable concomitant of licentious living. The plea of ignorance should no longer be available to shield those who bring disease and death in families, who ruin the lives of those whom they have sworn to protect.

The fathers of marriageble daughters should know that dissolute men make dangerous husbands. Mothers should know that a man who has lead an unclean life is not a safe husband for her daughter; that venereal disease is a common consequence of such a life is a prolific cause of feminine infirmities and inflammatory diseases peculiar to women which may result in dangerous disease and ultimate loss of her reproductive organs. While it is not contended that the exposure of existing evils should form a necessary part of the education of young women, yet they should know something of matters which so closely touch their health and domestic happiness and the future of their children. The public should recognize what the medical profession has long known, that venereal diseases are a social pest or plague which menaces not only the public health but the welfare of the family and the race. This instruction would have more weight and more persuasive force coming from a medical fraternity man whose right to speak authoratively on questions of hygiene cannot be questioned. The family physician is peculiarly fitted, not only by his professional knowledge, but through his close and personal relations with his patients to impart this instruction. Every physician should be a missionary in his own field. While the duty of reforming the morals of the community is not within the province of the physician individual reformation may be accomplished through his agency by instruction in matters relating to sexual hygiene and diseases of sexual life in his individual capacity, he can impart this instruction to the young men of his field. The intimate and confidential relation existing between the physician and his patient permit a large latitude in regard to all subjects relating to disease, the freedom with which his vocation permits him to talk on subjects ordinarily forbidden, allows him to discuss delicate matters regarded as peculiarly intimate, personal and even shameful without encroaching upon reservation of propriety and good taste; he can speak with tact but with sufficient plainness to be understood upon all questions relating to sexual morality, sexual life and its diseases without offending the succeptibilities of even the most modest woman; prudery, of course, can not be considered in matters of this nature and should be discouraged.

The true remedy, the most effective remedy available to modify or lessen the appalling evils, moral and physical, which flow from venereal diseases, is the general dissemination of knowledge respecting the dangers and modes of contagion of these diseases. It is by persuasive force of enlightenment by combating the dense ignorance which prevails among the laity, especially among the young, upon whom the incidence of these diseases most heavily falls that these evils can be diminshed such crimes which entail suffering and shame, disease and death upon the innocent should be no longer possible. All legislative, moral and sanitary forces should unite in preventing the commission of such shameful cruelties upon our race.

INFANTILE ECZEMA

BY DR. CURTIS R. DAY, PH. G., M. D. LECTURER ON DERMATOLOGY EPWORTH COLLEGE OF MEDICINE OKLAHOMA CITY, OKLA.

In the discussion of my subject I believe a better understanding can be had by first saying a few words about eczema in general.

It is often said that the line of demarcation in the differential diagnosis of eczema and the different forms of dermatitis is not easily told in words, yet the trained diagnostitian has no trouble in such differentiation.

That eczema is a dermatitis no one questions for a moment, yet it is a class peculiar to its self. This classification may not be made by the study of the malady from the standpoint of its history and clinical manifestations alone, but must be made from a histopathological point of view.

In the discussion of the etiology of eczema; Dr. Pusey, in his work on Dermatology says, in part: "It occurs in both sexes, at all ages, and in all classes of society. From their general exposure it is some what more frequent in males than in females.

"It is more frequent in infancy and during the active period of adult life. The disease is not hereditary in the sense that it can be transmitted from parent to child, but there are certain conditions which predispose to eczema that are hereditary.

Read before the Section on Pedatrics, Oklahoma State Medical Association, Oklahoma City, Okla., May 11, 12, 13,'09

"The disease is more apt to occur in individuals with fair, thin skin, than in those with dark, thick skin, for the reason that the thin skins are more sensative."

We are taught that there are two causes of eczema, internal irritation and external irritation. Applying this statement to the statement of Dr. Pusey, (and he no wise differs from other writers of reputation) might we not conclude that the lowered resisting power, the defective anatomical structure of the skin, has more to do with the etiology of eczema than any other one factor?

The manifestations of infantile eczema differs in no wise from other forms of eczema, only in the subject or individual affected. It however appears upon these little patients during their first and second years. In the majority of cases it is situated on the cheeks, chin, behind the ears and on the scalp, yet it may extend to any part of the body and limbs.

In the beginning the area involved may be very small and consist only of a slight vesiculo-pustular area covered with a crust of dried excretion, surrounded by an erythematous area.

Passing through the evolution of weeping vesicular, pustular and in some cases ulcerative conditions it spreads peripherally, with irregular, poorly defined lines if demarcation. Itching is a very prominent subjective symptom and at times is very severe. Should the affected area become of sufficient depth to involve lymphatic vessels we are likely to have enlargement of lympatic glands and possibly abscesses, from which large quantities of pus will be discharged.

A condition of the latter type may be found to have for its origin, pediculi, which should be easily recognized by the discovery of pediculi and their ova, and in all this type of conditions one should never forget to examine closely for pediculi.

Infantile eczema is found in all classes and conditions of society. In one case the child may be poorly nourished and cachectic while in another the baby may be fat and chubby. In the one case the child may be poorly nourished from the lack of a sufficient amount of wholesome diet, while in the other case there may be a lack of proper relation as regards digestion and assimilation.

Reflex irritation may explain the pathogenisis of some of them, yet it is not a matter of vital importance for the treatment will be the same whether the origin be gastro-intestinal or reflex irritation.

This brings us again to the question of etiology. Is eczema caused by irritation either external or internal, or is it due to the pathological condition of the skin its self; (the defective anatomical structure of the skin, if you please), and that the irritation what ever it may be is only an occasion for the outbreak of the malady.

I wish to call attention to a few of the pathological conditions of the skin, which might be considered as special etilogical factors in eczema. A hyperidrosis, wherein the epithelial cells are continually being macerated, resulting in excessive proliferation which leaves the deeper structures unduly exposed to external irritation and unfit to perform the natural excretory functions imposed upon them. The opposite condition, anadrosis with its excessive dry epedermis, ready at all times to crack and form deep fissures, will also be unable to do the work which nature demands.

Another important condition which should at all times be looked for is seborrhoea with its abundance of oily excretion; and the negative pathological condition, asteatosis, either of which will produce a dermatitis, the continuation of which we denominate eczema. Should there be a hyperkeratosis, the redundant epithelium, will arrest elimination thus adding material favorable to the production of a dermatitis, while a parakeratosis with the loss of its epithelium, leaves the underlying tissues without the protection nature intended they should have. Again a histo-pathological condition of the corium could be an etilogical factor in producing pathological condition of superficial structures, and the combination of such conditions might produce an eczema. Viewing the disease from this standpoint might we not expect, that eczema may yet be recognized as a symptom of some variety of structural defect of the skin rather than a disease per see.

This causes me to be of the opinion that more attention should be paid to the defective anatomical condition of the skin than is usually done, and by so doing we could doubtless learn more regarding the etiology of the disease and at the same time direct our treatment to the end that the resisting power of the skin be increased, for by so doing our patients would be less liable to repeated attacks. On account of this defect in the development of the skin it is of course very susceptible to irritation.

A lack of sufficient food only adds to this defect, while the over-fed infant must of necessity over burden all excretory glands of the body and we too often forget that the skin is the largest of such glands.

We are very prompt and very diligent in our efforts to discover any additional burden placed on the liver, kidneys or the gastro-intestinal tract and adopt methods for their relief, but too often neglect even the slightest consideration of any additional burden that may be placed on the skin, much less to attempt to discover any pathological or histo-pathological condition that may exist.

The laity are loth to believe that eczema can be cured, and will call attention to the fact that the patient in question, has had outbreaks of the disease since childhood. We recognize that certain individuals are of a bilious temperament, and why, because of the fact that there is a histo-pathological condition of the liver which renders its functions irregular, yet no one is continually calling attention to the fact that biliousness is incurable. We ask the question, why this difference of ideas with the laity? Our answer is that the profession has earnestly studied the one condition, and have been able to satisfactorily explain the pathology to the laity, while with the other we fail to carefully investigate and thoroughly study existing conditions, but join with the laity in taking it as a matter of course. Let us then study the condition of the skins of these patients, learn the defects, whether of glandular or structural origin, make a diligent effort to increase the development of the defective parts at the same time instruct our patients how best they may protect themselves from pathological conditions resulting therefrom.

If the skin of these patients, thus affected, can be strengthened, if its anatomical structure can be increased, that its resisting power may be normal, we need only to maintain such a condition to have positively relieved the malady.

In the case of these little patients it is necessary to give the affected areas all the protection possible. If the head is involved it should be protected by a cap and in most cases it is necessary to cover the hands with gloves to keep these little patients from scratching. The digestive organs should be thoroughly studied and the diet regulated to conform to what ever kind of defect exists, bearing in mind that it is necessary to establish perfect harmony between digestion and assimilation. Elimination must be carefully watched and normally performed. These measures should be carefully estimated with the view of building up and sustaining the normal condition of the skin. Local medication should be soothing and protecting. In the selection of the topical remedies, the local pathological condition should be carefully studied in order that only such measures be adopted as conform to the defect of the skin.

If the fault is with the glands, the development of the epidermis or the structural defects of underlying tissues, that fact must if possible, be known first, and the peculiar defective action of the part must be known or all measures will either be worthless or harmful. *Security Building.*

PELVIC DRAINAGE

BY DR. G. H. BUTLER, TULSA, OKLA.

It has occured to me frequently, that of all conditions, in which a great many practitioners "stop at the half way house," or

(Read before the Tulsa County Medical Society.)

try to move a mountain with jack screws, pelvic drainage is most frequent.

I shall not include in my observations, drainage from traumatism or from the bladder, but restrict myself to those cases of infection in women, in which the uterus is the portal of entrance.

Drainage is needed in pelvic infection, in the relative frequency of its occurrence; first from abortion or miscarriage, second from gonorrhoeal infection, and last from labor at term.

The man who can say positively—following the expulsion of a foetus from the uterus—that all membranes have come away, is either ignorant of the physiological processes of reproduction or is so wonderful in his diagnostic ability that he should be censured for not establishing "Temple of Health" No. 2.

Following such cases—the clinical history and symptomology of which, you are all familiar, arises the question, What is to be done?

"Nero fiddled while Rome burned" and too many of us are content to use vaginal douches, local applications, swabbings, etc., which only keep in abeyance, to a limited degree, the dangers, prolong pain, suffering, anxiety and finally, after imperiling the functions, if not even the existence of the organs of reproduction, bring the patient to the table anaemic, nervous, broken in health and spirit, with enough damage already done, to prevent the best results, following any line of treatment, or leave her to the smoldering fires of infection in a semi-convalescent state, to burst forth later, consuming the ovaries, tubes, uterus or all; mayhaps the patient herself.

The secret of sucess in this class of cases lies in one word DRAINAGE. The object of drainage in any location and for any condition, is to get rid of those products of inflammation, which, by their absorption, produce those symptoms we differentiate, by such terms as pyaemia, septicemia, puerperal fever, etc., and to accomplish the greatest good, to get the most perfect drainage, if follows that the least

there is to be brought away, the more nearly we will approach perfection.

In draining punctured or gunshot wounds, we use knife and scissors to remove all the dead or infected tissue we can; in draining the mastoid cells we use chisel and gouge and in draining the uterus, I want to try to impress it on you that the curette is the one remedy that gives results you like. In the uterus the curette is both knife and chisel more commonly, but less perfectly used, I believe, than either.

The sins of omission that are committed in the name of currettage are appalling. The sense of security, given patient and family, by the knowledge that something vigorous is being done, that the fever, the pain, the sleepless nights and the hollow eyes are soon to be over, when, indeed, only a dabbling in the interior of the uterus, has removed part of the infectious material contained therein, and perhaps done more harm than good, by opening up new channels for absorption, and brought disrepute to one of the most potent procedures in surgery. Better a uterus, untouched, than one imperfectly cleaned out.

Personally, I very much prefer a sharp curette. Being guided wholly by the sense of touch, whatever style of instrument is used, I have trained myself to the touch of the sharp instrument. I have never perforated, nor seen another perforated, a uterus, with such an instrument and too, it is hard for me to believe, that the clinging piece of membrane, to a large freely movable soft muscular sack, such as is the pregnant uterus, may be easily and completely removed by an instrument, whose rounded edge glides so easily over damp slippery tissue. Having finished the curetteage and washed out the uterine cavity well, the question as to draining is very much simplified, and if you will believe me is done in this manner:

Use iodoform gauze strips—those with

both edges selvidged preferred, and introduce the first part of the gauze up to the
fundus. Take time in this part of the work
to do it well and fold the strip upon itself,
laterally, keeping it well and firmly pressed
toward the fundus, until the cavity is full
to the inner os cervix, and then reverse
your procedure. Pack the cervix lightly,
picking up a long loop of gauze and carrying it into the cavity in contact with the
packing of the body. Two or three such
loops will be enough for the canal and you
will have a drain instead of a dam, which
you can very easily get by too firmly packing the cervix.

Such a dressing may remain from 48
to 72 hours but should be removed just as
soon as it becomes so saturated that it no
longer drains well.

I shall not burden you with a recital of
cases under this head, as the condition is
so common that you are all familiar with
the management of it.

Drainage of the pelvis, when the foci of
infection is extra-uterine, is based on the
same principles as that from intra-uterine,
but the procedure, of course, is different.
To illustrate, I will recite a case or two.
showing what may happen and how to deal
with it.

Case No. 1. A single woman, age 20
years, never pregnant, never had any serious illness, of good sturdy stock, was seen
by myself as consultant, on the 12th day
of an illness, the most prominent symptoms
of which were pain in the lower abdomen
or pelvis, nausea, loss of appetite, constipation, a temperature running from 101 to
103 and tenderness over the region of the
right ovary.

Bi-manual examination revealed great
sensitiveness in the posterior vaginal vault,
an induration in the region of the ovary,
some fixation of the uterus, and some rigidity of the right rectus abdomines. Fluctuation indeterminate.

A diagnosis of pelvic supuration was
made and operation confirmed same.

Having obtained permission to remove
the ovary, or tube or both, at my discretion, I entered the abdominal cavity
through the vagina and locating the ovary,
it was easy to trace the tube, and in the
tracing I found a pus sac, within the folds
of the broad ligament. It was opened,
after draging it down near the incision as
I could, and two or three ounces of very
foul pus was evacuated.

I thought it best not to remove the tube
at that time on account of the danger of
general peritonitis, so swabbed the cavity
out as well as possible with moist bichloride
gauze and while holding the sac well down,
by dressing forceps, used to catch it before
opening, packed the cavity with 10 per cent
iodoform gauze. The edges of the wound
in the vagina were brought together with
chromic gut and the gauze drain left in the
central incision for two days, when it was
removed and again lightly packed. It
being impossible, of course, to reintroduce
the gauze into the collapsed abscess cavity,
I was content to pack well around it,
bringing the strip out through the vaginal
wound, where it was invested with the plain
sterile gauze, with which the vagina was
packed.

Temperature went to normal within 18
hours and convalescence was rapid and uninterrupted. The tube and ovary were removed some months later by the abdominal
route. This case was one of undoubted
gonorrhoeal origin.

Case No. 2. In this case a different type
is presented.

Woman, age 32, the mother of two
children, was seen by me in July last year.
On the 10th of February, preceding, she
was delivered of a still-born child, instru-
mentally, after a very prolonged and difficult labor, following which, she had a
puerperal infection that came near costing

her her life and kept her in bed some eight or ten weeks. She made a fair recovery and removed to this city in May. With the exceptions of being obstinately constipated, having a good deal of pelvic pain, and difficult, painful menstruation, which had re-established itself after two months, her health had been fair.

When I first saw her, in addition to the symptoms mentioned, she was running a temperature from 100 to 102, having septic chills, was salivated, and her stomach badly upset from heroic doses of quinine, in an effort to cure her of malaria—from which her attendant thought she was suffering.

When I examined her I found a large mass in the right quadrant of the pelvis, tender on pressure, a firmly fixed uterus, retroverted, a prolapsed ovary and such pressure on the rectum that the introduction of a rectal tube was impossible and the introduction of my finger extremely difficult and intensely painful to the patient. Diagnosis of pelvic suppuration as the cause of the fever and advised that in operating for the relief of that condition it might become necessary to open the belly and possibly remove part or all the appendages. Advice was accepted by patient and husband, and as soon as I could get her in proper condition I performed as follows:

Plainly I had to deal with a case in which the fury of the volcanic fires had left ruin in their wake, and had again broken into flame, and it was with some misgivings that I undertook to try to save the woman's uterus and appendages. It looked like a case in which nothing short of total hysterectomy might restore her health. In making my vaginal incision, I made a larger one than for ordinary drainage and inserted into the lateral angles of the wound—one at either end—two strong silk sutures, that were knotted and held by haemostats, to act as tractors.

On entering the peritoneal cavity, I found the uterus so firmly adherent to the rectum, and the bands of adhesion so strong that it was necessary to use the scissors often, in freeing the parts. Hemorrhage was controlled by long haemostats, and later by hysterectomy forceps, until the uterus had been freed. I then turned my attention to the ovary and in trying to distinguish it, in the mass of adhesions with which it was tied down, I found two points that fluctuated. Opening them by thrusting closed, sharp pointed uterine scissors into them, guided by my finger, I evacuated quite a little pus, which was carefully mopped away as I could do it. I then dug the ovary out from its bed—followed by more hemorrhage—which was controlled by very hot gauze packs, and restored it to it's natural place. Then I tried to do the best packing I ever was called on to do. The thing to be hoped for was to so pack the pelvis that the uterus and ovary would be held in proper place, to introduce gauze between the freshly denuded surfaces, that there might not be more and perhaps equally troublesome adhesions form and that I might remove my gauze without pulling down the ovary or uterus. Having finished the pelvic pack, I curetted the uterus, packed it, introduced chromic gut instead of the strong silk I had in the angles of the wound, introduced, without tying two sutures of the same material lightly packed the vagina with plain gauze and put my patient to bed. She had been under the anaesthetic for one hour and twenty minutes and was some what shocked from the operation. She rallied well, the temperature was normal the following evening and did not again go above 99. The uterine drain was removed the second day but the pelvic gauze was left for five days, when it was removed. I replaced the pelvic dressing, using a much smaller quantity, which was allowed to stay four days when it was removed. the remaining sutures tied and the central incision allowed to heal spontaneously.

She made a good recovery, is entirely free from pain, her constipation is gone and she is enjoying better health than for years. I might add that she expects a visit from the stork within the next few months.

In this class of cases vaginal douches should not be used, on account of the danger of disseminating infective material.

The fact that a woman has her uterus scraped and some gauze crammed into it, or that she has had her vagina or belly cut open and some gauze pushed into her peritoneal cavity, does not necessarily mean that drainage has been done, for gauze may be so arranged that it hinders rather than assists in drainage and my observation leads me to believe, that the success in this class of work, is directly proportionate to the perfection of technic and skill of the physician. Properly done it often saves mutilating operations and gives as great a degree of satisfaction to physician and patient and as positive results as any practice I have ever done. I thank you, gentlemen.

RETROPERITONEAL SHORTENING OF THE ROUND LIGAMENTS

BY DR. W. E. DICKEN, PROFESSOR OF CLINICAL GYNECOLOGY EPWORTH UNIVERSITY MEDICAL COLLEGE OKLAHOMA CITY. OKLA.

Alquie', of Montpieliar, France, appears to have been the genius who first conceived the idea and proposed a plan of shortening the round ligaments to correct down-ward and back-ward displacements of the uterus. He called the operation, which he had only performed on animals and the dead subject: Utero *inguinoraphic,* which name was soon dropped for a shorter and better one.

The Academie de Medicine condemned the proposal of Alquie' in tota, both as regards the possibility of permanently correcting uterine displacements by shortening the round ligaments and as regards the practicability of the operation itself.

The Academie, however, passed a vote of approbation on Alquie' for his prudence in never having attempted his operation upon a living woman.

Deneffe, with the courage of the recent graduate, was the first to attempt the operation upon a living woman at Ghent, Belgium, in June, 1864.

(Read before the Medical Association of the Southwest at San Antonio, Nov. 9th, 1909.)

During his student days he had frequently practiced the operation successfully upon the cadaver, and immediately upon obtaining his degree, requested an opportunity to shorten the round ligaments upon the living woman, avowing his confident belief that he would be able to carry the operation to a successful conclusion, which was granted.

In the presence of the masters of his day, the operation was undertaken upon a patient suffering from prolapsus, and he failed to find either round ligament, although he opened up the entire ingunal canal on both sides. The patient recovered from the attempt but the masters were called to account by the Hospital Committee for permitting experiments upon patients committed to their care.

Thereafter the idea seems to have slumbered in the medical mind until Dec. 14th, 1881. William Alexander of Liverpool performed the first successful shortening of the round ligaments upon the living woman.

This operation has since been known as the "Alexander Operation" with which we are all familiar: and I might add, 'has almost become obselete except in selected cases.

In considering the most rational treatment of the displacement of the uterus it behooves us (1) to assure ourselves of the certainty of the diagnosis: (2) to determine accurately the degree of displacement: (3) to ascertain whether the displaced organ is reducable or non-reducable: (4) what are the apparent causes: and (5) is the disorder of place of the uterus associtaed with disease of the so-called uterine appendages?

So simple an element of diagnosis as the determination of the *degree* of the displacement is important, for on its finding rests often times the decision of the urgency of local treatment.

Is the uterus mobile and natural in this particular: or is it immobile and fastened in its abnormal posture? A satisfactory solution of this feature in diagnosis shapes materially our plan for management of the case.

Experience unmistakable proves that, while a displacement is occasionally the primary link in the chain of the pelvic disease, as a rule, the disorder of the uterus is only secondary to some recognized disease.

To secure success, in the treatment, this must receive proper consideration, and that too, early in the management. It may be an easy matter to replace the uterus, and possibly retain it in normal position, but such does not imply a cure or even a relief.

Taking this 'for granted then, we must take some time, if need be, to ascertain whether it is some impediment in the circulation of the womb and its adnexa, or from some other cause. If found that the trouble is of circulatory origin then if this cannot be relieved by mechanical or medical means, some surgical measures must be resorted to.

In my experience I have found that the uterus need not necessarily be misplaced to a surgical measure, to cause quite a disturbance in the circulation and on the other hand I have found a very aggravated misplacement of the uterus and seen the woman enjoy perfect health, without any symptoms of a disturbed function.

Now it would be absurd to resort to surgical measures in this case, just because of the displacement alone.

A complete and accurate diagnosis, then of the intra-pelvic condition—uterine and parauterine, are paramount for success, and from it the deduction of a rational treatment; and this is by no means always easy of accomplishment.

Fritsch of Bonn, Germany, asserts that no so-called displacement is abnormal and that retroversion is not unnatural.

Perhaps there is no part of the whole field of the subject of uterine displacement which has excited so much interest and discussion, nor which even today is so much sub-judice, as, what is the best surgical movement to be made in this direction.

The Alexander operation has its place in gynecologic therapy, but in my judgment its field is very limited—in fact so very limited that I have abandoned it almost all together and in its place have substituted a relief by mechanical supports or other simple measures. In other words any displacement which can be benefited by an Alexander operation or its modifications can likewise be equally improved without any operation whatsoever; simply more time is needed.

It is not worth while then, it seems to me, to give it further consideration. In the desire to extend the use of the principal of the operation to women with diseased appendages or having adhesions, various intra--peritoneal operations have been invented, which are known by the name of the inventor.

The operation of suturing the round ligaments to the uterus, or in folding the intra-abdominal portion of the round ligament upon itself in various ways, as was done first by Wylie, Dudly and Mann has long since been abandoned and is considered now only a matter of history.

Webster and Baldy conceived the idea of shortening the round ligaments by piercing the broad ligaments beneath the Fallopian tube, seizing the round ligaments and drawing its free position through the opening in the broad ligament and suturing it to the posterior surface of the uterus at or about the level of the internal os.

This operation has been stamped as a failure (1) because it depends for its strength upon the weakest portion of the ligament and (2) in order for it to be successful we must have intra-peritoneal adhesions between the round ligaments and the posterior surface of the uterus; and lastly it is anatomically incorrect as it fastens the round ligaments behind the uterus and at a point at least 2 cm. below that intended by nature.

Gilliam received the suggestion for his operation from Ferguson, who, in 1899, proposed to suspend the uterus by suturing the proximal third of the round ligaments to the anterior abdominal wall. Gilliam's operation has the merit of simplicity, but the fact that it divides the pelvic cavity into three segments (one external to each round ligament and one between the ligaments) any one of which may serve as a pocket in which the bowel may become incarcerated, this led Simpson in 1902, to propose the retropertoneal shortening of the round ligaments, at the meeting of the Southern Surgical and Gynecological Society.

At this meeting papers were also read by Drs. Ferguson and Geo. H. Noble, describing other methods of shortening the round ligaments by means of abdominal sections and fastening the ligaments to the anterior wall of the abdomen.

Since 1902, the retroperetoneal shortening of the round ligaments as proposed by Simpson has been carried out by various gynecologists in a slightly different manner, so that the technic of the operation will now be described as it is performed by myself, giving full credit to Simpson for the conception of the principals, and Kelly, Mann and Ill for the steps of the operation

The patient is prepared the same as for any abdominal section. The abdomen is opened through the right rectus muscle a little to the right of the median line. An incision two inches in length is usually sufficient, but a much longer one is sometimes better in order to see the complications met with. Whatever complications are present must be dealt with, by the separation of adhesions, and the removal of any thing that must be removed.

Then our round ligament is caught about 5 cm. from the cornu of the uterus, and provisional ligature of silk is passed under it. This point is about one-third distant from the cornu of the uterus to the internal abdominal ring. If the round ligament is long enough to permit, it is caught again at a point half way between the provisional ligature and the internal ring, and is held by means of an artery forceps.

This point is then sutured to the round ligament at its junction with the uterus by means of two chromicized cat-gut sutures. If the round ligament is rather short this part of the operation may be omitted, and with the cases I have operated upon the results seem to be the same; however, theroretically it is much better to double the round ligament back and suture it to the cornu of the uterus. As a result of these sutures, the uterus is held forward, by that portion of the round ligament which runs through the injunal canal; the proximal two-thirds of the round ligament now forms a loop, the middle of which is caught by the provisional ligature just described.

By pulling upon the provisional ligature, the anterior face of the broad ligament is exposed and the peritoneum covering it is caught just below the round ligament, making a hole large enough to admit the index finger.

If the operator stands upon the patient's right side, the next step of the operation is to open the sheath of the left rectus muscle. A blunt anerysm needle with a long curve, is then passed between the aponenrosis of the external oblique muscle and the rectus muscle. The needle is passed under the sheath of the rectus to the outer border of the muscle, and then penetrates the rectus and passes beneath the peritoneum to the internal ring.

The point of the needle is then made to follow the round ligament along the anterior face of the broad ligament to the rent in the peritoneum already described.

This can be done much easier if your assistant will elevate, rather than make lateral traction, upon the abdominal wall.

When the needle emerges through the rent in the peritoneum, it is threaded with the provisional ligature and the needle is withdrawn, bringing with it the provisional ligature.

Now all that remains to be done is to make gentle traction upon the provisional ligature and by so doing you bring the loop of the round ligament up through the broad ligament and the internal abdominal ring, beneath the pertoneum of the anterior abdominal wall to the outer border of the rectus muscle, then through the muscle and between it and the aponenrosis of the external oblique until it emerges in the abdominal incision.

If the peritoneum should be dragged in front of the round ligament it must be separated to permit of its retraction.

The loop of the round ligament is now sutured, by two sutures of chromicized catgut, to the under surface of the aponenrosis of the external oblique. I usually prefer interupted sutures.

The operator then passes to the opposite side of the patient and the other round ligament is treated in like manner. The abdominal incision is then closed, and the patient required to keep her bed for two weeks.

I cannot see how the retropertoneal shortening of the round ligaments could interfere either with pregnancy or labor, as the ligaments should develop during pregnancy as they do after the Alexander operation, and should not lead to dystocia: but my experience has been too short, and as it has only been two years since my first operation of retropertioneal shortening of the round ligaments, I am unable at this time to give you my final conclusions upon these points, but I shall endeavor to do so at some future time.

312, 313, 314 American National Bank Building.

EDITORIAL

DEATH OF MRS. EBEN N. ALLEN.

The many professional and personal friends of Dr. E. N. Allen of McAlester will regret to hear of his irreparable loss in the death of Mrs. Allen, which occurred in Little Rock, Ark., February 8th.

Mrs. Allen was a most highly cultured woman, a slendid type of the American mother and her death will be sadly felt by

Dr. Allen and her son and daughters besides' a host of friends in this and other states.

The profession extends to Dr. Allen its sincere sympathy in his bereavement.

NEED FOR BETTER REPORTING OF DISEASE.

The recent statement in the Muskogee County Medical Society that out of forty-three cases of typhoid reported fifteen deaths had occurred emphasizes the need for the profession to be more prompt in reporting this and other diseases on which report is demanded by the rules of the Commissioner of Health.

No one believes for a moment that that high a death rate prevails here or anywhere else on account of this disease and the conclusion that the cases are not reported or that many of the milder ones are not diagnosed is inevitable.

This is about the only solution of the matter and should call for a more strict observance of the rules by the profession.

Naturally many cases are not reported on account of forgetfulness and the pressure of other affairs and the fact that the law is new and not yet understood by physicians; so wide publicity should be given these requirements and all concerned should heed them.

Another phase of the question probably not considered by many, is the bad effect a reputation for typhoid and other diseases will have on emigration. Nowadays people read more than they ever read before and after a prospective citizen looks into property prices and possibilities, and the tax rate he investigates the problem of health and seeks the best and healthiest place for a home. It behooves us to at least make things look no worse than they are.

THE ANNUAL MEETING.

For the information of many enquirers it is announced that the next annual meeting of the Oklahoma State Medical Association will occur in Tulsa, May 10, 11 and 12, 1910.

FOR THE PREVENTION AND CONTROL OF TUBERCULOSIS.

To the Secretary of Each State and County Medical Society and Other Interested Members:

At the last meeting of the American Medical Association at Atlantic City the following report of Committee on Miscellaneous Business was adopted: "The committee recommends that the President of this Association appoint a committee of five members to inquire into the desirability and practicability of the establishing under the auspices of the American Medical Association of a fund for the assistance of physicians disabled by sickness, and for a sanitarium for the treatment of such members of the Association, as may be afflicted with tuberculosis or similar diseases; such committee to report to the House of Delegates at the next annual meeting of the Association."

As a basis for wise action the committee urges that the officers of State and County Medical Societies, and others interested in the subject, should at the earliest possible date, forward to the Secretary of the committee, Dr. A. C. Magruder, Colorado Springs, Colorado, answers to the following queries, with some account of any special cases that seem to illustrate the need for provision for disabled members of our profession.

1. Is there any provision by your State Medical Society, or local society, for the care of destitute and disabled physicians

and those dependent upon them? If so, how is such care provided?

2. What number of instances of special need for such assistance (or sanitarium treatment) have arisen in your locality within the last five years and what number of your members need such assistance now?

3. About how many members of your County Medical Society are at present afflicted with tuberculosis or similar diseases, or have, within the last five years died, or withdrawn from professional work on account of such disease?

It is earnestly requested that this matter be brought before each County and State Society at its next regular meeting, and that the desired information be furnished our committee at the earliest possible date.

Fraternally yours,
EDWARD JACKSON,
Denver, Colorado.
JEFFERSON R. KEAN,
Washington, D. C.
A. T. BRISTOW,
Brooklyn, N. Y.
H. B. ELLIS,
Los Angeles, California.
A. C. MAGRUDER,
Secretary, 305 N. Tejon St., Colorado Springs, Colorado.

INCREASE YOUR MEMBERSHIP.

The present membership of the State association compares most favorably with membership of other state organizations and this is a tribute to the men who believe they are aiding in the elevation and unity of the profession in the state by organization, but there are many men in the state who are not members and are of the material from every standpoint that goes to qualify them for membership. These men are not members for various reasons; some have not thought about it, others have some personal feeling against some man or men who are already members and are deterred from attaching themselves to the organization and there are others who advance the statement that they have not time to give to attendance. None of these arguments are good ones and it is the duty of every member to try to get such men inside. They should be prevailed upon to come in at once and swell the influence of our body.

Try and see if you cannot add one new member to your County Society. Many counties have scarcely half their legally qualified number of physicians enrolled and the field is prolific for good work.

Misunderstandings, which are more easily had on account of the peculiar nature of our profession, are so easily engendered that often five minutes talk dissipates them and the parties concerned wonder how such a little thing could cause a rupture. After they are explained and friends are made every one feels better over it.

Nothing is more disagreeable than a fight or constant bickering among physicians and the physicians who live in a community where they are reduced to the minimum is indeed happily situated.

Do your share toward elimination of misunderstandings. You can best do it by having the men inside your County Society. If a man is a little bad outside of one he is certainly less so on the inside and he can better be reached and criticised for his acts as a member than otherwise. GET HIM IN.

TO CONTRIBUTORS OF PAPERS FOR THE ANNUAL MEETING.

Please remember that your contributions are the property of the Oklahoma State Medical Association.

If in addition to the paper you propose to read you will have prepared a neat copy and hand it in to the Secretary at the time you read your paper you will save future worry and correspondence about it.

You should send at once to the Chairman of the Section under which your paper belongs the title of the same.

C. A. THOMPSON,

Secretary.

IF YOU WRITE A PAPER FOR THE ANNUAL MEETING.

Following is a list of the Chairmen of the various sections for the annual meeting to be held in Tulsa, May 10th, 11th and 12th, 1910:

Medicine, Dr. R. H. Harper, Afton.

Surgery, Dr. Chas. Blickensderfer, Shawnee.

Pathology, Dr. Elizabeth Melvin, Guthrie.

Eye, Ear, Nose and Throat, Dr. S. M. Jenkins, Enid.

Pediatrics, Dr. H. M. Williams, Wellston.

You can greatly facilitate the work of the above named Chairmen by writing them the title and abstract of your proposed paper and by so doing at once you will not be a cause of delay and rush at the last moment in the preparation of the program for the meeting.

It is earnestly recommended that you prepare two typewritten copies of your paper, one for your own private use and for preservation and one to be handed in to the Secretary at the meeting; this latter step will obviate a great deal of unnecessary correspondence after the meeting is over.

YOUR MEMBESHIP CERTIFI- CATE.

Membership certificates, which are virtually receipts for the money paid your County Secretary for membership dues, are now being sent out as rapidly as remittances are being received from the County Secretaries and as the reported names accumulate in quantity sufficient to warrant their handling.

If you do not receive your certificate or if there is an error in your initial or address kindly advise this office, return the certificate and a new one will be sent you.

BOOK REVIEWS

A TEXT-BOOK OF THE PRACTICE OF MEDICINE.

Ninth revised edition.

A Text-Book of the Practice of Medicine, by James M. Anders, M. D., Ph. D., LL. D., Professor of the Theory and Practice of Medicine and of Clinical Medicine. Medico-Chirurgical College, Philadelphia. Ninth revised edition. Octavo of 1,326 pages, fully illustrated. Philadelphia and London. W. B. Saunders Company, 1909. Cloth, $5.50, net; half morocco, $7.00, net.

W. B. Saunders Company, Philadelphia and London.

In this work the practitioner recognizes an old friend, one that is brought down to the present time by judicious additions in the way of the newer affections and an elaboration of all the latest points in diagnosis and treatment.

Many of the matters taken up will puzzle every one except the close reader and the consideration of these will show the infinite care and patience of the author in the preparation of the work.

The section on "Nervous Diseases" has been thoroughly revised.

The work is one of the best from the standpoint of diagnosis and treatment and in its portions devoted to the differential diagnosis of disease.

The work devotes considerable space to tropical and allied diseases and on this account will find favor with the profession in the South.

PRICE-LIST OF NEW AND NON-OF-FICIAL REMEDIES.

Cloth Cover.

1 Copy, postpaid	$0.50
2 Copies, postpaid	.90
5 Copies, postpaid	2.00

Over 5 copies (express collect), at 30 cents per copy.

Paper Cover.

1 Copy, postpaid	$0.25
2 Copies, postpaid	.45
5 Copies, postpaid	1.00
10 Copies, postpaid	1.70

Over 10 copies (express collect), at 15 cents per copy.

American Medical Association,
103 Dearborn Ave., Chicago.

PERSONAL

Dr. J. A. Nelson of Centrahoma has located in Pauls Valley.

Dr. W. G. Brymer of Comanche is attending the New Orleans Polyclinic.

Dr. E. Brent Mitchell of Anadarko has located in Lawton. Dr. Mitchell is doing eye, ear, nose and throat work.

Dr. Burgess of Walter is in the Lawton hospital for a mastoid operation.

Dr. W. M. Turner of the Turner and Lewis private hospital is in Chicago undergoing treatment for a rheumatic affection.

Dr. J. Hutchings White of Muskogee has resigned as local surgeon for the Midland Valley railway.

Dr. W. E. Floyd, Coweta, has moved to Muskogee and formed a partnership with Dr. W. T. Tilly.

The firm of Drs. Fite, Blakemore and Thompson, Muskogee, has dissolved by mutual consent and Drs. Blakemore and Thompson have formed a partnership.

COUNTY SOCIETIES

HASKELL COUNTY.

This county held its annual election for officers in January and selected:

President, Dr. S. E. Mitchell, Stigler.

Secretary-Treasurer, Dr. F. A. Fannin, Stigler.

Delegate, Dr. C. A. Turner, Garland.

BECKHAM.

The Beckham County Medical Society held its annual election of officers January 20th, and selected:

President, Dr. J. M. McComas, Elk City.

Vice President, Dr. H. K. Speed, Sayre.

Secretary-Treasurer, Dr. G. Pinnell, Erick.

This county starts out with practically all the old members enrolled.

CANADIAN COUNTY.

This county held its annual election for 1910 and selected:

President, Dr. D. P. Richardson, Union City.

Vice President, Dr. J. A. Hatchett, El Reno.

Secretary-Treasurer, Dr. James T. Riley, El Reno.

Censors, Drs. Thos. Lane, W. J. Muzzy and R. F. Koons, El Reno.

Delegate, Dr. R. F. Koons, El Reno.

Alternate, Dr. James T. Riley, El Reno.

Canadian county has for the past year been carrying out the program outlined for Post-Graduate Society work and considers much good has resulted from it and will continue the work during the coming year.

On January 8th Dr. John W. Duke, Guthrie, read a paper on "Insanity" before this society.

January 15th H. A. Dever read a paper on "Diseases of the Pancreas," the paper being thoroughly discussed after which an oyster supper, tendered by Drs. Hatchett and West, was enjoyed.

GARFIELD COUNTY.

This county held its election for officers for 1910 December 14th, 1909, at Enid and elected:

President, Dr. J. H. Barnes, Enid.

Secretary-Treasurer, Dr. Julian Feild, Enid

Censor, Dr. W. A. Aitken, Enid.

Delegates, Drs. G. A. Boyle and J. H. Barnes, Enid.

TILLMAN COUNTY.

This county elected officers December 28, as follows:

President, Dr. F. G. Priestley, Frederick.

Vice President, Dr. J. H. Hansen, Grandfield.

Secretary-Treasurer, Dr. A. B. Fair, Frederick.

Delegate, Dr. H. L. Roberts, Frederick.

Censors, Drs. J. D. Osborn, one year; J. P. Allen, two years; A. J. Hayes, three years, all residing in Frederick.

ELLIS COUNTY.

The officers elected for 1910 in Ellis county are:

President, Dr. H. W. Hubbell, Arnett.

Secretary, Dr. John F. Sturdivant, Arnett.

Treasurer, Dr. L. T. Green, Shattuck.

WASHITA COUNTY.

The annual election of officers for Washita county held at Cordell December 21, 1909, resulted in the following officers being chosen for 1910:

President, Dr. J. W. Kerley, Cordell.

Vice President, Dr. G. A. Dillon, Foss.

Secretary-Treasurer, Dr. A. H. Bungardt, Cordell.

Censors, two years, Drs. J. E. Farber; three years, J. H. Barnes, Cordell.

Delegate, Dr. Wm. Tidball, Sentinel.

Dr. J. H. Barnes delivered an address on "Eye Strain in Children," which was discussed at length by the members present.

CHOCTAW COUNTY.

The annual election of officers for Choctaw county for 1910 was held at Hugo the first Tuesday in December with the following result:

President, Dr. E. R. Askew, Hugo.

Vice President, Dr. J. S. Miller, Hugo.

Secretary-Treasurer, Dr. J. C. Ellis, Hugo.

Delegate, Dr. R. L. Gee, Fort Towson.

Alternate, Dr. H. H. White, Hugo.

The following program has been arranged for the meeting of February 1st:

"Croupous Pneumonia," Dr. R. L. Gee, Fort Towson.

"Hook-Worm Disease," Dr. J. C. Ellis, Hugo.

TULSA COUNTY.

January 8, 1910, Tulsa county elected the following officers for the ensuing year:

President, Dr. G. H. Butler, Tulsa.

Vice President, Dr. W. Q. Conway, Tulsa.

Secretary, Dr. W. E. Wright, Tulsa.

Treasurer, Dr. S. DeZell Hawley, Tulsa.

Delegate to annual meeting, Dr. W. Albert Cook.

Alternate, Dr. Fred S. Clinton, Tulsa.

ADAIR COUNTY.

The election of officers for 1910 in Adair county resulted in the selection of:

President, Dr. T. S. Williams, Stilwell.

Vice President, Dr. Calvin C. Barnes, Westville.

Secretary-Treasurer, Dr. Chas. M. Robinson, Stilwell.

Delegate, Dr. Jos. A.-Patton, Stilwell.

Censors, Dr. Oliver W. Farrar, Stilwell; Dr. G. W. Dickey, Chance, Dr. P. C. Woodruff, Stilwell.

HUGHES COUNTY.

For 1910 Hughes county elected the following officers:

President, Dr. A. L. Davenport, Holdenville.

Vice President, Dr. A. J. Hemphill, Holdenville.

Secretary, Dr. A. M. Butts, Holdenville.

Board of Censors, Drs. Mitchell, Scott and Howell.

Delegate, Dr. A. M. Butts.

OKLAHOMA COUNTY.

The annual election for officers in this county resutled in the selection of the following:

President, Dr. A. A. Will, Oklahoma City.

Vice President, Dr. M. Smith, Oklahoma City.

Secretary-Treasurer, Dr. W. R. Bevan, Oklahoma City.

Delegates, Drs. C. B. Bradford, E. S. Lain, M. Smith and J. F. Kuhn, all of Oklahoma City.

At this meeting the fact developed that Dr. J. T. Hensley, member of the Board of Examiners of Oklahoma, appointed as a homeopath, had been requested by a majority of the board to resign as a member. After discussion and Dr. Hensley had made a statement of his side of the affair a committee composed of Drs. A. L. Blesh, A. W. White and R. M. Howard drafted resolutions upholding Dr. Hensley and requesting him to retain his membership on the board.

The resolution was as follows: "Having observed in an evening paper a purported copy of resolutions presented to Dr. J. T. Hensley requesting his resignation from the Board of Medical Examiners of the state of Oklahoma; the said request coming from the President of and signed by three or four members of said board: Be it resolved by the Oklahoma County Medical Society in regular session, that we do most earnestly endorse the conscientious and faithful work of Dr. Hensley on the State Board of Medical Examiners and do most heartily support him in the fight he is making for clean medicine in this state.

"Be it further resolved, That we do most respectfully urge Dr. Hensley to retain his membership on said board.

"Be it further resolved, That a copy of these resolutions be published in the daily press and also spread upon the minutes of this society as a part of the official record."

Dr. W. T. Tilly, President of the State Board of Medical Examiners, was in Oklahoma City at the time and took strong exceptions to the resolutions and expressed himself freely and decisively in the daily press.

A petition was circulated calling for a special meeting of the county society to take the matter up. The meeting was called January 15 and as soon as the society was called to order a motion was made and carried to adjourn and no further action was taken on the question. Dr. Tilly, thus not having an opportunity to present his argument to the society.

COMANCHE COUNTY.

Selected the following officers for 1910 at the annual meeting:

President, Dr. L. T. Gooch, Lawton.

Vice President, Dr. E. Brent Mitchell, Lawton.

Secretary, Dr. D. A. Myers, Lawton.

Censors, Drs. Jackson Brashear, H. A. Angus and P. G. Dunlap.

Delegate, Dr. D. A. Myers.

At this meeting the following paper was presented and read:

"Carbuncle," by Dr. E. D. Meeker, Lawton.

The membership of this society has doubled since January 1st.

TEXAS.

The officers for 1910 for Texas county are:

President, Jas. M. McMillan, Goodwell

Vice President, Dr. Wm. H. Langston, Guymon.

Secretary-Treasurer, Dr. R. B. Hayes, Guymon.

GREER COUNTY.

The Greer County Medical Society held its January meeting at 2 o'clock p. m. on the 11th, in Mangum, Oklahoma.

"Cause and Treatment of Early Abortion," by Dr. James W. Scarborough, Mangum.

"Complications in Typhoid Fever," Dr. W. H. Ruthland, Mangum.

Case Reports.

Clinics, by all members.

KAY COUNTY.

The Kay County Medical Society held their January meeting in Blackwell on the 12th of that month and the following program was carried out:

"State Board Examinations and Reciprocity," Dr. Matthews, Braman.

"Nasal Catarrh and Its Treatment, Dr. Ezell, Newkirk.

A paper by Dr. Phillips, Newkirk.

Presentation and Discussion of Cases.

Election of officers for 1910.

ATOKA-COAL.

The officers elected for 1910 for Atoka-Coal county were:

President, Dr. J. B. Clark, Coalgate.

Vice President, Dr. Spangler, Phillips.

Secretary-Treasurer, Dr. T. H. Briggs, Atoka.

Board of Censors, Drs. Fulton, Atoka, Logan and Conner, Coalgate.

Delegate to annual meeting at Tulsa, May 10, 11 and 12, 1910, Dr. T. J. Long, Atoka.

Alternate, Dr. W. A. Logan, Lehigh.

The meeting which was held February 7th, devoted its entire attention to the subject of tuberculosis.

A paper on "The Prevention of Tuberculosis," by Dr. W. B. Wallace, was presented and will appear in some future issue of the Journal.

STEPHENS COUNTY.

The officers elected by the Stephens County Medical Society for 1910 are:

President, Dr. R. L. Montgomery.

Vice President, Dr. H. C. Frie, Duncan.

Secretary-Treasurer, D. Long, Duncan.

Censors, three years, S. H. Williamson, H. C. Frie, both of Duncan.

Committee on Public Health, Drs. C. E. Frost and S. H. Williamson, Duncan, and P. M. Haraway, Marlow.

GRADY COUNTY.

This county selected as officers for 1910 the following:

President, Dr. Walter Penquite, Chickasha.

First Vice President, Dr. W. R. Berry; Bradley.

Second Vice President, Dr. B. B. Ownes, Minco.

Third Vice President, ..., Chickasha.

Secretary, Dr. Martha Bledsoe, Chickasha.

Censors, Drs. S. O. Marrs, R. J. Gorden and R. P. Tye, Chickasha.

MAYES COUNTY.

The officers in Mayes county for the year are:

President, Dr. E. L. Pierce, Salina.

Vice President, Dr. J. L. Mitchell, Pryor.

Secretary-Treasurer, Dr. F. S. King, Pryor.

OKMULGEE COUNTY.

The officers of Okmulgee County Society for this year are:

President, Dr. Wm, Cott, Okmulgee.

Vice President, Dr. Perkins, Henryetta.

Treasurer, Dr. W. C. Mitchener, Okmulgee.

Secretary, Dr. W. G. Little, Okmulgee.

Delegate, Dr. H. E. Breese, Henryetta.

Censors, Drs. W. C. Mitchener and Warren Newell, Okmulgee.

PAYNE COUNTY.

The officers selected in Payne county for the year are:

President, Dr. C. H. Beach, Glencoe.

Vice President, Dr. L. A. Cleverdon, Stillwater.

Secretary-Treasurer, Dr. D. F. Janeway, Stillwater.

Delegate, Dr. J. H. Cash, Glencoe.

Censors, Drs. J. B. Murphy, Eli Hughes and J. H. Pickering, all of Stillwater.

KIOWA COUNTY.

Kiowa county selected the following officers to control it for this year:

President, Dr. G. W. Stewart, Hobart.

Vice President, Dr. M. E. Chambers, Gotebo.

Second Vice President, Dr. A. Barkley, Hobart.

Secretary, Dr. J. M. Bonham, Hobart.

Treasurer, Dr. A. L. Wagoner, Hobart.

Censors, Drs. A. Barkley and A. L. Wagoner, Hobart, and Dr. Holland.

Delegate, Dr. J. W. Stewart, Hobart.

A paper, "Oezena," was read by Dr. J. R. Dale and will appear in the Journal later.

LEFLORE COUNTY.

Officers for Leflore county are:

President, Dr. B. D. Woodson, Monroe.

Vice President, Dr. G. A. Morrison, Poteau.

Secretary-Treasurer, Dr. R. L. Morrison, Poteau.

Delegate, Dr. G. A. Morrison, Poteau.

Alternate, Dr. W. W. Bewley, Bokoshe.

WASHINGTON COUNTY.

This society held its annual election for officers January 7th, 1910, and selected:

President, Dr. G. F. Woodring, Bartlesville.

Vice President, Dr. H. C. Weber, Bartlesville.

Treasurer, Dr. J. V. Athey, Bartlesville.

Secretary, Dr. W. E. Rammell, Bartlesville.

Delegate, Dr. J. W. Pollard, Bartlesville.

After the election a banquet was indulged in at the Hotel Alameda.

ON THE DEATH OF MRS. ALLEN.

An expression from Pittsburg County Medical Society on the death of the wife of Dr. E. N. Allen.

The most sacred relation among men is that of husband and wife. This has received divine emphasis in the command: "What God hath joined together let not man put asunder."

The sacredness of this sweet and tender relation grows as the years go by until each looks upon the other as a part of his or her very existence. But some, by reason of the peculiar character of their labors, feel more acutely the helpfulness of a devoted companion. The physician probably stands first in this class. No man depends so much upon his wife for comfort and encouragement in the dark hours of trying circumstances, and without such help we are lost and grope in darkness.

We, the members of Pittsburg County Medical Society, realizing how typical was the marriage relation in the case of our fellow, Dr. E. N. Allen; realizing in what tender and high esteem he held his devoted wife; realizing as fully as it is possible for us to realize the irreparable loss and poignant grief he suffers, come now with assurances of our sympathy and love.

But words are empty things under such circumstances, and in our extremity we can but direct him to the precious promises of our blessed Redeemer for consolation and encouragement.

Resolved, That a copy of this expression be sent to Dr. Allen, and that the same be published in Oklahoma State Medical Journal and in the News-Capital of this city.

LE ROY LONG, Chairman,
J. A. SMITH,
J. O. GRUBBS,
Committee.
McAlester, Okla., Feb. 12, 1910.

PROGRAM

Of the Central Oklahoma Medical Association at Enid, Oklahoma, Tuesday, January 18, 1910:

Order of business.

Call to order at 10 a. m., Dr. E. S. Lain, President.

Address of Welcome, Dr. R. A. Field.

Response, Dr. A. L. Blesh, Oklahoma City.

Reading Minutes of Previous Meeting.

Reports of Committees.

Miscellaneous Business.

Election of Officers.

Papers.

Banquet in evening by physicians of Enid to visiting physicians and their wives.

PROGRAM.

1. Fractures, G. H. Thrailkill, Chickasha.

2. Post Operative Ileus, C. E. Bowers, Wichita.

3. Cholecystitis, J. F. Messenbaugh, Oklahoma City.

4. Pericolitis, J. F. Binnie, Kansas City.

5. Paper, A. A. Will, Oklahoma City.

6. The Role of the Pneumococeus in Surgery, A. L. Blesh, Oklahoma City.

7. Diabetes, G. A. Boyle, Enid.

8. Paper, D. W. Basham, Wichita.

9. Ectopic Gestation, E. D. Ebright, Enid.

10. Report of a Case, J. M. Cooper, Enid.

11. Chronic Gastritis, J. M. Postelle, Oklahoma City.

🔯 EXCHANGES AND ABSTRACTS 🔯

HEUBNER'S MUSTARD TREATMENT FOR CATARRHAL PNEUMONIAS IN CHILDREN.

Abstract from The Journal of the Medical Society of New Jersey, by Arthur Stern, M. D., Elizabeth, N. J.

Take a pound of mustard flour and add to it a quart and a half of warm water, stir until the odor of mustard is perceptible. A towel is dipped into this mixture, wrung out and wrapped around the child from head to feet, and then a woolen blanket is put over this. The neck must be well covered so that the mustard does not affect the eyes and lungs. The child stays in this dressing from ten to thirty minutes, or until the skin is red. It is then washed with lukewarm water, after which a lukewarm bath of five minutes' duration is given. Then a moist warm towel is put around the chest. The procedure may be repeated the next day, and in some cases it has to be repeated on two or three consecutive days before the temperature is normal and the respiration quiet. I have never seen any bad results from this method, only that some of the children become restless during the application and that after three or four applications the skin begins to peel.

THE PHARMACOPEIA, ITS HISTORY AND ITS IMPORTANCE TO THE MEDICAL PROFESSION.

The importance of the next Pharmacopeial Convention should be thoroughly understood by all medical societies and physicians. These conventions, as well as the national Pharmacopeia, originated in a proposition submitted to the Medical Society of the County of New York by Dr. Lyman Spalding in 1817. Dr. Spalding proposed that the United States be divided into four districts—Northern, Middle, Southern and Western—and that each district should hold a convention of delegates from the medical societies and schools situated within it, to formulate a pharmacopeia. The four district pharmacopeias were to be taken to a general convention to be held at Washington, composed of delegates from the four districts. From the district pharmacopeias the delegates were to compile a national pharmacopeia. This plan was adopted, the district convention for New England being held in Boston and the convention for the middle states in Philadelphia, June 1, 1819. No conventions were held in the Southern and Western districts, but delegates to the national convention were appointed. The first general convention for the formulation of a national pharmacopeia met at Washington, Jan. 1, 1820. The two pharmacopeias in the Northern and Middle districts were consolidated into one work, which was published in Boston, December, 1820, in both Latin and English. A second edition appeared in 1828.

The convention of 1820 provided for its own perpetuation and for future revisions, by instructing its president to issue notices in 1828 to all incorporated state medical societies and incorporated medical colleges and schools, asking each to vote for three delegates to represent the district at the general convention to be held at Washington in January, 1830, the convention to consist of twelve delegates. The second convention was held at Washington on Jan. 4, 1830, thirteen delegates being present. It provided for its perpetuation by instructing its president to issue a notice to incorporated state medical societies, incorporated medical colleges and incorporated colleges of physicians and surgeons, asking each to elect three delegates to attend a general convention to be held at Washington in January, 1840. The district plan of representation was given up and has never been resumed.

At the third convention, held in 1840, twenty delegates were present. A committee on revision and publication was appointed which published the second revision of the Pharmacopeia in 1842. This committee was instructed to ask the co-operation of schools of pharmacy in its work.

In the call for the fourth convention of 1850, incorporated colleges of pharmacy were included and were allowed to send three delegates, the same as medical colleges. This convention, which met at Washington in May, 1850, was composed of thirty delegates. Only two pharmaceutical schools were represented, all of the other delegates being from medical colleges and societies.

In 1860 the fifth convention was held, thirty delegates being present, four colleges of pharmacy being represented.

The sixth convention was held May 4, 1870, sixty delegates being present, seven pharmaceutical schools being represented. The fifth revision was published in 1873.

The seventh convention met May 5, 1880. One hundred and nine delegates were elected to represent ten medical societies, twenty-three medical colleges, eleven pharmaceutical colleges and the medical departments of the Army, the Navy and the Marine-Hospital service. Seventy-five delegates were present.

The eighth convention was held on May 7, 1890, 175 delegates being present, representing fifteen medical societies, twenty-three medical colleges, twenty-five pharmaceutical associations, twenty-three colleges of pharmacy and the medical departments of the three government services. The provisions made for representation in 1900 were the same as those for 1890.

The ninth decennial convention was held at Washington May 2, 1900. Forty-one delegates were present representing twenty-six medical societies, forty-four delegates from thirty medical colleges, fifty-three delegates from twenty-seven pharmaceutical colleges and fifty-seven delegates from twenty-eight pharmaceutical societies, the American Medical Association, the American Pharmaceutical Association and the three government services being represented by twelve members. The total attendance, as shown by the official report, was two hundred and seven, of which one hundred and fourteen were pharmacists and ninety-three were physicians.

The point to be emphasized in the above historical summary is that the convention was originally inaugurated and for many years carried on solely by the medical profession, and that it was not until 1850 that other than medical societies and medical colleges were authorized to send representatives. In that year, pharmaceutical colleges were for the first time given representation. Not until 1890 were pharmaceutical societies added to the list of accredited bodies.

The medical profession during the past thirty years has not given to the revision of the Phramacopeia the attention which its importance deserves. In spite of the fact that this book originated with the medical profession and was compiled and published primarily for its use, it has come to be regarded too much by physicians as a book which is of interest and value mainly, if not solely, to the pharmacist and in which the physician is not especially concerned. The attitude of the physician toward the Pharmacopeia as well as the lack of knowledge on this subject has been frequently commented on in The Journal. It is now time that specific and lasting reforms were effected. Two definite steps should be taken before the meeting of the next convention in Washington: (1) All incorporated State Medical Associations and Medical colleges entitled to representation should select the three best representatives possible and should see to it that they attend and take part. (2) Each County Society should devote at least one meeting during the winter to a discussion of the present Pharmacopeia and the formulation of suggestions as to its improvement.

There is, indeed, grave danger lest this work, which was primarily a reflection of the needs of the medical practitioner, should become a purely pharmaceutical rather than a medical compilation. There is also danger of its being controled by commercial interests. Such a result will be due solely to lack of interest and activity on the part of the medical profession. Active interest in this matter should be aroused and medical societies should see to it that they are properly and effectively represented in the coming convention, and that their delegates are instructed regarding the desires and opinions of those they represent. If every county society will devote one evening to the discussion of this question and will send its recommendations to Dr. Reid Hunt, chairman of the committee of the American Medical Association on the Pharmacopeia or to the Council on Pharmacy and Chemistry of the American Medical Association, their recommendations will be transmitted to the convention and will receive consideration.

Reprinted from The Journal of the American Medical Association December 4, 1909, Vol. LIII, pp. 1918 and 1919.
Copyright, 1909.
American Medical Association, 535 Dearborn Ave., Chicago.

ECHINACEA.

This drug, which when first introduced was a typical nostrum, is reported on by the Council of Pharmacy and Chemistry, Journal A. M. A., November 27. According to J. U. Lloyd (Pharm. Review xxii, pp. 9 to 14), its introduction to eclectic medicine was due to the efforts of Dr. H. F. C. Meyer to increase the sale of a secret remedy containing it which he called Meyer's Blood Purifier, for which very extravagant claims were made. When the identity of the plant had been determined by Lloyd it was put out under the name of echinacea angustifolia with similar claims as an almost universal antidote and cure-all. These claims were passed along into the more recent advertising matter and much of the eclectic medical literature, some of the statements being still more extravagant. All of these are based only on the clinical trials by unknown men who have not achieved any general reputation as reliable observers; no attempt has been made to verify them by accurate scientific methods, clinical or otherwise, though that could easily have been done. None of the eulogists seem to have thought it worth while to determine by the simplest control experiments whether the drug possesses any bactericidal or antiseptic properties whatever. With the above record and in the lack of any scientific scrutiny of its claims, the Council concludes that echinacea is not worthy of further consideration until more important evidence is adduced in its favor.

BROMALBIN IN EPILEPSY.

The defects of the inorganic bromides in the treatment of epilepsy and other convulsive disorders have long been recognized by medical practitioners. While the bromides have been extensively prescribed —because nothing better had been devised to take their place—their proneness to derange the stomach and to produce systemic disturbances has militated against their usefulness.

The "something better" appears now to be at hand. Reference is made to Bromalbin, an organic compound in which bromide is chemically combined with albumen. Bromalbin contains approximately 15 per cent of bromine. It is in the form of a light-yellow powder and is odorless and practically tasteless. It is insoluble in water, alcohol, acids and the ordinary solvents, but is slowly soluble in alkaline solutions.

Bromalbin was evolved in the chemical laboratories of Parke, Davis & Co. Before being offered to the medical profession at large it was subjected to thorough clinical test by leading practitioners throughout the country in a large number of cases in which bromine medication was indicated. Reports of its use in the treatment of epilepsy were highly encouraging, and the belief is expressed that it will prove equally efficacious in hysteria, neur-asthenia, reflex headache, insomnia, migraine, and other nervous affections.

The chief advantage of Bromalbin over the inorganic bromides appears to be in its adaptation to long-continued treatment. It passes through the stomach practically unchanged, consequently does not produce the gastric irritation common to the alkaline bromides. Slowly dissolving in the intestinal secretions, it is then absorbed, producing a gentle, prolonged systemic effect. Other advantages are: its more complete absorption, its comparative tastelessness, and the small likelihood that it will produce acne, dizziness, or other symptoms of bromism. It is marketed in powder form (ounce vials) and may be given in water, coffee, chocolate, syrups, wines or any beverage

not alkaline in character. It is also supplied in 5-grain capsules (bottles of 100), in which form, perhaps, it is likely to be most commonly used. There is wide need of a sedative such as Bromalbin promises to be, and fuller reports on the new agent will be awaited with interest by the profession.

STANDING COMMITTEES OKLAHOMA STATE MEDICAL ASSOCIATION.

Public Policy and Legislation—Dr. David A. Myers, Chairman, Lawton; J. H. Scott, Shawnee; J. A. Hatchett, El Reno; F. S. Clinton, Tulsa; Claude A. Thompson, Muskogee.

On Medical Education—Drs. B. J. Vance, Checotah; A. K. West, Oklahoma City; E. O. Barker, Guthrie.

On Scientific Work—Drs. Floyd E. Waterfield, Holdenville; P. A. Smithe, Enid; Claude A. Thompson, Muskogee.

On Necrology—Drs. C. S. Bobo, Norman; H. M. Williams, Wellston; M. A. Warhurst, Remus.

FOR SALE.

$1,250 cash gets property consisting of three-room dwelling house, barn, stables, pair of horses, good buggy, office furniture and fixtures; $4,000.00 practice gratis; will introduce. Reason for selling going to specialize in Texas. Address Dr. John T. Vick, Fort Towson, Oklahoma.

FOR SALE.

The Journal has tuition to the amount of forty-four dollars in the New York Polyclinic School and Hospital which will be sold at a reduction from the usual rates. Address The Journal.

BOOK REVIEWS.

THE PRACTICE OF GYNECOLOGY.

New (4th) Edition, Thoroughly Revised.

A text-book on the "Practice of Gynecology. For practitioners and students, by W. Easterly Ashton, M. D., L. L. D., professor of gynecology in the Medico Chirurgical of Philadelphia. Fourth edition thorough revised. Octavo of 1,099 pages, 1,058 original line drawings. W. S. Saunders Company, 1909. Cloth, $46.50 net; half morocco, $48.00 net.

This is unquestionably the most complete work ever prepared on the subject of Gynecology. The author prefaces it with the statement that he attempted to leave nothing for granted and perusal shows that he has carried out his statement in a most thorough manner. The only criticism of the book from a local surgeon being that it contained too much, but this attracts the busy practitioner who has to cover a wide range of investigation in his work and to him the book will be found to fill every requirement. In leaving nothing out Dr. Ashton goes so far as to present the operative and preparatory work step by step with cuts and illustrations which are of great help to the busy man.

The writer, in the short time the book has been in his possession has found it of inestimable value as a work of reference and one that covers the field in such a way that no information along gynecological lines cannot be readily found and explicitly considered.

FOR SALE.

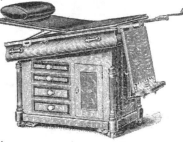

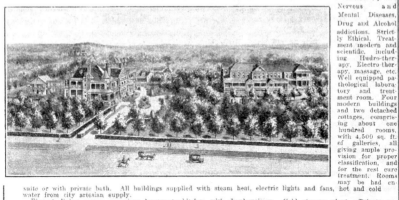

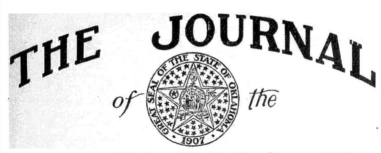

THE JOURNAL
of the
Oklahoma State Medical Association.

| VOL. II. | MUSKOGEE, OKLAHOMA, APRIL, 1910. | NO 11 * |

DR. CLAUDE A. THOMPSON, Editor-in-Chief.

ASSOCIATE EDITORS AND COUNCILLORS.

DR. J. A. WALKER, Shawnee.
DR. CHARLES R. HUME, Anadarko.
DR. F. R. SUTTON, Bartlesville.
DR. G. W. ROBERTSON, Dustin.

DR. JOHN W. DUKE, Guthrie.
DR. A. B. FAIR, Frederick.
DR. W. G. BLAKE, Tahlequah.
DR. H. P. WILSON, Wynnewood.

DR. J. S. FULTON, Atoka.

Entered at the Postoffice at Muskogee, Oklahoma, as second class mail matter, June, 1909.

This is the Official Journal of the Oklahoma State Medical Association. All communications should be addressed to the Journal of the Oklahoma State Medical Association, English Block, Muskogee, Oklahoma.

THE TREND OF MODERN THERAPEUTICS AND TREATMENT OF DISEASE.
BY A. B. LEEDS, A. B., M. D., CHICKASHA, OKLA.

A larger and more intimate knowledge of medical art, a more precise acquaintance with the nature and properties of materia medica., and a more rational application of therapeutic science shows us conclusively that there is a progressive advancement in this branch or field of medicine.

Upon our conception of the etiology of disease depends the selection of the therapeutic agents and the method of their employment.

The various incantations and mysticisms employed by the ancients for the purpose of appeasing the anger of the gods; the use later of the acids and the alkalies for coun-

(*Read Before Grady County Medical Society, September 3, 1909.*)

teracting the basic and acid character of disease; Homeopathy, exemplifying the reaction against the nauseating dosage of the earlier part of the nineteenth century; Eclecticism, endeavoring to obtain a smaller, definite and specific dosage; Christian Science, suggesting the lack of mental concentration and absolute abstention from drugs; the patent medicine, embodying with its shotgun feature, a lulling per cent. of alcohol and narcotics; the introduction of the vast array of synthetic chemicals, together with a plethora of new remedies, many of which were new in name only; the proprietary remedies, exploited for their palatability and thorough, yet empirical, incorporation of needed drugs; the reactionary therapeutic nihilism, so prevalent a few years ago; Osteopathy, suggesting disloca-tions of ligaments, muscles and pressure on blood vessels as a source of all diseases; Chiropractic, a side degree of Osteopathy, laying the blame on the pressure of the various nerves, due to the dislocation of the different vertebræ; the alkaloidal idea of active principles, suggesting the minute dose according to the symtomatology; and last, yet, perhaps the most scientific of all, the internal secretions, with the adrenal active principle as the dynamic element of life, and the accurate scientific conclusions, as elaborated and demonstrated by Sajous, together with the resulting more intelligent therapy, are all evidences of the changing conception of the etiology of disease and the endeavor to obtain a more rational theory.

In the treatment of disease, irrespective of any conventional classification, we realize that the etiological factors are either some inherent degenerative change or error of metabolism or some extraneous agent introduced into the system, and upon investigation, in every case, of these conditions, with their individual peculiarities, depends the successful treatment.

With the abnormal arrangement of the physiological phenomena as our conception of disease, we believe, with Butler, that "Symptomatic therapeutics is not only curative of a portion of disease, but preventive, besides, of ulterior morbid phenomena, complications and aggravations."

In addition, a thorough appreciation of the relation of the different temperaments, environments and climatic conditions, and a realization of the importance of careful and minute clinical observations, augmented by the accuracy and utility of laboratory methods, further suggest the efficacy of treating the symptoms, primarily, and the disease, as modified by the typical symptoms.

The similarity in symptomatology in the incipiency of many pathological conditions calls for an active and effective therapy at the earliest possible stage of the disease prior to the malady becoming firmly seated in the tissues affected, for in this manner many an infection can be jugulated before gross anatomical lesions have developed and the severity of the attack ameliorated and modified.

With specific medication, in only three conditions, viz: the salts of quinine and arsenic in malaria; mercury and the iodides in syphilis and the antitoxin in diphtheria, we are dependent, in all other pathological conditions, upon the maintenance of nutrition and the circulation upon antipyretic measures and upon elimination, by the intestinal tract, by the kidneys, by the lungs and by the skin.

Yet too much reliance can not be placed upon these specific remedies alone, for one of the worst cases of syphilis coming under my observation was thoroughly saturated, and had been for some time, yet anæmia and malnutrition were making greater ravages than the disease itself.

Lacking specific medication in the majority of the pathological and conditions, and not being able to depend entirely on what specific medication we possess, it is absolutely necessary for us to take into consideration every possible phase of each case if we successfully combat these pathological conditions.

We find that the therapy and prognosis are simplified, many times, by giving the exciting causes, of many pathological conditions, careful consideration.

Almost miraculous cures will, often, be, effected by eliminating the exciting cause of the use of alcohol, in cases, with obscure symptoms of doubtful origin, where we elicit the constant use of this agent, for, in this condition, we know that the use of alcohol has a peculiar corroding effect, on the cells and tissues; that there is an impairment of the growth, development and diminution of the functional activity of the cells of the body; that there is an increased strain placed, on the blood vessels, lessening the oxygen-carrying property of the blood, and that the abnormal increased activity of the liver and kidneys diminish nutrition.

A more intelligent and successful therapy is obtained in cases of Syphillis in both its acquired and inherited forms, with manifold and obscure manifestations, appearing at variable intervals, when due consideration is given these facts, and they are thoroughly understood.

A true appreciation of the effect of the lack of proper exercise, confinement in unsanitary surroundings, and the use of food, not adapted to the climate and work, simplifies the therapy in these cases.

Many headaches, backaches, eye and other abscure troubles could be simply explained and more successfully treated, if we unnderstood more thoroughly and more often took into consideration the intimate vascular and nervous associations of the sexual organs and the effect of their derangement upon the general system

The lessened normal vital resistance, in our growing youth, would be better understood and more easily corrected, if we considered, carefully the effects of the difference in the mode of living, not only, in the larger cities, but also in the smaller towns; the effects, upon the nervous and mental systems, of our present educational system, with its long hours and often unhygienic surroundings; the effects of the habitual errors of diet; the effects of the lack of intelligent instructions, regarding the sexual organs the effects of the mad rush for riches, which necssitates the entrance into commercial life, of your youth, at an early age, and the surroundings, of the factories, stores and offices, in which they work.

While we possess the advantages of the intelligent ideas of infection, immunity and etiological factors of pathological conditions as demonstrated, with the aid of the microscope and the latest laboratory methods, in the hands of such students as Pasteur and Koch, assisted by Ehrlich, with his side chain theory; Metchinkoff, with his doctrine of phagocytosis, Sajous, with his study of the internal secretions of the adrenals and the ductless glands; and Wright, by his elaboration of the Opsonic theory; the rapid advances made in general and, local anesthesia; our perfect asepsis and antisepsis; our modern dietitics, founded on the exact laws of nutrition and metabolism; psychotherapy, with definite and limited fields of usefulness; physical means of treatment, as hydro and electro-therapy, massage, and the principles of rest and exercise; organo and Serum Therapy, made possible by the recent chemical and bacteriological researches, and each of these have added their mite, in the development of the modern therapeutic treatment of disease, yet at the present time, the basis of the modern treatment of disease if the neutralization and elimination of the nitrogenous products of toxicity, that are either the cause of disease or have an influence in shaping their severity, circulating through the fluids of the body, the blood and the lymph.

We find that these nitrogenous products of toxicity are elaborated in all diseases, marked by increased catabolism and are due to the fact that the toxic products, which are formed in the intestinal canal, are not converted by the liver and other organs, into harmless products.

Examples of this condition, we find in autotoxemia with its faulty metabolism and impaired elimination; and in the infections and contagious and all other febrile diseases.

We are rapidly realizing that tonics and therapeutic agents, to increase the vital resistance of the cells and tissues, are more potent, in the treatment of tuberculosis, than many of the nauseating mixtures, usually used.

The rational employment of hot water, internally and externally, a more elaborate and liberal liquid diet, small normal saline enemata and symptomatic treatment will lessen the mortality and hasten the convalescence, in both typhoid fever and pneumonia.

There will be, in a short time, practically, no need for an antitoxin or specific treatment, for either typhoid fever or pneumonia, if we realize that every case of either of these diseases is an active focus of infection and contagion and will use as thorough and effective an isolation and quarantine, with the destruction of the dejecta and fumigation as is used with yellow fever.

The modern treatment of disease, which comprises, supplying the deficient normal constituents of the blood, stimulating the excretion through the emunctories, of the products of imperfect metabolism; destroying the effects of toxic materials and improving the nutrition, can be best illustrated by giving you the treatment, for typhoid fever, as suggested by Sajous.

This treatment is based upon the fact that Sajous has demonstrated, beyond a question of a doubt, that the leucocyties, owing to the ferments which they contain, are endowed with a most active transforming activity, capable of transforming and modifying toxic substances into food for the entire organism and by taking up the products of intestinal digestion, in the alimentary canal, and converting them into granulations, which they deposited in the tissues, they supply the entire organism with the agencies which combine with the oxidizing substance to insure the continuation of life and the efficacy of all organic functions:

We find that the bacilli of the typhoid group include the colon bacilli, and whether as a result of rapid multiplication of the latter or of the assumption, by it, of greater activity, it can assume any virulence of the typhoid bacilli irrespective of any infection, when the environment is suitable.

In the intestinal canal, which contains, constantly, the baccillus coli communis, the condition which renders possible such an assumption of virulence, by this germ, is the presence in the intestinal juice of an insufficient proportion of auto-antitoxin or protective substance.

Over-work, fatigue, loss of sleep, poverty, and immoderate exercise play a very important part in the development of sporadic cases and epidemics.

There is no doubt, in my mind, that these causes contributed more to the epidemic of typhoid fever, suffered by our soldiers during the Spanish-American war, than any impure water supply or deficient sewerage.

The efficiency of the British army medical service, although high, was unable to prevent the troops in South Africa, from suffering from typhoid fever, to a deplorable extent.

Fatigue was a very important factor in the pathogensis of these cases.

Typhoid fever may be caused, therefore, without infection of external origin when, either through hypo-activity or sluggishness of the adrenal system or through excessive utilization of the blood's protective substance (as during exhaustion, prolonged exercise and labor) the proportion of auto-antitoxin, in the body at large is inadequate.

This accounts for the development of typhoid fever in the so-called "spontaneous origin" group; this, also, explains the atypical cases, in which we are able to limit the febrile period to eight or fourteen days;

our inability, often, to demonstrate the Widal reaction test and the development of cases, extremely mild, after an experience, such as Chickasha has had, during the past six months, with the dust, mud holes, etc., resulting from the paving and grading work.

Most often the disease is caused by the ingestion of the typhoid bacillus with food or beverages, especially water derived from a contaminated source or in milk, contaminated in the handling that the dairies and on the wagons.

Some of the morbid phenomena, present, in this disease are but manifestations of a violent reaction of the body's protective resources.

In animals, immunized by gradually increased doses of living or dead typhoid bacillus a bacteriolytic or anti-toxin substance appears, in their blood and the accompanying marked febrile process continues until the pathogenic organisms, living and dead, and their toxins are destroyed.

The energy with which the protective functions are stimulated by the typhoid toxins and endotoxins is well known by the marked localized leucocytosis evoked, in favorable cases.

We find that the tumefaction of the intestinal, mesenteric and splenic lymph-apparatus is due to the excessive proliferation of the phagocytic endothelial cells, arising from the lymph spaces, lymph vessels and endothelial layers of the blood vessels.

These cells, we find, diffusely scattered through the swollen follicles and glands, in immense numbers or accumulated in large groups and manifesting pronounced phagocytic activity, as well as, multiplication or retrogressive changes.

The prognosis, in these cases, depends, greatly, upon the power of the small and the large phagocytes to offset the multiplication of the typhoid as well as their acting as a barrier to general infection.

If these phagocytes succeed, by ingesting the bacteria, laden cells, in ridding the lymphoid follices of the pathogenic germs, the amoeboid cells collect the local detritus and remove it and the lymphoid elements resume their normal functions, about the eighth to tenth day, by new epithelium growing into the area, from its periphery and fortunately for us, the cicatricial tissue formed is longitudinally disposed, and does not therefore, tend to cause constriction of the corresponding portion of the intestinal canal. The healing process terminates the fever.

But, if such is not the case, the epithelial elements become necrotic and slough, leaving a round or elliptical ulcer occupying a solitary follicle or a portion of Peyer's patch, which may reach down to the muscular coat and even through to the serous coat.

This may give rise to intestinal hemorrhage, owing to an erosion of an artery or vein; or perforation of the intestinal wall may be followed by peritonitis, a condition which may, also, be caused by an extension of the inflammatory process in the lymphoid tissues.

The essential object to be obtained, in the treatment of typhoid fever is the enhancing, not only of the bacteriolytic powers of the blood, as soon as possible, but to increase the protective agencies, so that the bacteria may be sensitized and their ingestion and digestion by the phagocytes, may be activated.

The administration of 5-grain doses of calomel every three hours, until liquid green stools occur, incites an active bacteriolytic and antitoxic process, in both the liver and the intestines, as we find that the green color is due to the biliverdin, a reduced or used-up protective agency.

Then, by provoking a flow of intestinal fluid, which contains auto-antitoxin, by the administration of either, a bottle of citrate of magnesia or a dose of epsom salts, you are able by the resulting flushing to rid the intestinal canal of the pathogenic germs. and their poisons, contained therein at that time.

Violent saline purgation should be avoided, however, since it reduces the defensive properties of the blood, by depleting, too freely, the blood of its serum and auto-antitoxin.

This should be followed by 1-10-gram doses of calomel, every three hours, until salivation begins, as in this way, the functional activity of the adrenal system is sustained and enhanced.

Upon the appearance of salivation. the intervals between the doses may be increased sufficiently to keep its action just within this symptom, the limit of safety.

To sensitize the bacilli and facilitate their ingestion by the phagocytes, an agent contributing auto-antitoxin, to the blood, must be used, in conjunction, with the calomel.

One-half grain dose of Iodine with 5 grains of ammonium iodide, night and morning, are sufficient to insure adequate sensitization of all pathogenic elements.

In cases, where there is an idiosyncrasy to mercury, 5 grains thryroid extract, three times a day, in conjunction with the iodine and iodides will be sufficient to increase, markedly, the defensive properties of the blood.

Another as important factor, in the successful treatment of typhoid fever, as in all febrile diseases, is to use saline solution, from the outset.

By its use, the osmotic properties of the body fluids are preserved and the efficiency of their defensive functions are increased, for though, the blood be rich in auto-antitoxin, with an abnormal viscidity, of the blood and especially the lymph, any action of the bacteria. and the poison derived from them, is limited, to a great extent, if it is not entirely prevented.

For owing to the smallness of the molecules of NaCl and its chemical inertia, it is, pre-eminently, the salt which maintains the osmotic equilibrium, between the tissues and the blood, for it insures the access of the plasmotic serum globulin to the diseased area and through the thyroidase which it contains, it sensitizes the bacteria, detritus, etc., thus facilitating their ingestion and destruction by the phagocytes; by holding the serum globulin, in solution, it insures its free circulation, as a constituent of the plasma, in all vessels, down to the minutest capillary net works distributed to the cellular elements, including those of the nervous system.

This enables the serum globulin-laden plasma to transude freely through the capillary walls, in order to reach the tissue cells and carry on the life process.

The free osmotic properties which the lymph, in the tissue spaces also owes to NaCl, insures the sweeping away, by the lymph current, of all the wastes derived from the cell.

During febrile diseases, with its normal supply of NaCl not being replaced by the ordinary floods, the body's supply becomes inadequate, very soon; the protective properties are hampered in proportion as the deficiency of the NaCl and this is a very fruitful cause of death, in all infections.

On the whole, the proportion of NaCl and alkaline salts to be administered should corresponding with the diminution of nourishment, which the disease, in one way or another, entails.

If the patient receives, in 24 hours. one-fourth of his usual amount of foods, the salts given should be three-fourths of the quantity excreted, taking into account the age. sex and size.

These salts may be added to milk, broths, or other beverages or foods.

When the salts cannot be administered, entirely, by the mouth, they should be given by enema, and if necessary, sub-cutaneously or endovenously, and very slowly.

The free ingestion of water preserves the normal specific gravity of the blood and other fluids and insures a low specific gravity of the urine, thus protecting the kidneys, notwithstanding the free elimination of acids and other wastes.

Any oedema, nephritis or liability to hemorrhage contra indicates the use of the saline solution, except in guarded doses.

The elevation of temperature, after its use, is not a contradiction because it is due to the fact that the blood is enabled to resume its bacteriolytic and antitoxic functions; the rise of vascular tension is but a normal outcome, as the muscular coat of all vessels and the cardiac muscle itself are also the seat of enhanced metabolic activity; the glycosuria is also but a proof of the sudden liberation of the adrenal system, as we find that the adrenal extractives provoke glycosuria.

With the diet one should have in mind the fact, that the intestine is the seat of lesions, which render the use of foods, that impose physical irritation or undue peristaltic action, upon the organ dangerous as they tend to promote local complications.

If the foregoing measures are carried out, cold baths are not only not necessary, but do not add anything to the treatment, and hot or lukewarm sponge baths are much more efficacious in enhancing the dissipation of heat from the skin.

Hemorrhages are best controlled by the use of small doses of ergot and morphine, as the contraction of the inestinal arterioles are produced, by the employment of these drugs.

Constipation is best overcome by means of large enemas of saline solution at 110 degrees, Fahrenheit.

We have a powerful prophylactic combination in thyriod extract, 2 grains and quinine, 2 grains, taken after meals, because the thyroid extract increases powerfully the bacteriolytic action of the blood and quinine drives the blood towards the capillaries, causing the intestinal mucosa and its lymphoid follicles to become congested with blood, rich in protective properties, and the digestive activity of the phagocytes.

With the blood and its cells, likewise, fully supplied with thyroidase, pathogenic germs are readily sensitized, thus augmenting greatly, their vulnerability to destruction by the phagocytes.

Iodine and the iodides can also be combined with quinine, preferably the hydrochlorate.

A very pernicious agent is alcohol because it reduces the blood's serum globulin and produces effects similar to those caused by fatigue.

None of the other agents, in our pharmacopœia, are sufficiently active to afford adequate protection in the disease.

September 3, 1909.

Read before Grady County Medical Society by

A. B. LEEDS, A. B., M. D.,
Chickasha, Oklahoma.

Drs. J. C. Mahr, State Commissioner of Health, J. M. Trigg of Shawnee, Oklahoma, and S. M. Crumbine, Commissioner of Health for Kansas have been appointed to represent the State of Oklahoma in the Ninth Decennial Convention for the Revision of the Pharmacopœia.

Dr. R. A. Allis, a graduate of the Indiana State University, Medical Department, has located in Waunette.

"THE RELATIVE PATHOLOGY COMPLICATING A DISPLACED UTERUS"

BY DR. G. N. BALLARD, M. D., OKLAHOMA CITY, OKLA.

Associate Professor of Gynecology and Clinical Gynecology at College of Physicians and Surgeons (Medical Department of the University of Illinois;) Surgeon to Marion Sims' Sanitarium, Chicago; Attending Surgeon at West Side Hospital, Chicago; Attendent in Gynecology at the West Side Free Dispensary.

The uterus occupies a position in the pelvis almost transverse to the perpendicular body. There is a slight anteflexion normally. The cervix points backward and the fundus forward. It is a movable organ necessarily so on account of the important organs with which it is supported. We might say that it is an organ of accomodation, as its movability allows room for a distended bladder or a distended rectum. Two conditions that often occur and must have extra room when so distended, even though this important organ is displaced. This displacement however is not pathological unless it be so long continued the the new position becomes permanent or fixed.

It may become permanently displaced backward from a neglected distention of the bladder, or forward from chronic constipation, or a repeatedly distended rectum.

Grossly considered the uterus is in relation posteriorly with the rectum, anteriorly with the bladder, latterly with the layers of the broad ligament.

It is held in position by the various ligaments radiating from it, the deposit of adipose tissue, and various grades of connective tissue which are found filling up every point of vantage about the organ not otherwise occupied. Muscle fibres enter into this as well. They can be found strengthening all the ligaments, being reflected from the most contiguous part of the uterus. These fibres can be traced in the tissue of these various ligaments to a greater or less distance from the uterus, being found throughout the tissue of the ovarian and around ligaments. This last statement is contrary to the teaching of many authors, but by a careful study of the tissue of the last named ligament you can satisfy your own curiosity and be convinced of the certainty of its existence.

Every author has his own idea as to the real support of the organ. If we weigh them all carefully, we can get some facts from each one, and conclude that they are all right, in part, and that there are, as enumerated above, many factors in its support. Any one of these may be disabled by disease or trauma and thus cripple the general support of the organ.

Despite the assertions of many authors to the contrary, I must say that any permanent deviation from the normal *does* produce symptoms. Many recent articles would lead us to believe that simple displacements were not productive of symptoms. I agree that some displacements produce only transitory symptoms while other seemingly simple conditions are the cause of symptoms of the most severe character.

They are all abnormal conditions and must produce more or less severe symptoms in proportion to the importance of the organs or tissue infringed upon. This is virtually true of all other organs, how can we make an exception of the uterus?

In the first place we have an organ supplied with blood vessels, nerves and lymphatics, properly adapted to its normal position. You may say that the blood vessels are so arranged that they adapt themselves to the enlarging and displacement of the organ during pregnancy. Granting that this actually does take place during this change of position, yet this is a physiological change of position only, and is provided for, while other changes in position are permanent, are pathological, and are not compensated for. Any abnormal permanent change in position lessens the caliber of the vessels, causes partial obstruction of the flow of blood and hence disturbs the vitality of the tissues supplied by them. The traction upon the nerves supplying these parts causes pain or a sense of uneasiness, and more or less general suffering. The circulation is not only interfered with by the traction exerted by the displacement but also by the pressure on adjacent organs and their nutrient vessels. This interference with the blood supply lowers the vitality of all tissue supplied by the vessels so effected, making them more susceptible to disease. The veins become varicosed. The walls of these vessels become inactive owing to the obstruction of the circulation through the nutrient vessels supplying them.

Any abdominal surgeon will agree with me that it is very common, in operating for displacements to find a varicose condition in the wall of the uterus as well as in the surrounding tissue. Let the displacement be extreme in any direction and we will have a general varicosity in the pelvis. This always produces symptoms not only in the pelvis generally but in the bladder and rectum, the two most important organs in close relation. The symptoms here mentioned are the ones most frequently overlooked, and it is for this very important fact that this paper is written.

I have seen so many women suffering with these symptoms and consulting one physician after another until it seems to me not out of place to study this commonplace subject a little, refreshing our memories as to the more common symptoms and studying carefully some new phases that present themselves to us in our different experiences.

The uterus may be disposed backward —(retroversion). This is a most common condition in women of all ages. It may be adherent in this position or it may be movable. If it is allowed to remain in this position too long it is likely to become adherent.

Normally all the ligaments of the uterus are as guy ropes; they are lax and not put on the stretch, as is sometimes supposed. They are not intended to hold the weight of the uterus for any length of time, but only to tether it within certain limits. If it become displaced beyond this certain limit for a time sufficient to overcome the intended strength of these various ligaments or any one of them, their power to recover it to its normal position is gone and it remains out of its normal limitation. Other ligaments and tissue entering into its support become overtaxed and their vitality is interfered with to the extent ofttimes of destroying their usefulness entirely.

In retroversion the folds of peritoneum between the bladder and uterus known as ultero-vessical ligaments, are put upon the stretch. Traction here lessens the calibre of the vessels. The blood supply is thus interfered with; their walls are weakened and a varicose condition is produced. Traction on the bladder causes an irritation, congestion follows and a final change of position is the result. The round ligaments enter into this general change and are affected in like manner. Their muscle fibers and blood vessels are stretched and lose their vitality even to the point of inability to fulfill their function.

The posterior reduplicated reflection of the peritoneum with its strengthening muscle fibers are also taxed beyond their strength and are lengthened and weakened. The larger blood vessels in the broad ligament and walls of the organ, by pressure or traction become over-filled and their walls weakened and a general varicosity is the final outcome.

The above conditions do not come on suddenly, but are of slow progress, hence the tendency of the patient to treat them lightly at first. The rapidity of the advancement of these abnormal conditions are enhanced by trauma to the pelvic outlet, which removes another help to the general support.

If the latter condition is present, the loss of the support of the vaginal walls occur. A dragging downward of the bladder and rectum takes place. These walls are already increased in thickness by the engorged blood vessels. Mingled with the foregoing abnormalities we find all the blood vessels of the pelvis engorged, heavy, and assisting in the displacement of the organs contained within, in the direction of least resistance, which is in the line of the vaginal outlet.

The bladder and rectum are both displaced in proportion to the severity of the relatively existing pathology. The severest symptoms now are referable to these relative organs.

The bladder symptoms most commonly found are, frequent urination, scalding of urine during its passage, its irritation of the external parts, an amoniacal odor, inability of the patient to empty the bladder without the assistance of the hand, dribbling of urine while on the feet, relief of this latter symptom when reclining.

An illustrative case I wish to report is as follows: Mrs. C., age 42, children 6, miscarriages one, at three months. Family history negative. She had a severe laceration of the perineum four years ago—unrepaired, extensive prolapse of entire vaginal wall. A cystocele and rectocele had developed to a marked size. Constipation and dribbling of urine were prominent sypmtoms. The latter symptom was so annoying as to isolate the patient from society.

She had been treated in a palliative way for four years, even the galvanic and farradic currents had been used. No vaginal examination had been made and hence no accurate diagnosis could be made.

I often wonder how it can be possible that such a plain case as this, able to give such a clear history, could be mistaken for an ordinary case of cystitis. From the treatment given the diagnosis evidently was one of cystitis. Is it any wonder that such cases are compelled to consult different medical men? I would not want to say that any graduate of medicine would not know the cause of the most marked symptom in this case if he had made an examination. But I do censure such carelessness in arriving at a diagnosis. We must dismiss the prevalent idea that all bladder troubles are simply cystitis, due to some chemical change in the urine. I make it an invariable rule to make a vaginal examination when such symptoms present themselves, unless I can dismiss them by exclusion. It is true that cystitis does occur if this condition obtains for too long a time. To treat such symptoms lightly and without carefully weighing them is to say the least not strictly honest surgical practice.

After taking a complete written history of the case with her description of her symptoms I was convinced what I would find on examination, which I did by making a vaginal exploration. I found the perineum lacerated to the bowel, leaving only the thickness of the bowel wall and vaginal mucous membrane separating the vagina from the rectum.

The mucous membrane of the vagina was thickened and its folds were very prominent and pouching. The posterior portion was protruding from the now wide open vaginal outlet. On further examination, per rectum, I discovered that the bowel was drawn down with it and hence formed a rectocele. Any effort at stool caused the protrusion to become more prominent. The anterior wall of the vagina was also protruding through the anterior portion of the vaginal outlet. A closer examination proved this to be followed by the bladder wall, forming a true cystocele. This latter condition was extensive enough to prevent the bladder emptying itself and hence the decomposed residual urine. Wearing the corset aggravated the most annoying symptom—the dribbling of urine. It was for this symptom in particular that she consulted me. In addition to the above there was a sub-involution of the uterus, thickened vaginal walls and an extensive bilateral laceration of the cervix. The displacement of the vaginal walls was out of proportion to that of the uterus.

The diagnosis being fully established, we will all agree that no palliative treatment could cure such a condition. The only relief was to be accomplished by surgical interference—a plastic operation. I did a colpoperineorraphy and an anterior colporrhaphy considering this sufficient as the displacement of the uterus was slight. A retroversion pessary is being worn and the symptoms formerly existing have completely disappeared. I repaired the cervix by doing a tracheloplasty, a modified trachelorrhaphy, removing the greater portion of the vaginal cervix. In doing all of this plastic work I have lessened the weight of the uterus, supplied the lost perineal support, and added the temporary artificial support until involution has been accomplished, and the blood vessels regained their tonicity. The normal vitality will soon be restored and then I will remove the artificial support (the pessary) and the organ now practically with its near normal supports will adjust itself to its normal position and so remain.

Case No. 2 illustrates another phase of a retro-displaced uterus. Mrs. P———, age 24, married 4 years, began menstruating at 14, regular but very painful. She suffered from constipation which grew worse from puberty until the age of 18, when by exposure to cold and wet, at the time of her menstrual flow, an inflammation was induced after recovery from which she was never healthy. A constant weight and pressure was felt in the pelvis. Backache, low down, was almost constant and aggravated when standing. Diarrhœa now took the place of constipation and any kind of food taken into the stomach excited peristalsis and a thin fluid evacuation occurred. This symptom grew worse until the patient was reduced in flesh from 135 to 85 pounds. All palliative remedies and modes of dieting had been exhausted without any permanent relief.

After an exhaustive written history had been taken I made a thorough examination of all the vital organs and found them practically normal.

A pelvic examination revealed a retroverted uterus, bound down by adhesions on either side of the rectum to the extent of about two inches. This constricted the bowels to less than half its caliber. Above the constriction the bowel was dilated to twice its normal diameter. So far all treatment had availed nothing. As a new departure I concluded to break up the adhesions and place the uterus in normal condition by shortening the round ligaments. I expected this to relieve the irritation, hoping that by so doing to remove the cause of the hypersensativeness of the bowel and thus stop the excessive diarrhœa.

The operation was successful, my hopes were more than gratified by the complete recovery of the patient, without return of the bowel symptoms. It took a few months for the bowel walls to gain their normal vitality and activity, but it was finally accomplished and health virtually restored.

It is not common to recommend a laparotomy for chronic diarrhœa, but here is one case where the results of the radical work done allowed the accomplishment of the desired end. My firm belief is that had not this extensive work been done, removing the source of the irritation palliative treatment could never have accomplished the results thus secured.

These illustrative cases are used only to show the importance of our extending wide our examinations in order to make sure of our diagnosis. Superficial exploration and careless and thoughtless examinations are the source of many of our best patients drifting from us and trying other isms, pathies and even practors.

The varicosities enumerated are usually complicated with that most annoying condition known as hemorrhoids. How many times are these dilated vessels amputated without taking into consideration what the real cause is.

Pressure from a retrodisplaced uterus is so frequently the primary cause. What will be necessary in such case? It is plain to be seen that the removal of the pressure will be necessary. We know without this one procedure that the removal of the now existing hemorrhoids will only be transatory. That which had produced such condition if allowed to remain will be the cause of more similar pathology. It will be necessary to restore the uterus to its normal position and then we may expect a removal of the hemorrhoids to be a permanent success.

CONCLUSION.

1. That uterine displacements *do* produce symptoms immediate or remote.

2. Disturb the normal uterine position and you add to it the bladder or rectal complications.

3. Pelvic varicosities are very much aggravated by uterine malpositions.

4. The cause removed the effect removed, permanent relief may be expected.

LARYNGEAL TUBERCULOSIS

BY DR. H H. WILSON, SHAWNEE, OKLA.

The subject of Laryngeal Tuberculosis would seem to be one as little discusseu as any particular brand of medicine, due possibly to the fact that it is usually associated with and secondary to lung phthisis, the gravity of the latter outweighing the former to such an extent as to almost overshadow the throat complications, for we rarely see death resulting from the laryngeal form.

Very little was known of the pathology of tuberculosis of the upper air passages until about the date 1825 A. D., when Matthew Baillie reported the results of his research and investigation, and there appears to have been very little added to his find-

ings since that time unless perhaps it be in the matter of treatment.

The primary form, I believe should claim the attention of the physician rather more than the secondary for it is here that it can be successfully combatted if recognized early and the proper treatment instituted. Not, however, that the destruction to tissue and life are not just as great, but the site affords us means of combatting it by topical applications which is not possible with lung phthisis. In considering the primary form we must acknowledge the conditions as being such, only, when it appears prior to and independently of lung involvement; otherwise there is no such affection recognized or extant, for it has been demonstrated to the satisfaction of all laryngologist of authority that there be

---

(Read Before the Pottawatomie County Medical Society, March 10, 1910.)

a pretubercular condition of the cervical lymphatic glands and tonsils of sufficient per cent to explode the theory of a primary laryngeal tubercular condition arising from a tubercular baccilli nidus within the laryngeal mucosa or muciferous glands or the parts.

Statistics would seem to establish the fact that of all hypertrophied tonsils eneucleated at various times and by numerous individuals examined with the view of ascertaining the per cent containing tubercular bacilli, that six is about the percentage arrived at by practically all investigators, and the cervical lymphatic glands furnish a rather higher per cent either by way of the blood or lymph channels or directly through the tissue spaces, and too, by the latter route without leaving any traces of their passage.

The local condition of the larynx is perhaps as great an etiological factor as the tubercular bacilli, especially in the primary form. An enumeration of the many and varied conditions and circumstances favorable to its development will at least lead us to that conclusion. Local conditions that invite tuberculous involvement are usually, however, brought about by a general or systematic condition and other phenomena incident to our physical economy.

The physiological changes in the nerve and blood supply in the female larynx at puberty as also during gestation furnish a striking example of what slight changes, either pathological or physiological may invite or render the parts susceptible to tubercular bacilli invasion. These two predisposing causes are of greater moment than all others combined when considering the primary variety. Any deviation from the normal in the larynix of the girl at the beginning of her menstrual period, as evinced by the many symptoms of laryngeal disease, should be looked upon with a great deal of circumspection and invite a thorough examination of the parts, and the throat symptoms that appear during the period of gestation are no less important.

Any predisposing cause effecting the onset of phthisis pulmonalis may also be said to favor the laryngeal form, and quite a few are attributed to the latter that would not materially effect the former. Age, sex, occupation, previous local disease and acute and chronic laryngitis are chief among the predisposing causes. The greater per cent of cases are developed between the ages of twenty and forty. The female is the victim in the ratio of about two to one in that of the male. Diphtheria and scarlitina claim their proportion of causes; tobacco and alcohol cannot be second in the category predisposing causes. The adynamic fevers and in fact any systemic disease that tends to lower the vitality will render the advent of laryngeal tuberculosis more prone.

The diagnosis is not difficult save in the first, or stage of infiltration, the infiltrate being not unlike that of any other form of laryngitis except in the case of catarrhal inflammation in its several stages. The infiltrate in the latter is always bilateral and uniform, while in the former it is usually unilateral and is never uniform, though we may have a mixed infection of syphillis and tuberculosis that would render the diagnosis more difficult and indeed, could not be cleared up without the theraputic test. And again, we may have the pear-shaped epiglottis that is said to characterize tuberculosis in the syphillitic infection. But in the stage of infiltration of the two conditions as appearing separately we need not confound them when we consider the difference in the duration of the two. In syphillis we would expect the infiltrate to give way to an ulcerative condition in from a few days to two weeks, while in that of tuberculosis the duration may be from one to six months. In the ulcerative stage of the two infections there need not be a mistake in the diagnosis by one who has observed them. There would seem to be some stress laid upon the particular site of the two as a diagnostic feature, but personally I have failed to note or appreciate that difference. The ulcer itself in each case furnishes a striking dissimilarity; a tuberculous ulcer is superficial, is coated ever with a thin much-purulent exudate of a grayish yellow color, is not sharply defined, and rather moderately indurated, while that of syphillis is sharply defined, excavated, notably indurated and as a rule has a coating of a dirty grayish or brown exudate.

New growths pachydermia and lupus may be confounded with tuberculous infiltrate but on careful inspection differential diagnosis is usually very readily made. The ulceration of lupus is very similar in character to that of tuberculosis. In the former, however, we are generally able to detect the presence of all three stages, viz: The infiltration, ulceration and cicatrization, a clinical picture that we are never able to observe in the tuberculous ulcer. The throat symptoms of lupus are always secondary to skin involvement which makes the differential diagnosis clear.

The onset of a throat lesion in individuals who are suffering from pulmonary phthisis naturally suggests the diagnosis, but even here we should not take too much for granted, bearing in mind especially the prevalence of syphillis in some form in the human family. Primary tuberculosis of the larynx, while it is recognized by all laryngologists of authority, is not a very common occurrence and I do not believe that we are justifiable in arriving at a scientific conclusion in any given case without having given the patient the benefit of the tuberculin test, and in extremely suspicious cases we should not content ourselves with one, but give the second or the third and

the latter with an increased amount, sufficient to clear up all doubt.

The results obtained from treatment depends largely upon circumstances, as ninety-nine per cent of all cases are secondary to lung envolvement, and it would be akin to folly to attempt to permanently relieve any given case by topical applications without affording the patient all the means possible to combat the primary malady by climatic conditions, where it is possible to do so, and other recognized stipulated auxiliaries pertaining thereto.

Serum therapy has its advocates; personally I have had no experience with it and what ultimate results may be obtained by such medication remains to be seen. But I do know that by the judicious topical applications of such theraputic remedies as are employed today by the laryngologists of the country much may be achieved in the way of mitigating the pain and sufferings of our tuberculous patients, and a cure may be expected in the primary form in practically all cases. The various modes of application in vogue today embrace inhalations and sub-mucous injections, but in so far as medical treatment is concerned, the one really effective procedure is the direct application of the various pigments. Both, the method of using, and the drugs to be employed, demand careful consideration. The applicator best suited may be said to be one that combines strength, elasticity and delicacy, yet of sufficient size to admit of a firm grasp. The remedies should be well rubbed into the tissues, and at such intervals as seem best suited to the given cast.

Lactic acid is no doubt the remedy par excellence in the ulcerative stage; the strength to be employed should be determined by the laryngologist as best suited to the individual case. Usually, however, we begin with a twenty per cent sol. and gradually increase to the full pharmaceutical strength. It is best as a rule to employ the weaker sol. with oft-repeated applications for in the use of the stronger we are apt to mistake the over stimulation of the drug for advancement of the disease and thereby compromise all the beneficial results obtained by the medication. Lactic acid in full strength exerts a cauterizing effect on an abraded surface with one formation of a thin scab, which scab is thrown off in from one to two weeks. Under the scab, healthy granulations are seen to spring up and interference by repeated applications prior to the cleaning off of the surface is unwholesome to say the least. Under its judicious use we may confidently expect to relieve to a marked degree the suffering incident to these throat lesions. Formalin is likely of as much therapeutic value as the former drug, especially is it seriviceable in the stage of infiltration, where it is not advisable to use the acid.

In strength varying from three to ten per cent rubbed well into the mucous membrane overlying the infiltrate at intervals varying from one to three days will in many instances cause an absorption of the infiltrate in the secondary form and a cure can confidently be expected in practically all cases of primary origin. By the judicious employment of the above remedies we can in most instances render our patients fairly comfortable and where they are given the benefit of climatic advantages combined with a suitable regimen, etc., a cure can be had in many cases. Ulceration of the cartilaginous structures may be relieved by surgical means but it is a procedure, I believe that it is not jutifisable unless the conditions and circumstances are such as to enable us to hope for an ultimate recovery of the lung involvement.

In advanced cases where there is considerable destruction of tissue and beyond relief, a spray of cocaine sol. should be resorted to as also the hypodermic use of morphia to relieve the excruciating pain that sometimes accompany these conditions.

OZENA

BY DR. J. R. DALE, HOBART, OKLA.

This short paper will take up a very interesting subject, owing to the fact that there is considerable confusion as to the cause of the disease.

Ozena is derived from the Greek, meaning a stench.

Some authors claim it to be but a symptom, and this symptom being associated with atrophic rhinitis, the stench in syphilis, in glanders, coryza caseosa, in necrosis of the bone, and in suppurative processes of the accessory sinuses. Other authors again give ozena a place as a disease under the synonym of rhinitis caseosa, rhinitis chronici foetida and fetid coryza. This is the condition I desire to discuss which is asso-

(*Read Before the Kiowa County Medical Society, February* 15, 1910.)

ciated with chronic atrophic rhinitis, and not the kind due to syphilis, tumors or necrosis of bone, as they have their own place in surgery with their own treatment.

I would like to touch lightly on the etiology with the different theories, and then on the pathology. It is mostly found between the ages of five and twenty years. In females it is twice as common as in males.

Barring out the scrofulous, syphilitic and tuberculous, it is found mostly in the strong and robust.

There being three principal cause theories, viz.: The inflammatory, neuropathic and the bacterial, I will take them up separately under

"Pathology."

Grossly speaking, we find atrophy of the osseous and membranous tissue of the turbinated bodies, the glands of the pituitary membrane becoming atrophied up to a total loss of the glandular tissue. To bring this about we have the epithelium undergo cloudy swelling up to fatty degeneration. These cells are exfoliated in great numbers. We have overproduction of connective tissue, which contracting interferes with the blood supply. Thus nutrition is interfered with and the whole tissue is changed into an entirely new structural element. The cells changing to cuboidal flat cells or pavement epithelium, a deeper tissue being fibrous, it makes a tough leathery surface, more like the cutaneous surface than a mucous membrane.

So we come to the inflammatory theory, that atrophy follows the hypertrophic condition Zuckerkandl distinguishes three stages of atrophy. The mildest stage, the turbinated bodies shrunken but slightly; next, the bone is reduced in size, and finally, **the** turbinated bodies showing but a small projection. He explained the odor due to degeneration of the pavement cells epithelium formed.

The nerotrophic theory is based on the trophic changes, interfering with function of the pitutory membrane, and saprophytic bacilli becoming lodged on the surface, hence the stench.

Now we come to the microbiotic theory, which I look on as the most favorable one. Belfanti claims that it is the pseudo-diphtheritic bacillus that causes the condition. This bacillus is associated with the bacillus necrosis. The reason I think it is due to bacilli pseudo diphtheria is that the condition improves under the anti-diphtheritic treatment. I will cite a case.

Mr. S. L. in May, 1908 came to me for relief for ozena. He had been to Oklahoma City and had taken a prolonged course of treatment, and while considerable improvement had taken place, the scales and odor had come back as bad as ever.

On inspection the alae of the nose was wide, the turbinated bodies being greatly atrophied and shrunken, and covered with a yellowish greenish scale which extended on down and over the vault of the naso pharynx. The stench was unbearable. I treated him for three months with the ordinary methods, antiseptic, etc. Also used the cotton plug, with air space the size of a lead pencil to breathe. While I did temporary good, later on he was as bad as ever after a month from the time of treatment.

He came back, so I commenced giving the anti-diptheric serum injections. I gave 1,000 units at an injection, giving four of them a month. I kept it up for two months. In the meantime I built up the lower turbinates some by injecting into the bodies sterilized vaseline. He has not been troubled with scales forming to any extent since, and no odor has ever occurred.

Gradenigo reports out of thirty-seven cases he has cured sixteen of them by the use of the anti-diphtheric injections. That is the crust, and the odor was stopped.

I have had but little experience with ozena, having only three cases where the patients consented to the cost of the serum method. All these three cases are apparently well.

I thank you for your attention.

(*Read Before Kiowa Medical Society, February 15, 1910.*)

Dr. Benton Lovelady is spending some time in the East doing Post-Graduate work. He will visit the principal hospitals of the East and spend some time with the Mayo's before returning to the State.

WHY STATISTICS ARE IMPORTANT

BY DR. C. L. REEDER, COUNTY SUPERINTENDENT OF HEALTH, TULSA, OKLA.

Prior to the act of the Oklahoma Legislature creating a State Board of Health, the Superintendents of Health of the several counties of Oklahoma met in convention and organized under the name of the "Association of County Superintendents of Boards of Health."

In order to realize effective service a legislative committee was selected to aid in securing the best possible laws regarding a health department for the State. This committee labored continuously in conjunction with the president of the State Board of Health, and the statutes of the most modern legislation of the different States of the Union were investigated and personal inquiry was made of the boards of health of the States having the best laws, and from this data the present health laws of Oklahoma resulted.

A bureau of vital statistics was undertaken by the New State Health Commission, employing the most modern and up-to-date methods, and while it has in some instances worked hardships and has been a matter of annoyance to the busy practitioner of medicine, yet we must all fully-realize the importance of this great work.

In compiling information for a bureau of vital statistics for this State it places a great deal of work upon the county superintendent of health of each county, and all without remuneration. Therefore, it is well to understand that the burden of reports does not alone fall upon the practitioner of medicine. It is required of the superintendents of health of each county in the State to make the following report:

First, the report of each death and birth. Second, the report of all contagious and infectious diseases. Third, a report of all public nuisances. Fourth, a report of all marriages legalized and completed in the county. Fifth, a report of all divorces in the courts of the county, giving all data as to the number of children, if any, and ages and disposition made of them by the court, the ages of the divorced couple and names given by them.

While all this information may appear extreme, yet in the years to come the records of the Bureau of Vital Statistics will have become the most valuable records in the State and may determine the disposition of immense fortunes and estates hereafter. While it is not an easy matter to secure all information desired, yet it is a matter of business to search the records for marriage licenses and court records for divorce proceedings, but it is impossible for the county superintendent of health to secure valuable information from the practicing physician, as that depends entirely upon the promptness, courtesy and integrity of the individual doctor, and if the doctor fails to make his report within a reasonable time, if he permits the matter to rest from time to time, until even a report that he may render at a later date is valueless, as it is largely a matter of memory with the doctor.

While I am not undertaking to criticise the practitioner of medicine for incomplete returns, yet it would be a great service to the State if the necessary data for all reports was secured at the time. Under the requirements of the law the State of Oklahoma will eventually force prompt and complete reports, under heavy penalty, but the disposition of the present health commission is to act in harmony with the medical profession and jointly develop and

(*Read Before the Tulsa County Medical Society, November 6, 1909.*)

maintain a bureau of vital statistics that will be a credit to the State, however, in the returns from the practitioners of medicine in the classification and causes of death, if the attending physician would render with his report explanation in detail for the following causes:

Abortion, cellulitis, childbirth, convulsions, hemmorhage, gangrene, gastritis, meningitis, miscarriage, peritonitis, phlebitis, pyæmia, septicæmia and tetanus, it would, be of untold value to the Health Commission, and would often prevent tedious correspondence. as the Health Commission of Oklahoma have adopted the international classification given by the Census Office, and if the practitioner of medicine would make the initial report in Washington it would place the report of the Bureau of Vital Statistics in much better standing.

The superintendents of health are supplied with official instructions and classifications of causes of death, and copies of same will be mailed to any practitioner of medicine upon request.

While, we as residents of the county of Tulsa, recognize that our county is at least the equal of any county in the State, yet it remains an established fact that our reports to the Bureau of Vital Statistics rank very much below a good many counties. Now this is not on account of intentional negligence on the part of the physicians, but rather thoughtlessness, and in this paper I desire to impress upon the mind of every doctor in the county the importance of a prompt and complete report in order that Tulsa County may rank first in the office of the State Board of Health, as she justly deserves.

In concluding this paper, I consider it just to recognize and compliment Dr. Wright, superintendent of health of the city of Tulsa, for his very efficient administration, as the reports from his office are prompt and in splendid condition. The good people of Tulsa should feel proud that the city commission have organized and adopted by ordinance the best health law of any city in the State, and while some foolish citizen may deliberate and argue over the price of a garbage can, yet the future of the city will convince all that the first consideration in any community must be the matter of health of its people.

MORPHINOMANIA

DR. CHAS. BLICKENSDERFER, SHAWNEE, OKLA.

The increasing number of resorts for the treatment of the various drug habits is a sad commentary upon the social conditions and relations maintained by a civilized people permitting it. It is also a reflection, in many instances at least, upon the careless methods employed in the treatment of some of the commoner forms of disease.

It is for us to seek and remove the causes leading up to this state of affairs. and by a proper education of the on-coming physician, fit him as adequately for the prevention and treatment of these cases as we do for those diseases daily encountered by the general practitioner. Speaking from my own personal observation, until recently, that is to say; within the past ten years, it was an exceedingly uncommon thing to encounter what was known as a "morphine or opium eater." These unfortunates were looked upon by members of the laity and also by a large per cent of the medical men with feelings of distrust mingled with those of fear. It was a condition dealt with from an intellectual distance and as such received that consideration prompted alone by ignorance.

With the growth of knowledge relative

to the great and splendid uses of opium and its derivatives, the advent of cocaine, and a familiarity with its many virtues, has grown also the number of victims addicted to their inordinate uses. They furnish an ever increasing clientele for the quack and imposter. But the knowledge of the general practitioner has not kept pace with the conditions outlined above, so that as a general rule he is both incapable and unwilling to assume the care of such a case falling into his hands. Because of his lack of knowledge of the number of such cases, their symptomatology, and the pernicious effects of the continued and ever increasing dosage of such drugs, he is careless in their legitimate application, thereby becoming an unwitting agent for increasing the number of addicts. Before passing the causes operating to increase the number of drug victims, it would be unfair not to mention their hypodermatic administration. This has, of course, been one of the most potent factors in the increased use of these drugs.

By morphinomania, is understood that condition in which an individual feels compelled to use morphine as a means of stimulating his physical and intellectual faculties to the production of comfortable or pleasurable sensations or to enable him to perform his accustomed duties with a degree of satisfaction not otherwise obtained.

Morphine, while it relieves pain in most instances, is capable also of producing in some a sense of intellectual and physical well being, an inebriation of the senses combined with much pleasure, a condition known as Euphosia. This effect of the drug is more marked in hypochondriacs, neurasthenics, and those who are easily depressed mentally. The method of administration is almost always by means of the hypodermic needle, and is self administered. Those who take the drug by the mouth rarely suffer from the baneful effects of it

to the same extent as do those who take it by the injection method.

The mania for morphine is usually acquired through its use in the treatment of some ailment, fancied or real. From its continued use the body becomes accustomed to it, and the constant craving makes the habitue a slave to the drug. The daily amounts must be increased to produce that degree of stimulation required by the individual in order that he may feel adequate to the social, professional, or other demands made upon him.

Physicians, dentists, druggists, professional nurses, and that class of the laity known as neurasthenics are most susceptible and in the order named.

The symptoms are to be divided into three classs: Somatic, Psychic, and the symptoms of Abstinence. They are not immediate but usually appear in about six to eight months or even later. Of the first class may be mentioned the following: From the lessened secretions there is dryness of the mouth, constipation, and insufficient salivation of the food. Later the constipation may give way to diarrhœa. The pupils are contracted, usually equal, and react slowly to light. Later on Miosis is replaced by Mydriasis. It not infrequently happens that the pupils are widely dilated, due to the combination of atropia with the morphine. One such case fell into my hands, in which the individual had had glasses fitted by the optician to correct the errors of vision due to an ever increasing mydriasis caused by the rapidly increasing doses of atropine. He had begun taking morphia 1-4, atropia 1-150, for the pains of an acute appendicitis with recurring attacks. For about ten years he had averaged from four to six grains daily, with a corresponding amount of atropine. The nutrition is seen to suffer, the fatty tissue disappears, the skin becomes yellow, dry and wrinkled. The hair becomes gray prematurely and the teeth carious. There is anemia and general cachexia supervenes. The heart becomes weak, the pulse intermittent and slow. The appetite is capricious, the individual often developing great hunger just after having taken his accustomed dose. He may eat anything to which he may have access, going for hours afterward eating practically nothing. These excesses and irregularities are often accompanied by acute attacks of gastric and intestinal disturbances, for the relief of which morphine is again resorted to. The urinary secretion is usually lessened, and may contain albumin. In some there is seen a frequent desire to urinate from cystic irritability. This is frequently simulated, the patient being desirous to absent himself in order that he may secretly take his accustomed dose. There is loss of sexual desire, with impotence in men, and cessation of the menstrual flow in women. Knee jerks are diminished or absent. There is increased susceptibility to cold, and diminished sensibility to touch and pain, and concentric limitation of vision. The perspiration is usually diminished, but it is sometimes markedly increased. There is headache, localized and vague shooting pains, neuralgias, and paresthesias. In the advanced stages of intoxication, keeping pace with the ever increasing marasmus, there is fever of an intermittent or remittent type, sometimes resembling typhoid, but more often simulating the different types of malarial infection. Obstinate insomnia adds to the rapidly increasing defection of the individual, for the relief of which recourse is had to the rapid increase in size and frequency of the dosage. Death, from marasmus, unless caused by some intercurrent disease, closes the scene.

Of the psychic symptoms may be mentioned intellectual torpor, loss of memory, loss of will power. There is almost total perversion of the ethical sense. The impairment of the moral character, loss of self control and diminished mental energy and force are always marked. There are simple, elementary illusions and hallucinations of all the senses. The unfortunate votary of morphine neglects his personal appearance, his principal and most important care being to obtain a sufficient quantity of morphine to supply his wants To do this he will stoop to any method, however, reprehensible or degrading. It might perhaps be interesting to note the manner in which this drug is carried and used. In the earlier stages of a chronic intoxication before the morphinist has withdrawn from or been dropped by his associates he customarily carries a small vial with a wide mouth with a capacity of from four drams to an ounce. In this he makes a solution containing more than enough for his daily requirements. He always makes more than enough because of the constant fear that something will come up during his daily routine of life that will require larger doses than before. Or, he carries an ordinary teaspoon, a hypodermic syringe, some matches, a vial of water, and the morphine in the form of some of its salts. By placing a dose of the morphine in the spoon and adding some water it quickly goes into solution by aid of heat or from a match and can then be drawn into the syringe and injected. It is astonishing to note the cleverness shown by come of these individuals in taking their injections. I saw one, a patient of mine, take out his syringe while seated at a table in a dining room of a large hotel, take water out of his drinking glass, load his syringe, and take his injection without being observed by the waiters or any of the guests. It is characteristic of an individual addicted to the use of morphine that he is notoriously unreliable and untruthful. A well-developed psychosis is usually the result of abstinence.

The symptoms of abstinence are not usually manifested short of five or six hours following the withdrawal of the drug. The patient grows restless, yawns, stretches himself, complains of being chilly and has frequent desire to urinate. There is cystic uneasiness, and an increased flow of saliva. The skin itches, and there is nausea, vomiting and increased anxiety. The bowels become loose, and unless controlled by the drug, the condition passes quickly into one of serious diarrhœa. The vomiting and diarrhœa, with a cool clammy skin, resembles cholera morbus. There is a great need of warmth, profuse perspiration, and great muscular weakness. The pulse becomes irregular, intermittent, the volume and tension variable. The reflexes are increased, and there is general sensorial hyperesthesia. The patient complains of neuralgic pains in his limbs and viscera, muscæ volitantes and hallucinations. One of my patients complained several days of "that hellish smell," "if I only could get rid of that damnable smell." With these there is complete loss of appetite, agrypnia, arousal of the sexual desire, and there may be delirium and epileptiform or choreic attacks. Collapse may follow resulting in death. During this time the patient begs, screams, and prays for morphine. One, a patient of mine who was being treated by gradual withdrawal, would cry, wring her hands, beg for morphine, and declare that, "my flesh is being torn from my bones." Another says, "My legs reach from here to St. Louis, and my head is in the Gulf of Mexico. Every time I close my eyes I begin to stretch out."

"The patient who has once experienced the anodyne influence of the drug—as captivating to his sense as though it was a draught of fabled Lethe—readily yields to it upon the slightest occasion, as, for instance, to alleviate trivial indispositions for which, in ordinary circumstances, he would ridicule the idea of medical treatment. With repeated indulgence—often promoted by a casuistic reasoning of which by degrees the subject is scarcely conscious, or by persistent and intentional deception—comes the craving, which knows no restraint, and which can be quieted only by complete mental and physical regeneration or the merciful release of death. Dependent for fancied happiness upon his extraneous resource, the blind idolater of personal ease pursues his *ignus fatuus* heedless of consequences, in his mental and moral degeneracy apparently lost to all finer feelings or to manlier resistance in the presence of his insidious, blighting temptation. Meanwhile physiological torpor demanus an ever increasing amount of the drug that the system may be sufficiently impressed. Psychical emotions, anxiety, anger, mental anguish, or, indeed, the most puerile pretexts, continue to furnish occasion for indulgence, and the facilities afforded by the modern method of hypodermic injection unhappily serve to stimulate a longing for momentary exhiliration or the alluring oblivion which may obliterate the past but which reason cannot suffer to ignore the future when the mind recalls the overwhelming testimony of experience. Should amelioration be now attempted and the drug withheld, more distressing symptoms still are developed. Depression and exhaustion are manifested at once, followed by increasing melancholia, attended by horrible visions and anxieties that no mental energy—such as remains of it—can dispel. The pulse is scarcely perceptible; the patient is in a state of nervous tension, occasionally evinced by paroxyms of despair; and in the deprivation endured the poor wretch, with out-stretched hands and imploring expression, begs, screams, for morphine, laudanum, or other habitual form of opium; at last breaking down utterly in a fit of passionate weeping when denied the solace craved. It is, indeed, an appaling spectacle of human misery which, could it be witnessed by those in whose imagination the first subtle effect of opium awaken dreams of elysium, might well persuade the victim to forswear a gratification for which so tragic a fate is reserved."

TREATMENT.

The treatment of this malady requires the utmost patience and kindness on the part of the physician. The services of a nurse of unquestioned integrity and character are invaluable, for the patient is wholly and altogether unreliable, and cannot, for a single moment, be depended upon to assist in maintaining the abstinence necessary to his cure. The daily minimum amount of the drug must be ascertained and divided into six or eight doses of equal size and be given at regular intervals. This amount is usually much less than that habitually taken, for they usually take much more than is required to produce the necessary stimulation. It has been my custom to then thoroughly clear out the bowels by means of salines and to stimulate the skin and kidneys in order to rid the system, as much as possible, of the accumulated toxins. The gradual withdrawal of the drug is then begun. This may be more or less rapid, according to the size of the daily amount habitually taken by the patient, his general condition and the effects produced by the withdrawal. Great care must be used during this time to conserve the strength of the patient. Alcohol in the form of good brandy, whisky, or wines, is often useful for this purpose, especially during the most active period of withdrawal, for at this period the appetite is gone and nausea and vomiting prevent, to a great extent, the giving and assimilation of food. These patients feel the need of heat externally and should be kept in well heated apartments. A warm bath at night with a cold sponge and massage in the morning will both relax and stimulate him. The injections necessary should be timed to come at the same time as the baths and diet periods, for when thus combined insomnia is not so pronounced and the desire for food not wholly abated, thereby conserving the energy of the patient. For agrypnia trional, bromides either alone or combined with chloral may be tried, though, as a rule chloral should be avoided, for we have to deal with a weakened musculature generally, and the exhibition of chloral hydrate may cost the patient his life on account of its depressing effect upon the heart. Rest in bed, nourishing diet, and good wine in liberal doses are essential. The giving of food should be timed, to come immediately after the injections of the drug, for there is usually an aversion to food during the periods of abstinence. Nourishment should consist of a good quality of milk, wine, brandy, soft cooked eggs, and such other forms of diet as are easily and quickly digested and assimilated. The intense desire for morphine which is evidenced at times during the intervals between the injections is often largely psychic, and the patient can often be quieted by injections of plain water. Upon learning of this deception his confidence is increased. At other times an injection of a solution containing a tablet of strychnine may be used for the same purpose, the patient being allowed to see the tablet enter into solution, under the belief, however, that it is morphine. In the course of ten days to four weeks, withdrawal will be complete, and the patient under the influence of restored normal conditions regains his appetite, and, as all his functions are normally re-established, he begins to enjoy a sense of well-being. Sleep comes again, and with it rest of both mind and body. These individuals usually regain their flesh rapidly, and, as their strength returns, the causes which in the first place rendered them morphinists must be removed. Otherwise relapses are inevitable. The after-treatment is important in the prevention of relapses. A sojourn in the country or a sea voyage is beneficial, the patient in the meantime being under the care of the physician. After a cure, morphine should not be given as a remedial agent except under the most extreme circumstances, for the dangers of a relapse are so great that a single dose thus given may, and often does cause a return to the habitual use of the drug. Of Levenstein's cases, out of 82 males, 61 relapsed; 28 females, 10; of 32 physicians, 26. The high per cent of relapses thus given, shows the necessity of prolonged after-treatment and a full return to the natural conditions of a normal life, before entrusting the interests of the patient to his own resources.

EDITORIAL

THE NECESSITY FOR EARLY DIAGNOSIS OF ABDOMINAL SURGICAL CONDITIONS.

Perhaps in no particular class of human affections is the need for early diagnosis of acute abdominal troubles as great.

The ability of the family physician, will of course, never reach that acute state of development attained by the skilled surgical diagnostician, but he should strive to attain that degree of skill that will enable him to make a "surgical diagnosis," that is, one that will enable him to say to his patient and the family, "here is a condition which I believe to be so and so, I am not positive that this is the case. It may be some other of the following conditions which closely simulate the trouble named, but at any rate this patient should be immediately removed to the hospital or a surgeon called and a line of action determined. Whatever the conclusions I believe this patient should have that abdomen opened and time is the most important factor in such conditions."

How often has the scene of death by procrastination been presented to the view of the consultant and attendant in our hospitals?

Scarcely a surgeon, in fact none, but who can recall many cases of neglected and postponed operation for acute inflammatory and infectious conditions in which the patient could not have been easily saved by early operation.

Many men still cling to the idea that medical treatment is indicated in many surgical affections and point out this and that successful result of medication as against surgical interference; they are usually of that class wherein the statement is made by friends of the patient "that everything was done in power of medical skill, but to no avail," and their recoveries from acute abdominal troubles are due not to the treatment, but to that tendency of human flesh to recover, even under most adverse circumstances and the fact that many have recovered from non-surgical interference should not deter an honest man from trying to save a larger percentage of his clientele.

A 48 or 72 hour diagnosis of a burning fire in a building would probably disclose a pile of brick remaining and the same delayed diagnosis of an internal fire of the human economy often gives the same end results and when a practitioner is guilty of trying to smother his fire with a hand sprinkler he is of not as much use as the volunteer neighbor who brings his bucket into action.

The day of idly sitting by the bedside and allowing your patient to grow hourly worse should be over, if you try to quiet his vomiting and pain with medicines and they are due to appendicitis, gall bladder disease, ovarian or tube inflammation, obstruction or one of many other conditions sole y amenable to surgical treatment you are culpable and no longer deserve the work of that patient or any other.

AN HONEST AND INTELLIGENT PRESS, OUR GREATEST AID.

A vast amount of good information to the public has been made through the medium of the weekly magazines who have the moral stamina and financial means which place them above the sordid and grasping in journalism.

This especially applies to two publications in our country: The Ladies' Home Journal and Collier's Weekly. In the former publication for April appears from the pen of one of our greatest surgeons Dr. W. W. Keen, on vivsection and from time to time appear other articles affecting the general public, which can not be reached in a more effectual manner.

The people as a rule are very indifferent to the dangers of infection and contamination, except where they are closely and personally concerned. Very few of them even know and most of them do not care what vivisection means and the lurid appeals of the vivsectionist press, which it must be said is most active, is more likely to attract their attention and excite a maudlin sympathy based not on reasoning and common sense, overlooking the great good such work has done and will continue to do to the human race and as a consequence enlist their aid in a matter of which they know nothing and which requires the mind and training of an earnest investigator to appreciate.

Dr. Keen places the medical side of the question to the people, shows them by strong illustration the good and need for such work and goes far toward educating the public on this question. The article will be read by thousands and glanced through by the million readers of the Ladies' Home Journal and in the end be productive of a conclusion based on common sense and not one produced by the hysterical work of a set of cranks.

THE ANNUAL METTING AT TULSA, MAY 10, 11 and 12, 1910

Preliminary Program

Section on the Practice of Medicine, R. H. Harper, Chairman, Afton, Okla.

1. Address of the Chairman.

2. "The General Practitioner, Esau despised his Birthright"—Chas. W. Fisk, Kingfisher.

3. "Poliomyelitis Anterior"—J. Donohoo, Afton.

4. "Broncho-Pneumonia, Etiology and Treatment"—Leonard S. Willour, Atoka.

5. "Diagnostic Relationship Between Internal Medicine and Special Surgery" —Jacob Block, Kansas City, Mo.

6. "The Prevention of Disease"—T. F. Renfrow, Billings.

7. "Cases of Neuritis"—Eugene J. Wolff, Waukomis.

8. "Thermogenesis"—G. H. Thrailkill, Chickasha.

9. "Cases of Amœbic Dysentery with Hepatic Abscess"—Ellsworth Smith, St. Louis, Mo.

10. "Diffuse Dilitation of the Esophagus, with Report of a Case"—C. C. Conover, Kansas City, Mo.

11. "Diagnosis and Treatment of Diabetes"—Harry E. Breese, Henryetta.

12. "Membranous Pericolitis"—Jabez N. Jackson, Kansas City, Mo.

13. "The Slow Hearts; Their Significance, with Special Reference to Heart Block, Louis H. Behrens, St. Louis, Mo.

14. "Malaria; Atypical Forms,"—R. K. Pemberton, Krebs.

15. "Clinical Significance of Uterine Hemorrhage"—J. A. Hatchett, El Reno.

16. "Arteriosclerosis"—W. A. Tolleson, Eufala.

17. "Early Diagnosi of Tuberculosis"— Sea A. Rilly, Oklahoma City.

SECTION ON SURGERY, CHARLES BLICKENSDERFER, CHAIRMAN, SHAWNEE

1. Address of the Chairman.

2. Paper, Subject unannounced—Geo. W. Cale, Jr., St. Louis, Mo.

3. "Post-Operative Exudates,'—W. E. Dicken, Oklahoma City.

4. "Open Treatment of Fractures by Internal or Direct Splints"—Herman E. Pearse, Kansas City, Mo.

5. "Treatment of Fractures of the Elbow"—C. T. Harris, Konowa.

6. "Clinical Notes on Fractures and Dislocations of the Upper Extremity"—M. E. Preston, Denver, Colo.

7. "Hernia"—A. C. Scott, Temple, Texas.

8. "Cause and Treatment of Inguinal Hernia," W. J. Frick, Kansas City, Mo.

9. "Gall Bladder Surgery"—W. C. Graves, McAlester.

10. "Report of a Case of Intestinal Obstruction"—J. C. Watkins, Hallett.

11. "Concussion"—B. F. Fortner, Vinita

12. "Management of Fractures of the Extremities"—J. A. Foltz, Ft. Smith, Ark.

13. "Surgical Treatment of Bone Tuberculosis"—Report of Two Cases"—L. H. Huffman, Hobart.

14.—"Local Anesthesia"—Leigh F. Watson, Oklahoma City.

COUNTY SOCIETIES

McCURTAIN COUNTY.

———

The officers for McCurtain County for 1910 are:

President, Dr. A. S. Graydon, Idabel; Vice-President, Dr. W. H. McBrayer, Haworth; Secretary-Treasurer, Dr. W. B. McCaskill, Idabell; Delegate, Dr. W. H. McBrayer, Haworth.

CLEVELAND COUNTY.

———

The annual election of officers in Cleveland shows the following elected:

President, Dr. John Dice MacLaren, Norman; Vice-President, Dr. J. A. Davis, Norman; Secretary-Treasurer, Dr. Albert C. Hirschfield, Norman; Censors, Drs. C. S. Bobo, R. D. Lowther and Robt. E. Thacker, Norman.

KAY COUNTY.

———

This County elected officers as follows on March 9th, at the annual meeting held in Ponca City:

President, Dr. W. A. T. Robertson, Ponca City; Vice-President, Dr. G. H. Nieman, Ponca City; Secretary, Dr. A. S. Risser, Blackwell; Treasurer, Dr. A. S. Nuckols, Ponca City; Censors, Drs. H. M. Stricklen, Tonkawa, Allen Lowery, Blackwell, and H. H. Panton, Ponca City; Delegate, Dr. A. P. Gearhart, Blackwell.

POTTAWATOMIE COUNTY.

.The Pottawatomie County Medical Society held its annual election of officers on March 10, in Shawnee. The following officers were elected:

President, Dr. T. D. Rowland, Shawnee; First Vice-President, Dr. J. E. Cullum, Earlsboro; Second Vice-President, Dr. F. L. Clarkson, Shawnee; Secretary-Treasurer, Dr. G. S. Baxter, Shawnee.

Program of Annual Meeting
of
Pottawatomie County Medical Society
Thursday, March 10, 1910
Shawnee, Oklahoma

President's Annual Address—Dr. J. M. Byrum, Shawnee.

Paper—Scarlet Fever—Dr. J. E. Cullum, Earlboro.

Paper — Laryngeal Tuberculosis—Dr. H. H. Wilson, Shawnee.

Paper—Report of Case of Hydrocephalus—Dr. H. G. Campbell, Asher.

Paper—Obstetrical Surgery and Repair of Laterated Perineum—Dr. J. M. Trigg, Shawnee.

Paper—Infant Feeding—Dr. R. M. Anderson, Shawnee.

Paper—Prevention of Malaria—Dr. G. S. Baxter, Shawnee.

Paper—Work of the State Board—Dr. A. M. Butts, Holdenville.

'A Kick from Venus—Dr. W. B. Pigg, Shawnee.

Bovine Tuberculosis—Dr. E. H. Troy, McAlester.

Tuberculosis of Bones—Dr. A. A. West, Guthrie.

The Medical Profession in the Work of the State Tuberculosis Association—Dr. H. H. Williams, Wellston.

The National Tuberculosis Crusade—Dr. J. A. Walker, Shawnee.

Banquet.

DEATH OF MRS. J. C. W. BLAND.

The Professional friends of Dr. J. C. W. Bland of Red Fork will regret to learn of the loss he sustained in the death of his wife who succumbed to pneumonia in February.

The Tulsa County Medical Society adopted the following resolution of the occasion, and the Journal extends to Dr. Bland the sympathy of the state-wide profession on his loss.

"The Grim Reaper has come to the home of one of the members of this Society and claimed the companion and wife. Many of you were doubtless surprised or shocked today when you learned of the death of the wife of Doctor J. C. W. Bland. Those of you who attend the Medical Society meetings will recall that he only recently presented a paper upon pneumonia. Consequently it is a strange coincidence that his wife should be a victim of the disease of which he so intelligently wrote.

"It is but right and proper that we should acknowledge the Sovereignty of the Arbitor of Human Destinies and out of a sympathy for our brother practitioner and his family, and with due deference to the memory of the departed dead, I move Mr. President, the adoption of the following resolution:

"Be it resolved by the Tulsa County

Medical Society, That the usual program be dispensed with, and that this mark ot respect and token of our appreciation be transmitted to Dr. Bland and his family, and that a copy of these resolutions be spread upon the minutes of this Society and that a copy be furnished the press."

Dr. A. D. Young, Secretary of Epworth University, Oklahoma City, and Lecturer on Nervous Diseases in that school will take an extended course of study in New York and other Eastern cities after the Commencement of Epworth, May 13.

BOOK REVIEWS

EXAMINATION OF THE URINE.

The New (2d) Edition.

Examination of the Urine: A Manual for Students and Practitioners. By G. A. DeSantos Saxe, M. D., Instructor in Genito-Urinary Surgery, New York Post-Graduate Medical School and Hospital. Second Edition, enlarged and reset. 12mo. of 448 pages, illustrated. Philadelphia and London:

W. B. Saunders Company. 1909. Cloth, $1.75 net.

This work is in compact and accessible form and will be found useful to the busy man who wants his directions tersely written.

It is simply and well written, avoiding many of the complex theoretical propositions found in such works.

Contains a good chapter on Indican and tests for its detection and application in the practice of medicine.

A VALUABLE BOOK FOR THE PHYSICIAN.

The Propaganda for Reform in Proprietary Medicines; Sixth Edition: Containing the various exposes of nostroums and quackery which have appeared in The Journal of the American Medical Association. Price, Paper, 10 cents; Cloth, 35 cents. Pp. 292. Illustrated.

This book presents in convenient form most of the exposures that have appeared in The Journal of the American Medical Association showing fraud either in the composition of various proprietary preparations or in the claims made for such preparations. Not all of the products dealt with, however, are such as are or have been—used by the medical profession. Many preparations of the "patent medicine" type have been subjected to analysis and the results of such examinations appear in this volume. The book will prove of great value to the physician in two ways: 1, It will enlighten him as to the value, or lack of value, of many of the so-called ethical proprietaries on the market; and 2, It will put him in a position to answer intelligently questions that his patients may ask him regarding the virtues (?) of some of the widely advertised "patent medicines" on the market. After reading the reports published in this book physicians will realize the value and efficiency of simple scientific combinations of U. S. P. and N. F. preparations as compared with many of the ready-made, unstable and inefficient proprietary articles.

THE PROPAGANDA FOR REFORM IN PROPRIETARY MEDICINES.

This is the title of a new volume just issued from the press of The American Medical Association, Chicago.

This little work is the result of the investigations of the Council on Pharmacy and Chemistry of the A. M. A., which was organized in 1905. A great deal of the work performed by this Council and its sub-committees, has from time to time appeared in the columns of the Journal and here the work is put before the reader complete and in a compact form.

The average physician going to his office and opening his mail receives all kinds of literature stating the claims of various remedies, sometimes samples are enclosed and they keep coming to his desk; often they are lead into prescribing in this way, mixtures and preparations that have no merit beyond the wold claims of the advertiser and the Council on Pharmacy and Chemistry having invited all manufacturers to place in their hands samples of their products, or bought them in open market have subjected them to the close examination of the chemist. If the goods are what they are represented to be they are favorably passed upon and if not comment is made as to their short comings and the difference between the claims made for them and the actual findings is noted.

The work should be purchased by every physician; its pages investigated and there can be no question that the information contained will be found of great benefit to the reader.

EXCHANGES AND ABSTRACTS

THE URINE IN DIABETES.

W. Lintz, Brooklyn (Journal A. M. A., March 12), says that the urinary findings in diabetes not only give the diagnosis of the disease but throw light on the etiology and aid the surgeon and physician when their work is complicated with diabetes. Certain mistakes, however, must be avoided. The sugar test may fail unless a twenty-four hour sample is taken and it may disappear and be replaced by uric acid and phospates. The turbidity of diabetic urine is noticeable and it is of practical importance as it is due to the growth of yeast cells which may cause, by fermentation, complete disappearance of glucose if the qualitative and quantitative examination is not made sufficiently early. Many other substances than glucose will reduce the various copper solutions, among which may be mentioned as most frequent, conjugated glycuronic acid, alkapton, creatinin, uric acid in excess, blood and lactose. A point that he had not seen mentioned elsewhere is that occasionally the urine of menstruating women will reduce the copper solution, on account, as he is fully convinced, of the presence of blood in the urine. This is an important point. Blocking of the secretion of the mammary glands may also produce lactose in the urine and the fermentation test will reveal the difference. It is surprising, Lintz says, how easy it is to eliminate the above-mentioned reducing substances by the simple Fehling test provided it is properly done, i. e. after boiling the solution and adding the urine drop by drop. Reboiling is not necessary, warming will do. If the reduction is rapid we may be pretty certain of the presence of glucose, but if it is slow and the precipitate yellow, instead of red, the fermentation test will verify. While the specific gravity of diabetic urine is usually high, it may be low if the absorption of nitrogenous material from the digestive tract is low. The quantity also is not invariably high. The total nitroge nof the urine should be increased on account of the greater ingestion of protein, but it becomes pathologic when the body albumin is also excreted with the high sugar output. The greater the nitrogen loss the more the patient suffers. A high ammonia value means a severe case and the ammonia determination gives an accurate estimation of the acidosis present. We can predict the onset of coma by the urinary findings. The finding of beta-oxbutyric acid or diacetic acid in the urine should always serve as a danger signal. The increase in the ammonia output is equally important. A sudden diminution or disappearance of glucose, together with turbidity from hyaline granular casts and the appearance of albumin in urine previously free from it, are also danger signals. Lastly, he mentions the Cammidge reaction as a valuable indication of pancreatic disease which may be present in diabetes though he has had no experience with it in this disorder.

CANCER ON THE LIP.

Delay in operating for cancer of the lip is deprecated by E. A. Babler, St. Louis (Journal A. M. A., January 8), who especially condemns any trifling with palliative measures in these cases. He says that the secret of success lies in early and complete removal of the growth on the lip and the glands in the sub-mental and sub-maxillary fossæ. The technic which he says seems best is given as follows: "For two or three days before operation the patient is given a mouth-wash and the teeth cleansed three times daily. Under ether anæsthesia, a collar incision is made and the glands in the submental and submaxilary regions, together with the adipose tissue, are excised. Drainage is provided for through two small supplemental incisions. The wound is then sutured and protected with gauze pads, which latter are held in place by an assistant while the growth on the lip is being removed and the parts sutured. In my own cases the entire wound surfaces are swabbed with Harrington's solution and then with salt solution before being sutured. The rains are removed on

the second day. The patient is permitted to leave his bed on the fourth day." The conclusions which Babbler feels justified in offering from his study of the subject are given as follows: "1. The causes of failure in the treatment of cancer of the lip are (1) late recognition of the disease, (2) the patient's refusal of early operation, and (3) incomplete operative technic. 2. The common practice of treating persons of persistent "fissure" or "crack" of the lip in a patient 30 years of age or over, with pastes, caustics or powders, is to be deplored. The fissuer or crack should be excised and immediately subjected to microscopic examination. 3. The secret of success lies in early recognition and prompt excision of the growth, together with contents of submental and the submaxilary fossæ. The character and completeness of the primary operation determine the success or failure of the treatment. 4. Moles and warts, especially when so situated that they are subject to more or less constant irritation, should be excised, lest they become malignant."

PARATYPHOID FEVER.

H. F. Hoskins, Weyers Cave, Va. (Journal A. M. A., March 19), describes an epidemic of 35 cases of paratyphoid fever occurring in the spring and summer of 1909. It originated in a family of 8 and the cases were scattered over a radius of 3 miles, under such conditions as to render it unlikely that the spread of the infection was due to any other cause than flies. Each family had its own water supply independent of the rest. The incubation period varied from 1 to 2 weeks' though in over half the cases the time was from 9 to 11 days. The prodromal symptoms were abdominal distress and usually constipation and increased in severity so that the patient quickly consulted a physician. In half the cases there was bronchitis and constant headache, chilliness of feet and legs, and feeling of heat elsewhere. Temperature ranged from 100 to 104 F., and to 105 F. in 6 cases. The morning remissions were more marked than in typhoid. The pulse was rapid, from 120 to 155. Delirium was present in 3 cases. Neuromuscular pains were complained of in about three-quarters of the cases but soon disappeared. Constipation was the rule though diarrhæa, sometimes profuse, occurred in several cases. The stools were at first normal, later greenish or yellowish and watery. The urine was acid, scanty, and highly colored. Rose spots were present in about three-fourths of the cases, and tympanites. not specially marked, in four-fifths. Enlarged spleen existed in 17 of the 35. There was nausea and anorexia in the majority. The tongue was heavily coated and the odor similar to typhoid. Hemorrhage was rare. Peculiar features of the disease were its prevalence in children, only 6 of the patients being adults, and the horrible illusions experienced by the patients, even when not delirious. The special sypmtoms are reviewed in detail. The sequels were less numerous and severe than those of typhoid. The diagnosis was made by its more abrupt onset than is the case in other fevers, severe initial headache, the quick rise of temperature and the serum reaction with paratyphoid B. which gives a typical agglutination. The prognosis is good under ordinary typhoid treatment and sterilization is equally necessary, with subsequent disinfection of the quarters. In the beginning of the disease, calomel in doses of from 2 to 4 grains followed by castor oil in children, seems to render the disease milder. Mouth toilet is important, washing out with a saturated solution of boric acid was used every 2 or 3 hours. Good nursing is the most important factor in the treatment and prevention of the spread of the disease.

The bacteriologic and agglutination tests are detailed. The latter were positive. No positive reasonable explanation of the cause of the spread of the disease can be given.

ANIMAL EXPERIMENTATION.

The advantages of animal experimentation to the animals themselves are well shown by V. A. Moore, Ithaca, N. Y. (Journal A. M. A., March 12), who points out that what we have learned about the diseases of animals and our ability to prevent the economic losses sustained on their account, is mainly due to animal experimentation. In the United States there are, according to the Year Book of the Department of Agriculture, 1907, exclusive of poultry, cats and dogs, domestic animals valued at $4,331,230,000, permitting an export trade in animals and animal products of $254,798,329. The acquisition of this great wealth in animals has been possible because of the somewhat successful methods which have been learned and applied for controlling and preventing epizootic diseases. The number of infectious diseases to which domestic animals are liable and the suffering and loss which they formerly occasioned are too generally unrecognized. The fact should not be lost sight of that these diseases are liable to be introduced even after they have been successfully controlled and this calls for constant vigilance and study. Moore shows how the preventive vaccine against anthrax has enabled farmers to keep live stock in many localities where it would be otherwise impossible; how the contagious pleuropneumonia of cattle has been eradicated and the spread of glanders has been very much reduced. The Pasteur treatment of rabies, so effective in man, can also be effective in treating the dogs themselves. Hog cholera is also a disease which we have learned to control by animal experimentation, as are also

Texas fever, and tuberculosis to a large extent. Moore thinks it probable that if attention had not been called to this latter disease in cattle it would have become a more universal and destructive plague among these animals than any other that has yet visited the animal kingdom. Other diseases are mentioned which have lost much of their terror by this work. In spite of everything that has been done and the benefits obtained, the demands for further investigation are still pressing, and in order to make diagnoses, prepare antitoxins and vaccines with which to better the condition of animals, it is necessary that animal experimentation be continued. Needless suffering need not be inflicted and, in fact, what is necessary is far less than the animals are liable to in their natural lives. In most cases the experimental animals have a more comfortable life and a far easier death than those that enjoy their natural freedom. Men and women are allowed wantonly to shoot and trap innocent animals simply to gratify an appetite for brutal pleasure or to supply means for their personal adornment and comfort. Why then should we hesitate, on account of a misguided sentimentalism, to sacrifice a few that thousands of others may be protected from disease and suffering?

PUS TUBES IN THE MALE.

W. T. Belfield, Chicago (Journal A. M. A., December 25), says that these conditions in the male are generally unrecognized, and he defends the use of the name he had given them by describing the clinical anatomy of the parts, showing the analogies with other tubal suppurations. He describes the symptoms, the vesical and rectal tenesmus, the abdominal pain simulating appendicitis, the toxemia causing the neurasthenic symptoms, and the impotence and sterility which are the results. The surgical treatment of these conditions and its advantage over the medical treatment are pointed out. He has operated for draining and medicating the vas ampula, and vesicle 149 times in 107 patients by vasotomy, usually in the office under cocaine anæsthesia and often without medication, also protecting the epididymis from infection, or if infected from pressure infection, as free drainage is afforded through the vas incision. In the technic of vasotomy three features are important: (1) Fixation of the vas, which otherwise may drop into the scrotum; (2) raising the vas through the skin cut for accurate manipulation; (3) exploration of vas for obstruction by sounding with a silkworm thread. When resection is performed a silkworm or catgut thread is passed into the lumen and out through the wall of each cut, and the ends tied above the skin, the thread serving as an axis splint securing exact apposition of the cut end. This method of anastomosis, devised by Mayo, should, he thinks, supersede all others. His experience has taught him the value of accurate vaccine therapy, especially with autogenous vaccine, as a constitutional aid to the local treatment. He summarizes his paper in the following conclusions: "1. Pus infection of the seminal tract plus occlusion of the ejaculatory duct soon converts vesicle, vas and finally epididymis into a closed abcess. 2. Vasotomy is the simplest and least objectionable means of evacuating pus, relieving tension and medicating vas and vesicle. 3. Among the effects of these infections on the urinary organs are bladder irritation and obstruction of the ureter with consequent kidney lesions. 4. Impotence, sterility and sexual neuroses in the male are frequent results of pus infections of the seminal tract and amenable to appropriate treatment thereof. 5. Vaccine therapy, accurately applied, is the most valuable internal measure against the infections which produce pus tubes in the male."

....*NOTICE*....

ANNUAL MEETING AT TULSA, MAY 10, 11 AND 12TH., 1910

County Sectetaries Send in Report and Remmittance for Your Membership.

Contributors, Make Two Copies of Your Paper.

If You Are Not a Subscriber For Your State Journal Hand Your County Secretary Fifty Cents and Become One.

If You are a Delegate and Cannot Attend the Annual Meeting Have Your Alternate Properly Authenticated in Order to Avoid Confusion in the House of Delegates.

If Some of Your Old Members Have Not Renewed Persuade Them to do so at Once.

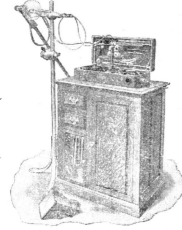

STANDING COMMITTEES OKLAHOMA STATE MEDICAL ASSOCIATION.

Public Policy and Legislation—Dr. David A. Myers, Chairman, Lawton; J. H. Scott, Shawnee; J. A. Hatchett, El Reno; F. S. Clinton, Tulsa; Claude A. Thompson, Muskogee.

On Medical Education—Drs. B. J. Vance, Checotah; A. K. West, Oklahoma City; E. O. Barker, Guthrie.

On Scientific Work—Drs. Floyd E. Waterfield, Holdenville; P. A. Smithe, Enid; Claude A. Thompson, Muskogee.

On Necrology—Drs. C. S. Bobo, Norman; H. M. Williams, Wellston; M. A. Warhurst, Remus.

FOR SALE.

$1,250 cash gets property consisting of three-room dwelling house, barn, stables, pair of horses, good buggy, office furniture and fixtures; $4,000.00 practice gratis; will introduce. Reason for selling—going to specialize in Texas. Address Dr. John T. Vick, Fort Towson, Oklahoma.

FOR SALE.

The Journal has tuition to the amount of forty-four dollars in the New York Polyclinic School and Hospital which will be sold at a reduction from the usual rates. Address The Journal.

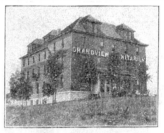

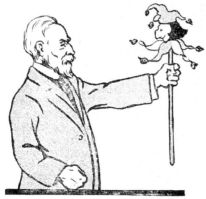
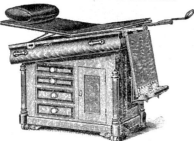

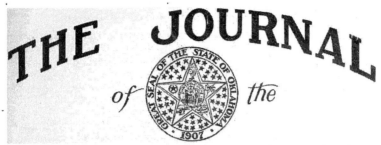

Oklahoma State Medical Association.

VOL. II.   MUSKOGEE, OKLAHOMA, MAY, 1910.   NO 12

DR. CLAUDE A. THOMPSON, Editor-in-Chief.

ASSOCIATE EDITORS AND COUNCILLORS.

DR. J. A. WALKER, Shawnee.   DR. JOHN W. DUKE, Guthrie.

DR. CHARLES R. HUME, Anadarko.   DR. A. B. FAIR, Frederick.

DR. F. R. SUTTON, Bartlesville.   DR. W. G. BLAKE, Tahlequah.

DR. I. W. ROBERTSON, Dustin.   DR. H. P. WILSON, Wynnewood.

DR. J. S. FULTON, Atoka.

Entered at the Postoffice at Muskogee, Oklahoma, as second class mail matter, June, 1909.

This is the Official Journal of the Oklahoma State Medical Association All communications should be addressed to the Journal of the Oklahoma State Medical Association, English Block, Muskogee, Oklahoma.

COMATOSE PERNICINOUS MALARIA.

BY DR. CHARLES SUMNER NEER, VINITA OKLAHOMA

With Report of Cases.

The fact that coma may occur in the course of malaria as a result of the localization of the parasites in the brain is well known, but the frequency of this event, even in our own latitude, I believe is hardly realized by many physicians. In the Journal of the American Medical Association for July 1908, I reported three of these cases and gave a general consideration of the subject of comatose malaria. Since that time I have observed five additional cases, the history of which I will give here.

The cases in which comatose malaria occur are usually those in which estivo-autumnal malaria has existed for some time without proper treatment. Actual trombi of malarial organisms are formed in the capillaries o fthe brain. After death this blocking of the capillaries with malarial plasmodia may easily be demonstrated by placing a small fragment of the brain tissue under a cover glass.

When the coma comes on suddenly it resembles apoplexy. When it comes on gradually there are usually preceding disturbances of the sensorium such as somnolence, delirium, restlessness and melancholia.

The skin is usually flushed and often has an ecteric tint. The soma sometimes resembles natural sleep. The patient may move the limbs about restlessly and may respond in some measure to stimuli. There may be twitching of the limbs or face. In two of the cases of my service there were generalized convulsions

The eyes are often open and frequently the balls roll from side to side. The pupils are usually equal and react to light until late in the attack. The tendon reflexes are usually intact. In one of my cases there was a marked exaggeration of the knee and ankle reflexes, with Babinski's and Oppenheim's phenomena on both sides. Another case showed a well marked Babinski on the right. Cases have been recorded in which symptoms of focal disease of the brain persisted after the attack.

The patient may emerge from the coma after a few hours but is apt to become comatose again within 12 or 24 hours or the coma may continue over a period of 3 or 4 days until recovery or death. In two cases reported here, considerable mental hebetude persisted several days after recovery from coma.

The temperature is irregular. Sometimes it is subnormal, and it is usually not high.

The diagnosis of this condition resolves itself into the old problem of the differential diagnosis of the comatose state. In rare cases where the previous history of the patient can be obtained, a fairly positive diagnosis of comatose malaria can be made from the symptoms alone. However, in the great majority, a blood examination is necessary. I would here insist upon the importance of placing dependence upon the examination of the fresh specimen rather than the stained smear. In almost all of the cases reported here, large numbers of hyaline bodies were found and very often 2 or 3 organisms in a single blood cell. I have seen an excellent microscopist fail to find plasmodia in a stained specimen, when an examination of the fresh blood showed them in numbers.

The conditions for which comatose malaria is most likely to be mistaken are cerebral apoplexy, sunstroke, and uraemia.

Aside from the blood examination the main points to be considered in distinguishing it from apoplexy are the age and general appearance of the patient, the splenic enlargement, and the higher temperature in malaria, (though this is not to be relied upon).

Malarial coma may sometimes simulate sunstroke quite closely, and exposure to heat may aggravate or precipitate a malarial paroxysm. Cardamitis lays down the rule that, with a temperature above 104 F. the coma should be attributed to insolation rather than to pernicious malaria.

The examination of the urine alone does not give sufficient data for a diagnosis between comatose malaria and uraemia. In both there are albuminuria and cylindruria. The history, the general apperance of the patient and the temperature must be considered, and examination of the blood may be absolutely necessary The prognosis in malarial coma is very grave. The writer in Nothnagel's System says: "Even after energetic treatment with quinine the mortality is large. Moreover cases that show from the beginning a mild form may succumb in spite of the early administration of specific therapy." Craig states that the great majority of the fatal cases of malaria are of the comatose form. Of the eight cases of this series, six died, a mortality of 75 per cent. In all of these the quinine was started very soon after admission to the hospital. The treatment consists in the administration of quinine hypodermically. It may be given as the hydrochlorate, the bisulphate or the muriate of quinine and urea. Osler advises 30 grain doses of the bisulphate hypodermically or 10 to 20 grain doses of the quinine and urea muriate every 2 or 3 hours. Craig advises small doses; 8 grains of the hydrochlorate repeated until 24 grains have been given. Stimulants are often required, and of these strychnine is probably the most useful.

Cases 1, 2 and 3 were previously reported in the Journal of the American Association. All of these were fatal. The five cases whose reports follow, were observed by me in the early fall of 1908 while house surgeon in the Frisco hospital, Springfield, Mo.

Case 4—Patient A. E., age about 30, Mexican, laborer, was brought to the hospital unconscious, from Clayton, Okla., Sept. 13, 1908, at 3 p. m.

History—No satisfactory history could be obtained as the brother of the patient who accompanied him could not speak English.

Examination—Well developed and well nourished man. The skin had a decidedly yellow hue which was partly physiological.

The face was flushed and warm. No edema. The lips showed a herpetic eruption. The lungs and heart were negative, the pulse regular and increased in frequency. The abdomen was soft and flat. The spleen was palpable one inch below the ribs and very hard. The temperature was about 102 F. at the time of admission. The patient was unconscious but the coma was not deep, rather resembling a natural sleep. He would move his limbs about restlessly at times, and irritation of the hands or feet always produced movements. The eyes were open much of the time, and had a natural expression. The eyeballs would sometimes oscillate slowly from side to side. The pupils were equal and reacted normally to light. The knee jerks were present but somewhat sluggish. there was no paralysis and no Babinski.

The blood (fresh specimen) showed very many estivo-autumnal parasites. As

many as three hyaline bodies were to be found in a single cell. The urine showed a large trace of albumin and granular casts.

Further Course—The coma continued until 10 p. m. of the 13th when he began to regain consciousnes. He asked for water and by the morning of the 14th seemed entirely clear. The temperature was normal and he said he felt good. He remained clear all day, though the blood still showed many parasites present, notwithstanding the hypodermic injections of quinine. About midnight he became drowsy again, and by 2 a. m. of the 15th he was again in coma which was deeper than it had been in the previous attack. He did not emerge from it. The pulse became weak and thready, the breathing stertorous, and he died at 11:30 p. m., 22 hours after the second onset of coma.

Treatment—Ten grains of quinine bi-muriate were given hypodermically every 4 hours from the start, and quinine was given by mouth.

Case 5. Patient—A. G., Greek, laborer, age about 40 was brought to hospital at 2:30 a. m. Sept. 13, 1908.

History—No history could be obtained.

Examination—At the time of his admission patient was delirious, and was inclined to get out of bed and wander around. The temperature was 101 and the pulse 102. He was muscular and fairly nourished. The skin was sallow. No edema. The lungs and heart were negative. The spleen was palpable but not greatly enlarged. The pupils were equal and reacted to light. The knee jerks were present but rather sluggish. The plantar and cremasteric reflexes were sluggish. No Babinski. No paralysis. The urine was not obtained.

Blood examination at 10 a. m. on the 13th showed estivo-autumnal parasites (crescents).

Further Course—During the morning and afternoon of the 13th he was fairly quiet but vomited several times and complained of some headache. At noon and at 6 p. m. there was no fever. At 9 p. m. he had a general convulsion followed by unconsciousness. The temperature taken soon after the convulsion was 104, the pulse 140. The patient remained in deep coma, hiccoughing part of the time and sweating freely. Toward the last the reflexes were abolished, and the pulse became very weak and frequent. He died Sept. 15 at 9:15 p. m.

Treatment—Quinine was given in large doses by mouth. and after the onset of coma quinine bimuriate was given in 10 grain doses hypodermically. Treatment was not begun in this case so promptly as was to be desired owing to his having come to the hospital during the night.

Case 6. Patient—P. B., laborer, age 36, entered hospital Oct. 1, 1908.

History—Family history negative. Patient had always been in good health. During the two or three weeks previous to his entering the hospital he had noticed slight shortness of breath on exertion. He stated that he had been having chills off and on all summer. For the two weeks preceding his admission he had been working in Arkansas, and had been having a chill every day.

Examination—Well developed man of average appearance. Skin slightly yellow. Lungs negative. A loud systolic murmur was to be heard over the entire front of the chest, with its maximum intensity over the right 3rd costal cartilege. The murmur was heard well in the left axilla or behind. The pulse was regular and fairly full. There was no difference in time or size of the pulse of the two radials. Blood examination showed a very large number of malarial organisms of the estivo-

autumnal form. The urine showed a specific gravity of 1,008, a faint trace of albumin and many fine granular casts.

Further Course—Patient entered the hospital in a semi-comatose condition, being unable to give any account of himself at the time of his entrance and for several days thereafter. His temperature was normal and the pulse 88 at the time of entering. A few hours after admission he attempted to walk and fell in a kind of fainting attack. He seemed greatly confused afterward. The temperature taken by rectum a little later was found to be 104 F., the pulse 120. The temperature the next day was normal but went up the following day to 102 F. He vomited frequently and was stupid and slightly delirious for 5 or 6 days, although he had no fever after the fourth day following his admission. Eight days after entering hospital he was entirely clear and expressed himself as feeling very well.

Treatment—Four ten grain doses of quinine were given daily by mouth.

Case 7. Patient—A. J. M., laborer, age about 40; was admitted to hospital Oct. 9, 1908, at 2:30 a. m. in a semi-conscious state.

History—Patient would answer questions in an uncertain way but could give no clear account of his illness. He said he had been having chills for about two weeks.

Examination—Rather poorly nourished man. Skin rather cold. The temperature at time of admission was 92 F. The pulse 70. The lungs and heart were negative There was a cataract in the right eye and a defect in the pupil of the left. The abdomen was soft and flat. The spleen was not palpable. The reflexes were equal and active. Examination of the blood showed a moderate number of estivo-autumnal parasites.

The urine was turbid and showed a

large trace of albumin, and a moderate number of coarse and fine granular casts. No diazo.

Further Course—At 9 a. m. patient seemed a little clearer. The temperature was 98.6 and the pulse 104. During the afternoon, however, he sank into a deep coma. The respiration became stertorous and the pulse weak. The temperature at 3:30 p. m. was 102. Coma continued until death at 7:30 p. m. The temperature at 5 p. m. was 105.

Treatment—Quinine bimuriate was given in 10 grain doses hypodermically and stimulants were given symptomatically.

Case 8. *Patient*—J. B. E., age 26, brakeman, entered hospital Oct. 13, 1908, at 7 p. m., delirious.

History—Parents living and healthy, patient had always enjoyed good health and had been in the employ of the railroad 7 years. He had been having fever about 2 weeks. He did not remember having had a distinct chill but would have fever every other day. He had taken some medicines but did not know what it was.

Examination—Slender, somewhat anemic appearing young man. Heart and lungs negative. Spleen greatly enlarged, coming about 3 inches below the ribs. Abdomen seemed sensitive over the spleen but no where else and it was not tympanitic. The skin was clear and there was no edema.

Blood examination showed large numbers of estivo-autumnal plasenmdia, mostly hyaline bodies. Many cells contained more than one parasite. The urine contained albumin but no casts were found. There was no diazo reaction. The pupils were equal and reacted to light. All reflexes were present.

Further Course—At the time of his admission he was very delirious and had somewhat the appearance of a delirious typhoid patient in the 3rd week. The temperature was 100.2 F. and the pulse 100. He remained quiet all night and the next morning appeared clear. The temperature remained at 100 F. all day, and at 4 p. m was 101. Coincidently he became stupid, could hardly be gotten to swallow anything and would not talk. The eyes remained open and the unconsciousness was not complete but he could be aroused only with difficulty. This condition continued nearly all night, but the next morning (the 15th) he was clear, although he was still unable to remember how long he had been sick, etc. At noon on the 15th the temperature was 98.8 and after that was never above normal. The sensorium gradually cleared and he left the hospital a few days later.

Treatment—10 grain doses of quinine by mouth and hypodermically were given.

C. S. NEER, Vinita, Okla.

MEXICO FROM A DOCTOR'S STANDPOINT.

BY A. K. WEST, M. D., DEAN OF THE MEDICAL DEPARTMEMT EPWORTH UNIVERSITY, OKLAHOMA CITY, OKLA.

The land of the Montezumas holds much of interest for the sightseer in general. The purpose of this paper, however, is to deal only with topics medical or of allied interest.

First—Let us consider the climatology. There is a prevalent impression that the Republic of Mexico is a hot country, which is a very natural conclusion after noting its position on the map with reference to latitude as it lies largely within the tropics. However, this is entirely erroneous. Climate depends upon other conditions than latitude and location, altitude playing a most important part, as well as air currents and humidity.

Now, the topography of Mexico is in a general way about this: A low fringe of land bordering the Gulf of Mexico on the east and the Pacific Coast on the west, leading up to the foot of high mountain ranges which border the sea coast on either side and between these ranges is a vast plateau of varying altitude, so that the climate of Mexico is divided by the Mexican authorities into three distinct zones separated one from the other by very few miles but by a wide difference in altitude. We have first the "Tierras Calientes" or hot lands. This is a narrow fringe of land lying adjacent to the sea coast and rising up to the foot of the mountains on either side, bordering the Gulf of Mexico on the east and the Pacific Ocean on the west. This is the only typical tropical country there is in the Republic, and in square miles it is comparatively small. The vast central plateau, varying in altitude from 3,000 to 6,000 feet for the greater part, is known as the "Tierras Templadas," or temperate regions, while nestling among the mountains adjacent to the snow covered peaks are the "Tierras Frias," or cold lands; these have an elevation of 7,000 feet and upward, and in certain localities a half day's ride on the railroad will transfer one from the cold lands to the tropics. The rainfall on the Gulf is greater than on the Pacific coast the temperature being about the same on either side and, as stated before, is humid, hot, and favorable to the growth of the luxuriant vegetation which is considered typical of that country. Here we also find the condition favorable for the development of the so-called tropical diseases. The temperate regions have more rainfall, more sunshine, and a temperature varying from 40 to 80 degrees. The mean temperature between winter and summer is very slight, not more than five to ten degrees. The cold lands vary from the temperate only

in the lower mean temperature which usually varies from the frost line, about 35 degrees, to the maximum of 70 degrees, with practically no variation between summer and winter of the mean temperature. It is therefore evident that the greater portion of the Republic of Mexico, leaving out the hot lands, is a very salubrious and certainly one of the most pleasant climates to live in to be found in the civilized world. Indeed, if man could live by climate alone, my recent experience would lead me to emigrate to the high plateaus of Mexico. So much in a general way for the climate.

It will be seen from the foregoing that a sharp line of demarcation is likely to be found between the regions of certain diseases which we may glance at for a moment.

In the hot lands malarial fevers continually ravage the population but stop suddenly at the foot of the mountains as soon as we get away from the heavy rainfall and breeding places of the mosquito. As in the temperate regions of the United States there are localities in the higher zones where there has been an occasional outbreak of malaria, chills and fever of a mild form, while in the higher regions malaria is practically unknown. Likewise in the hot lands we have the focal zone of yellow fever where it is continual the year around, but never spreads beyond the sea coast region on the low lands. Epidemics of yellow fever, however, even at the tropics are at the present time permanently abolished owing to the work of the sanitary authorities following the lead of Dr. Walter Reid and the Yellow Fever Commission, and while sporadic cases continue to occur they are immediately screened and for the last six years they have been able to control and completely prevent epidemics even in the hot lands. Other diseases of the temperate regions are practically those to be found in the United States, with one or two curious exceptions.

For instance, Typhus Fever, which is with us an exceptionally rare disease is continually present in all the larger cities of Mexico and adds considerable to the death rate of the population, However, the sanitary authorities are making strenuous efforts toward protecting the people against its ravages, and at the present time a representative of the Carnegie Institution, Dr. Rosenberg, is at work in the City of Mexico, supported by, and using the laboratories of the Superior Board of Health in carrying on a series of experiments looking toward the discovery of the aetiology and method of propagation of this dread disease. I had some curiosity while in the City of Mexico to visit the Typhus wards in the hospital but felt it would hardly be wise.

Another curious discovery made by myself, which was very gratifying, was that small pox, a disease which has been generally thought to be endemic in Mexico is now practically a thing of the past. The City of Mexico, Guadlajara, and San Louis Potosi, cities ranging from 100,000 to 500,000 people have not now a single case of small pox. This is due to the compulsary vaccination act which went into effect some ten or twelve years ago, all children being presented for vaccination before the end of the fourth month, under pain of a heavy fine being levied against the parents. It is indeed a noticeable fact that a very large per cent of the adult population in any of the forementioned cities are typically pock marked, while the children show no evidence of ravages of the disease. When I think of the trouble that we liberty loving Americans have in enforcing so valuable a sanitary measure, it appeals to me that after all the autocratic

government of Mexico has some advantages.

Tuberculosis seems to be much less prevalent in Mexico than in the United States. However, there are a few cases to be found in all the largest cities, but I was told by native physicians that it rarely developed in the country, nearly always originating among the poorer classes living around the suburbs of the large cities where the habitations are dark, poorly ventilated, and poorly-lighted, many of these people living, the whole family including the dog and the pig, in one room with a dirt floor, and the only reason, it would seem to me, they are able to live at all is that they spend practically all hours of the day in the open air, only sleeping in their adobe huts at night. In the great Hospital General, of which I shall have occasion to speak a little later, is a magnificent ward for Tubercular patients, which is built and equipped in keeping with the most advanced ideas along the line of Tubercular Sanitoria. The patients of this ward are being treated now by static electricity. I saw several tubercular patients taking the treatment while in the hospital and only inquired into the method far enough to find it is only in the experimental stage and the physicians are more or less divided in opinion as to whether it had any real efficacy.

Another idea worthy of note is that nearly all Americans among the laity seem to have the idea well fixed that Pneumonia in Mexico is peculiarly fatal. Two of the American physicians also informed me that the disease was much more fatal there than in the United States, one of them declaring that the mortality was as high as eighty per cent. This, however, led me to inquire into the subject, also to study the hospital records and get the opinion of the native physicians, and I am convinced that the mortality, if higher at all, is only slightly more than in the United States. The records of the Hospital General indicate a mortality of about 25 per cent, which is possibly 5 per cent higher than hospital records on an average in the United States, and this record we well know to be entirely too high for the average patient in private practice.

Another subject which attracted my attention somewhat, which may be of a medical or social nature according to our view point, is that of alcoholism. The Mexicans have no liquor problem. The native fermented drink as pulque is very commonly imbibed by all classes. As a beverage I should class it as being very closely akin to hard cider, having possibly an alcoholic per centage of two or three. This beverage is the juice of the maguy plant which belongs to the palm family. It is the same plant that is cultivated as an ornament in this country under the name of "century plant," owing to the story that it blooms once in a hundred years, which is indeed true, for the plant blooms only once at all, the plant has this curious life history, after attaining its full growth it throws all its vital energy into the process of reproduction throwing up a great flowery stalk later to be covered with seed pods, upon the ripening of which its whole plant withers and dies, sacrificing its life to the great physiological duty of reproducing its kind. The blooming process, however, takes place after the plant matures and a large seed stock is thrown up in the center, or body, something like the head of the cabbage, from which this seed stalk is to be developed, this is cut out leaving a bucket like opening of the top of the plant which is filled with the sap sent up from the roots at this critical period of the life of the plant, and is poured out in large quantities, the

bucket like depression being filled several times before the plant gives up its fight and withers away and dies. The process is analogous to that seen in many of our own plants, noticeable in grape vines at the time the sap rises in the spring, the wounded vine will continue to bleed, as we call it, for several weeks in its effort to throw sap out through the terminal branches. This juice is collected and is allowed to ferment naturally, without the addition of any foreign substance. However, the natives flavor it to suit the individual taste, and onions and red pepper are the chief condiments added to it. The plant pulque, while not particularly palatible to the American taste, is regarded as a great delicacy by practically all the natives, and the preparations containing onions and pepper, which are sold at a higher price and greatly in demand, is absolutely noxious and disgusting to the Americans, as the smell in fact is exactly analogous to that of the swill barrel at the back door of a second class restaurant or hotel. From this same material is distilled, with the addition of various substances, two or three different strong alcoholic beverages, mescal, tequila and some others. These are all strong fiery brandies containing between 40 per cent and 50 per cent alcohol that are for sale at every grocery store and the prices are ridiculously low, the price of an ordinary drink being only about three cents Mexican money which is equivalent to a cent and a half in gold, though some of the cheaper brands may be had for about half that amount. It is therefore possible for a man to get on a glorious drunk for about ten cents in American money, but the striking thing is that none of them get drunk, and very few hang around the drinking places as loiterers, such as we are accustomed to see in this country. Drinking to excess seems to be distinctly the exception and I was informed that in the wards of the hospital the diseases, scirrhosis of the liver, Bright's disease, locomotor ataxia, and certain other chronic degenerative processes which we are accustomed in this country to attribute very largely to alcoholism, is comparatively rare. There is nothing that is analogous to our saloons in the smaller towns in Mexico. In the larger cities they have the saloon but it occupies a much less important position due to the fact that gambling houses are not allowed to be run in conjunction with them, and to the fact that they play no important part in local politics, for the reason that they have no legal politics in Mexico, but this is another matter, and as the habit of social drinking does not obtain, it robs them of most of the baleful influences which surround the institutions in America, or rather the United States.

Sanitary laws and government originate in the Superior Board of Health of the Republic of Mexico. I spent some time in the company of Dr. Edwardo Liseago, who has been for twenty-four years president of this Superior Board, and can not proceed without acknowledging my indebtedness to him for much of my information touching things medical, and expressing my admiration for his personality, as well as his culture and scientific attainments. He is also Dean of the National Medical College of the City of Mexico, and to this man and his co-workers during the last quarter of a century Mexico is indebted for the vast improvements along sanitary lines, and especially is the republic indebted to him for his efforts and success in stamping out small pox, in stamping out yellow fever epidemics, in establishing water and sewerage system for the city of Mexico, in building the great Hospital General for the city of Mexico covering forty acres of ground, maintaining thirty odd additional buildings and wards, and taking care of and having a capacity of between fifteen hundred and two thousand beds; in fact, this hospital to my mind is as nearly perfect as any institution I ever knew of for the treatment of the sick, or that I have ever seen in my own country or any other. Its chief advantage, as I see it, consists in the fact that each ward is a separate building, all one story, thoroughly lighted and ventilated, it being erected in a beautiful garden, the plats of ground covered with carefully mown grass, beautiful tropical verdure, flowers and native fruits, rendering it possible to have full ventilation and sun light. The climate, of course, makes this arrangement possible in Mexico, which would be impossible in a temperate or northern climate. In the first place no heating plant is maintained as they have no need of any artificial heat. The water supply, electric light and sewerage is equal to the best and the arrangement of the wards, furniture and equipment are patterned after the better class of hospitals in our own country. Operating rooms and amphitheaters which are used as part of the teaching department of the medical college are in fact indentical, so far as I could see, with such institutions in Chicago and New York. This great institution has inclosed within the same wall what is known as the department of mechano-therapy, hydro-therapy and electro-therapy. It is therefore possible for any physician having a patient in the general hospital to prescribe any of these physical methods of treatment and the prescription is filled by experts in the several lines, that is, Swedish movements, Osteopathic movements, ordinary massage, and any system of physical culture or exercises are supplied in one department, any sort of a bath from a plunge in a beautiful swimming pool to a Russian vapor may be had, and in the department of electro-therapy any of the various light treatments, vibrator treatments, electric current treatments, of any kind whatever may be prescribed by the physician in charge and the treatment given by an expert in that line. This particular aspect, I believe to be more complete, and better adapted to the needs of the patients than anything I had ever seen. There are, of course, a number of other hospitals in the City of Mexico which are far from being on a plane with the Hospital General which I have just mentioned. It is quite impossible to make some of these older institutions strictly sanitary on account of peculiarities of their ancient structure, and, while most of them are being improved from time to time, the best results will never be obtained except as new hospitals are built from the ground up.

The Hospital of Jesus has an historical interest which I must mention in passing. It was founded by Cortez, and a certain portion of land set apart by him from his original grant to maintain the institution for all time. This institution has been in operation without a break for now almost four hundred years, a period of service which makes all our American hospitals look like mere beginners. I am not familiar with the means of support of all the hospitals but presume all of them have an endowment of some kind. The Hospital General is supported by a Federal appropriation, as well as an appropriation from the City and State. It is recognized as part of the equipment of the National Medical School, which institution has an annual appropriation from the National government of $175,000, about one half of which goes for teacher's salaries, the rest for incidental expenses

of the medical college building proper and the hospital. Sanitation generally throughout Mexico is upon a higher plane than I expected to see. Even in the small towns streets are well paved with cobble stones which as a rule keep remarkably clean, and everywhere I find the city ordinance strictly enforced concerning this matter of street cleaning. In the larger cities asphalt is now being used to a limited extent. It varies somewhat in different places, but the general rule seems to be that the down town or business district is kept clean by the police department from general taxation, while in the residence district each one is required to sweep and sprinkle his sidewalk and half the street once or twice each day. The sanitary officer, I was told by an American who used to live in the city of Guadlajara, never failed to remind him if he ever missed a single day cleaning his sidewalk and half his street, so that it is the habit to have the house servants attend to this as a part of the ordinary duties required of them, with the result, as I have before stated. The streets taken as a whole are cleaner and better kept than in towns of like size in the United States. The primitive method of sprinkling and cleaning the streets in the smaller towns are almost laughable. For instance, in a city of 125,- 000 I saw the street cleaning gang at work, —indeed took some kodak views of the procedure,—the water was brought in a barrel carried on the shoulders of two men, an ordinary quart cup was used to dip the water out of the barrel and then it was skilfully sprinkled over the dusty street, while following the sprinkling brigade came the sweepers, eight or ten in number, with little hand brooms and, while the work was done slowly, it was done very much better than is possible with our machine sprinklers and sweepers. It seems that the only reason this primitive method is adhered to is a financial one, as it is much cheaper to sprinkle the streets in this way in a country where the usual wages for such labor is about fifteen cents a day, gold, than it is to do the work by machinery and horse power.

Now, just a word about medical schools of Mexico and medical educator: There are six medical colleges in the republic of Mexico, turning out between 150 and 200 graduates each year. It will therefore appear that the percentage of graduates to the population is distinctly less in Mexico than in the United States. There is no uniforimty of standard in these schools, and each does not necessarily recognize the work of the other. The National school, which, by the way is the oldest medical school in America by many years, being established three hundred and fifty years ago, and being in continuous operation ever since, has a high requirement for admission equivalent to the entrance requirements of our first class colleges in this country, which is strictly enforced. It requires five years of study for graduation the first two years of which are given almost entirely to text book and laboratory work, the second two years to didactics and clinics, and the fifth year practically as a hospital interne, though a certain amount of class work is required in the last year. The equipment of this old school is up to date in every respect, the library and museum being far above the average to be found in American schools, their laboratories are also well equipped and well manned, anatomical, physiological, pathological, chemical, pharmacal and bacteriological are well equipped and well manned. At the time of my visit there were about three hundred students in this school. I understand that other medical colleges are in a measure equal to this one,

though Dr. Liseaga, the Dean, informed me he could not accept the work done by other colleges in the Republic except upon examination. The advanced class standing is only given by examination, and the work of no other school is taken for granted. I see no reason why not, and I am sure the fact is that the graduates of this school are the equals of any turned out in the United States. Most of the graduates of this school, however, do not enter into general practice. The army, navy, and various official positions absorb the greater part of their graduates. Medical education is entirely free. Students pay absolutely no fee of any kind. The general practitioner presents to me the saddest picture of anything I saw in Mexico. In the first place there is no punishment for practicing medicine without a diploma or license. The physician without a diploma recognized by the Mexican authorities has no standing at law, but likewise there is no penalty for his praticing. He cannot collect his bills by law and cannot exercise any legal right as a physician, but he can maintain an office, advertise, play on the prejudices and ignorance of the population, in fact play the quack ad libitum without fear of interference from the civil authorities, and this seems to be the class of physicians who do most of the general practice in the Mexican towns and cities. The cultivated Mexican physicians nearly all hold some official position, and among the fakirs Americans easily head the list, though there are physicians of practically all nationalities. Illustrative of the low level in which the practice of medicine generally has sunk, you will notice every drug store has what they call a Free Dispensary, with the name of three or four, or more, physicians marked opposite certain hours, indicating when patients may meet them at the dispensary. All who are able, of course, come and are treated free at the dispensary by the physician, without charge, care being exercised, however, by the druggist to collect in advance for dressings and appliances prescribed by the physician? Just the nature of this partnership or the rake-off the doctor gets, I was not able, of course, to find out, but the system I can only mention for the purpose of condemnation, and can only blush that there are many graduates of our own American schools engaged in this low class of practice among these ignorant people. For the benefit of any young physician who thinks of going to Mexico to make his fortune practicing medicine, I would admonish him to give up the idea. The only positions which seem worthy of acceptance are salaried positions with mining, railroad or other corporations, with the opportunity of private practice when not engaged in the business of the company. Under the present conditions I see no possibility of a reputable physician making a living unless he adopts the advertising quack dispensary methods which are commonly in vogue, and I hardly think a self-respecting physician would be satisfied with that life. I think the medical and superior authorities of Mexico are sadly derelict in their duties toward the common people and the mass of the population that they do not immediately enact laws fixing a severe penalty for this class of unlicensed practitioners. I do not mean to say absolutely all the foreign physicians practicing medicine in Mexico are practicing illegally, but clearly a majority of them are: many of them having no diplomas and many of the diplomas are from schools which are not recognized and are not validated by the Superior Board of Health. Fees of the better class of physicians are somewhat lower than in the United States. One of my acquaintances, who has lived in Mexico for the past eleven years, informed me that he paid his physician $3.50 a visit, Mexican money, for attention in his family, and that this physician was regarded as being very high priced. I think the usual fee among licensed physicians is about $3.00 Mexican money, or $1.50 gold. The fakir, of course, gets what he can. Among the natives obstetrical work is done almost entirely by midwives who do not pretend to be physicians, therefore obstetric fees are a negligible quantity.

Comparatively speaking, there is very much less surgical work done in Mexico than in the United States, due to the fact that a very much larger per cent of the population are unable to bear the expense of the major surgical operations. Outside of the hospitals where the work is done free there is little surgery. Of course, there are a few men who do private surgery in the large towns, but nothing to compare with the amount of work done in cities of like size in the United States, and I do not happen to know of any man in the City of Mexico who has developed a leadership or a position of prominence in surgery.

In conclusion, it has appealed to me that the admirable things in a medical way which I saw in Mexico, were the work of Dr. Liseaga in leading and directing sanitation and health legislation, the system of free hospitals, and the standard of medical education. And the one thing to be condemned most severely is the absence of some law to protect the ignorant masses against charlatans and fakirs who pose as men of science.

A LEGAL DECISION OF INTEREST TO THE MEDICAL PROFESSION.

BEING AN OPINION BY JUSTICE DUNN OF THE OKLAHOMA SUPREME COURT.

KERNODLE v. ELDER.

(Supreme Court of Oklahoma, May 12th, 1909.)

1. *Physicians and Surgeons (Sec. 14.—) Action for Malpractice—Evidence.*

In an action against a physician for malpractice in the setting and treatment of a fractured limb, where there is no guaranty of cure or contract for extraordinary skill or care, and where the evidence fails to show that the results are not such as usually and ordinarily result in such cases where treated by an ordinarily skillful physicians using ordinary care, then there is a failure of proof, and plaintiff is not entitled to recover.

2. *Appeal and Error (Sec. 1176)—Reversal.*

Where in such a case it is apparent from the record that the claim of plaintiff cannot be sustained, on reversal the court will not remand for new trial, but will direct a disimssal.

Error from Probate Court, Logan County; J. C. Strang, Judge.

Action by James B. Elder against J. D. Kernodle. Judgment for plaintiff, and defendant brought error to the Supreme Court of the territory. Case transferred to the Supreme Court of the State, and, on death of plaintiff, the action was revived in the name of Sarah M. Elder, administratrix. Remanded, with instructions.

Cotteral & Horner, for plaintiff in error. Lowry & Lowry, for defendant in error.

DUNN, J.—This action was begun by James H. Elder filing his petition in the probate court of Logan county, territory of Oklahoma, on June 5, 1905, wherein he alleged that on or about the 1st of February, 1905, he fractured the bone of his right hip joint, and that the defendant, holding himself out as a physician and surgeon, and being in the general practice of medicine for hire in Logan county, was employed to set such fractured bone and to attend to his said injury. The defendant was charged with having negligently and unskilfully diagnosed the difficulty in that he dressed and bandaged plaintiff's limb as if the break were between the knee and the hip, and as though the fracture were in the vicinity of the knee, and that by reason of this error on his part the fracture itself was left wholly unattended and uncared for. That this was careless, negligent, and unskilful on the part of the defendant, and that by reason thereof plaintiff suffered great pain, and that the broken bone has knit together improperly in such manner as to leave plaintiff crippled and lame, and to render him a permanent cripple for life. Damages were prayed for in the amount of $1,000. To this petition defendant answered by filing a general denial, and on the trial thereof before a jury a verdict for damages in the amount of $500 was returned. Judgment was rendered thereon, motion for new trial filed and over-ruled, and the case was taken to the Supreme court of the territory of Oklahoma by petition in error and case-made, and is now before us for our consideration by virtue of our succession to that court, under the terms of the enabling act and schedule to the Constitution. After the argument and submission of this case, which stood on the docket of this court as J. D. Kernodle v. James B. Elder, the death of the defendant in error was suggested, and the action has been revived in the name of J. D. Kernodle against Sarah M. Elder, administratrix of the estate of James B. Elder, deceased.

A motion to dismiss was filed on the grounds that the case-made was not properly a part of the records of this court, and that the motion for a new trial was overruled, at the request of plaintiff in error, and also the petition in error was not filed within one year. This motion was overruled on the 25th, of June, 1907, by our predecessor and the ruling will not be reviewed here.

Plaintiff in error relies upon the proposition to secure reversal, which is, "that the verdict and judgment are not sustained by sufficient evidence." To this issue thus raised, both parties have filed very full briefs, and the court has had the benefit of an able oral argument on the part of counsel, all of which have had our best attention and consideration. The record of the trial as presented here is unusually free of irrelevant or immaterial matter. The issue before the court and the jury was closely adhered to by counsel, and the instructions of the court are exceptionally lucid and comprehensive. All of these things tend to render it easier for us to determine the precise proof in the case, and to ascertain and determine whether or not the verdict rendered was in fact legally sustained by the evidence.

Let us first notice the law governing the responsibility of physicians and surgeons in cases of this character. The general rule is quoted in Volume I of Whitthaus & Becker's Medical Jurisprudence, Forensic Medicine and Toxicology, at page 30, wherein the authors of this work adopt the rule as laid down in Shearman & Redfield's work on the Law of Negligence.

"Although a physician or surgeon may doubtless by express contract undertake to perform a cure absolutely, the law will not imply such a contract from the mere employment of the physician. A physician is not an insurer of a cure, and is not to be tried for the result of his remedies. His only contract is to treat the case with reasonable diligence and skill. If more than this is expected, it must be expressly stipulated for. The general rule, therefore, is that a medical man who attends for a fee is liable for such want of ordinary care. diligence, or skill on his part as leads to the injury of his patient. To render him liable, it is not enough that there has been a less degree of skill than some other medical man might have shown, or a less degree of care than even himself might have bestowed; nor is it enough that he himself acknowledged some degree of want of care; there must have been a want of competent and ordinary result. But a professed physician or surgeon is bound to use not only such skill as he has, but to have a reasonable degree of skill. The law will not countenance quackery; and, although the law does not require the most thorough education or the largest experience, it does require that an uneducated, ignorant man shall not, under the pretense of being a well-qualified physician, attempt recklessly and blindly to administer medicines or perform surgical operations."

The rule as adopted by the Supreme Court of Oklahoma Territory is announced in the case of Champion v. Kieth, 17 Okla., 204; Pac. 845, wherein, on the authority of numerous cases cited, Mr.

Justice Pancoast, in a well-considered opinion, says of the practicing physician: "He is never considered as warranting a cure, unless under a special contract for that purpose. His contract, as implied by law, is that he possesses that reasonable degree of learning, skill, and experience which is ordinarily possessed by others of his profession; that he will use reasonable and ordinary care and diligence in the treatment of the case which he undertakes; and that he will use his best judgment in all cases of doubt as to the proper course of treatment. He is not responsible for damages for want of success, unless it is shown to be the result of want of ordinary skill and learning, such as ordinarily possessed by others of his profession, or for want of ordinary care and attention. He is not presumed to engage for extraordinary skill or for extraordinary diligence or care, nor can he be made responsible in damages for errors in judgment, or mere mistake in matters of reasonable doubt or uncertainty."

In order for plaintiff to recover in this case, it is absolutely essential that two conditions be shown to exist: First, it must appear from the evidence that the plaintiff sustained and suffered legal detriment or damage; and second, such detriment or damage may not be referable solely to the accident with which he met, but it must be shown on his part that considering the accident which he suffered, and his employment of a physician, still he is left in a condition worse than was his right to demand and expect, if his physician was ordinarily skilful and gave him proper care. In the case at bar Plaintiff complains of two things as constituting his detriment or damage: First, that his fractured limb was from an inch to an inch and one-half shorter than it had been; second, that the fractured and injured part was still painful, and that it was necessary, in order to use it, to call to his assistance a crutch or cane. Of course, if plaintiff's limb within a proper time had been restored in the treatment secured to a perfect limb, as it was prior to the time when broken, he could not recover from the physician who treated him, notwithstanding lack of skill shown or negligent care bestowed. So, in our judgment, it would follow if in the concensus of opinion of men schooled and learned in the science of surgery, well acquainted with the facts controlling and surrounding, and results attending, such an accident as this, the limb, after treatment, if no unnecessary pain was occasioned or time consumed, was in as good a condition as an ordinarily skilful physician, using ordinary care, could in the usual and expected course of events produce, then the plaintiff has failed to show that he has suffered such damage or detriment as the law will compensate him for: for while it may not be physically and actually perfect, it is in that condition in which the limitations of human skill leaves a limb, fractured as it was.

This being true, the plaintiff has not suffered legal damage. He is not damaged. Getchel v. Hill, 21 Minn. 464; Feeney v. Spalding, 89 Me., III, 35 Atl. 1027; Stern v. Lanng, 106 La., 738, 31 South 303; Hesse v. Knippel, Mich., N. P. (Brown) 109; Tomer v. Aiken et al., 126 Iowa, 114, 101 N. W. 769; Craig v. Chambers et ux., 17 Ohio St. 254; Ewing et al. v. Goode (C. C.) 78 Fed. 442.

In the case last cited, Ewing et al. v. Goode, Taft, Circuit Judge, said: "It is well settled that in such an employment the implied agreement of the physician or surgeon is that no injurious consequences shall result from want of proper skill, care, or diligence on his part in the execution of his employment. If there is no injury caused by lack of skill or care, then there is no breach of the physician's obligation, and there can be no recovery. Craig v. Chambers, 17 Ohio St. 253, 260. Mere lack of skill, or negligence, not causing injury, gives no right of action, and no right to recover even nominal damages. This was the exact point decided in the case just cited. In Hancke v. Hooper, 7 Car. & P. 81 Tindal, C. J., said: "A surgeon is responsible for an injury done to a patient through the want of proper skill in his apprentice; but, in an action against him, the plaintiff must show that the injury was procured by such want of skill, and it is not to be inferred." Before the plaintiff can recover, she must show by affirmative evidence: First, that defendant was unskilful or negligent; and second, that his want of skill or care caused injury to the plaintiff. If either element is lacking in her proof, she has presented no case for the consideration of the jury. The naked facts that defendant performed operations upon her eye, and that pain followed, and that subsequently the eye was in such a bad condition that it had to be extracted, established neither the neglect and unskilfulness of the treatment, nor the casual connection between it and the unfortunate event. A physician is not a warrantor of cures. If the maxim, "Res ipsa loquitur," were applicable to a case like this, and a failure to cure were held to be evidence, however slight, of negligence on the part of the physician or surgeon, causing the bad result, few would be courageous enough to practice the healing art, for they would have to assume financial liability for nearly all the "Ills that flesh is heir to."

On this proposition the Supreme Court of Ohio, in the case of Craig v. Chambers, supra, held, in the syllabus, that: "The implied liability of a surgeon, retained to treat a case professionally, extends no further, in the absence of a special agreement, than that he will indemnify his patient against any injurious consequences resulting from his want of skill, care, or diligence in the execution of his employment. And, in an action against the surgeon for malpractice, the plaintiff, if he shows no injury resulting from negligence, or want of due skill in the defendant, will not be entitled to recover nominal damages."

Should it be shown, however, by the evidence, that the limb which plaintiff had was not such a limb as a physician of ordinary skill and using ordinary care and diligence should have left him with, after treating it, then the burden is upon plaintiff, in order to sustain the verdict in this case, to show by the evidence that this result was brought about through lack of skill on the part of the physician, or through some wrongful or negligent act of omission or commission on his part. Neither of these conditions should be supported merely by theory, conjecture, or inference, but they should be based upon tangible, substantial evidence which the court and jury may grasp and understand. A physician employed in a case such as this, it should be remembered, as was said by Justice Upton (Williams v. Poppleton, 3 Or. 139,) "is obliged by his calling constantly to enter the abode of others, and frequently to undertake difficult cases, and to perform critical operations in the presence of those who are ignorant and credulous. He is liable to have his acts misjudged, his motives suspected, and the truth colored or distorted even where there are no dishonest intentions on the part of his accusers. And, from the very nature of his duty, he is constantly liable to be called to perform the most critical operations in the presence of persons united in interest and sympathy by the ties of family, where he may be the only witness in his own behalf. It is the intention of the law to protect the physician or surgeon as well as the patient. * * * A fracture or dislocation, or both combined, may be so complicated that no human skill can restore it. Or the patient may, by disregarding the surgeon's directions, impair the effect of the best conceived measures. The surgeon does not deal with inanimate or insensate matter, like the stone mason or bricklayer, who can choose his materials and adjust them according to mathematical lines but he has a suffering human being to treat, a nervous system to tranquilize, and an excited will to regulate and control. Where a surgeon undertakes to treat a fractured limb, he has not only to apply the known facts and theoretical knowledge of his science, but he may have to contend with very many powerful and hidden influences, such as want of vital force, habit of life, hereditary disease, the state of the climate. These or the mental state of his patient may often render the management of a surgical case difficult, doubtful, and dangerous, and may have greater influence in the result than all the surgeon may be able to accomplish, even with the best skill and care." This being true, he should not be condemned except the evidence requires and justifies it.

With these observations and the law before us, we now turn to the evidence upon which the plaintiff relies for recovery, and find that it shows briefly the following facts: About four months prior to the filing of his petition in this case, plaintiff, who was a man of 56 years and of fairly good health and activity, fell on the ice and fractured the femur of his right leg at or near the neck. He called in the defendant to treat him, and the defendant arrived in about two hours after the accident.

placed the plaintiff under the influence of chloroform, and made an examination. Plaintiff and a number of other witnesses, members of his family and neighbors, testified that the defendant informed him and them that the limb was fractured at a place above the knee and between it and the upper part of the femur, perhaps about the middle. It also appears that defendant applied what the physicians term a "Buck's extension," which consisted of, in this case, a splint in the shape of a board, attached to the limb on the under side, to which was fastened a rope which extended to a window frame, with a 5 1-2 pound iron attached, for the purpose of tiring and extending the muscles to bring the broken parts of the bone in apposition. This occurred on the 1st day o fFebruary, 1905; the doctor remained with the plaintiff all of that night and on the morning of the second day thereafter he returned, bringing with him what is commonly known as a "Hodgin splint," an appliance which he had made, consisting of an iron rod, bent much in the shape of a hairpin, the two sides laced together with webbing or cloth, and of about the length and shape of the leg. Into this the limb was placed with the foot near the top, the open end being toward the body, the inside about 10 inches shorter than the opposite piece. This entire frame was then swung about two inches clear of the bed, allowing the limb to lie in this splint, which was attached to a pulley from the ceiling or window ledge by ropes or cords. That in this condition plaintiff remained in bed about three weeks, during which time he was waited upon by the physician. Plaintiff testified that his limb was left by this treatment in a weak or stiff condition in the hip, which interfered with its use, that it hurt him in walking, and he stated: "I cannot use it as well as I could before it was hurt; it is stiff, and the muscles won't expand;" also that he could not walk without the use of a cane or crutch. This is the proof of the damage on which he relies to recover. On his examination by his counsel, being requested by his counsel, to stand in his natural position with his back to the jury, he stated that the reason he did not put his right heel to the floor, upon being requested to do so, was that he could not. On being asked how far his heel was from the floor, he stated it was about two inches, whereupon his counsel stated, "It may feel that way, but I guess it is about an inch." Plaintiff also stated that since the treatment by defendant he had applied to Messrs. Sharp and Stagner, local physicians, for treatment. Dr. Stagner, one of these physicians, called by plaintiff, testified that he made an examination of his limb at his own and at Dr. Sharp's office, and was present when the same was examined with the X-ray. That the examination revealed an impacted fracture of the neck of the femur, the result of which he stated necessarily shortened the limb. He further stated that in a case of this character it was very likely that treatment would not produce the best results, and that the limb would be shorter than its normal length. That some of the authorities claim this shortening to be inevitable, as the bones of old persons do not knit as well as those of young people, and that the union is more likely to be fibrous. That he would not regard 81 per cent of bad results as being much too high a per cent in cases of this character.

Dr. Sharp, the other expert called on behalf of plaintiff on this proposition testified as follows: Q. In treatment of fractures in the neck of the femur, how about shortening of the limb; is that a good re-

sult?

A. In many cases it is.

Q. Is it not a fact that there are eminent authorities who say that, in patients above 50 years of age, the shortening of the limb is inevitable?

A. I think there are a number of authorities who make that statement. The foregoing presents substantially all the evidence given by the experts called on the part of the plaintiff upon the question of the shortening of the limb. From them it appears that the injured limb was from one to one inch and one-half shorter than the other, and from this evidence no other inference can be drawn than that this was as good a result as could be reasonably expected, considering the age and condition of the plaintiff. At all events, there is an absolute lack of any evidence showing that in cases of this character, under any kind of treatment, the limb is ever perfect afterwards or equals in length the uninjured limb. In this case the burden was not upon the defendant to show that plaintiff's limb was in as good a condition as medical science and skill could place it after its injury, but the burden was upon the plaintiff to show that it was not. This, in our judgment, he totally failed to do. The defendant, however, voluntarily assumed the burden of showing that the result which was attained by the treatment were all that could have been expected under the conditions.

The plaintiff was able to get around on his limb by the use of a cane or crutch. It was, as we have seen, from an inch to an inch and one-half shorter than the sound one. The condition was presented to a number of physicians called by the defendant, and they were interrogated upon the proposition as to whether or not such a result was practically all that medical science could promise. We note a few of their answers to this question.

The defendant himself testified: Q. Would there likely be a perfect recovery in a fracture of that kind, Doctor, under any kind of treatment that medical science could give it?

A. In a man of Mr. Elder's age, the latest statistics say there are absolutely none that are perfect.

Q. In what way would there be any imperfection?

A. There would be a shortening of the limb, and consequently a lameness. He further stated that the statistics in cases of this character show that of young and old, taken together, 80 per cent get a bad result.

Dr. Morse, who for 18 months was shown to have been on the house staff of surgeons in the Cook County Hospital, in Chicago, after he had graduated, testified to having had many cases of this character, and deposed as follows: A. It seems, so far as I know, it is an unknown thing in the profession to get a good result, and a good result is one in which there is no abnormal condition; it is practically never obtained in hip bone fractures.

Q. What are the ordinary results?

A. I should say that, after a period of six months or within a year the ordinary case, if not too feeble, will get out with crutches first, and then with a cane, and then they will be fortunate if they can get along either with or without a cane.

Q. And are these the results that are expected and anticipated in the best hospitals?

A. They are.

Dr. Morse further testified on this same subject as follows: A. Sometimes if they get a bony union and good apposition of the bones, particularly where they are strong, I mean where the patients are strong, they can get along with practically very little limp or without even a cane, but this is only in exceptional cases; the majority of them use the crutches for a period of months, and sometimes never get along without a crutch, and in some instances never get out of their wheel chair.

Q. What about the shortening of the limb?

A. The degree of shortening varies from three-fourths of an inch to two inches, with more or less tenderness remaining all their lives.

Q. Then inability to get along without the use of a crutch or cane, a permanent shortening of the limb and a decided halt in their gait the remainder of their days, these are some of the results of a fracture of this kind?

A. Yes, sir, they are among the most common results.

Dr. Reed testified as follows: Q. Have you had information and know, Doctor, either by observation, experience, study, or reading, the liability of shortening of the limb by a break in the neck of the femur?

A. I have.

Q. What is the likelihood or probability of that?

A. We always expect to get shortening.

Q. Under the most approved and proper methods of treatment?

A. Yes, sir.

Q In a person as old as the plaintiff here, what about soreness in the parts?

A. There would probably be tenderness for a long time.

Q. What do you mean by a long time, Doctor?

A. Several years.

Q. What about the ability to get around after an injury of that kind and at his age?

A. The results are never perfect in a man of that age; the period of getting about varies in different patients. I would consider, if he was ever able to use the limb in walking by putting his weight on it, that it would be as good or better tnan the average result.

Dr. Hill testified: Q. On fractures in the neck of the femur, what is the probability or likelihood of a shortening of the limb in a person as old as the plaintiff, here?

A. It is practically inevitable, and it is expected in every case.

Q. What about the soreness, Doctor, and how long continued?

A. That would depend upon the immobility of the joint, but ordinarily it would last a year or two; depends upon the amount of inflammation at the time of treatment.

Dr. Barker testified: Q. In a person of this age, Doctor, and his apparent condition, what would you say as to the probability of a shortening of the limb?

A. I would say there would be a very remote possibility of getting a result without a shortening of the limb to some extent.

Q. What about soreness in the parts, and what might you expect in that regard?

A. He could expect trouble for the balance of his life in some way or another. If he didn't get union, he would have a limb that would be almost useless; if he got union, he might expect trouble in the way of soreness and things in that line, and the probability is he never would get entirely over it, so he would always have trouble. Q. Why is it that there is such a large per cent of bad results in the treatment of a fracture of this character?

A. Well, in the first place, it is on account of the location of the injury; it is impossible to keep them there if you do get

them; then a great many are mixed fractures, part intracapsular or extracapsular, difficult both of diagnosis and treatment; then in that location you may not get union at all on account of the intervention of muscles; the blood supply may be deficient, or a disease of the bone may develop and arrest the knitting process especially in the aged; in fact, some physicians question the advisability of trying to get union at all under some conditions because the patient will suffer less not to have union, although the leg may not be so useful; so it is the nature of the trouble and the location that causes so many bad results.

Dr. Melvin testified: Q. Now, under the best treatment that is known to medical science, what do you say as to the probability of a shortening of the limb from a fracture of the femur?

A. It is a very probable; indeed, I do not believe there would be more than five or ten out of a hundred that would not have shortening.

Q. Suppose the fracture is in the neck of the femur, is the liability to shortening greater or less?

A. It is more apt to have shortening if it is in the neck.

Q. Is it always possible to get a union of the bone with a person as old as the plaintiff?

A. No, sir.

Q. What about soreness in the parts; what might be expected in that regard?

A. Well, a great deal would depend upon the amount of lymph thrown out and the callous formation; it would naturally press on the nerves and cause a great deal of pain that might last for a number of years.

Dr. Ralph Smith testified to practically the same effect as the other physicians, and the testimony of them all, as is seen, supports the theory that the plaintiff, considering his age and the character of the fracture, without reference to the character of treatment given him by his attending physician, had as good a limb as he had a right to expect or demand, and, in the absence of evidence showing that an ordinarily skilled physician, exercising ordinary diligence in his treatment, would or should have produced a different and a better result, then plaintiff can not be said to be damaged or to be entitled to recover. There is no contention made on the part of the plaintiff that defendant was not possessed of skill sufficient to entitle him to hold himself out and to treat cases of this character, unless this claim could be predicated upon the contention of plaintiff that defendant made an erroneous diagnosis, and that the adoption of the splint heretofore mentioned and the manner of its use was an indication of such a want of skill. The conclusion to which we have come relieves us of the necessity of minutely detailing the evidence bearing upon this question, for reasons we have heretofore stated; but we will say that there was no physician called on either side who, when asked, did not testify that the Hodgin splint was such an apparatus as was recognized by the profession as standard and was used generally for cases of this character, either for a break in the shaft, or in the neck of the femur, while many of the physicians testify that this splint was considered as one of the best apparatuses of its character known to the profession and was in use in the best hospitals. The defendant testified that the limb of the plaintiff was attached to this frame, and that the extension was such that this was necessary to raise the foot off the bed in which the plaintiff lay in order to relieve him of being pulled down into the bed by the force of the same. Plaintiff testified that his limb was not attached to the apparatus, or that, if it was, the attachment was re-moved, and that by reason of this his limb came out of the splint, and that it was necessary to replace it on occasions. Some of the physicians testified that it was a matter of judgment as to whether or not, without being attached, there would be sufficient extension to overcome the contraction of the muscles; but the general net result, and only rational conclusion to be drawn from the testimony of all of the physicians is that the plaintiff received treatment such as was recognized to be proper, and that the result was practically all that could be looked for.

There is no other higher or better method known to our law or practice to determine disputed questions of fact than by the verdict of 12 jurors. Where a cause of action is shown to exist, and they are permitted to hear all the relevant, competent, and material evidence offered. and the instructions of the court are proper, a verdict reasonably supported by such evidence is not to be lightly regarded or set aside by an appellate tribunal. These observations are fundamental, but there are no classes of cases, perhaps, which go to juries, or indeed, with which lawyers and courts are called upon to deal, where results are so uncertain and so frequently unsatisfactory as cases involving damages against physicians for alleged ills to which the human flesh is heir to. It is nearly always the defendant's judgment which is on trial; and on the hearing the jury and the parties are all sitting and speaking after the fact, while the unfortunate physician when he acted was perhaps required by the conditions to grope, deliberate, and often speedily act, and always before the fact. After he had acted and the results are different than he desired or expected, and different than were expected or desired by the patient, if a suit is brought, the physician is confronted with all of the after-acquired knowledge, and his responsibility is weighed from that standpoint rather than from the true one. A preponderance of the evidence in cases of this character is sufficient to sustain a plaintiff's cause. No more should be required and no more is required; but it should be certain on the part of the court and jury that they are acting from actual evidence before them, properly referable to the cause, and that the judgment, when against the physician, is based upon such evidence and not upon bias, conjecture, or inference.

In keeping with these general observations, attention is called to the language used by Chief Justice Thayer in the case of Langford v. Jones, 18 Or. 307-323, 22 Pac. 1064, 1070: "The practice of leaving the jury to determine such cases has been permitted often, when the responsibility was really upon the court. It is wrong and unjust to the medical profession to pursue such a course it tends to encourage the institution of suits against its members when no grounds exist therefor. A physician, in the treatment of disease, or in the performance of surgical operations, does not always achieve that success he desires. Circumstances often intervene over which he has no control, and render his treatment unsatisfactory. This is more especially so with surgery. It frequently happens, in the reduction of a fracture or dislocation, that from some cause, for which the surgeon was in no wise responsible, the parts of the broken bone have not properly united, have been found not to be in perfect apposition, or the dislocated joint to be enlarged, or that muscular action of the limb has become suspended, or the limb become crooked and sometimes, in consequence of important nerves having been severed at the time of the fracture, a loss of sensation of the parts is occasioned, resulting in a permanent numbness, and amputation becomes necessary. In a majority of such cases the party injured by the casualty will claim damages against the surgeon who attended upon him, and have no difficulty in having an action instituted to enforce it, predicating his cause upon alleged negligence in the reduction of the fracture or dislocation, or of insufficient support to the broken parts, or of too tight bandaging, or upon some other pretext, but relying mainly upon the deformity of the limb as the ground for a recovery; and generally, through the sympathy, prejudice, or stupidity of a jury, succeed in mulcting the defendant in damages. The average juror knows very little about such matters. If he has sufficient discretion to understand them in the outset, he will lose it by the time he has heard the expert testimony and the summing up of the counsel. A trial court should never allow a case of malpractice to be submitted to a jury unless the plaintiff has fairly shown, by competent proof, that the defendant is guilty of the charge alleged against him.

In the concluding remarks of the court in that case it said: "The judgment appealed from will be reversed. Ordinarily such a disposition of a case is followed by an order remanding it to the court below for a new trial; but, under the peculiar circumstances existing in this case, such order will not be made. It will be remanded, however, with directions to dismiss the complaint."

In the case of Ewing et al. c. Goode, supra, Judge Taft said: "The condition of the plaintiff can not but awaken the sympathy of every one, but I must hold that there is no evidence before the court legally sufficient to support a verdict in her favor. I should deem it my duty without hesitation to set aside a verdict in her favor. I should deem it my duty without hesitation to set aside a verdict for the plaintiff in this case as often as it could be rendered, and, that being true, it becomes my duty to direct a verdict for the defendant."

In the case at bar, with all of the evidence before us on which the plaintiff could possibly predicate the hope of recovery, and there being a total want and absence of the necessary elements to entitle him to recover, the cause is accordingly remanded to the county court of Logan Co., with instructions to dismiss the same.

KANE, C. J. AND TURNER, WILLIAMS, AND HAYES, jj., CONCUR.

ACUTE POST-OPERATIVE DILATATION OF THE STOMACH.

BY J. E. GILCREEST, M. D., GAINESVILLE, TEXAS.

The late literature on acute dilatation of the stomach only dates back a few years. An article in the 1907 year-book on Surgery says acute dilatation in its most severe type is a rare condition and usually proves fatal within a few days. As a post-operative complication of surgical conditions it has received but scant attention until the past year, and, in the absence of post-mortem, is frequently overlooked just as appendicitis was 25 years ago.

Many of us can remember when we saw patients die of what we called peritonitis, locked bowels, etc. We now know that nearly all these cases were appendicitis and could have been saved by a timely operation. So for many years we have seen our laparotomy cases do well for a day or two and then have enormous distention of the abdomen and commence regurgitating a dark green fluid, and finally die when we could not see why they did not get well. I am fully convinced that many of those cases were post-operative dilatation of the stomach and would have recovered under appropriate treatment. This condition is not confined entirely to abdominal sections, but may occur in almost any medical or surgical illness. Synonyms:—Acute dilatation of the stomach has been called acute gastroduodenal dilatation, gastromesentericleus, arteriomesenteric obstruction of the duodenum, acute gastric paresis, etc., each different observer embody-

ing in the name his own idea of the etiology. Rokitansky described this condition in 1842, and Brinton in 1859 recognized the condition, and believed it to be of paralytic origin.

Occurrence.

Acute post-operative dilatation of the stomach is recognized today by the majority of surgeons as a condition different from a chronically dilated stomach met with in every day practice which is caused by stenosis of the pylorus due to cancer, ulcers, tumors and inflammatory conditions. The chronic cases will go on for years, and when the stomach becomes over-distended it is relieved by vomiting. Acute dilatation comes on quite suddenly and may follow any surgical operation where a general anaesthetic has been given. I do not think there has been a case reported where a general anaesthetic has not been given. While it may occur after any operation it has been observed more frequently after operations on the gall bladder and its ducts. W. J. Mayo says that he has observed it more frequently after gall bladder operations.

Etiology.

Thompson in discussing the etiology divided the cases into 5 groupes:—

1. Those in which dilatation occurs without any cause being apparent.

2. Where, after death, some other lesions were found.

400 JOURNAL OF THE OKLAHOMA STATE MEDICAL ASSOCIATION.

3. Those where some gross indiscretion of diet seemed to be the chief cause.

4. Those in which dilatation followed an injury.

5. Those that followed a surgical operation, no other lesion being demonstrable at the autopsy.

The scope of this paper will permit only a mere mention of the many views that have been advanced by different writers on the causes of acute dilatation of the stomach. When we remember that the root of the mesentery extends from the left lateral aspect of the second lumbar vertebra downwards, crossing obliquely the spinal column, aorta, vena cava inferior, and third portion of the duodenum, ending at the right iliac fossa. we know that the duodenum is flattened where the mesentery lies over it, and when the intestines are drawn downwards from any cause, the tension over the duodenum may be increased sufficiently to obstruct the passage from the stomach through it. In a large per cent of the cases that come to postmortem, the duodenum is compressed by the mesentery sufficient to close off the lumen at this point; but it has been shown that this compression is not absolutely essential in the production of acute dilatation of the stomach. Whether the dilated stomach primarily causes the occlusion by crowding the small intestines into the pelvis, thus tensing the mesentery so that it constricts the duodenum; or whether the duodenum is primarily constricted by the mesentery. causing a gastric dilatation: whether a primary motor insufficiency of the stomach walls or a pronounced enteroptosis should be reckoned as factors; whether or not much importance should be accorded to a long lax mesentery; whether postoperative vomiting and the crowding of the intestines into the pelvis: whether a primarily dilated stomach may compress the duodenum, and—finally—whether the an-

aesthetic is a factor in causing the dilatation, —all are unsettled points. According to Albrecht the duodenum alone may be dilated without the stomach. He says that at autopsy it can be shown that pressure on the duodenum is unable to force anything to the left of the mesenteric band; moreover, that the contents of the small bowel cannot be forced into the duodenum. In Baumler's case the construction of the mesenteric root was so marked that circular necrosis of the mucosa was found. While authors are divided as to whether dilatation of the stomach is primary or whether it is proceeded by occlusion of the duodenum, Thoma believes the former is more probable, since cases of gastric dilatation are found without any enlargement of the duodenum. However, it is well to remember that dilatation of the duodenum may accompany that of the stomach.

The experiments of Cannon and Murphy demonstrated that the splanchnic nerves are inhibitors of gastric and intestinal peristalsis and they concluded that strong impulses through these nerves may be regarded as a cause of gastric and intestinal inactivity. All of the experimental results favor the necessity of an innervation factor in the production of acute dilatation, and this factor is most logically explained as paralysis of the vagus nerves or stimulation of the splanchnic nerves.

The cause may be direct or reflex. There are certain surgical factors which directly produce post-operative peristaltic inactivity, trauma, cooling and exposure of the viscera, the presence of wicks, the development of peritonitis, overstretching of the bowel, etc. Whether the source of diminished peristalsis is of central or peripheral origin, it seems impossible to say Cannon and Murphy concluded that the diminished peristalsis, as the effect of handling is not necessarily the consequence of reflex inhibitions from the spinal cord, but can be entirely explained as a disturbance of the local mechanism in the wall of the gut. The occurrence of acute dilatation so frequent after operations on the biliary tract, and the fact that recurrence may take place until the drainage has been removed, suggests that the wicks may be a cause of local paralysis. Whether the cause is from paralysis or pressure on the duodenum by the root of the mesentery, are points not definitely settled. The findings at autopsy are important; the stomach is usually enormously enlarged; it may reach to the pubis. In a case reported by Albrecht the greater curve measured 27 inches, the lesser 7 inches and the pyloric opening 2 inches. Evidently the majority of the reported cases were not recognized or they would have come to autopsy.

Symptoms and Signs.

Vomiting a bile-stained fluid is usually one of the first symptoms. At first it may be free, but more often will be regurgitated in small quantities. This may be a continuation of the post-anaesthetic vomiting, but more frequently comes on from the second to the fifth day after the operation. This late vomiting, in the absence of a reasonable cause, should always be looked upon with suspicion. Conner and others have spoken of enormous quantities of the vomitus. My observation is that the vomiting is persistent and uncontrollable, but not profuse. More frequently it is regurgitation of bile looking fluid with but little odor. The continuation of vomiting of large quantities would indicate intestinal obstruction more than paralytic dilatation of the stomach.

Pain is not a constant symptom and 's seldom acute, but is better described as an intense fulness, and pressure in the epigastrium.

The stomach may be enormously *distended* while the lower abdomen remains flat, but usually the intestines fill with gas soon after the trouble begins. The contents of the stomach usually consists of gas and a dark bile-stained fluid. The quantity ejected far exceeds the amount taken in; showing that the condition causes hypersecretion of the stomach.

Thirst is usually a constant symptom, and, after vomiting freely or washing out the stomach, water will be tolerated well for a while, but comes back in an hour or two, and usually much more fluid than was taken in. Enemas will often move the bowels and cause the expulsion of gas but does not relieve the distressed feeling in the epigastrium.

Murphy says the most pronounced symptoms are cyanosis, rapid respiration, frequent emesis in small quantities, sunken eyes, and a relaxed doughy skin with epigastric distention and large flat area in the hypogastrium.

The *temperature* is not usually high and will often be found subnormal. The *pulse* and respiration are accelerated, and, as the process advances there is cardiac weakness, the pulse becoming rapid and small, respiration superficial and the general appearance indicating collapse.

The amount of *urine* is much reduced, amounting at times to almost complete anuria.

These symptoms usually continue until death which occurs on the 4th to the 6th day, unless relieved by mechanical means.

The *diagnosis* is not difficult if we keep in mind the symptoms. The prognosis in recorded cases is bad; the mortality from 60 to 72 per cent. However, this represents the mortality of unrecognized and untreated cases. If the cases are recognized early and treated at once the prognosis is good. With timely and appropriate treatment 80 per cent or more should recover.

Treatment.

It is of the utmost importance in the treatment of acute dilatation of the stomach to differentiate it from peritonitis; a failure to do this often leads to a fatal termination. The modern treatment of peritonitis demands that the toxic intraperitoneal exudate be kept away from the open lymphatic stroma by using the Fowler position (head high, pelvis low). To reverse this in a case of beginning peritonitis would be to gravitate the toxic exudate towards the diaphragm, which would favor the absorption of the toxins before the organism had time to call into play its complicated mechanism of immunization. The treatment of acute dilatation is diametrically opposite to that of peritonitis. The intestines are already drawn in the pelvis, tightening the head of the mesentery over the duodenum. The Fowler position would be the surest way to increase the imprisonment of the bowels and draw a tighter band over the duodenum.

Granting then that the treatment of the two conditions are opposite, is it possible to differentiate these two conditions? The distention of the bowels from gas after laparotomies always commences in the hypogastric region. The distention from acute dilatation of the stomach commences in the epigastric region, but may finally distend the whole abdomen. The efficacy of treatment will depend on the stage at which it was begun. The first indication is to empty the stomach with the stomach tube, wash it out with warm normal salt solution, repeating this as often as necessary to keep the stomach empty. This cleanses out of the stomach the irritating bile, and pancreatic secretions and promotes peristalsis. Purgatives as a rule are useless, but stimulating enemas do good by emptying the lower bowels, and often cause the expulsion of gas. Paralysis is temporary and is caused by over-dis-

tention of the stomach and bowels, and passes off as the distention is relieved. The foot of the bed should be elevated, but the extreme Trendelenburg or knee-chest position, as advised by some, makes the patient very uncomfortable, and I can not see that it does the good claimed for it. In my opinion the best results have come from a moderate elevation of the pelvis, and the free use of the stomach and rectal tubes. Rectal feeding should be resorted to as soon as the patient begins to need supporting. Morphine in very small doses hypodermically is often necessary to rest the patient. Strychnine, adrenalin and normal salt solution should be used as necessary to prevent prostration. No operative procedures have been crowned with brilliant results, and are usually contraindicated.

I shall report in detail the last case I treated, which was a typical one. Mr. R., age 35, usual weight 150 lbs., height 5 ft. 10 in. He was an habitual drinker, and was intoxicated when he entered the Gainesville Sanitarium April 2, 1909. He was then suffering from an acute attack of appendicitis. This attack was the third within the past six months. At this time he had been sick about ten days and was slowly recovering. He was kept in bed and given liquid diet and rectal feeding until his pulse and temperature had been normal several days.

An appendectomy was performed at 2 a. m. April 11th. The appendix had perforated and was buried in adhesions. It was removed and the wound closed without drainage. He had no shock but that night his temperature went to 103 degrees, and pulse 120. Pulse and temperature gradually went down and, at 4 p. m. the next day were about normal and remained so until the evening of the third day when he reached a pitcher of water on the washstand near his bed and drank a large quantity. That night he vomited several times. When I saw him the next morning he was regurgitating a very dark fluid and had a distressd fulness of the stomach but the lower abdomen was not distended. His bowels had moved on the morning of the third day, and flatus had passed freely.

I had my associate, Dr. Garrett, to see him and we made a diagnosis of acute dilatation of the stomach. I had feared sepsis from the old diseased appendix and had kept him in a medium Fowler position, so I changed his position at once, elevating the foot of his bed about 15 inches. The stomach tube was next passed and a quart of dark bile-stained fluid ran out, giving him great relief. I then washed the stomach by running in and out if it a pint of warm normal salt solution, repeating this until the fluid came out moderately clear which took about 6 or 8 washings. He was given an enema which moved his bowels again and caused some gas to pass. He did quite well the remainder of the day, but that night he grew worse and the next morning was in about the same condition. The stomach tube was used again with the same result as on the first occasion, only that the relief did not last as long. Vomiting commenced again in about 4 hours time. I then emptied and washed the stomach every 2 or 4 hours for 4 days and nights before the regurgitation of dark fluid ceased. During this time he was given, by the drop method, 11 ounces of normal salt solution with 1 ounce of liquid peptonoids every 4 to 6 hours. When the distention was greatest, the stomach could be distinctly outlined, reaching 2 inches below the umbilicus. During this dilatation period his pulse never ran over 110, but was very weak at times.

He had strychnine hypodermically, and digitalis and adrenalin by rectum as they were indicated. As soon as the regurgitation ceased he began to take nourishment and retained it well, and made a good recovery. I believe had I washed this patient's stomach every 2 hours from the beginning it would have shortened his convalesence.

Conclusion.

Acute dilatation of the stomach occurs much more frequently after operations done under general anaesthesia than is generally supposed. Many cases are mild and recover without any treatment. Others more severe often die without a diagnosis until they reach the post-mortem table. I am sure that I have several times seen this condition when I did not recognize it. The best results are obtained by frequent irrigation of the stomach with warm water or normal salt solution and elevation of the hips.

Examination of this patient's stomach contents by Dr. Garrett showed:

Total Acidity—50 degrees.

Free Hydrochloric Acid—40 degrees.

Pepsin—present.

Bile—present.

Odor—Stale and somewhat offensive, but not fecal.

Pancreatic Juice—Not examined for, but constant presence of bile in stomach contents would indicate its presence.

Read before the Marshall County Medical Society, Nov., 1909, and North Texas District Medical Society at Ft. Worth Dec., 1909.)

. EPISTAXIS.

BY W. ALBERT COOK, M. D., TULSA, OKLA.

(Read before the Tulsa County Medical Society February 5, 1910.)

In the selection of a subject I have endeavored to choose one which might be of interest to all of you, as well as the specialists. Epistaxis is liable to be met with at any time, and none of you know how soon you may be called upon to check what might possibly be a fatal hemorrhage. Epistaxis occurs at all ages, although it is more prevalent during childhood and advanced age than it is in middle life and occurs more frequently in men than in women.

The causes of epistaxis may be classed as idiopathic, vicarious and traumatic.

Idiopathic.

A hemorrhage may occur anywhere in the nasal fossae, but ninety per cent occur on the nasal septum, directly from the anterior artery of the septum, which is a branch of the superior maxillary, or it may be from one of the superficial branches of the anterior artery. The nasal septum is covered with a very thin mucous membrane, the arteries in this locality are poorly protected and on this account are more often the seat of erosion and ulceration than any other part of the nasal fossae. Epistaxis may also be encountered in connection with typhoid, malarial and pneumonia fever, and while it is usually one of the prodromal symptoms of typhoid fever, I have seen some severe cases occur during convalescence. An attack may be brought on by violent exercise, causing a rush of blood to the head in plethoric individuals, and may also occur in connection with diseases of the heart, kidneys and pregnancy; may also follow the ingestion of large doses of quinine and may occur spontaneously in cases of haemophilia.

Cases occur in elderly people due to degenerative processes in the walls of the blood vessels; also, in phosphorus poisoning, gout and syphilis, and in cases of aenemia.

Vicarious.

Under this head we include those curious cases, in which hemorrhage from the nose is substituted for the normal menstrual flow. In the same way, a nasal hemorrhage at the menopause may be regarded as to a certain extent vicarious. B. Frankel has collected a number of cases of vicarious menstruation, which bring out some exceedingly interesting points. Thus, in the case of Kussmauls, there was periodical nasal hemorrhage in a woman with a total absence of the uterus, while in a case reported by Fricker, violent hemorrhage recurred at intervals of six weeks, in a girl of nineteen who had never menstruated, resulting finally in the death of the patient. Still another case was observed by Sommer, in which monthly hemorrhage occurred from the nose in a woman during the whole period of the fifth pregnancy, while Obermeier reported an instance in a woman in whom regular menstruation occurred once at the age of fifteen after which she had a monthly recurrence of nasal hemorrhage lasting three or four days, ceasing only when she was pregnant. Joal lays special stress upon the intimate relation which he believes to exist between the sexual apparatus and the turbinated bodies. He believes that many cases of epistaxis in young persons come from masturbation, congestion of the turbinated bodies at the time of the catamenial flow, or some other form of irritation affecting the sexual apparatus.

Traumatic.

Most cases of the traumatic variety are caused by external violence, such as blows on the nose, causing fractures most frequently of the septum, operations upon the turbinate bodies and the removing of osteoid spurs in the nasal septum.

The bleeding is usually from one side only, although if the hemorrhage has continued for sometime, there may be a clot in the side where the hemorrhage originated, blocking up the anterior nares on that side, damning up the blood so it will pass around behind the septum and drop from the other nostril, which might lead you to believe that you are encountering a second hemorrhage. The blood is usually arterial, and clots easily except in cases of haemophilia. A great many cases of epistaxis are relieved by the congulation of the blood in the anterior nares which gradually fills the nasal fossae until the clot covers the seat of bleeding. This condition is favored by the patient sitting in a stooping position with the head well forward, while if the patient sits in an upright position or lays on his back, the blood will run down into the pharynx and is either swallowed or expectorated by the patient, leading him to believe that he has a hemorrhage, either from the lungs or stomach.

The most common means of arresting a nasal hemorrhage by the laity is the placing of some cold metallic substance, or a piece of ice on the nape of the neck, or folding a piece of brown paper and putting it under the upper lip.

Some cases may be relieved by simply applying pressure directly over the bleeding point, by pressing the nose on that side firmly down against the septum. In cases where the bleeding point can be located and does not respond to simple means of treatment, the point should be touched with the galvano cautery or silver nitrate, chromic acid is recommended, but it is difficult to limit its action, and a great many cases of perforations have resulted from its use. One very efficient haemostatic, which we can find in most every household is peroxide of hydrogen. By spraying the nose with this it forms a flocculent, creamy mass, which fills up all recesses of the nasal fossae, and will afford instant relief in the majority of cases.

Adrenalin chloride is the most popular haemostatic agent that we have today, and when applied to the nose in the form of a spray, or on lint or gauze checks, the bleeding by its powerful action contracting the walls of the blood vessels.

In severe cases, ten drops of adrenalin chloride one to two thousand solution is recommended to be injected into the upper lip on the side on which the hemorrhage is located. A great many astringent sprays. principal of which are alum and tannic acid, have been recommended, but their efficiency is limited, and you can do more in controlling a hemorrhage with a two or four per cent solution of cocaine than with the aforementioned remedies. The most popular treatment for obstinate cases is packing the nose with a long, narrow strip of plain sterilized or iodoform gauze an inch wide and eighteen inches or two feet in length may be packed into the nose by carrying the gauze as far back into the fossae at the beginning as possible and then packing the rest firmly against it. In some cases this stops the bleeding anteriorly, but there may be some bleeding which will drop into the throat, or pass around behind the septum, and drip from the other nostril, and in these obstinate cases it is best to remove the packing and block the posterior nares. This is best done by passing a small size French rubber catheter through the nose back into the pharynx, and grasping the end with a long pair of forceps, and bring the point of the catheter forward through the mouth and tie a string around the eyelet, then drawing the catheter back out of the nose, now we have one end of the string coming out of the nose and the other out of the mouth. To the end of the string extending from the mouth firmly fasten a piece of gauze or cotton firmly compressed about the size of an English walnut; then grasp the nasal end of the string with one hand making firm tension which will draw the plug back through the mouth into the vault of the pharynx, following the plug with the other hand and directing it into position and pressing it well up into the posterior nares. The nasal end of the string should be left protruding leaving the string on the tampon long enough so that it will extend out of the mouth and tie to the nasal end of the string. The anterior nares may be packed, and a clot will soon form between the anterior and posterior plugs which completely fills the cavity.

This will stop the most obstinate cases, but it is objected to by some on account of the pressure in the region of the orifices of the eustascian tubes, setting up otitis media or sometimes mastoiditis or meningitis.

A free hemorrhage from the nose may relieve vascular tension and prevent possible hemhorrhage in other undesirable situations especially in the brain. If the bleeding has been so profuse that the patient shows the constitutional effects of the loss of a large amount of blood as extreme pallor, and a small rapid thready pulse, frequent attacks of syncope, and convulsive twitching of the muscles, then subcutaneous injections of warm normal saline solutions are to be given in quantities varying from eight ounces to two pints. Such patients are to be kept in bed and restlessness controlled by morphine, and be given a light fluid diet. As recovery takes place tonics containing iron are to be give.

W. ALBERT COOK, M. D.,
Tulsa, Okla.

GALLSTONES

No article on "Gallstones" can be looked upon as complete which does not take up the treatment by sodium succinate. Thousands of physicians have testified to its value, and its use is steadily increasing every year.

The treatment is simple: 5 grains of the chemically pure sodium succinate administered before each meal and on going to bed, and the treatment is continued for one year. Long before the expiration of that time the paroxysms have been steadily decreasing in frequency and severity until they cease, and every trace of bile vanishes from the urine.

The one condition necessary for success is that the succinate should be of standard quality. This may be supplied by others but is *is* certainly supplied by the Abbott Alkaloidal Company. This is not a remedy for the paroxysms. H. M. C. is indicated in these, and some cases *must* have the knife, but sodium succinate cures the cholangitis upon which the disease depends, and the symptoms dissappear under its use. Whether gallstones are dissolved or not we do not know, because the patients are so mean that they won't die and let us have a chance to hold an autopsy to prove this interesting question. Instead of that, the great majority persist in getting well.

Samples of sodium succinate with literature will be mailed free on request to interested physicians.

THE HIGH INCISION IN ABDOMINAL CESARIAN SECTION.

LEIGH F. WATSON, M. D., OKLAHOMA CITY.

The short, high incision was first suggested by Drs. Davis and Markoe of New York, and has been employed at the New York Lying In Hospital in 239 Cesarian sections.

This incision has many advantages over the method in general use, and in selected cases a maternal mortality only slightly higher than normal labor and assures the safe delivery of every child alive at the beginning of the operation.

I have seen the child delivered in 45 seconds by this technic, but Dr. Markoe from personal experience of 57 sections, emphasizes the fact that there is no more necessity for haste in performing a Cesarian section than any other abdominal operation, he states that 3 minutes is the usual time required to deliver the child.

Bleeding from the uterus never requires the use of an elastic ligature, even with the low incision, besides it is harmful to the child whose vitality is often already lowered.

The high incision in the uterus gives less hemorrhage than the low, in eclampsia the uterine incision bleeds slightly, in one case Dr. Markoe waited several minutes before closing the uterine wound and during the entire period not over 1-2 ounce of blood was lost.

The Cesarian section cases that show a mortality are those that have undergone prolonged exhausting labor, repeated applications of forceps, or other intrauterine manipulations.

The cases operated on before or at the onset of labor that have not been subjected to repeated examination or attempts at delivery by unskilled attendants are practically without mortality.

In central placenta previa with a rigid cervix and a viable child Cesarian section is the operation of a choice, giving both mother and child a better chance than any other method of delivery.

McPherson gives the following indications for Cesarian section:

1. Deformed pelvis.

2. Placenta previa.

3. Eclampsia with a firm, undilated cervix, and complicated or not with the two previous causes mentioned.

4. Neoplasms of the uterus, such as fibroids, carcinoma, etc.

5. Vaginal deformities, such as marked contraction from scars, tumors, etc.

6. An excessively large child.

To these might be added a desire for children in case of doubtful viability by other methods.

While it is customary at the New York Lying In Hospital to allow patients to go into labor until the os dilates sufficient for free lochial drainage, the cases that were operated on before labor set in apparently drained as well as those that went into labor before operation.

In describing the technic Dr. Davis (2) says: The abdominal cavity is opened by a median incision 12 cm. (5 in.) in length, extending from above downward to the umbilicus.

The fundus of the uterus is found directly under this wound.

If dextro torsion, which is frequently present. occurs. the uterus is manually adjusted so that the anterior uterine wall faces forward.

The abdominal cavity is then walled off by means of three or four moist gauze pads, wet in salt solution.

This leaves only a small area of the uterus exposed to view.

An assistant now places a hand at either side of the abdominal wall, near the wound and well backward, so regulating his pressure that the uterus remains in place during the process of being emptied, and afterward until the deep sutures are tied.

A median incision, which begins well up at the fundus and extends downward so that it is a little longer than the abdominal incision, is made.

This incision should be made carefully so that the amniotic cavity is not opened.

Should the placenta be found situated directly under the wound, it is better to cut or tear directly through it.

If, however, the membranes present, it has been found advisable to sweep the hand quickly between them and the inner surface of the uterus in order to prevent adhering of the membranes.

The lower extremity of the child, which is most readily found, is grasped and practically a breech extraction is done, the after coming head being delivered by the Smellic-Veit maneuver.

The cord is clamped and cut by an assistant, and the child carried from the room in order to avoid confusion while establishing respiration.

A double tenaculum is now placed on either side of the uterine wound at its upper angle to prevent the uterus from slipping down into the wound, the uterus is emptied of any clots that may have formed, also of the placenta, and with as little delay as possible the deep interrupted sutures of heavy chromic cat-gut are placed; each suture is inserted about one centimeter distant from the edge of the uterine wound, carried down to the endometrium, and passed through the opposite side in reverse order.

After these sutures are placed, being tied as they are put in, a continuous suture of fine cat-gut is used to bury the first row of sutures, and bring the peritoneum into apposition.

The sponges are now removed, and the abdomen closed in layers in the usual manner.

Patients who have been delivered by Cesarian section should be operated on at the onset of labor in subsequent pregnancies because of the liability of the uterus rupturing through the old scar.

Lobenstine has shown that thinning of the uterus in the scar line of a previous section may occur during labor regardless of the method of closure or suture material employed.

Occasionally in repeating Cesarian section on the same patient it will be impossible to locate the scar of the former uterine incision, when the scar is visible it should always be excised.

Advantages of the high incision:

1. No danger of ventral hernia.

2. No adhesions, uterus is one to three inches below lower end of abdominal incision.

3. Minimum shock, because of the non-delivery of the uterus from the abdominal cavity and slight handling of visceral peritoneum.

4. The abdominal scar after a few weeks is not over 7-10 cm. (3-4 in.) in length.

1. McPherson, J. A. M. A., August 22, 1908.
2. Davis, Lying-In Hospital Bulletin, December, 1905.

CHRONIC GASTRO-INTESTINAL AUTO-INTOXICATION.

BY DR. J. M. POSTELLE, OKLAHOMA CITY, OKLAHOMA.

Published by request of Central District Society meeting in Guthrie, Okla., Oct. 1909.

Mr. President and Gentlemen of the Oklahoma Central Medical Association.

I have chosen this subject as the most important one that all classes of practitioners have to deal with. From time immemorial the conscientious doctor has been bluffed, his skill outwitted and his patience taxed with the chronic grumbler, the hypochondriac and the "won't get wells," on this same class of patients the quack or the charlatan have fatted. If this class of human ills could be eliminated the quack would vanish.

It is very hard to study the etiology of any given disease when there is no apparent pathological findings and from this very reason chronic auto-intoxication has been very much neglected. One of the discouraging features in the study of these troubles is the lack of laboratory facilities and the constant observation the clinican should have over his patient. Most physicians turn homeopath in treating chronic auto-intoxication treat the symptoms paying but little attention to the underlying cause. The symptoms in these troubles are so varied we are prone to classify them under a head of some known disease; with a known etiological factor, losing sight altogether of the true cause. A man is not naturally a hypochondriac or neurasthenic, if he is such, he has a right to be, he is intoxicated with a definite chemical compound that he has manufactured himself and appropriated unintentionally to his own use.

We have a very definite idea of the etiology of nearly all the diseases affecting the human body because of the scientific study of the unvaried train of symptoms and the constant pathological findings in each disease. In the auto-intoxicated it is different, we have no definite line of symptoms but a conglomerate mass of everything in one patient at different times. The etiology lies with the gastro-intestinal secretions and the pathology with the changes that take place in their transit through the intestinal tract.

Pathology.

A study of the gastric and intestinal secretions together with the intestinal flora should be made in each individual case of auto-intoxication. The stomach is usually at fault, a hyperacid condition with a diminished motor function is usually found, the acid condition of the stomach overbalances the alkaline secretions of the pancreas and the intestinal contents remain acid throughout, this pathological change provides an excellent culture media for the protoleitic bacteria and in the process of fermentation through the action of these on the poorly-prepared peptones we have formed in the gases the sulphoethers and the aromatic bodies such as the indols, skatols, and phenols these bodies are always found in the urine of the auto-intoxicated *and* give a good index to the cause of the conditions present. In normal digestion we have the intestines besides peptones, aromatic substances and ptomaines, these ptomaines are ordinarily excreted by the feces, if their quantity is too great a diarrhœa is brought about by their local irritation and they are swept out and the condition is called actue enteritis or enterocolitis or in the child simply diarrhœa. In the chronic auto-intoxication we have a pathological digestion and a constant manufacturing of ptomaines and toxic substances.

As long as all the emunctories are working and the antitoxic glands bring in their defenses the patient gets along without a great deal of trouble, the deleterious matters are neutralized, these defensive organs must sooner or later suffer from excess of work, then we have secondary reaction of the existing lesions and the resulting functional disorders. The nitrogenious bodies furnish the most toxic substances particularly the ptomaines.

The toxic substances are absorbed into the blood eliminated through the various channels of elimination. After fatigue of these organs are brought about we have an irritation of the heart, the blood vessels, the vascular glands and the nervous system, then it is we have the multiplicity of symptoms.

Symptoms.

It is from the multiplicity of symptoms that first arouses our suspicion as to the condition of the patient.

General Appearance.

The skin is often pale and sometimes yellow, the expression of the face is sad, the eyes often sunken with more or less yellow conjunctives, the lids are often puffed, the lines in the face bespeak long anxiety and fear, the skin is frequently covered with yellow or brown spots and is usually dry, the hair on the body is usually over developed dry and broken.

Objective Symptoms.

The papillæ of tongue are usually swollen and prominent, the tongue is red anteriorly and coated yellow or brown posteriorly.

The breath is often of an aromatic odor. The abdomen especially in children is prominent and often tense, the liver can nearly always be palpated easily. The veins over abdomen are well defined and most patients have hemorrhoids.

Subjective Symptoms.

Most patients suffer from anorexia or from irregular appetites, some have bulimia and eat gluttonously, some have polydipsia or unsatiable thirst. Most all of them complain with diffuse tenderness over stomach and bowels, many complain with pain in limbs and back, but the exact location they can never determine. Often these patients are treated for rheumatism when none exists. Paroxysmal sick headaches or migraine are very common, it is nearly always accompanied with pyrosis, nausea, and eructations followed by vomiting of a strong acid stomach contents. Usually the headache disappears with the vomiting and the patient sleeps soundly.

Vertigo, dyspnœa and palpitation of heart are very common symptoms. In the profoundly auto-intoxicated we find mental disorders up to the point of illusions, delusions and hallucinations.

Diagnosis.

Usually the gastro-intestinal symptoms predominate so markedly that the diagnosis is evident, but not always so. In any event one should not depend on symptoms alone. Where it is possible and it should be made possible to examine the feces with the microscope, by this method we can determine the degree and kind of indigestion present, whether fatty, carbo-hydrate or nitrogenous. In the chemical examination of the urine we have an index that will not fail. We cannot find the ptomaines in the urine, it would be ideal to have some simple way of finding these bodies and isolating them. We could then handle them chemically and find their true antidote, however we have in the sulpho-ethers and aromatic bodies which develop parpalelly with the intensity of putrefaction which serves as an index to the amount of the intensity of the ptomaines present.

Owing to the fact that it takes considerable time to extract the sulpho-ethers from the urine and no little chemical skill it is hardly practical to employ it in general practice.

The aromatic bodies, indol, skatol, and phenol are easily found, give the same index as the sulpho-ethers and take but a few minutes to make the analysis.

The following chemicals and technique and three minutes time is all that is necessary to find these bodies:

Indican—Equal parts of urine and a solution of two parts ferric chloride in 1,000 parts of C. P. Hcl. about one dram each in a test tube is sufficient, shake vigorously and add 15 or 20 drops of chloroform, shake again, if indol is present it will be shown by a blue precipitate at the bottom of the test tube.

Skatol—About one dram in a test tube of urine C. P. Hcl, and 10 per cent solution calcium chloride in H_2O—shake vigorously a few minutes and add about 20 or 30 drops of amyl alcohol (fusil oil) shake lightly as the fusil oil will emulsify if shaken vigorously, set aside for a few minutes and the skatol will collect at the top of the solution as a brown precipitate.

Phenol—Add one dram each of urine and .C. P. Nitric acid in a large test tube and boil. Cool solution by immersing tube in cold water, after the solution is cool add 15 or 20 drops of U. S. P. Chlorine water, if a trace of phenol is present the solution will become cloudy, the cloudiness will be in proportion to the amount of phenol present up to the degree of a black solution when a large amount is present.

The test for indican is all that is necessary and when found present is absolute proof that ptomaines are being absorbed into the blood and that an auto-intoxication is present.

Any druggist can put up these solutions and the physician should keep them on hand in stock bottles in his office or laboratory. In all disturbed processes these analyses will be found of incalculable value in making a diagnosis.

Treatment.

Since we have found in the large majority of cases that gastro-intestinal auto-intoxication is caused by the bacterial action on the nitrogenous substances in the intestinal tract causing putrefaction and the absorption of the ptomaines we would first reduce or withhold altogether the proteid foods such as meat and eggs, stimulate the channels of elimination and protect and rest the antitoxic organs of the body. Modify the culture media in which the bacteria live, by feeding the patient on a lacto-farinaceous diet which is practically anti-putrefactive. This is done by feeding the patient soured milks containing pure lactic acid baccilli. Lactic acid is known to be one of the best intestinal antiseptics directly opposed to the growing protolytic bacteria. Diminish the number and vitality of protolytic bacteria by means of germicidal medicines of which calomel stands at the head of the list, next would be placed menthol. Menthol can be given in from 1 to 5 gr. doses three times a day, until its full antiseptic effect has been obtained.

Next of importance is the evacuating of the protolytic bacteria and their toxines by means of intestinal lavage. This is done by placing the patient on his back, hips well elevated, introduce into colon by means of a colon tube irrigator 1-2 to one gallon normal salt solution at a temperature between 116 and 120 degrees F. Fill the colon with this solution then allow it to run out through the tube, repeat several times until the colon has been well irrigated. This heat stimulates portal circulation besides removing the toxines from the intestinal canal.

The diet has more to do in the successful treatment of these conditions than all other remedies combined, forbid all meats, eggs, pastries, condiments, and fruits, but let him eat freely of cereal foods including bread, butter and the lactic acid soured milks, when in a large majority of cases a speedy recovery ensues.

EDITORIAL

WORK FOR THE ANNUAL MEETING

There is much work for the next annual meeting of the State Association to take up. Among the most needed matters to be considered and for which plans should be started and matured are:

Physicians Liability Insurance.—In several states the question of insuring members of the State Association has been advocated, discussed and after much work and time put into execution and at a rate far below the average cost of such protection where bought from corporations in such business. The plan is worked out mutually and the cost is so trifling when the benefits are considered that we can hardly afford not to take the matter up and have it in our own state.

Regulation of the Sale of Fireworks.— Many of the Eastern cities have ordinances regulating the sale of fireworks; that is prohibiting their sale absolutely. The wisdom of these regulations is evidenced in the fact that the usual holiday casualty has almost disappeared from those localities. The State Medical Association is the only body that can consider these matters, present the arguments and data calling for enactment of prohibitive regulations and we should do it.

Aid for Infirm and Disabled Physicians. —Fortunately we are not often called upon to witness any real suffering in our professional ranks, but many other state societies are considering the matter of raising a fund to be used in such instances and also taking other means to alleviate any suffering in the profession that may come to their attention.

Oklahoma is nothing if not progressive and this statement applies to all professions and lines of business, and we can well imitate our Eastern brothers by taking some steps to establish such a feature.

LEGISLATIVE QUESTIONS AND MATTERS PERTAINING INTIMATELY TO THE MEDICAL PROFESSION.

The State Medical Association should have a Legislative Committee composed of men who are peculiarly fitted by nature and endowment for such work. A man may be a splendid surgeon, a good physician, a true man in every respect yet fall short in his ability to secure legislation for the good of the profession; he may be all this and yet unable to say more than a few words in support of some good measure under consideration.

It has occurred to the Editor also that the Committees of the State Medical Association, often named annually can hardly have an adequate idea of their duties and functions in the short time allotted them and that it would be well to perpetuate these bodies in such a way that there would always be a majority on them who had had previous experience and information on the questions at issue and thus have united action of all members.

Such Committees should place their wishes and conclusions before the county societies and individual members as often as needed, ask their support and they would have it almost unitedly.

The profession must have more unity of action on part of its membership than has heretofore existed in order to receive its due and it seems that this concert of action can only be had by following some such line of action as above indicated.

ONE WAY TO HELP YOUR JOURNAL.

The Editor recently received a circular letter, such as is usually sent to physicians by manufacturers and purveyors of preparations for sale to the Medical Fraternity, calling attention to the virtues of their product and inviting a trial of it.

They were advised that a good way to place their product before the Oklahoma profession would be to use the columns of the Journal for such a laudable purpose as it reached all the better class of physicians in the state; practically all of the Regular profession.

Now in this there are two objects:

If they sell physicians their wares and advertise we should have a little of their advertising appropriation. That is very

just reciprocity.

If the goods are not as represented the Journal has a way of discovering that fact and after a time the physician will be warned to refrain from using an unethical preparation.

Of course we do not propose to ask all advertisers to use our columns; we would degenerate into a monthly advertiser if they did, but we have some space which may well be utilized by them and a few lines keeping a reputable product before the profession which uses it seems to be demanded and due us.

We plead guilty to having used preparations from time to time which were misrepresented to us, but no longer than we knew of the misrepresentation.

The Council on Pharmacy and Chemistry of the American Medical Association have done a great deal of good work in showing the merit or lack of merit of many preparations and their work is now in progress and from the results they are getting will continue for a long time.

The busy physician can have no idea of the various nostrums he is called upon to use by the detail man and circular letter and only by being a stickler in the use of those remedies that are found to be right can he assist the Council in their good work.

BOOK REVIEWS

BOOKS RECEIVED.

INTERNATIONAL CLINICS. Volume I. Twentieth Series, 1910. By various Authors, containing seven colored plates and forty-six illustrations. Bound in cloth. J. B. Lippincott Company, Philadelphia and London.

This work contains three articles on

syphilis by Homer F. Swift, Hideyo Noguchi and B. Sachs; the first two considering the serum diagnosis of syphilis and the last the serum diagnosis of syphilis of the central nervous system. The three articles combined are exhaustive and thorough.

The remainder of the volume is devoted to various subjects of medicine and surgery the leading one being "The Diagnostic Value and Therapeutic Effects of the Bismuth Paste in Chronic Suppuration", by

Emil G. Beck.

The success attained by Beck in this method of treating conditions, which have heretofore proved hopeless to the surgeon and physician such as tubercular abcess cavities and sinuses warrants a close study of Dr. Beck's article.

DISEASES OF THE STOMACH AND INTESTINES.

Diseases of the Stomach and Intestines. By Robert Coleman Kemp, M. D., Professor of Gastro-intestinal Diseases, New York School of Clinical Medicine. Octavo of 766 pages, with 279 illustrations. Philadelphia and London: W. B. Saunders Company, 1910. Cloth $6.00 net; Half Morocco, $7.50 net.

MODERN SURGERY.

The New (6th.) Edition, Greatly Enlarged.

Modern Surgery; General and Operative. By J. Chalmers DaCosta, M. D., Professor of Surgery and of Clinical Surgery in the Jefferson Medical College, Philadelphia. Sixth Edition, Greatly Enlarged. Octavo of 1502 pages, with 966 illustrations, some in colors. Philadelphia and London: W. B. Saunders Company, 1910. Cloth, $5.50 net; Half Morocco, $7.00 net.

POCKET THERAPEUTICS AND DOSE-BOOK.

Pocket Therapeutics and Dose-Book. By Morse Stewart, Jr., B. A., M. D. Fourth Edition, Rewritten. Small 32mo of 263 pages. Philadelphia and London: W. B. Saunders Company, 1910. Cloth, $1.00 net.

W. B. Saunders Company,
Philadelphia and London.

FOR SALE—A $3,000.00 practice well established and good collections in the City of Sapulpa. A complete modern office, furniture and equipment, a good horse and buggy. Address The Journal.

PROGRAM OF THE EIGHTEENTH ANNUAL MEETING OF THE OKLAHOMA STATE MEDICAL ASSOCIATION, TULSA, OKLAHOMA, MAY 10, 11 AND 12TH, 1910

SPECIAL NOTICE.

Registration,

Every physician, whether visitor or member, should on arriving report to the registration Committee and secure a badge, which will be furnished on verification of membership.

Dues.

The annual dues of the State Association are $1.50, payable through your county society. If you have not paid your dues do so at once and receive your membership certificate.

Delegates.

Each local society is entitled to one delegate for each 25 members or fraction thereof. Each delegate should be provided with credentials signed by this County Secretary and countersigned by the President of the County Society.

If a delegate is unable to attend the meeting he should provide his alternate or proxy with such certificates in order to avoid confusion.

Contributions.

Are the property of the State Association and should be handed to the Secretary in the original or by copy, preferably, on arrival.

Membership.

If you know of good men in your county who are not affiliated with your county society persuade them to join at once.

2:00 P. M. Tuesday, May 10th, 1910.

Preliminary meeting, Grand Opera House, 2nd. St. between Boston and Cincinnati.

Invocation, Reverend A. F. Smith, Tulsa.

Address of Welcome, Honorable Loyal J. Martin, Mayor of Tulsa.

Response, Dr. LeRoy Long, McAlester.

Address of Welcome from the Tulsa County Medical Society, Dr. Charles L. Reeder, Tulsa.

Response, Dr. John B. Rolater, Oklahoma City.

President's Address, Dr. Walter C. Bradford, President Oklahoma State Medical Association, Shawnee.

Announcements.
8:30 P. M.

Meeting of the House of Delegates, Grand Opera House, 2nd St. between Boston and Cincinnatti.

8:00 A. M. Wednesday, May 11, 1910.

Meeting of the House of Delegates, Grand Opera House.

9:00 A. M. Wednesday, May 11, 1910.
SECTION ON SURGERY.

Chas. Blickensderfer, Chairman, Shawnee.
Knights of Columbus Hall, between 1st and 2nd St. on Boston.

1. Address of the Chairman.

2. Paper, subject unannounced, Geo. W. Cale, Jr., St. Louis, Mo.

3. "Post-Operative Exudates," W. E. Dicken, Oklahoma City.

4. "Open Treatment of Fractures by Internal or Direct Splints," Herman E. Pearse, Kansas City, Mo.

5. "Treatment of Fractures of the Elbow," C. T. Harris, Konowa.

6. "Clinical Notes on Fractures and Dislocations of the Upper Extremity," M. E. Preston, Denver, Colorado.

7. "Hernia," A. C. Scott, Temple, Texas.

8. "Cause and Treatment of Inguinal Hernia," W. J. Frick, Kansas City, Mo.

9. "Gall Bladder Surgery," W. C. Graves, McAlester.

10. "Report of a case of Intestinal Obstruction," J. C. Watkins, Hallett.

11. "Concussion," B. F. Fortner, Vinita.

12. "Management of Fractures of the Extremities," J. A. Foltz, Ft. Smith, Ark.

13. "Surgical Treatment of Bone Tuberculosis," report of two cases, L. H. Huffman, Hobart.

14. "Local Anesthesia," Leigh F. Watson, Oklahoma City.

15. "Some Interesting Observations in Connection with Appendicitis," LeRoy Long, McAlester.

9:00 A. M. Wednesday, May 11, 1910.
SECTION ON PEDIATRICS.

H. M. Williams, Chairman, Wellston.
Grand Opera House.

1. Address of the Chairman.

2. "Laryngeal Diptheria," A. B. Montgomery, Checotah.

3. "Cretinism, with report of case," J. E. Hughes, Shawnee.

4. "Report of some cases found among the Dependent Children of Oklahoma," Carl Puckett, Pryor.

5. "Cerebral Meningitis," F. B. Erwin, Norman.

6. "The Empyemata, with special reference to Differential Diagnosis," D. E. Broderick, Kansas City, Mo.

7. "Disease of the Respiratory Tract," Winnie Sanger, Oklahoma City.

8. "Hygiene of Infancy and Childhood," W. G. Little, Okmulgee.

9. "Pneumonia of Children," C. S. Petty, Guthrie.

10. "Report of Cases of Infantile Paralysis," J. C. Mahr, Oklahoma City.

9:00 A. M. Wednesday, May 11, 1910.
SECTION ON DISEASES OF THE EYE, EAR, NOSE AND THROAT.

S. M. Jenkins, Chairman, Enid.
Robinson Hotel Parlors.

1. Chairman's Addresses, "Hypopion."

2. "Diseases of the Middle Ear," C. E. Orelup, Enid.

3. "Tuberculosis of the Tonsil," Robert A. Kooken, Ft. Worth, Texas.

4. "The Prevention of the Ophthalmias of the Newborn," Milton K. Thompson, Muskogee.

5. "Bacteria of the Eye," J. H. Barnes, Enid.

6. "Subject to be announced, Flavel B. Tiffany, Kansas City, Mo.

7. "Eye Diseases from the standpoint of the General Practitioner," G. A. Boyle, Enid.

8. "Otitis Media Catarrhales," D. W. Miller, Blackwell.

9. "Conservative Intranasal Surgery," H. Coulter Todd, Oklahoma City.

2:00 P. M. Wednesday May 11, 1910.
SECTION ON THE PRACTICE OF MEDICINE.

R. H. Harper, Chairman.
Grand Opera House, 2nd St. between Boston and Cincinnati.

1. Address of the Chairman.

2. "The General Practitioner," "Esau Despised His Birthright," Charles W. Fisk, Kingfisher.

3. "Poliomyelitis Anterior," J. Donohoo, Afton.

4 "Bronchc-Pneumonia, Etiology and Treatment," Leonard S. Willour, Atoka.

5. "Diagnostic Relationship between Internal Medicine and Special Surgery," Jacob Block, Kansas City, Mo.

6. "The Prevention of Disease," T. F. Renfrow, Billings.

7. "Cases of Neuritis," Eugene J. Wolff, Waukomis.

8. "Thermogenesis," G. H. Thrailkill, Chickasha.

9. "Management of Cardiac Compensation," Ellsworth Smith, St. Louis, Mo.

10. "Diffuse Dilitation of the Oesophagus, with report of a case," C. C. Conover, Kansas City, Mo.

11. "Diagnosis and Treatment of Diabetes," Harry E. Breese, Henryetta.

12. "Membranous Pericolitis," Jabez N. Jackson, Kansas City, Mo.

13. "The Slow Hearts, their significance with special reference to heart block," Louis H. Behrens, St. Louis, Mo.

14. "Malaria, Atypical Forms," R. K. Pemberton, Krebs.

15. "Acute Pancreatitis, with special report of a case," Arthur S. Risser, Blackwell.

16. "Clinical Significance of Uterine Hemorrhage," J. A. Hatchett, El Reno.

17. "Arteriosclerosis," W. A. Tolleson, Eufaula.

18. "Early Diagnosis of Tuberculosis," Lea A. Riely, Oklahoma City.

2:00 P. M. Wednesday, May 11, 1910.

SECTION ON PATHOLOGY.

Elizabeth Melvin, Chairman, Guthrie.

Address of Chairman.

Medical Education of the Laity, J. M. Postelle, Oklahoma City; Subject Unannounced, L. A. Turley, Norman. Robinson Hotel Parlors.

5:00 P. M. Wednesday, May 11, 1910.

Seeing Tulsa trip, auto ride over city. Cars will start from Robinson Hotel at 5:00 P. M. sharp and from Grand Opera House at 5:05 P. M.

8:00 P. M.

Hyeckka Club Musical, Grand Opera House.

10:00 P. M.

Tulsa County Medical Society banquet, for the doctors and their wives or sweethearts. Robinson Hotel.

8:00 A. M. Thursday, May 12, 1910.

Meeting of the House of Delegates, Grand Opera House.

Election of Officers.

9:00 A. M. Thursday, May 12, 1910.

SECTION ON OBSTETRICS AND GYNECOLOGY Knights of Columbus Hall, between 1st and 2nd St. on Boston, G. H. Thrailkill, Chairman, Chickasha.

1. Address of the Chairman.

2. "Metritis," J. B. Bryce, Snyder.

3. "Causation of Puerperal Mania," John W. Duke, Guthrie.

4. "Modern Trend of Obstetrics," A. B. Leeds, Chickasha.

5. "Non-Surgical Pelvic Diseases," Winnie M. Sanger, Oklahoma City.
Sanger, Oklahoma City.

6. "The Value of Antiseptics in Obstetrics," E. P. Miles, Duke.

7. "A Case Requiring Herniotomy and Lipectomy," Charles Nelson Ballard, Oklahoma City.

8. "Pathological Conception," Paul D. Vann, Chickasha.

9. "Obstetrical Surgery and Repair of Lacerated Perineum," J. M. Trigg, Shawnee.

10. "Eclampsia," G. A. McBride, Ft. Gibson.

11. A Paper, subject not announced, D. N. Wadsworth, Tulsa.

12. "Extrauterine Pregnancy, Diagnosis and Treatment, with case reports," I. B. Oldham, Muskogee.

9:00 A. M. Thursday, May 12, 1910.

Information Bureau.

Paul Clinton, Robinson Hotel Lobby; J. Burr Gibson, Brady Hotel Lobby; Headquarters, Robinson Hotel.

Meeting Places—Grand Opera House, 2nd St. between Boston and Cincinnati; Knights of Columbus Hall, Boston St., between 1st and 2nd St., rear Central National Bank, opposite Reeder Bldg.; Parlors Robinson Hotel.

Exhibit Hall—Knights of Columbus Hall, Boston St., between 1st and 2nd Street.

Hotels—Robinson Hotel, Corner 3rd and South Main; Brady Hotel, Corner North 1st and Main; Frederick Hotel, Corner

Second and Boston; Crescent Hotel, Cor. Frisco R. R., and Main St.

Rooming Houses—Shirley Apartments, 2nd St., between Cincinnati and Detroit; Shields Rooms, 2nd Street, córner Cincinnati; St. Regis Hotel, North Main Street; Crescent Rooms, Main and Frisco Track; Rorrabaughs Rooms, 3rd Street between South Main and Boulder; Robinson Hotel Annex, Corner 3rd and South Main.

Cafes—Subway Cafe, 2nd Street, between Main and Boston; Quick Lunch, South Main St., between 1st and 2nd Streets; Waldorf Cafe, South Main St., between 3rd and 4th Streets; Bismark Cafe, South Main St., between 1st and 2nd Streets; Ferndale Cafe, 3rd St., between Main and Boston; Thos. Drug Co., 2nd St., between Main and Boston; Chocolate Shop, 3rd St., between Main and Boston; Oil Flyer Cafe, North Main St., between 1st and 2nd Streets.

Place of Registration.

Lobby of Grand Opera House, 2nd Street, between Boston and Cincinnati.

Meeting Places of Sections.

HOUSE OF DELEGATES. Place, Grand Opera House. Time, Tuesday, 2:00 P. M. and 8:00 P. M. Wednesday 8:00 A. M. Thursday 8:00 A. M.

SECTION ON SURGERY. Place, Knights of Columbus Hall. Time, Wednesday 9:00 A. M. and 2:00 P. M.

SECTION ON MEDICINE. Place, Grand Opera House. Time, Thursday 9:00 A. M.

SECTION ON GYENECOLOGY AND OBSTETRICS. Place, Knights of Columbus Hall. Time, Thursday 9:00 A. M.

SECTION ON EYE, EAR, NOSE AND THROAT. Place, Robinson Hotel Parlors. Time, Wednesday 9:00 A. M.

SECTION ON PENDIATRICS. Place, Grand Opera House. Time, Tuesday 2:00 P. M.

SECTION ON PATHOLOGY. Place, Robinson Hotel Parlors. Time, Tuesday 2:00

TULSA, OKLAHOMA.

BY FRED S. CLINTON, CHAIRMAN ENTERTAINMENT COMMITTEE.

THE PIONEER.

The first authenticated settler in the Territory embraced within the present incorporated City of Tulsa was a full-blood Creek Indian named Archie Yahola, who came here from Georgia in 1836, as the King or Town Chief of the Tulsa Lochapokas. His splendid physique and superior mind gave him a powerful prestige in addition to the position to which he was elevated by his people. He was justly considered a guide, philosopher and friend among his followers. He died in 1850 and is buried in the southern part of the City near the old amphitheater erected by the members of his clan for the practice of their religious rites. His name or fame is not emblazoned on the pages of history, but his affectionate memory is enshrined within the hearts of his tribesmen.

In the springtime when the bracing breezes swayed the myriads of multi-hued flowers, it was his coveted privilege to stand upon one of the hills of our City and view the red torch of day, in russet mantle clad, gradually mount the heavens, shooting his fiery shafts across the virgin soil of a coming commonwealth, afterwards to be gemmed by a cosmopolitan City called Tulsa.

As he watched the sun mount higher and higher, kissing away the dewdrops from the fragrant flowers and shedding his luminous and life giving rays throughout this great new empire, there was presented a pleasing picture to this prince of pioneers.

At eventide he turned his gaze to the westward to behold the hills clothed in azure and purple as the golden orb of day lazily sank to rest. As the glory of the parting day left him to contemplate the beauty of the approaching night, when the countless candles lighting the sky burst upon his vision, he might have turned in poetic fancy to Milton's lines,

"how glowed the firmament
With living sapphires; Hesperus, that led
The starry host, rode brightest, till the moon,
Rising in clouded majesty, at length
Apparent queen, unveiled her peerless light,

And o'er the dark her silver mantle threw."

As his clay curtained couch is not marked by any monument, this tribute is proposed to the first,

"pioneer;
Old Druid of the West;
His offering was the fleet wild deer,
His shrine the mountain's crest.
Within his wild wood temple's space
Where erst, alone of all his race,
He knelt to Nature's God."

As he journeyed from the wave washed shores of the great Atlantic to guide his people in their new found home, this sweet sentiment seems appropriate to an old

"pioneer:
Columbus of the land;
Who guided freedom's proud career
Beyond the conquer'd strand,
And gave her pilgrim sons a home
No monarch's step profanes,
Free as the chainless winds that roam
Upon its boundless plains."

His brother, Che-ya-ha, succeeded him in 1850. Tulsa Fixico was the next successor to the Kingship, and during the Civil War, while Captain of Company I of the Indian Home Guards, was killed. He was the father of Joe Tulsa, the great ally of Chitto-Harjo, or Crazy-Snake. O-kel-essa Micco came next into power, and was followed by Waitie Beaver the present Chief.

Time veils all personality and the merciless march of the fast fleeting years soon engulfs pioneers. These Indians have been mentioned that they may not be forgotten in their own land.

While Archie Yahola slept and dreamed of the trophies of the chase and of the happy hunting grounds, the buffalo, coyote, deer and antelope moved across the trackless prairies and over the eternal hills to be practically lost forever. The missionary and railroad, the great harbingers of civilization, made manifest through their powerful agencies, the destiny to which each was attached by selections. Should the din of modern industry and the activity of a determined people to work out their commercial salvation, awake the slumbering spirit of this pioneer he would find that distance had been discounted by the steam and electric railways; that time and space had been annihilated by the telegraph and telephone and that cold storage and transportation facilities had placed with-

in reach of every Tulsan perishable products of all seasons and climes at any time of the year. If he sought a position at any central down town district he would see the great buildings fashioned out of brick and stone, mortar and concrete. He would hear the clang of the street car bells, the rumble of the buggies or carriages and the clatter of horses' hoofs upon the splendid pavements, and the honk-honk of the "goggle-eyed grunting machine," the patter of the pedestrian's feet on the sidewalks as they scurried to and fro, betokening the close of the day. Looking to the north he would see the Midland Valley train threading its way through the prairie until it would stop on account of the block signal. He would observe the clouds of black smoke from the great engine gradually rise and gracefully float out over the city to join the other elements of incomplete combustion, forming the foundation for one of those beautiful sunsets which require certain atmospheric conditions to complete it's gorgeousness.

The day has departed and night's candles are shut out by the gathering clouds, but someone starts the machinery and that mysterious, unseen and subtle fluid, chained by Franklin, begins to blink at every dark corner and soon a flood of light comes into view from the arc lamps.

No prophetic ken could have delved into the future and foreshadowed this great progress.

Name.

It is natural that some interest should attach to the meaning and origin of the Creek Indian word "Tulsa." It is not descriptive. That is, it does not mean any animal or stream, etc. It is simply the name of a former Creek clan. Anciently, clans or secret societies existed among the Creek Indians out of which, in the march of progress, a constitutional form of government was framed, and these clans sent their representatives to the councils of the Creeks. There was a time when this oligarchic government was very strongly established among the Creeks, or Muscogees, because the members of clans were not allowed to intermarry and representatives were hereditary. However, upon the adoption of the constitution in 1867 and the inauguration of the House of Kings and Warriors an elective form of

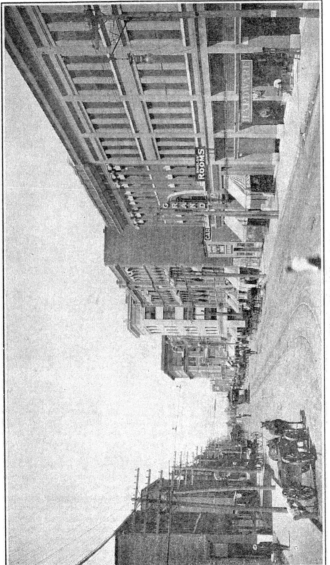

TULSA STREET SCENE.

government succeeded the hereditary custom. The Creek Nation was divided into forty-seven "towns" or communities, each of which selected a member as Town Chief who sat in the House of Kings, and two or more members to sit in the House of Warriors. Three of these forty-seven towns formerly bore the name of Tulsa; they were Tulsa Lochapoka, Tulsa Canadian and Tulsa Little River. They have practically dropped the name of Tulsa and are known by their last names. These names are descriptive of the place of residence or the object from which they derive their name. Lochapoka means "turtling place," or where they fish and kill turtles, and was brought with them from Alabama. Canadian and Little River have reference to the location of the towns on these streams.

It was a custom among the members of these towns to have an annual meeting place called a "busking ground" where some of their religious rites were practiced. Before they could eat green corn they would attend these annual meetings and take certain medicines which had an emetic affect. This was followed by a final cleansing bath in some nearby stream, after which they took a short sleep, ate of the first green corn of the season and at night time commenced their "stomp" dance. Some leader with a sort of war whoop, like a bugle call, would spring into a previously prepared ring in the center of which had been built a fire, and with a sort of shuffling gait proceed to encircle this fire, singing in a gutteral tone a monosyllabic song. One by one the men and women dropped in behind this leader, each joining in the song, after their leader, whose voice was heard above all the others. Many of the women wore on the tops of their feet terrapin shells in which had been placed pebbles, producing a kind of rythmic shifting sound. As the flickering flames in the darkness of the night silhouetted against the trees and other surroundings, the moving forms of the participants, and an occasional wild war whoop pierced the night air, giving a strange weirdness to the scene and aweing the uninitiated spectator. It was the establishment of the busking ground of the Tulsa Lochapokas on a prominent elevation near the outskirts of the City, that gave to Tulsa her name.

Location.

Tulsa is located in Oklahoma on the St. Louis and San Francisco Railroad, 425 miles southwest of St. Louis; 251 miles south and west of Kansas City, and 121 miles east of Oklahoma City in the valley of the Arkansas River.

It is the county seat of Tulsa county, the third richest and third smallest county in the State.

Population.

In 1900 the population was 1,390, in 1910, 25,240.

Temperature.

The mean average temperature is 60 degrees Fahrenheit.

Rainfall.

The mean annual rainfall is 36 inches.

Topography.

Tulsa is situate on the northern and eastern bank of the Arkansas River. On the North and West it is skirted by a range of hills. The hills on the West are divided by the Arkansas River. On the South is found the fertile valley of this river and on the East the great broad prairies of Tulsa County. Two small streams pass through the City from North to South which give most excellent natural drainage, and when one takes into consideration the numerous small hills throughout the City, there is not a more perfectly drained area of inhabited land anywhere.

Elevation.

The City is about 700 feet above the sea level. Its location secures a maximum amount of available sunshine during the entire year. The range of hills which bound it on the North and West form a wind break and makes the City reasonably free from storm.

Character of Soil.

The soil within the City and over a large portion of the County consists of a chocolate colored sandy loam, varying from one to six feet in depth. Its productivity is unquestioned. Cotton, corn, wheat and oats may be seen growing by each other. Flowers and fruits of large variety and excellent quality are produced in season. It is estimated that 2,000,000 bushels of corn and 12,000 bales of cotton were produced in the County last year.

Shale ridges extend through the City from the northwest corner to the southwest corner in an approximately straight line. There is also a half-moon shaped shale ridge paralleling the northern edge of the City and

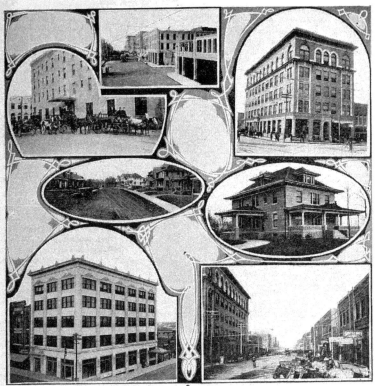

SOME TULSA OFFICE BUILDINGS AND RESIDENCES.

circling the northwest corner. The subsoil drainage of the City is excellent, and in those places where no ledges of stone or clay or shale are present to prevent the proper percolation of water through the soil, one may rest assured that the well water, if kept sanitary or free from outside contamination, may be drunk with impunity.

Water Supply.

Much of the drinking water of the City may be had from dug or bored wells, and a great deal of it is of most excellent quality. There are also mineral springs in and near the City which afford a considerable supply of drinking water, and this has given rise to a new industry, that of bottling and supplying this pure water not only locally but to neighboring towns. The local water works, owned and operated by the City, furnishes an abundant supply for fire protection and sanitary use. The large settling basins and modern treatment of the water give a clear product.

Sewerage.

There is a complete system of sanitary sewers extending throughout the City 14 miles in length. There are over 17 miles of storm sewers ranging from twelve inches to seven and one-half feet in diameter.

Fuel Supply.

Natural gas, coal, wood and crude oil.

Gas.

Tulsa is the center of the Mid-Continent Oil and Gas field. The Bird Creek district, including both the Cherokee and Osage; the Glenn Pool, the Red Fork, Taneha, Sapulpa, Mounds and Twin Hills districts of the Creek Nation, are all in Tulsa's trade territory, and she is the basis of oil and gas supplies. There are about 100 producing gas wells in this territory and each average, as a conservative estimate, about 5,000,000 cubic feet, which would aggregate 500,000,000 cubic feet of gas a day. As the field has not been fully developed, one may better understand and appreciate the possible use to which this gas may be put and what an inestimable heritage of priceless comfort and convenience is to those fortunate enough to reside in Tulsa. Since the inauguration of the present plant, which was the first complete one in the territory or state, the pressure has been so uniform that not a single accident has been recorded, and while other cities have shivered in cold there has never been a time when Tulsa did not enjoy the luxury of ample fuel supply. The recent arrangement on the part of the Commercial Club with the Osage and Oklahoma Gas Co., to furnish gas for factory purposes, insures the future destiny of this City among the greater cities of the southwest.

Domestic Gas.

At sixteen cents per thousand cubic feet, in unlimited quantity and with unvarying pressure is a luxury few cities enjoy, and three cent gas for manufacturing purposes is really cheaper than the cost of wages to a man to shovel coal into the boilers.

Oil.

As the districts enumerated above are in Tulsa trade territory, one may find in this area from 2,500 to 3,000 producing oil wells, the daily production from which is about 90,000 barrels, or practically one-half of the production of the entire Mid-Continent field.

Coal.

Tulsa's commercial rivals frequently advise prospective investors of capital of the short life of gas and unwittingly warn them of Tulsa, forgetting her real coal resources. In Tulsa County there was mined during the past year, over 100,000 tons of coal for export. This gives employment to between 600 and 800 men, most of whom have families. During the six to eight months activity in the coal districts, approximately $200,000.00 is put in circulation each year. The headquarters of the various coal mining companies operating in contiguous territories are in Tulsa. Coal extends from the extreme northern boundary to the extreme southern boundary of the county, at depths of ten feet in the North and fifty feet in the South. This is known as the first vein and is the only one being worked at the present time. The thickness of the vein at Collinsville is twenty-two inches, at Dawson thirty inches, and at Scales thirty-six inches. Oil men have reported a vein five feet thick at a depth of two hundred and forty feet, but this has never been worked. The supply is practically unlimited and has scarcely been developed at this time.

Wood.

Along the small streams in the County and in the great Arkansas bottom, will be found for some time hence, wood enough for any reasonable fuel demand.

Building Material.

Ample shale for the manufacture of paving, building and face brick is found along the Northern boundary of the City. A good quality of building stone is secured East and South of the City. In the Arkansas river bed is found some of as fine and sharp sand as may be desired. Beyond the river is located a large crusher which prepares a good quality of stone for concrete work. Near this is being promoted a plant that will furnish a high grade of Portland Cement. At the foot of these hills is said to be a good grade of potters clay. In these same hills thousands of barrels of lime has been kilned and used for domestic building.

Pavements.

For heavy traffic some of the streets are paved with brick, but twenty-two miles of asphaltum pavement adorn and beautify the City, and the good work is being rapidly pushed, as ten miles are under construction.

EDUCATIONAL INSTITUTIONS.
City Schools.

Seven modern school buildings are distributed over the city. The high school building consisting of twenty-one rooms and built at a cost of $55,000.00 is centrally located. The north side school has eleven rooms and there are four ward buildings of eight rooms each. Each building is modern in every par-

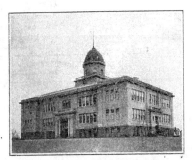

TULSA HIGH SCHOOL BUILDING.

ticular, having splendid light, good ventilation, automatic heat regulation and the best sanitary apparatus obtainable. The estimated value of buildings and ground is over $275,000.00. There are eighty-five teachers employed in the city schools. The school term is thirty-six weeks of actual work. The grade work covers a period of eight years, depending upon the age and ability of the pupil. The teachers are all selected with a view to their proficiency and adaptability to the particular work in hand. The schools are liberally supplied with apparatus such as maps, globes, charts, reference books, and helps for teachers. The high school course requires four years and an average of 60 per cent. on rigid examination for passing each subject. There are eight teachers in this department, nearly all of whom hold degrees from the best colleges and universities. There are two hundred and forty-nine pupils in attendance and twenty-one in the class of 1910. The total enrollment in the city schools for the year is three thousand four hundred and twenty. This is a gain of one hundred and six per cent, in three years, fifty-four per cent. in two years and a gain of over twenty-five per cent. of the number enrolled in school a year ago. The graduates of the high school are placed on an accredited list of the various western colleges and universities, which means that they are admitted to the Freshman classes without further examination.

Henry Kendall College.

The Henry Kendall College is beautifully located about a mile and one-half East of the business center of the City, and in close proximity to the eastern terminus of the street railway, on a prominent elevation. In a campus of twenty acres a group of buildings have been symmetrically arranged, and the following have been completed: Administration building at a cost of $54,000.00; three dormitories, the largest costing $26,000.00; the president's home cost $5,000.00. The faculty consists of twelve members. Entrance to college fifteen credits, of which ten are required and five elective. The preparatory and collegiate departments require four years each. There are five courses of study consisting of, Classical, Scientific, Music, Art, and Elocution. Degrees of Bachelor of Arts and Bachelor of Science are conferred. The college has an invested endowment of $92,500.00. Pupils enrolled last year 176.

The Holy Family Parochial School.

Has an enrollment of three hundred pupils which includes thirty boarding school pupils. They give a business and musical course. The school is in charge of Mother Superior Jerome, who is assisted by eight Sisters of the order of Divine Providence.

Tulsa Business College.

Has an enrollment of one hundred pupils. The course comprises bookkeeping, shorthand and typewriting.

The Hospital Training School For Nurses.

The Tulsa Hospital Training School for Nurses is conducted in connection with the Tulsa Hospital, and has an enrollment of ten pupils. A complete course of instruction is given by a competent corps of teachers.

County Schools.

Tulsa County has an area of 522 square miles and a greater taxable valuation than any county of equal area in the State of Oklahoma. It has the remarkable taxable valuation of more than $1,000.00 for every man, woman and child living within its boundaries. It is divided into twenty-nine school districts, ranging in size from nine to forty-two square miles each, which conform to the topography, population and width of their respective locations. The county had a scholastic population of six thousand three hundred thirty-three in the first school census taken in January 1908, which number is now greatly increased. There are sixty-nine white and five colored teachers employed, outside of the City of Tulsa, with salaries ranging from $40.00 to $75.00 a month. The revenue for school purposes is derived from accruing rents of the leased school lands of the State, fines collected by the County, interest on the $5,000,000.00 appropriated by Congress and direct taxation. Notwithstanding the extra expense of starting the schools the first year, the average tax levy in the districts is less than five mills on the dollar.

following have churches erected: First Baptist Church; First Presbyterian Church; First Christian Church; First Methodist Episcopal Church; First M. E. Church, South; Tigert Memorial; United Presbyterian Church; Holy Family Church; Protestant Episcopal Church;

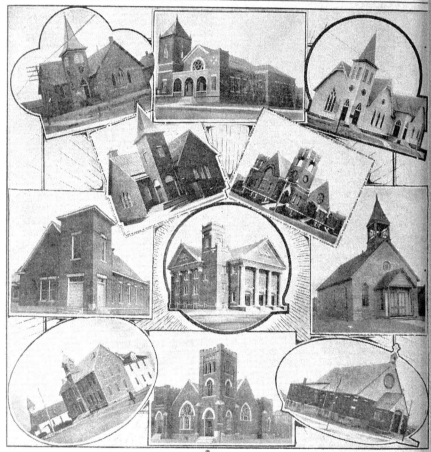

SOME TULSA CHURCHES.

Churches.

There are thirteen churches with a combined membership of 4,500 and a property valuation approximating $250,000.00. The Colored Baptist Church. Among these churches may be found some of beautiful architecture and with all modern conveniences. The Lutheran body has purchased a valuable lot and will build in the near future. The Christian Science Church, although strong, is without a building and worships in the Boswell Building on South Main street. The Salvation Army through the generousity of wealthy oil men, will soon be possessors of a fine hall in the city and a magnificent home in the country.

Lodges.

There are eighteen lodges with a membership aggregating several thousand. Among these having the largest membership, or being the longest established are the Masonic, Elks and Odd Fellows.

Clubs.

There are five Women's Clubs in the City, and their object is intellectual advancement corporated in 1906 and owns, maintains and operates The Tulsa Hospital which has grown from a fifteen to a forty bed capacity. It is of stone and brick construction and located at the West End of South Fifth street. It is equally open to all reputable physicians and is the emergency hospital for the railroads and cares for proper City and County patients usually acceptable in a small hospital in this locality.

The Northside Hospital.

It is a commodious frame structure beautifully located on North Eighth and Cheyenne streets. While a private institution it is open to other physicians. It has a capacity of fifteen beds.

The Physicians and Surgeons Hospital.

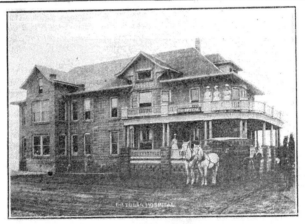

TULSA HOSPITAL.

and civic improvement. The Hyeckka Club is a musical organization consisting of fifty members, including the best talent in the City, and it is affiliated with the State and National federations. The Tuesday Book Club has twenty-five members, the Women's Club has thirty members. The Ruskin Art Club, the Kendall Bible Study Club, the Country Club are well supported. There are twenty-one other clubs whose purposes are purely social.

HOSPITALS.

Tulsa Hospital.

The Tulsa Hospital Association was in-

Is a frame building located on South 13th and Carson avenue. It has a capacity of twenty beds and is open to other physicians.

None of the above hospitals knowingly accept contagious diseases such as the eruptive fevers, tuberculosis in advanced stages or other cases usually excluded from well conducted small general hospitals.

Banks.

There are eight banks, three National and five State, having an aggregate paid up capital of a half million dollars, with over four million dollars in deposits. All of Tulsa's banks are prudently managed.

Fire Department.

The Department is completely organized, and has twenty men all fully paid. The stations are all well located. The alarm system consists of twenty-nine Gamewell boxes, the equipment for three stations. In addition to a complete equipment otherwise, a new seventy-five H. P. auto hose wagon and pump has been added, bringing the department down to date.

The Press.

There are three daily papers. The Daily Democrat and Tulsa Post are published in the evening and the World in the morning. There are numerous other publications.

Post Office Receipts.

1900	$ 2,954	1904	$ 9,733
1901	3,427	1905	17,017
1902	4,544	1906	23,482
1903	7,158	1907	34,714
1908	41,451	1909	53,928.61

Quarter ending March 31, 1910 . . . $16,878.52

Railways.

There are four railway systems consisting of the St. Louis and San Francisco including the Arkansas Valley and Western; Atchison; Topeka and Santa Fe; Missouri, Kansas and Texas, and Midland Valley Railroad, giving eight outlets and thirty-four daily passenger trains. Through connection with points East and West, North and South may be had. There are seventy-five counties in the State of Oklahoma, and seventy-five per cent of the county seat population is reached from Tulsa without change of cars thirty-five county seats are accessible; with but one change thirty-two county seats may be reached; with two changes two county seats may be reached. There are only six county seats in the State without railroad facilities.

STREET RAILWAYS.

The Tulsa Street Railway Company.

Has in operation a complete trolley car system, and when the present contracts for extension are completed there will be about twelve miles of trackage.

Union Traction Company.

This Company has four and one-half miles of track completed and in operation. It contemplates extension and the operation of an interurban system at an early date.

Factories and Wholesale Houses.

There are seventy-six factories and wholesale houses located in and adjoining the City, 10,250 employes.

Health.

With two hundred twenty days of sunshine, an equable temperature, ample annual rainfall, potable water, remarkable natural drainage, supplemented by sanitary and storm sewers Tulsa may be regarded as a healthy place of residence. The mild and short winters and cool nights of the summer months attract many people from the torrid South and frigid North, from the dry West and crowded East. Many of the acute diseases, such as pneumonia, scarlet fever, diphtheria and typhoid fever, appear much milder than in the North. The application of knowledge gained in other cities and the adoption of modern methods of sanitation will do much to prevent the establishment of some of the diseases which have become entrenched in older communities and each year exacts their tribute to the folly and unwisdom of a penny wise and pound foolish government.

Health Department.

Under the efficient direction of Doctor W. E. Wright, City Superintendent of Health, with the collaboration of others a splendid system of reports and intelligent collection of valuable data have been inaugurated. This information has been presented to the City officials and they in keeping with the spirit of progress have authorized the purchase of an Incinerator Plant, the picture of which is exhibited in connection with this article. This is the modern method of garbage disposal and Tulsa is glad to have the world know her physicians and citizens recognizing and realize that the greatest resources of any community is health and happiness.

The Department of Health of the City of Tulsa is divided into three working sections:

Department No. 1, covers the reports of Births, Deaths, Contagious Diseases etc., the care of the poor, sick, the establishing of quarantines and other health and sanitary regulations.

Department No. 2, provides for the inspection of Dairies, Bakeries, Hotels, Cafes, and other places where milk and food is sold, also for the inspection of all food stuffs and live stock shipped into the City.

Department No. 3, provides for the collection and disposal of the garbage, trash, dead animals, and other surface waste.

During the past year, as a result of thorough inspection and grading of the Dairies furnishing milk to the City of Tulsa the sanitary conditions have been greatly improved. Proper disposal of manure; properly constructed barns and milk houses, thorough sterilization of utensils, and other sanitary measures have been insisted on and obtained.

diseases, under the direction of the City Health Officials is rigidly enforced. Sixty-eight cases of small pox were cared for at the Contagious Hospital during the seasons of 1909 and 1910, with only two deaths.

Commercial Club.

Is incorporated and has attractive and useful features not embraced in any other Club in the State. This Club is systematiz-

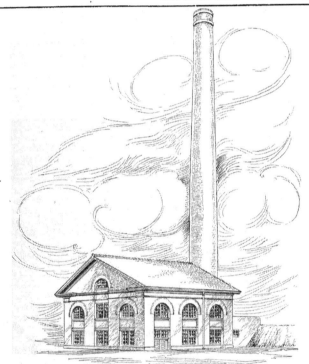

TULSA INCINERATOR PLANT.

A systematic method of garbage collection and disposal has been instituted, requiring each householder to provide himself with a covered garbage can. The garbage is collected daily in closed, especially constructed wagons. The trash, manure, dead animals and other surface waste is also collected in the same systematic manner.

The placarding, quarantining and fumigating of all communicable and contagious

ing and unifying the efforts of her citizens for commercial, moral and educational achievement. It has a membership of six hundred with two salaried secretaries and a Public Affairs Commissioner.

Boosters and Builders.

The progressive citizens of Tulsa desired to have the future City construction illumined by the torch of experience of the past, and to that end, March 13th, 1905, sent the One

Hundred Club, in a special complete vestibuled train of four coaches, on a visit to the North and East, as purveyors of knowledge. During the journey of thirteen days upon this train, for the first time in the history of the world, so far as is known, there was published a daily newspaper, 15,000 copies of which were distributed each day.

On April 13th, 1908, the Booster Club, having on board the five Pullman coaches 113 citizens of Tulsa, invaded the East, and after nineteen days systematic study returned home. These journeys were primarily to secure a broader information, and secondarily to exploit the resources of this City and State. Many citizens contributed toward the fund to make this trip possible, and others gave of their means and accompanied the train.

To those who have contributed of their mind, time and money to place the City of Tulsa upon the map and make it a good place to live in, the eastern portion, if not the whole State, owes an everlasting obligation. Their brains have planned, their money has supported, their hands have wrought many of the notable achievements, sometimes at great personal sacrifice. It would be impracticable, in a brief resume such as is contemplated in this article, to mention the names of all those entitled to notice, and the writer feels that in the fullness of time their imperishable names will be inscribed upon the deathless scroll of fame, for they are inseparably interwoven into the woof and warf of one of the most magnificent little cities in the world. Men who have so unselfishly served their neighbors, men of such lofty ideals and high purposes can not be lost to the impartial historian.

Reflections.

The building of a City such as Tulsa, though in the midst of a vast and resourceful empire, has not been free from struggle, but the threatening clouds that gathered about the human landscape have always parted at the right time, and through the rift has shone with resplendent glory, the sparkling stars of hope. Tulsa today, though full of magnificent achievement, is only prophetic of a greater destiny. Over her homes now floats Old Glory, and a free people with local self government, exultantly raise this emblem of progress so that the breezes of the North, South, East and West may kiss it and the sun of all the earth reflect it.

The whole world is flooded with sunshine and if we could gather the sunbeams from the people we meet, we could weave them into a great shaft of light with which we could dispel the gloom that settles about many others who have an obscured vision. These people who see things darkly have a mission to perform; it is through their shadows that the warm effulgent glow of light is made manifest. The rising sun, without clouds to reflect its burnished rays, would not be half so glorious; the setting sun, without the purple and the gold, would not be half so beautiful. Few people express their admiration for the sun at meridian height, if he sits enthroned in a cloudless sky, for beauty is revealed largely, not only through conception of ideals, but by comparison with those things with which we have knowledge.

The writer wishes the reader God speed upon the great sea of life, and trusts that as you sail in the greatest of all ships, Friendship, your haven at last will be some sunny clime of your own choosing, a port safe and secure from storms, or tempestuous scenes, where the deep tranquil waters afford the safest of all landings.

"I hear the muffled tramp of years
Come stealing up the slopes of time;
They bear a train of smiles and tears
Of burning hopes and dreams sublime."

INDEX, VOLUME 2.

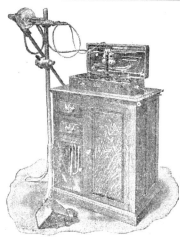

STANDING COMMITTEES OKLAHOMA STATE MEDICAL ASSOCIATION.

Public Policy and Legislation—Dr. David A. Myers, Chairman, Lawton; J. H. Scott, Shawnee; J. A. Hatchett, El Reno; F. S. Clinton, Tulsa; Claude A. Thompson, Muskogee.

On Medical Education—Drs. B. J. Vance, Checotah; A. K. West, Oklahoma City; E. O. Barker, Guthrie.

On Scientific Work—Drs. Floyd E. Waterfield, Holdenville; P. A. Smithe, Enid; Claude A. Thompson, Muskogee.

On Necrology—Drs. C. S. Bobo, Norman; H. M. Williams, Wellston; M. A. Warhurst, Remus.

FOR SALE.

$1,250 cash gets property consisting of three-room dwelling house, barn, stables, pair of horses, good buggy, office furniture and fixtures; $4,000.00 practice gratis; will introduce. Reason for selling—going to specialize in Texas. Address Dr. John T. Vick, Fort Towson, Oklahoma.

FOR SALE.

The Journal has tuition to the amount of forty-four dollars in the New York Polyclinic School and Hospital which will be sold at a reduction from the usual rates. Address The Journal.

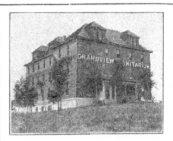

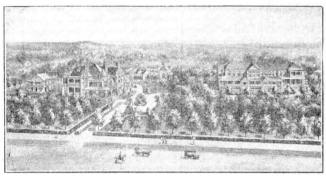

www.ingramcontent.com/pod-product-compliance
Lightning Source LLC
Chambersburg PA
CBHW071357050326
40689CB00010B/1673